The Path of Modern Yoga

"This is a detailed, comprehensive, and rich examination of the history of modern yoga, showing clearly—and with new insight—how 'postural yoga' is thoroughly enmeshed in the culture of health, fitness, and athletics. Goldberg has provided us with an important perspective on how different aspects of 20th-century 'body culture' shaped the practice of *asana* during the modern yoga renaissance."

JOSEPH S. ALTER, PH.D., PROFESSOR OF SOCIAL SCIENCE AND ANTHROPOLOGY AT YALE-NUS COLLEGE IN SINGAPORE AND AUTHOR OF *YOGA IN MODERN INDIA* AND *MORAL MATERIALISM*

"In *The Path of Modern Yoga,* Elliott Goldberg has laid out a clear road map—with detours into philosophical musings—of the path of modern yoga from its origins in the early 20th century to its current state of practice in the early 21st century, especially noting the profound influence of my teacher, B. K. S. Iyengar. Although more could've been written about the openness and love with which Iyengar gave of himself, if you want to know about yoga and how it got to be what it is today, this is the book to read."

JOHN SCHUMACHER, FOUNDER AND DIRECTOR OF UNITY WOODS YOGA CENTER, DESCRIBED BY *YOGA JOURNAL* AS "ONE OF 25 ORIGINALS SHAPING YOGA IN AMERICA"

"This is a deep history of the birth of modern yoga. There is dogged research on and profound insight into the main protagonists. Their contributions are shown to be both unique and tempered by the spirit of the times in the West as well as in India. As a result, this story of modern yoga is equally intimate and expansive. Now we practitioners of yoga can muse over where we really come from."

NORMAN SJOMAN, PH.D., STUDENT OF SANSKRIT, ARTIST, AUTHOR OF *THE YOGA TRADITION OF THE MYSORE PALACE,* AND COAUTHOR OF *YOGA TOUCHSTONE*

"Goldberg's 'detective work' is impressive. In his investigation into the writings of British journalist Louise Morgan, he has uncovered her critical role in the transformation of the 'Sun Salutation' into an 'Elixir for Women'—a missing link in the development of modern yoga as a practice for women as well as men. Although at times irreverent, *The Path of Modern Yoga* is filled with wisdom and understanding into the culture and experience of yoga."

STUART RAY SARBACKER, PH.D., PROFESSOR IN THE SCHOOL OF HISTORY, PHILOSOPHY, AND RELIGION AT OREGON STATE UNIVERSITY AND THE COAUTHOR OF *THE EIGHT LIMBS OF YOGA*

"Combining original historical research with a compelling narrative, *The Path of Modern Yoga* profiles some of the most significant—and in some cases surprising—personalities to shape modern yoga practice. Goldberg's reflections and insights will further understanding, both popular and academic, of yoga and its place in the contemporary world."

SUZANNE NEWCOMBE, PH.D., ASSOCIATE LECTURER FOR THE OPEN UNIVERSITY, LONDON, AND RESEARCH OFFICER AT INFORM AT THE LONDON SCHOOL OF ECONOMICS AND POLITICAL SCIENCE

THE PATH OF
MODERN
YOGA

The History of an
Embodied Spiritual Practice

ELLIOTT GOLDBERG

Inner Traditions
Rochester, Vermont • Toronto, Canada

Inner Traditions
One Park Street
Rochester, Vermont 05767
www.InnerTraditions.com

Library of Congress Cataloging-in-Publication Data

Names: Goldberg, Elliott, 1943– , author.

Title: The path of modern yoga : the history of an embodied spiritual practice / Elliott Goldberg.

Description: Rochester, Vermont : Inner Traditions, [2016] | Includes bibliographical references and index.

Identifiers: LCCN 2015047711 (print) | LCCN 2015049188 (e-book) | ISBN 9781620555675 (hardback) | ISBN 9781620555682 (e-book)

Subjects: | MESH: Yoga—history | Exercise | History, 20th Century

Classification: LCC RM727.Y64 (print) | LCC RM727.Y64 (e-book) | NLM QT 11.1 | DDC 613.7/046—dc23

LC record available at http://lccn.loc.gov/2015047711

Printed and bound in the United States by Versa Press, Inc.

10   9   8   7   6   5   4   3   2   1

Text design and layout by Virginia Scott Bowman
This book was typeset in Garamond Premier Pro and Myriad Pro with Basilia used as the display typeface

To send correspondence to the author of this book, mail a first-class letter to the author c/o Inner Traditions • Bear & Company, One Park Street, Rochester, VT 05767, and we will forward the communication, or contact the author directly at **elliottgoldbergyoga.com**.

The physical signs of perfection in hatha yoga are a slim, lithe body; a luminous face (a manifestation of self understanding and acceptance); sparkling eyes; a sonorous voice; increased gastric fire (good digestion); vitality (not just absence of disease); mastery over sexual urges; awareness of anahata, *the inner sound (a sign of great calm); and purity of the* nadis, *the channels through which* prana, *the life force energy, flows.*

—SVATMARAMA, *HATHA YOGA PRADIPIKA,*
CHAPTER 2, VERSE 78

Contents

PART I

Divesting Yoga of the Sacred
Yogic Physical Culture and Health Cure

PART II

Making Yoga Dynamic
The Sun Salutations as Yogic Exercise

PART III

Making Yoga Sacred Again

Yogic Embodied Spirituality

Foreword

Surely the most consequential and curious development in modern yoga is its emphasis on *asana* (postural practice). Although taking this strand of modern yoga as its subject, Elliott Goldberg's *The Path of Modern Yoga* is not by any means a survey of trends in postural yoga in the 20th century. It is instead a reconstruction of the course of modern postural yoga as a transformation from a set of primarily religious practices within traditional Hindu settings to an exercise regime deeply influenced by Western physical culture and health care and finally to an embodied spiritual practice that renews the spiritual aspirations of premodern forms of yoga within refined postural training.

Goldberg tells this *grande histoire* of modern yoga by reconstructing a complexity of interwoven trajectories of the pioneers of modern postural practice that presents a new and deeply human perspective on the history of modern yoga. He interprets this intertwined network of life stories with impressive psychological sophistication and a good portion of humor. He blends in often surprising cultural and social circumstances—usually Western trends—to elucidate the larger contexts of personal achievements.

Goldberg also provides insightful interpretations of historical developments that lead us to a deeper understanding of the meaning of modern postural yoga. Academic studies on the history of *asana* have largely treated the yogic postures as a form of exercise, one largely influenced by Western gymnastics. Only a few attempts have been made to reconstruct historical perspectives on yogic practices generated by the experience of dwelling within *asanas*. Goldberg's reading of the achievements of the pioneers of modern postural yoga leads us closer to our actual experience of body-centered forms of yoga than any other historical study.

Research on the history of modern yoga has recently flourished. I am certain that *The Path of Modern Yoga* will be accorded the place of prominence within this field of study that the book so richly deserves. But *The Path of Modern Yoga* also appears at a moment of widespread interest in yoga history within the general public as well as academia. Luckily Goldberg creates a multifaceted, in-depth, and sweeping history that is scholarly but not academic. And unlike the usual academic treatise, his work is elegantly written, making it extraordinarily pleasurable to read. In short, it is a work of literature. Thus, his research findings, engagement with recent scholarship, and insights are accessible to a large audience.

Goldberg writes the sort of history that not only illuminates the past but has an implicit practical goal for the future: in this case, to inspire a change in yoga practice—to push it toward being more existentially and spiritually meaningful. For this reason, not only readers interested in learning about the history of modern yoga (as well as the history of modern India and of modernity as an intercultural phenomenon) but also yoginis and yogins who want to deepen their practice stand to profit greatly from reading this remarkable book.

Karl Baier

Karl Baier holds a doctorate in philosophy and heads the Department for the Study of Religions at Vienna University, Austria. He published a highly influential two-volume study, *Meditation und Moderne* (Meditation and Modernity), which among other things contributes to our understanding of the emergence of modern yoga, and has published two seminal lectures, "On the Philosophical Dimensions of Asana" and "Iyengar and the Yoga Tradition," which illuminate the nature of our experience in *asana*. Karl has been practicing yoga since the late 1970s, and in 1992 he received a teacher's certificate from B. K. S. Iyengar. He has taught the history and philosophy of yoga in several European Iyengar yoga teacher-training programs.

Acknowledgments

The Path of Modern Yoga couldn't have been written without the generous help of many people around the world over more than a dozen years. Among these are a handful of people who played a critical role in the book's creation. Since May 2000, Norman Sjoman has unfailingly answered my questions about yoga. Since April 2004, Ramu Rao, my "uncle," has translated key texts for me and, with charm and wisdom, explained Indian culture to me. In April 2006, Mark Singleton, Elizabeth De Michelis, Suzanne Newcombe, Benjamin Smith, and Klaus Nevrin, fellow participants in the Modern Yoga Workshop at Cambridge University, generously welcomed me into the emerging field of modern yoga scholarship and encouraged my work. Since November 2006, Stuart Ray Sarbacker has championed my work. From July 2008 to July 2013, Suzanne Newcombe, my godsend in the early and middle stages, made countless smart, insightful, and invaluable suggestions for improving the manuscript. From December 2015 to March 2016, Nancy Ringer, my godsend in the very last stage, made countless smart, insightful, and invaluable suggestions for improving the manuscript. In February 2016, Karl Baier graciously wrote the complimentary foreword.

I'd like to thank the people who provided me with published materials and background information on the people that I write about (presented here in the order in which they are featured in this book):

On Shri Yogendra—Armaiti N. Desai and Jack McKenzie (both at the Yoga Institute)

On Swami Vivekananda—Eric Shaw and John Schlenck (the latter at the Vedanta Society of New York)

On Swami Kuvalayananda—Manmath M. Gharote, Subodh Tiwari, Malti Shanbag, and Nigol Koulajian (all at the Kaivalyadhama Yoga Institute)

On K. V. Iyer—Vasantha and K. V. Karna, K. Rauhineya Iyer, Kartheek Karna, Jan and Terry Todd (at the H. J. Lutcher Stark Center for Physical Culture and Sports), Anantha Rao, Madhava Rao, David L. Chapman, Mark Singleton, Michael Murphy, Ramu Rao, Daniel Freund, and Shashidhar Rao

On S. Sundaram—V. Balaji (at the Girinath Yoga Centre), Vishwanath Iyer, and Hari Shankar R.

On Bhavanarao Pant Pratinidhi—Roxanne Gupta

On Eugen Sandow—David L. Chapman

On T. Krishnamacharya—Mark Singleton and Elizabeth Kadetsky

On Louise Morgan—Mark Singleton

On Apa Pant—Roxanne Gupta

On André Van Lysebeth—Atmatattwa (at *Yoga Magazine*)

On Swami Sivananda—Swami Sadasivananda (at the Sivananda Yoga Vedanta Center, New York)

On Indra Devi—Phillip Oliver and Audrey Youngman

On B. K. S. Iyengar—B. K. S. Iyengar (at the Ramamani Iyengar Memorial Yoga Institute), Suzanne Newcombe, Norman E. Sjoman, Eric Shaw, Hector Guthrie, Marian Garfinkel, Bobby Clennell, and Joan White

I'd like to thank the people who provided me with images of the people that I write about:

Of Shri Yogendra—Armaiti N. Desai, Ms. A. N. Desai, Arvind Maherchandani, and Jack McKenzie (all at the Yoga Institute)

Of Swami Vivekananda—Swami Nishpapananda (at the Vedanta Society of St. Louis)

Of Swami Kuvalayananda—Malti Shanbag (at the Kaivalyadhama Yoga Institute)

Of Bernarr Macfadden—David L. Chapman

Of K. V. Iyer—Michael Murphy, Ronne Iyer, and Shashidhar Tokanahalli Nagabhushan Rao

Of Maxick—David L. Chapman

Of Eugen Sandow—David L. Chapman

Of S. Sundaram—Vishwanath Iyer and Hari Shankar R.

Of Louise Morgan—Moira Fitzgerald (at the Beinecke Rare Book and Manuscript Library)

Of Matthias Alexander—Luke Chatterton (at the Society of Teachers of the Alexander Technique)

Of Apa Pant—Benegal Pereira

Of Swami Sivananda—Nazly Botas (at the Sivananda Yoga Vedanta Center, New York)

Of Indra Devi—Larry Payne (at Samata International)

Of B. K. S. Iyengar—Stephanie Quirk and B. K. S. Iyengar (both at the Ramamani Iyengar Memorial Yoga Institute) and Emory Elizabeth Johnson (at Penguin Random House)

Of B. K. S. Iyengar and T. Krishnamacharya—Paul Harvey (at the Centre for Yoga Studies) and Stephanie Quirk and B. K. S. Iyengar (both at the Ramamani Iyengar Memorial Yoga Institute)

I'd like to thank the people who provided me with images from newspapers and magazines that illustrate the achievements of the people that I write about:

From *Physical Culture*—David L. Chapman

From *Strength*—David Rosado (at the Photographic Services & Permissions office, New York Public Library)

From the *News Chronicle*—Gary Johnson (at the Newspaper & Current Periodical Reading Room, Library of Congress)

From *Das Kunstblatt*—Randy Kaufman (at the Photo Service office, Bauhaus-Archiv/Museum für Gestaltung)

PART I

Divesting Yoga of the Sacred

Yogic Physical Culture and Health Cure

1

SHRI YOGENDRA

Rejecting the Role of Yoga Guru

The Disciple Meets His Guru

In 1916, after having been a devoted high school student at Amalsad English School in Degam, a village in Gujarat, eighteen-year-old Manibhai Haribhai Desai (1897–1989)—who would change his name to Shri Yogendra in 1923—went off to St. Xavier's College in Bombay, a Catholic institution that's one of India's oldest colleges. Once away from home Mani succumbed to depression. He lost all interest in his studies. He was listless, distracted, and withdrawn. He was beset with feelings of sorrow and hopelessness. He couldn't turn to his parents for solace—his mother had died when he was three, and his forbidding father, his sole caretaker, wasn't one to "indulge" in "love and care."[1] The principal of the college, Father Alban Goodier, who would later become archbishop of Bombay, intervened, but to no avail. As Yogendra's biographer Santan Rodrigues, a Goan poet of Portuguese descent, melodramatically sets the scene: "It was night and darkness all around. Where was the light to end the worldly ills that cast a gloom over [Mani]?"[2] That light would take the form of a guru.

Many of us are familiar with the narrative of the *guru-shishya* (master-disciple) relationship. The earliest prescriptions for seeking spiritual guidance appear in the Upanishads: "Let [a man devoted to spiritual life] give no thought to transient things, but, absorbed in meditation, let him renounce the world. If he would know the Eternal, let him humbly approach a Guru devoted to Brahman and well-versed in the scriptures." The guru accepts the aspirant as a disciple: "To a disciple who approaches reverently, who is tranquil and self-controlled,

2

the wise teacher agrees to give that knowledge, faithfully and unstintingly, by which is known the truly existing, the changeless Self."[3] The disciple then moves into the guru's ashram or household, where he lives together with other aspirants.

Over a period of years the disciple serves his guru with devotion and obedience, and the guru, in turn, gives his knowledge generously, without restraint. He elucidates the scriptures and, perhaps more importantly, argue Swami Prabhavananda and Frederick Manchester, in their translation of the Upanishads, "teaches by his life—by his daily acts, by his most casual words, sometimes even by his silence. Only to be near him, only to serve and obey him in humility and in reverence, is to become quickened in spirit."[4]

By means of this personal interaction, the disciple eventually masters the knowledge that the guru explains and embodies, thus achieving liberation. The disciple, now himself a master, sets off on his own.

Very little of this iconic sequence of the events, however, jibes with the story of Yogendra's relationship with his guru. It can be said that meeting his guru was the most auspicious event of Yogendra's life: his spiritual life was awakened. But the unfolding of Yogendra's relationship with his guru, while ultimately being a chronicle of the quickening of his soul by the soul of another, more nearly resembles a mad love affair.

When Mani's roommate, Ambalal, learned that the yogin Paramahamsa Madhavadasaji (literally, Supreme Swan, Servant of Krishna) of Malsar was about to give a discourse at the Madhav Baug, a community and religious center in Bombay, he "hoped that Mani lost in his own world would use this 'happening' to get over his troubled mind."[5] Although highly suspicious of *sannyasis* and *sadhus* (terms used interchangeably in India in the early 20th century to refer to non-Muslim ascetics who forsake the world for the contemplative life), Mani gave in to his roommate's pleading. "On the night of Saturday 26th August 1916 Ambalal and I set out for the *dharamshala* of Madhav Baug," recorded Yogendra in a graphic account written only a few months after the event. "I had mixed feelings even as I was going there. [However,] as soon as I saw Paramahamsaji I felt that here was a man—a great man. My early thoughts of belittling *sadhus* disappeared. All my earlier misgivings seemed to go away, as our eyes met. There was a feeling of complete understanding and I felt humble and greatly drawn to the Master. Madhavadasaji's eyes were glued on me. . . . I prostrated myself at the feet of the Master."[6]

As we read Mani's words (his misgivings disappeared "as our eyes met" and "there was a feeling of complete understanding"), we realize that it was love at first sight. And not just on his part. His most telling observation—"Madhavadasaji's eyes were glued on me"—shows that the attraction was mutual.

The following day Mani went to meet with Madhavadasaji in private. His sense from the previous night that they had taken to each other was confirmed: "There seemed to be an immediate and kindly bond between the two of us."[7] The guru "initiated me into the trance experience—*samadhi*. He praised my body and pure nature and appreciated the discipline and self-control."[8] (Addicted to physical culture, Mani had made himself into a powerful wrestler in high school. "Bursting at the seams with muscles and energy," he was hailed as a local Mr. Universe for his strength and athletic physique.)[9] After a sleepless night and an especially distracted day at college, Mani went again to see Madhavadasaji the next night. "The teacher seemed to be already waiting for me," Mani recalled. "Appreciating my pure nature he taught me some *kriyas* [yogic cleansing techniques]. That night I slept at his place."[10] The following day, after going back to his lodgings to pay off his bills and leaving with only the clothes on his back, Mani, "trembling in my ecstasy," returned to the Madhav Baug.[11]

> On seeing me in this excited state, the Master enquired as to what had happened. I could not utter a single word but seemed to be overwhelmed by sadness. Madhavadasaji noticing my total renunciation asked me to stay with him and requested me to write to my father.[12]

Courted by the Guru: The Letters

Alarmed to learn by mail that his son wanted to take the path of a yogin, Mani's father, Haribhai, rushed to Bombay to retrieve Mani. As his sullen son sat nearby, Haribhai told Madhavadasaji that he was taking Mani home. It was not that Haribhai wished for Mani a life of leisure, gaiety, and wealth instead of one of practice, austerity, and poverty. A petty official (he was the village schoolmaster), Haribhai badly wanted a similar but better position for his son:

civil servant. By expanding the participation of Indians in the British Raj, the Indian Councils Act, passed by the Parliament of the United Kingdom in 1909 to appease Indian demands for self-governance, had increased the need for civil service jobs for Indians. A prestigious and secure job, the civil servant was the highest rung of the Indian bureaucracy. Haribhai was determined to have Mani go to London to take the civil service examination.

Haribhai's hopes for Mani were by no means totally unselfish. To lead a life of renunciation, a *sannyasi* breaks all formal ties with society, forsaking not only worldly ambitions and pleasures but also responsibilities. Haribhai wanted Mani to marry and perpetuate the family name and to care for him in his last days (he believed his salvation depended on his son offering the *tarpana,* or water sacrifice, for the peace of his dying soul).

Upon arriving home Mani pined away for Madhavadasaji. Biographer Rodrigues describes the situation with his usual flair for histrionics: "The bonds between the Master and the student could not be snapped by distance in miles or even overwhelmed by stronger family ties. At home Mani continued to be aloof and had strange moods which the father found difficult to fathom. The only joy seemed be the postman's knock on the door. The letters which came from the Master speak volumes."[13] Indeed they do. Madhavadasaji's epistolary courtship of Mani was a kind of ravishment to which the swoony teenager submitted. It's impossible to discern who was more out of control. For both Madhavadasaji and Mani, each equally beside himself with longing, it was head-over-heels love.

Madhavadasaji's rhetorical strategy in his three letters to Mani, all written in September 1916, was to alternately set Mani's heart aflutter with reassurances of his love (or something of the sort) and then calm Mani's agitation with invocations to find contentment through God.

In the first letter Madhavadasaji was all reassurances and invocations, the pattern (like in a dream or fairy tale) repeated three times. "Dear Mani, who is tormented by the fire of separation. . . . He [Madhavadasaji, referring to himself in the third person] received your letter that is full of the sad feelings of a severed heart. The feelings of the heart appear like tears which have fallen on this letter. The letter was opened with the same eagerness as it was written." "There is no reason for sadness. . . . Your utterance should be 'What my Lord does is all for the good.'" "The image of your pure personality has played a magic on me and has drawn me towards you." "May God quieten your mind and give you happiness and satisfaction as He is the only hope that may create no further difficulties." "Whatever you write in your madness of separation is very pleasant for me, for to the lover whatever writings are communicated in whatever form are like nectar only and so remain happy, happy and happy. . . . Do not worry. You are far and yet you are near me, that is what I think." "It is not necessary to feel sad. Be constantly remembering God (Sri Krishna). You will thus gain peace."[14]

In the second letter Madhavadasaji ratcheted up the special nature of their love (it's simply divine) and began entreating Mani to join him. "Your post card was received today. Just as much as your heart and mind are attracted to me so also am I getting drawn to you. This is the law of nature." "In case you cannot come here in your person then my body and soul will run to you. I keep thinking when shall I see my Maniya. Your divine look has made a place in my heart. I lose myself when I receive your letter and I exclaim 'Come Maniya come, come quick. If you do not come I shall come.'" "Start seeing God in all things. Separation is just to cause glimpses of the divine. Radhaji's separation from Srikrishna was ultimately for union." "One who is mad after God [Shri Krishna] indeed God is mad after him. As you cannot write everything in a letter so also can I not. This is enough. I will send the incommunicable message through my heart."[15]

In the third letter Madhavadasaji implied that Mani's father was interfering with their correspondence, forcefully told Mani to leave his father (he finally came out with it), and rapturously declared the karmic nature of their love. "Your two letters received. Replies were written yet you write that you did not receive my reply. So this letter is sent via registered post. Find out who took the two letters sent in envelopes." "Reading this, come away. . . . Make your mind strong and adamant and abandon your father." "Be quiet! My dear Mani be quiet! Start the medicine of chanting the name of God (Sri Hari)." "Write quickly. I am even more worried than you. I do not know God's work but I know through His love that in the last life you were mine and I was yours. We had great love and so I write this."[16]

Mani's exhilaration over the prospect of reuniting with Madhavadasaji, sparked by the letters, alternated with his despair over the possibility of permanent separation. These "strange moods" alarmed members of the community.[17]

They were, after all, Indians, whose skepticism of love extends most famously to their view of marriage as an alliance between families in which the husband and wife only come to find romantic love after many years (but, conversely, whose conspicuous idealization of romantic love can be found in their myths and movies). "How could the simple folk grasp the significance of the attachment to the Master?" asks Rodrigues, implying that they couldn't understand the ardor of spiritual awakening kindled by a guru.[18] What the community couldn't comprehend, though, was the depth of Mani's need to be loved: Madhavadasaji's love for Mani had intoxicated the joyless boy's yearning heart. The love that Madhavadasaji proffered was simple, pure, faithful, and unconditional. "Dear Mani, come and overcome the confusion of the world," Madhavadasaji wrote.[19] Who among us could resist this entreaty? Certainly not an eighteen-year-old boy with deep feelings of abandonment and unworthiness.

"Well meaning neighbours thought that the young lad had gone mad," Rodrigues writes. "Well aware of the father's sacrifice for Mani they wanted to retrieve this brilliant young man from this insane plight." They proposed "various rescue measures," including "that the young man be put in chains till he returned to his senses."[20] Facing the fact that he no longer held sway over his son, Haribhai at last relented and gave Mani permission to join Madhavadasaji.

In *The Inner World: A Psycho-analytic Study of Childhood and Society in India,* Sudhir Kakar describes the consequences for Indian children, especially boys, of the "second birth" when, at age four or five, they come of age. For boys, the "second birth" is an abrupt separation from a world of the mother's "unchecked benevolent indulgence" into the man's world of "absolute obedience and conformity to familial and social standards."[21] "In spite of . . . 'extra-maternal' sources of comfort and guidance provided by the very structure of the extended family," writes Kakar, "the Indian boy's loss of the relationship of symbiotic intimacy with his mother amounts to a narcissistic injury of the first magnitude." As a result, Indian men have "a heightened narcissistic vulnerability, an unconscious tendency to 'submit' to an idealized omnipotent figure, both in the inner world of fantasy and in the outside world of making a living; the lifelong search for someone, a charismatic leader or a *guru,* who will provide mentorship and a guiding world-view, thereby restoring intimacy and authority to individual life."[22]

Yogendra said that his discipleship with Madhavadasaji was "prompted by an intense craving for knowledge of much different magnitude than the mere academic encumbrance, while searching for an expression of myself."[23] But when we consider the brevity of the time when unconditional motherly love was lavished on Mani, the finality of his loss, and the abruptness of his entry into the world of rules and responsibilities established by a stern and emotionally distant father, we can't help but think how much more intense than the average Indian boy's must have been the teenage Mani's yearning (perhaps hidden, even from himself) for a relationship "like that of the communion between mother and infant," in which he could find the "soothing of disappointments by a 'guru-mother's' love."[24]

Kakar's insights into the *guru-chela* relationship, however, only take us so far. To complete our understanding of the psychological dimension of this bond, we must also recognize the needs of the guru. Only then can we identify a key characteristic of the master-disciple relationship: its mutual ardor.

Moony relationships, ignited by love-at-first-sight meetings, between master and favored disciple are not uncommon. When the eighteen-year-old Swami Vivekananda met his guru, Ramakrishna Paramahamsa, in 1881, according to Vivekananda's disciples, the master, his eyes welling up with tears, cried out, "At last you have come!" The boy didn't know what to make of this man who, as if always knowing and loving him, was filled with joy to see him. "Reason tells me that he is mad," Vivekananda thought, 'but the heart is attracted to him!'"[25] The ardor on the master's part and ambivalence on the student's part would remain unabated for the next five years (until the master's death). "Sri Ramakrishna's love for Noren [Norendra Nath Dutta was Vivekananda's birth name] was such that if Noren failed to come for some days to visit him he would become inconsolable. He would sit, weeping alone. He would pray and pray to the Divine Mother with a sorrow-laden heart, begging that She would make it possible for him to come." Vivekananda would always show up, regarding Ramakrishna "differently as different moods came upon him."[26]

When the seventeen-year-old Paramhansa Yogananda and his fifty-five-year-old master Yukteswar Giri met in 1910, as recounted in Yogananda's *Autobiography of a Yogi,* they went gaga over each other. While shopping at the bazaar in Varanasi (Benares), Yogananda spotted "a Christlike man in the ocher robes of swami" in a lane. Yogananda continued on his way for ten minutes, then went running back to find the man. "I reached the narrow lane. My quick glance revealed the quiet figure, steadily gazing in my direction. A few eager steps and I was at his feet. 'Gurudeva!' 'O my own, you have come to me!'" Yukteswar cried out repeatedly, "his voice tremulous with joy. 'How many years I have waited for you!'" "We entered a oneness of silence," Yogananda remembered, during which he realized that they were fated to be together—again. "Dramatic time! Past, present, and future are its cycling scenes. This was not the first sun to find me at these holy feet!" As they walked along hand in hand, Yogananda assessed his newly found guru, finding him athletic, vigorous, and handsome ("his dark eyes were large, beautiful"), yet tender: "Strength mingled subtly with gentleness." Yukteswar led Yogananda to his temporary residence (he was in town to visit his mother for a few days). "'I give you my unconditional love,'" said Yukteswar, as they made their way to the balcony overlooking the Ganges. "'Will you give me the same unconditional love?' He gazed at me with childlike trust. 'I will love you eternally, Gurudeva!'"[27] Perhaps surprisingly, these mutual pledges of undying love gradually led to a relationship of hard-won constancy and reciprocal affection, in which a churlish young man learned valuable life lessons from a guru's sensible guidance.

Living with the Guru: The Apprenticeship

Upon arriving at Madhavadasaji's ashram in Malsar in late 1916, Mani immediately settled into the routine. Along with the other disciples, he awoke at about 5:30 a.m., took his ablutions at the Narmada River, participated in a period of worship in the small temple (the disciples were mostly Vaishnavites, believers in Lord Krishna, an avatar of Vishnu), and ate breakfast, usually consisting of milk and *chapatti* (a flatbread made of wheat) and sometimes supplemented with sweets and bananas. Afterward they watched as people came to see Madhavadasaji, seated on his *vyaghracharma* (tiger skin) on a dais, for guidance with their problems (fig. 1.1). Most of these people came from nearby villages, but some came from long distances, even from cities. Their issues were mainly personal, not spiritual, often revolving around family matters. Evidently Madhavadasaji provided a satisfying mix of advice, comfort, and blessings. Following these counseling sessions, he read his mail and dictated replies to his amanuensis.

When Mani first arrived the other disciples warmly welcomed him as one of their own. But within days of his arrival there was no hiding his special status. After dealing with the correspondence, Madhavadasaji invited Mani to accompany him for a daily walk, "sometimes in the pasture-land where cows (donated to the ashram) used to graze. Madhavadasaji being very fond of cows patted the little ones lovingly as they strolled by."[28] On these bucolic walks and on evening boat rides, Madhavadasaji instructed Mani on how to help others.

Madhavadasaji kept Mani increasingly close to him. "The great love between the *chela* and the *guru* called for newer ways to disseminate information," Rodrigues notes. "The close rela-

tionship demanded a no-barrier and no restriction [*sic*] tutorship. So why keep [Mani] at a distance?" They began to sit together to eat. "Paramahamsaji never trusted his beloved student to eat with others and so they shared a common plate. Trustworthy as the inmates of Malsar were, Madhavadasaji knew that Mani's unconventional life and bearing had aroused jealousy. He did not want any untoward incident to take place."[29] What aroused their jealousy, no doubt, was the special attention the master lavished on Mani from the start. Madhavadasaji had provoked in his other disciples the very response that he could use to rationalize his doting on Mani.

Gradually "Mr. Muscle-man" (as Rodrigues calls him) shed his wrestler's body. In losing his muscular physique, Mani was casting off the masculine ethos of wrestling—strength, fierceness, and competitiveness. Within a month he attained the slim figure conducive to the gentle discipline of hatha yoga, with its placid movements, acquiescent extensions, and rhythmic breathing. Madhavadasaji himself taught Mani the techniques of the yoga postures. "Under the guidance of the greatest Yoga expert," Rodrigues writes, "the two drank at the fountain of Yoga knowledge, perfecting each movement."[30]

Much of the yoga training was related to the application of yogic natural health cure to patients in the ashram's sick ward. Mani accompanied Madhavadasaji as he made his rounds. During these visits Mani developed his diagnostic skills and learned which hatha yoga treatment modalities—*asanas* (postures), *pranayama* (breath control), purificatory techniques, *mudras* (seals), *bandhas* (locks), diet, or

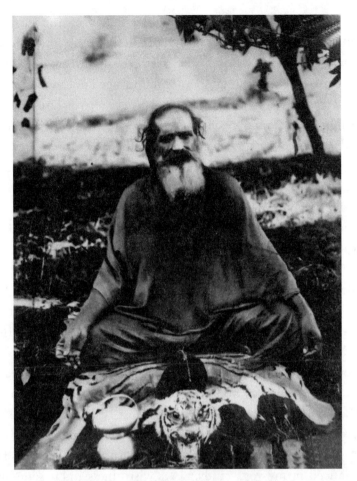

Figure 1.1. Paramahamsa Madhavadasaji seated on his
vyaghracharma (tiger skin), circa 1915
(With the kind permission of the Yoga Institute)

some combination of these—to apply to various illnesses. Learning and observing progressively gave way to resolving and acting: Mani was assigned his own cases to handle.

Two examples of the cases treated by Mani during his apprenticeship reveal the nature of the yogic medical protocols of this time as, respectively, scarily misguided and impressively intuitive. The first case involved a wealthy woman from Bombay seeking help at the ashram for pulmonary tuberculosis, thought to be a disorder of the esophagus and stomach cured by removing mucus. The treatment procedure—the purificatory practice *vaso-dhauti,* in which the throat, esophagus, and stomach are cleansed by having the patient partially swallow a four-fingers-wide cloth—nearly proved fatal. The cloth became lodged in the woman's throat. She was in danger of suffocation. An attendant ran for help to Madhavadasaji, who turned the matter over to Mani. The quick-witted Mani gave the panicked woman a little hot water and *ghee* (clarified butter) to sip, dislodging the cloth. The second case involved a depressed twenty-four-year-old man, the son of a Bombay Hindu knight, staying at the Forest Lodge in Matheran, a nearby hill station. Mani promptly dismissed the private nurse, to whom the young man had become overly attached. Cagily replacing her companionship with his, Mani was able to treat the young man with "long walks, a few simple Yoga practices and counseling."[31] After six weeks, his depression lifted.

In addition to teaching yogic health cure, Madhavadasaji took Mani to his underground retreat (Madhavadasaji prayed separately from his disciples), where the master taught Mani meditation (fig. 1.2). "It was the inner sanctum where the Master used to meditate twice a day, and to be allowed to enter here," Rodrigues observes, "was a great honour indeed."[32] (Only Mani and one other *chela* had this special privilege; they were always instructed separately.) "Our associations grew so intimate, as I advanced in my yoga study, that neither of us could dream of separation without remorse or agony," Yogendra reminisced fifteen years later. "The love he bore to me was inexpressible."[33]

In early 1918, about a year and a half after his discipleship had begun, Mani told Madhavadasaji that he was leaving. Madhavadasaji responded by offering him his *kamandalu,* or begging bowl, the sign of *sannyasa* (the life of renunciation). He had used it to feed thousands of his followers. Handing on the bowl symbolized delegation of leadership to Mani. Mani declined this enormously flattering enticement to stay.

In this offer to Mani the (quite understand-able) needs of the guru are fully revealed. Madhavadasaji knew from the moment he set eyes upon this splendid youth that he had found not another follower but a successor—someone "to whom he could disclose the secrets of the great Yoga culture with absolute confidence," someone who could grasp and pass on all his teachings.[34] Who could blame him for being delirious with joy from the get-go? "To him," Yogendra recalled, "I was *the* student he was waiting for during his whole life-time."[35] And what a long wait that was! Madhavadasaji was said to be 118 years old in 1916. (He would die five years later from malaria.) How crushing it must've been to him to have Mani reject his offer of succession.

Yogendra addressed the reasoning for his departure in a poignant letter to Madhavadasaji written just two years later (in February 1920) but seemingly composed looking back from the distant future, many decades hence, for it contains a wistfulness and wisdom usually only achieved with a great passage of time. The letter was an after-the-fact request for Madhavadasaji's approval of Yogendra's venture in America (see chapter 4).

It is due to some trifle misunderstanding that we were separated from each other, but that has nothing to do with our mutual love. I have chosen my own way to help humanity and you have yours. However, none is responsible for truth as it is *swa-dharma* [one's own right action or true path]. I deeply regret not to have seen you before I left India, but my love for you is still untarnished.

The enclosed cutting will show my activi-

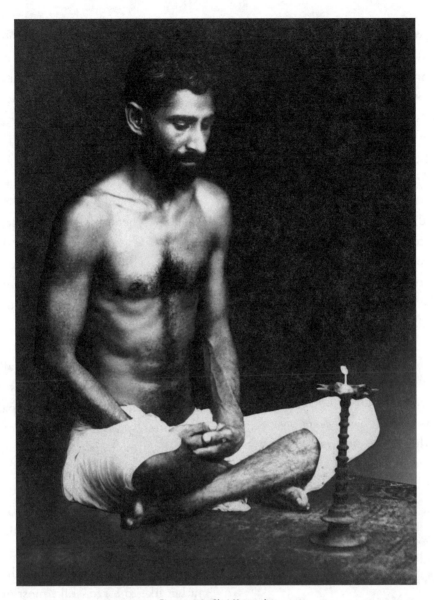

Figure 1.2. Shri Yogendra
sitting in meditation, circa 1930
(With the kind permission of the Yoga Institute)

ties here and my love for you. I still remember my days of old with you when I used to sit undisturbed in concentration. I know they were prosperous days for body, mind and spirit. Oh, how I wish I could get them back.[36]

There's nothing over-the-top about this letter, except its precocious nostalgia for a recent past that may have seemed to Yogendra more distant than his childhood, perhaps because more idyllic and dreamlike, or that may simply have been an expression of respect and obligatory flattery.

The letter expresses neither a consuming hunger for approval nor a burdensome guilt over his act of abandonment. It's a kind and considerate letter, especially for a twenty-three-year-old. Its calmness stands in contrast not only to Madhavadasaji's courtship letters to Yogendra but to what would become Yogendra's major work, *Yoga Asanas Simplified,* an intemperate book filled with rants.

A more candid clue to the reasons for Yogendra's decision to leave Madhavadasaji, though, may be found in his assessment of yogins, written in a letter to his friend Popat in late 1920, shortly after he had received his guru's blessings for his trip to America:

> No doubt it was a great surprise to me to receive Maharajaji's letter a few days back. He apparently seems to agree with my mission and sends his heartiest blessings for success.
>
> I know the nature of Yogis. They are mostly two-sided. Once they are tender and lovable while the next moment they are harsh and strict.[37]

But there was another reason—one deeper than a misunderstanding or his guru's mood swings—that explains why Yogendra broke his close bond with Madhavadasaji and rejected the role of guru for which Madhavadasaji was grooming him: Yogendra was forming a new identity—one that would both satisfy and put him at odds with not just his spiritual father but also his biological father.

The First Hatha Yoga Teacher

When his son returned home, Haribhai learned that Yogendra had not rejected the role of heir apparent to Madhavadasaji to become a civil servant after all. Yogendra wanted to become neither a guru nor a civil servant but something new under the sun: a yoga teacher—someone who provides instruction in yoga exercise to worldly students (to help them maintain and improve their health) during the day and then goes home at night. Although two years later Yogendra would write that he'd chosen his way to help others, his path to becoming a yoga teacher seems to have been just as much determined as chosen.

Yogendra clearly didn't have the makeup for being a spiritual father figure, a role that demands continually looking after one's followers. As Rodrigues bluntly puts it: "To fall in the modern tradition of *guru* for all seasons and climes was not Shri Yogendraji's line."[38] Yogendra was temperamentally incapable of taking absolute responsibility for disciples, or perhaps just unwilling to take authority over all areas of their lives. He would admit as much in a letter to a student in 1929: "Of course you have overestimated me in believing me to be your *guru,* which title is full of responsibilities and unless one is prepared to take upon himself all eventualities [for others], it is something one would rather like to forgo." Like most of us, Yogendra preferred to fully extend himself only to his friends and family.[39]

There was another reason Yogendra rejected the role of guru: its isolation from everyday life. Yogendra was no more capable of developing and consolidating an identity as a reclusive yogin than he was of becoming an engaged member of secular society with a traditional career. He'd transmuted this ambivalence about his place in society—which in previous eras (in the less fluid premodern world) might've led to marginalization but which was perfectly suited to an era (in the more departmentalized modern world) when the Indian middle class was beginning to consume spiritual guidance as a service—into an existential stance, a hard-won philosophy that would be held by others, he believed, were they only as brave as he was. On the title page of his first book, *Prabhubhakti* (Devotion to the Lord), a collection of reflections published in 1917, he proclaimed his heroic view of himself with a quote from Ralph Waldo Emerson, the American transcendentalist: "It is easy in the world to live after the world's opinion; it is easy in solitude to live after our own; but the great man is he who in the midst of the crowd keeps with perfect sweetness the independence of solitude."[40]

In aspiring to the job of yoga teacher, Yogendra sought a quasi-spiritual role perfectly suited to someone who, by his nature, wasn't capable of fully living within or withdrawing from society. But there was also yet another explanation—one not related to his psychological makeup—for his taking this path: his embrace of the new beliefs about yoga then current in India, which conflicted with the traditional beliefs held by Madhavadasaji.

"I find all religions uniform," Yogendra said.[41] By this he meant, in part, that they're simply different means of realizing the same truth: "Truth *is,* and is *One.*"[42] Madhavadasaji seems to have shared this view. During his leisure time at the ashram, after writing *Prabhubhakti,*

Yogendra composed *Hrdayapuspanjali* (Prayers from the Heart), published in 1918, a book of poems inspired by his musings while taking solitary walks about the nearby hills and plains. Both books were on the theme of the spiritual uniformity of all religions. With Madhavadasaji's permission—an indication that the guru was receptive to the reformist views of Hinduism espoused by Yogendra—the first and probably the second book were sold to devotees who attended the ashram.*

Yogendra picked up this approach to religion from the key figure in the introduction of yoga to the Western world, Swami Vivekananda, who, in the late 19th century, championed tolerance of religious diversity (his cagey strategy for elevating Hinduism to the level of the other major religions) because all religions, while having different paths, ultimately share the same quest: to comprehend the nondual reality underlying everyday existence (his slyly provocative way of saying that all religions, if they are true religions, conform to the Vedantic doctrine that identifies *atman,* the individual self, with *brahman,* the ground of reality).

Yogendra also followed Vivekananda in finding traditional yoga constraining. Adopting the spiritual leader's view, propounded in his seminal book *Vedanta Philosophy,* published in 1896, that yoga is a scientific and direct method for apprehending "the One out of which the manifold is being manufactured, that One existing as many," Yogendra was dismissive of a yoga informed by classical Hindu study and ritual and even belief and faith (and, by implication,

---

*Yogendra earned enough money from these sales to repay his father, who financed the publication of the first and probably the second book.

of all the formal religious paths that he, influenced by Vivekananda, claimed to tolerate!).[43]*

This view of Hinduism, with its emphasis on realization (the direct perception of religious truths, which is attained not by belief and faith but by experience), challenged Madhavadasaji's very identity as a spiritual guide to ascetics. In a December 1920 letter to Madhavadasaji, Yogendra tactfully explained their differences: "You have one way to work and I have the other."[44] Yogendra's way was to encourage people not to withdraw from society and join a sect but to partake of life's myriad experiences. Perhaps using a physical culture metaphor, he wrote: "Experience I found is an exercise for the soul. It is a realization for broader circumferences. Who would be [so] foolish as to run away from it and let the soul shiver in timidity?"[45]†

In a letter written to Popat about a year later, in March 1922, the twenty-five-year-old Yogendra expanded on his differences with Madhavadasaji by waxing indignant about a swami in America who advised a man—an idealistic, penniless American about to set sail for India in search of spiritual development—to become a Hindu renunciate: "These people take a sort of pride in turning men into *sanyasins* and this I really hate."[46]‡

Why should a man be tied to a certain order when he wants to be universal? Does it require one to be a Jain, a Buddhist, a *sanyasin* or a friar to find and realize higher truths of life? A man to be a real devotee of Truth needs to be a non-conformist. He must be neutral or else he is nothing. As soon as he gets into a certain order, it becomes his centre and they are his circumference. Anyway why should he give up this world physically when he has to realize the Infinite through it? The whole question of becoming something is very funny. Look at the numberless limits he draws on himself by doing so.

It is why I kept myself neutral and have become a free man, by not entering into any order though I was often forced to do so. Why should I register myself as something and leave the other? I must be able to say I am everything and that really I am. I must belong to none, They must all belong to me. This is the true spirit of a free man.[47]

Yogendra seems to have been influenced in his beliefs about "the true spirit of a free man" less by Vivekananda and more by Emerson and other 19th-century American transcendentalists, who held that an individual has no need for

---

*In taking up this contradictory position, Vivekananda had been influenced, in turn, by the leaders of the Brahmo Samaj, an Indian society founded in 1828, who, in turn, had been influenced by the missionaries of the Unitarian Mission in Calcutta, formed in 1821. Unitarians advocated the substitution of rational faith for mechanical ritual and otherworldly beliefs.

†Based on an interview with Yogendra's son, Jayadeva, scholar of modern yoga Elizabeth De Michelis argues that Yogendra's "*guru,* Sri Madhavadasji of Malsar, had in fact been very receptive to the Swami's message" (De Michelis, *History of Modern Yoga,* 183). This seems to be only partially true. De Michelis doesn't provide any supporting details.

‡While remaining skeptical of spiritual leaders all his life, Yogendra was especially wary of yoga gurus. Forty-five years later, in 1967, when he was seventy years old, he bemoaned the current state of yoga in which "floating spiritually-inclined schismatical students of yoga" on a "spiritual shopping spree" are given "grandiose promises" by opportunistic gurus "catering" to them with "simulated spirituality," such as "transcendental meditation" (Yogendra, "Right Approach to Yoga," 162–63).

the intercession of organized religion in transcending the everyday world because each individual has a divine spark within that can access the Divine. Yogendra believed that freewheeling experience (not ritual and study or even, apparently, seated meditation) in the profane world (not a separate sacred place) is a central precondition to unadulterated self-realization (in the Eastern sense of the attainment of the highest religious experience: enlightenment, liberation, realization of the god-self within)—that, in other words, self-realization is accessible (*more* accessible!) to nonrenunciates, who are independent of the intrusive trappings of religion.

2

SHRI YOGENDRA

Creating the Profession of Yoga Teacher

The Yoga Class

The First Yoga Class

In late 1917 Shri Yogendra (then still called Manibhai Haribhai Desai, his birth name) was asked by his guru, Paramahamsa Madhavadasaji, to translate *Gitanjali,* a volume of mostly devotional song poems by Bengali poet Rabindranath Tagore,* from Bengali into Gujarati. Despite having no knowledge of Bengali, Yogendra managed to translate the book (by learning the Bengali alphabet) in ten days. Delighted with the result, Madhavadasaji told Yogendra to seek Tagore's permission to have it published. After Tagore's consent was received, Yogendra's translation of *Gitanjali* was published in early 1918.

In late 1918, after Yogendra had left Madhavadasaji's ashram to return home, his translation of *Gitanjali* caught the attention of the vice chancellor of Bombay University, R. P. Masani. Masani invited Yogendra to visit him at his home in Versova, a fishing village on the Arabian Sea in Bombay, where a large, prosperous Parsi community resided. In December 1918

---

*Tagore was a renowned writer whose works helped introduce the West to India's spiritual heritage. His Bengali *Gitanjali* was published in 1910. In 1912 he published a collection of English poems, also titled *Gitanjali;* about half of the poems in this volume are translations by Tagore of his earlier Bengali volume of the same name. He was awarded the Nobel Prize for Literature in 1913, becoming the first non-European recipient.

Yogendra traveled there to meet with Masani.

The modern history of Versova, like that of the other towns in Bombay's "Suburban District," is closely linked to the history of the cotton industry in Bombay. Beginning with the founding of its first fabric mill for spinning cotton in 1851, Bombay's cotton industry (the European factory system transplanted to India, where making brightly colored, hand-decorated products from chintz, muslin, calico, and other cottons had long been an artisanal craft) greatly expanded in the second half of the 19th century, spurred by the outbreak of the Civil War in America in 1861, which reduced American exports to England (the result of the disruption of cotton production in the South), and by the opening of the Suez Canal in 1869, which facilitated shipping coarse cotton yarn to England from India. (Having created the first modern export-oriented economy, England imported raw cotton, cotton yarn, and plain cotton fabric for its textile industry and exported clothes, bedding, and other cotton goods, even to India.) By the end of 1895 there were seventy cotton mills in Bombay.

During this period, in which the modern Indian middle class was formed, the bulk of the Indian professional classes consisted of the intelligentsia.* "The increase in the number of Indian lawyers and public servants, doctors and teachers, writers, scholars, and members of other recognized professions," observes historian B. B. Misra, "was due to educational, judicial, and administrative development rather than to technological or industrial progress."[1] In Bombay, however, a sector of the Indian professional class emerged that was engaged in industry and trade as a result of the technological and economic changes in the cotton textile industry. The cotton mills were mainly supplied with capital, owned, and managed by Indians, not the British. Bombayites also founded and worked in banking, cotton pressing, shipping, insurance, reclamation, stock, and other businesses related to the founding of the cotton industry.

The rapid growth of the cotton mills was sustained by a large migration to the city of mainly Marathi-speaking workers, who lived in *chawls,* multistoried one-room tenements (which still exist; the slums of today's Mumbai, a cosmopolitan port city that's home to Bollywood and the Bombay Stock Exchange, are the by-products of the cotton boom). Not wanting to live in the crowded inner city, and not allowed to build houses in the European districts, the Indian middle class moved into small towns in northern parts of Bombay, where developments consisting of bungalows and rows of houses were built for them starting in the late 19th century. The bungalows of Versova (which have sadly vanished), in particular, were well known for their charm.

Following his meeting with Masani, Yogendra encountered a cosmopolitan Parsi consulting

---

*In India at the turn of the 20th century, with the poor making up the vast majority of people, the small group of educated, home-owning professionals with a high income and standard of living was the elite. Yet in contrast to maharajahs, the landed elite (owners of large properties who employed agricultural labor), international merchants, and prosperous industrialists, these professionals were not the wealthy. To differentiate them from the "lower class" and the "upper class," I use the term "middle class."

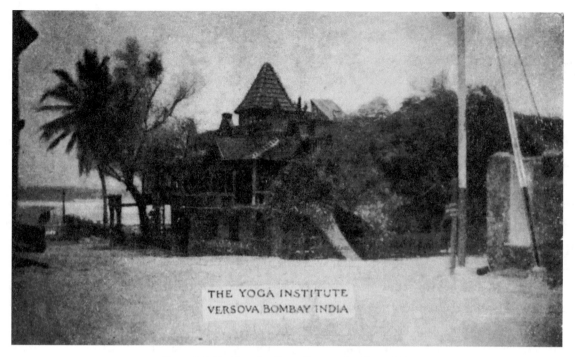

Figure 2.1. The Yoga Institute, Versova, Bombay, 1918
(From *The Householder Yogi,* by Santan Rodrigues)

engineer in his early fifties, Homi Dadina, the son-in-law of "The Grand Old Man of India," Dadabhai Naoroji, the renowned nationalist political leader who had died the previous year. Plagued for nearly twenty years by obesity, dyspepsia, hyperuricemia, prostatic hypertrophy, piles, and rheumatism (conditions caused, one suspects, by a lavish diet), Dadina expressed his frustration with the treatments provided by doctors in India, England, and Germany, which provided only temporary relief. Yogendra recommended to Dadina a natural treatment for his ailments: yoga. "Bowled over" by "the yogin's ways and manners" and eager to try his yoga treatment, Dadina invited Yogendra to stay on in Versova for two weeks at Dadina's large beachfront home, "The Sands," which had been his father-in-law's residence.[2]

After informally teaching yoga to Dadina and a few other men on the beach, Yogendra founded the Yoga Institute in Dadina's house (fig. 2.1). The first batch of students enrolled for a regular course on December 25, 1918. The instruction held that Christmas morning on Versova beach was a momentous event that marked the first step in the formation of modern hatha yoga. "This was a red letter day in the history of Yoga," proclaims Yogendra's biographer, Santan Rodrigues. "For the first time Yoga was taught to the man of the world."[3]

In founding the Yoga Institute, Yogendra had relocated the center of hatha yoga instruction from the realm of the sacred, the ashram, where renunciates withdrew from ordinary society to seek spiritual liberation, to the realm of the secular, the yoga center or institute, where students exercised together to improve their health. He had made an essentially religious experience into a secular experience. The means of this subversion of the hatha yoga tradition was its radical—but now axiomatic—form of instruction: the yoga class.

Goals of the Yoga Class

Physical Health

Yogendra defined yoga as "a comprehensive practical system of self-culture." By this he meant that its "interchangeable harmonious development" of the body, mind, and spirit "ultimately leads to physical well-being, mental harmony, moral elevation and habituation to spiritual consciousness."[4] It galled him that this invaluable training wasn't readily available to those who might benefit from it. "Theoretical Yoga was sprinkled in and throughout most of the ancient texts belonging to the various metaphysical schools and the theological traditions representing the pre-Aryan and Aryan culture," he wrote, "but the inestimable technique of practical training both for the body and mind always remained a secret."[5]

Following Swami Vivekananda, Yogendra believed that everyone, no matter what their beliefs, could benefit from yogic training because, as Rodrigues makes plain, "for him Yoga was never a religion. He always went about it in a very scientific way, demystifying it, de-linking it from religion, salvaging it from the forests and the withdrawn ascetics."[6] Yogendra capaciously declared:

> Above all, [yoga] is the only practical, scientific and catholic culture that is not limited to any sex, race, nationality, religion or creed. One may continue to be a Hindu, a Christian, a Mohamedan, a Russian or an American, a Socialist or a Fascist, a Theosophist or a Freemason or whatever one happens to be or styles himself and he can still follow Yoga and receive the fullest benefit. It does not require one to disown his beliefs, creed, religion or heritage.
>
> Further, the yoga technique is applicable to all grades of aspirants so that the sick and the healthy, the good and the bad, the intelligent and the ignorant, the believer and the nonbeliever can profit equally by its practice.[7]

Based on these beliefs, Yogendra advocated indiscriminately exposing people to yogic training as a means of attaining spiritual consciousness. Yet, to a great extent, the transcendent path that leads from "physical soundness" to "moral behavior" to "mental purity" and culminates in "spiritual realization" isn't at all what he taught.[8] And with good reason. It largely wasn't what his Indian middle-class clientele wanted to learn. (And, as he frankly admitted in his candid moments, it wasn't what he believed could be taught. "We are all unfamiliar with the Truth," he wrote to a student in 1929. For this reason, he contended, a sage "guiding" others toward knowledge of ultimate reality "is like the blind leading the blind."[9]) His students didn't turn to him—propelled by a feeling of deep uneasiness about their lives, which, they sensed, was caused by their own attachment to temporary things—for help in alleviating their suffering. They largely wanted to learn what Yogendra promoted as "yoga physical education": that portion of hatha yoga—postures, breathing, purificatory exercises—that enables one to preserve or obtain good health. "What yoga physical education . . . aims at," Yogendra explained, "is physiological soundness—pure radiant health conducive to immunity against disease and the promotion of longevity."[10]

Yogendra's yoga classes were a grand popularization of hermetical hatha yoga health practices, an effort to bring yogic health exercises—*asanas, pranayamas, bandhas,* and *mudras*—to a broad audience. He triumphantly proclaimed: "It should now become clear to the rationally-inclined seeking after good health through physical education that, for healthful living of an ideal type, no better system of physical culture has ever been investigated than the great science of the ancient yogins. The jargons of metaphysics and association of various religious traditions never disturbed its technique; the secrecy of ages about its practice has been lifted . . . ; and the various yoga processes are now available to the public . . . and may, with great benefit, be incorporated in the daily personal hygienic duties."[11]

Not that the members of the middle class didn't need some convincing to take up yoga to support their good health. They largely perceived of yoga as a form of self-punishment, long practiced by renunciates. This indictment was by no means entirely incorrect. In his chronicle of the yogic tradition of self-mortification in *Sinister Yogis,* scholar of South Asian religions David Gordon White describes the eyewitness account of Jean-Baptiste Tavernier in *Six Voyages,* circa 1676: "Tavernier plunges into a detailed cataloging of the various yogi or fakir penances to which he had been privy, which are illustrated in a remarkable lithographed mon-

tage of yogis arrayed in small groups around a cluster of shrines in a forest setting. The illustrated penances include what Tavernier takes to be a live burial, as well as yogis standing suspended by a cord for years at a time; maintaining arms upraised for years at a time, during which the fingernails grow to incredible lengths; and so on."[12]

Yogendra himself held that the very origin of yoga was bound up in the "various primitive efforts" that condemn the body in the name of spirituality.[13]

In all such efforts, the idea of defying the forces of Nature seems to have been so predominant that even acts of highest penance and self-torture were followed.

From the oldest Indian and even non-Indian spiritual records, we are able to gather that there was an age when the standard of spiritual superiority was measured by the amount of self-mortification one could undergo. This seems to be the beginning of a spiritual era, and Yoga . . . is as old as the spiritual civilization itself for the earliest practices of Yoga consisted of bodily penance (*tapas*).[14]

In giving this historical account, Yogendra was making it clear to the business- and professional-class skeptics—whose knowledge of yoga was gained primarily by seeing the ancient self-punishing practices carried on by yoga ascetics in the streets, a part of daily life in Indian cities—that he well understood their concerns about taking up yoga. This enabled him to reassure them that yoga had evolved over the centuries into an "elaborate and perfect programme of body-culture. . . . Let it therefore be again emphasized for the knowledge of those who know nothing or very little of Yoga culture that, unlike other spiritual systems that discard bodily health, Yoga has placed a definite value on body-culture."[15]

By tradition, the conditioning *asanas* of hatha yoga were practiced in the service of the meditation postures: they provided enough suppleness and strength for the yogin to remain in a meditative posture—usually the lotus posture—with steadiness and ease for a long time. By eliminating the distraction of having to hold the body still through effort (with the back, neck, and head in balance, the body, in effect, holds itself still), the meditative posture enables the yogin, who might otherwise fall prey to fatigue, restlessness, or outside disturbances, to meditate on the endless. Of the eighty-four postures that comprise many hatha yoga schools, four to six are generally recommended for use in meditation. The rest are the brief stretching exercises that condition the body to make the meditative postures endurable.

In the somewhat different interpretation held by Yogendra (and others), the conditioning postures were added to yoga as an aid to meditation by providing overall good health, not a sturdy foundation for holding a meditative posture. Yogendra believed that yoga's multifaceted system—consisting not only of conditioning postures but also of breathing and purificatory exercises, thereby making for "a complete scheme of knowledge, care, training and control of the external as well as the internal organs of the body"—was developed "for assuring *permanent* good health and, thus, for undisturbed meditation."[16]

The goal of practicing the conditioning postures in Yogendra's classes, however, was good health as an end in itself. In his writing, Yogendra argued that the reason why the "care of the body must primarily serve as a preventive against and immunity from disease is because physical indisposition and invalidism are regarded as a sin (*dehapapa*) . . . which obstructs mental, moral and spiritual progress in the rhythm of human evolution not only of one's own self but also of others who form the society."[17] But his students were primarily concerned with keeping or attaining good health solely as a means of staving off or relieving poor health. They eagerly took up yoga physical education to keep their bodies in good condition or remove bodily impediments (illness, injury, or disease) not to unite with God but simply to lead longer and healthier lives.

Moral Health

"The schools which first started, in the 1920s, to elaborate modern postural yoga practice [the modern yoga that foregrounds the postural exercises] in India used it to construct a sort of indigenized (and 'spiritualized') version of British [physical] education," posits modern yoga scholar Elizabeth De Michelis in her groundbreaking work *A History of Modern Yoga*. "Yoga-inspired routines of physical exercise would train the body, and a yoga-inspired self-control and morality would further 'character building.'"[18] De Michelis probably has gymnastics (or calisthenics) in mind as the model exercise of British physical education imitated by yogins. But between 1850 and 1880 religion was replaced by organized team sports, not gymnastics, as the primary means of character building in Britain and its colonies. Prayer was replaced by football, cricket, and other team sports as the locus of training in manliness. The chapel, where one learned control of one's passions, was replaced by the playing field, where one learned fair play (the "greater good" that served to thwart the dangers of unbridled competition in a time of rapid development of industry in Britain). "Typically enough," observes historian George L. Mosse, "the saying that the Battle of Waterloo was won on the playing fields of Eton dates from 1889 and not from the time of Napoleon."[19]

In any case, the first-generation pioneer hatha yogins rarely promoted yoga as a means of building character; their emphasis was preponderantly on its health benefits. Even Yogendra's passing examination of "moral health" is tied to physical health. "No one can be philanthropic with jaundice," he quoted Dr. George W. Crile, the famous American surgeon, as saying, "and no one suffering from Graves' disease can be generous."[20] "In the absence of pathologic morbidity . . . ," Yogendra concluded, "the high level of physical well-being gradually leads to an appreciation of moral traits and also to actual moral behaviour."[21] For Yogendra, hatha yoga as an "aid to moral life" derives not from cultivating particular attitudes or behavior but simply from attaining "positive and sedate health of the body."[22]

Mental Health

Members of the Indian middle class sought not spiritual liberation, which would facilitate transcending the emotional strains of everyday life, but help in coping with the emotional strains of everyday life. To accommodate their need, Yogendra formulated a hatha yoga that would enable them to empty their minds of all thoughts not in order to experience the ineffable mystery of divinity but to find relief from agitation. Accordingly, his classes culminated not with meditation but with *Savasana,* Corpse Pose, the ne plus ultra of bodily relaxation and revitalization—a state arrived at only after a period of exertion through exercise (see chapter 5).

Beauty

Yogendra didn't disapprove of Indians taking up physical exercise to pursue beauty. He recognized the value of the "agreeable and aesthetic nature" of calisthenics and other light gymnastics. But he not only pointed out that these disciplines lack hatha yoga's contribution to "the vital development of the internal organs" attained through "calculated movements of the body capable of maximum internal reactions," he also argued that hatha yoga exercise is superior to them in its ability to develop and enhance beauty—not in the contemporary sense of slimness, muscularity (he came to find muscular display repellent), sexiness, or youthfulness but in the sense of "grace, ease and rhythm."[23] Yoga exercises, Yogendra asserted, "urge towards poise and control of the body."[24] "The elasticity of the muscles and the suppleness of the body" gained through *asana* practice "contribute largely to graceful carriage."[25] Unable to acquire the wealth and/or status of royalty, the British, or the indigenous upper class, middle-class Indians could nevertheless mimic their bearing.

Form of the Yoga Class

Perhaps the most subversive aspects of Yogendra's transmission of knowledge of the physical aspects of yoga—what would've most upset "the great yoga master, His holiness Paramahamsa Madhavadasaji, under whom," Yogendra proudly proclaimed, "[he] received his secret traditional training in practical Yoga"—weren't its goals but the features it shared with forms of adult education programs, which first flourished in the West in the mid-19th century, including not only classroom instruction but also lectures, dramatic performances, and debates.[26]

Class Session

Traditionally, after a man is accepted for yoga training, his life resembles that of any novitiate joining a religious order: he submits to arduous ascetic conditions necessary to transform his life. Yogendra recognized that "there are today only a very few who would be eager to learn Yoga under conditions which may be imposed upon them" at hermitages.[27] "It was evident then that the orthodox tradition of imparting yoga education at the hermitages by requiring students to [permanently] leave their homes—no matter how essential or best—would fail to inspire the modern man," he wrote. "On the contrary, the strict adherence to yoga requisites might even be regarded as operose, anachronic, and even repulsive."[28]

So Yogendra created something novel: the yoga class session, a period of an hour or so, which pupils could attend and then leave. This tenuous agreement between yoga teacher and student was a fundamental and far-reaching departure from the sacred contract between guru and *chela*.

Open Class

While gurus, who were supported by varying degrees of charitable contributions, "taught not because they were paid but because they considered it their duty to impart their knowledge to the deserving; and the students were accepted not because they subscribed their fees in kind but because they were found fit for such studies," Yogendra, as a yoga teacher, would no more screen his students for their values, temperament, learning, goals, and so on than a lecturer would grill attendees before letting them take a seat at a lyceum or, for that matter, a department store clerk would interrogate customers before making a sale.[29] Whereas "the yoga technique [was] zealously guarded by the venerable yogins who handed over this sacred treasure-chest of knowledge to the most deserving disciples only," Yogendra indiscriminately dispensed his yoga expertise to anyone who showed up for a class.[30]

Urban Experience

Yogendra knew that his students had no desire to "retire into solitude" in remote places "wherein the masters dwelt," having abandoned "all their earthly attachments in search of Truth."[31] Proud of their worldly achievements, they wanted to stay in or near urban centers and spend their spare time improving their health in order to more fully enjoy their lives.

Whereas gurus "living in the solitude of mountains were hardly accessible" and had to be sought out, Yogendra made it possible for the middle-class residents of Bombay to take a hatha yoga class in their own community.[32] (He believed that the "modest huts, the solitary forest homes and caves carved in rocks . . . wherein the masters dwelt" were, in fact, purposely and perhaps perversely often made "inaccessible as a challenge to the devout."[33]) In this way Yogendra brought yoga back to city, where, as Asian religion scholar Geoffrey Samuel and world religion scholar Karen Armstrong point out, it had originated during the growth of cities and early states in the sixth and fifth centuries BCE as, in all likelihood, a method for relieving the stress felt by city dwellers cut off from the repetitive rhythms and connectedness to community of rural life and overwhelmed by a rapidly changing market economy, a social system in which they largely had to make their own way.[34] Whereas these ancient urban followers of yoga found solace from their suffering by meditating in a seated *asana,* the modern urban followers of yoga, turning to yoga during another period of great change and instability, found relief largely by performing conditioning *asanas,* which had been added to hatha yoga in the late Middle Ages for use in physically training the body for long periods of meditation.

Social Experience

There's a tradition in India of the householder yogin, one who practices yogic meditation in a designated area of the privacy of his home. The *Shiva Samhita* (*The Collection [of Verses] of Shiva*), a hatha yoga treatise probably composed between 1300 and 1500 CE, eloquently advocates this approach. "The practice should be done privately, avoiding company, and in seclusion," the Hindu god Shiva tells his consort Parvati. "For the sake of the community, ordinary outside matters should be carried on. All the proper duties of his karmic status should be performed. When these are done without

attachment there is no fault. . . . Remaining in the midst of the family, always doing the duties of the householder . . . [but] with sense-desires controlled, he attains liberation."[35]

Yogendra knew that most Indian middle-class residents of Bombay, who were affable and urbane, had no interest in taking up hatha yoga as a private, solitary religious experience. They wanted to practice hatha yoga as a social experience—but one far different from that which bound members of yogin orders, whether groups of disciples living in ashrams or wandering bands seeking alms. For those who had no interest in practicing yoga in isolation as a spiritual search or in joining ascetics living together and pursuing a common religious goal, he made available a place designated for practicing *asanas* to keep fit and healthy and relieve tension in the company of like-minded people. Participants performed the exercises in unison. Afterward students could share their experiences with each other. (Previously one would no more gab with someone about one's yoga practice than one would gab about one's spiritual revelations, or, for that matter, one's toilet habits.) Even if fellow students never spoke to one another, they could feel a connection, if only because they'd been put through the same paces and shared the common value of putting their spare time to productive use. (Yogendra's first students probably had an especially strong bond because they were mocked by outsiders— passersby who "cackle[d] away in derision."[36]) Then the students scattered, going off to their homes or workplaces.

In this manner Yogendra moved yoga practice not only from the sanctum in temples and the streets but also from the small, simple, elegant sacred space in houses to the classroom in yoga institutes (albeit, at the start, to an outdoor class on the beach at Versova).

Leisure Activity

The belief in leisure as compensation for hard work developed in middle-class industrial societies of the 19th century. In India the Indian professional class emulated their overlords, the British, in pleasure as well as business, eagerly taking up British leisure pursuits. In Yogendra's formative years, in the early 20th century, middle-class Indians spent their leisure time on activities that provided them with not only lively enjoyment (e.g., going to the movies or watching cricket matches) but also personal regeneration (e.g., attending lectures or taking family holidays at hill stations, the Indian version of health resorts). Yogendra presented hatha yoga as a form of physical culture in opposition to sports and other recreational activities involving physical exercise: unlike these other pursuits, hatha yoga could be "adopted conveniently to the daily life of every person in such a precise measure as is essential to the maintenance of the day-to-day good health."[37] Hatha yoga, Yogendra contended, was a kind of working at play that provided physical and mental renewal. Not to mention that it was nationalistic (because it derived from India's ancient cultural heritage) and "sedative" (it led to "sublimation," whereas most non-yogic physical education was "orgastic" and led to "animality").[38]

Service to Be Bought and Sold

"Are not there at every moment on the market, alongside wheat and meat and so on, also prostitutes, lawyers, sermons, concerts, theatrical performances, soldiers, politicians, etc.?" Karl Marx asked as a way of pointing out that services, like goods, are also commodities.[39] In turning yoga into a physical education routine, which enabled Indians to save or acquire fitness and good health, Yogendra transformed yoga from a spiritual quest into a service for middle-class Indian consumers. In becoming a yoga teacher instead of a guru, he became a purveyor of yoga to middle-class Indian consumers. In establishing the first hatha yoga center, the Yoga Institute, he took yoga out of the sanctified space, the hermitage, where no profits are made, and put it into the commercial space, the marketplace, where yoga could be bought by and sold to middle-class Indian consumers. In so doing, Yogendra lumped esoteric *asana* training, stripped of what he called its metaphysics, with the sermon, concert, or theatrical performance; the guru, transmuted into the yoga teacher, with the prostitute, lawyer, soldier, or politician; and the ashram, metamorphosized into the yoga center, with the whorehouse, courtroom, church, or theater. In other words, Yogendra made yoga into a commodity. This commodification was an integral aspect of the formation of modern yoga. Without it, very few of us would be practicing yoga today.

It was decidedly not his guru's custom of accepting contributions—sometimes cash (usually silver) or kind (occasionally fruit)—from the devotees from nearby villages and distant cities made in gratitude for his guidance or, for that matter, any Bombay professional's commercial activities that provided Yogendra with the business model for transforming the traditional transmission of yoga technique from guru to *chela* into a service with exchange value. It was the successful operations of new businesses, namely, gymnasiums, founded by Westerners with new professions, namely, physical culture teachers—in particular, the gymnasiums owned by Eugen Sandow.

Forerunners

In the first half of the 19th century, in response to members of the Western middle class increasingly finding themselves afflicted with ailments (such as anemia, dyspepsia, constipation, neurasthenia, corpulence, and insomnia) produced by an urban life that was frantic yet sedentary, stressful yet pampered, a health movement developed. By the 1860s it was flourishing. During the last decades of the 19th century, great numbers of the middle class were, for example, staying at sanatoriums to receive natural treatment, such as hydrotherapeutics, for chronic illnesses; flocking to outdoor areas designated for gymnastic exercises for adults; fasting to rid their bodies of toxins; participating in physical recreation as part of the curriculum of YMCAs; and vacationing at seashore, springs, and mountain resorts to restore vitality (the European elite had been traveling to health spas to pursue health and pleasure since the late Middle Ages).

Gradually, the need to improve health became intertwined with the desire to mold bodies. "In response to this desire," writes David L. Chapman, author of books on bodybuilding, "several entrepreneurs opened gymnasiums dedicated to building the body beautiful."[40] The renowned showman bodybuilder Eugen Sandow (1868–1925) opened his first Institute of Physical Culture in London in 1897. Trained by Sandow, the institute's instructors demonstrated and described exercises to the mostly white-collar patrons. "It was a healthful and fashionable retreat from the grinding routine of urban life," Chapman remarks.[41]

Before he had the strong body and athletic physique that so impressed Madhavadasaji, Yogendra had been a sickly and weak teenager ("the spirit and mind appeared strong and willing, the flesh had yet to muscle its way into activity"). He regained good health and built a strong, sculpted body under the guidance and training of Gulababhai Desai, his principal at Amalsad English School. The teenaged Yogendra became so enamored with physical exercise that, with a friend, he purchased equipment and started a gymnasium, which was attended by fellow students. Perhaps it was this early experience of Western physical culture, Rodrigues speculates, that was the "fore-runner of his involvement in Yoga and the mission to improve the health of his fellow people."[42]

During this period Yogendra also avidly acquired knowledge about the latest developments in physical culture through extensive reading on physical education and home exercise routines ("Delsarte's System of Expression, Kleen's Medical Gymnastics, Sandow's Body-building Exercises, Müller's My System, Macfadden's Physical Culture, Gulick's Exercises for the Busy Man, Camp's Daily Dozen and scores of short courses of home exercises without apparatus for the average person of mature age"[43]).

Thus, through his experience and self-education, Yogendra was inspired to create the new profession of yoga teacher just as much by the "irregular physician" and exercise instructor as by Madhavadasaji, and he was inspired to open the Yoga Institute just as much by health resorts and adult exercise facilities—critical elements in the modern commodification of beauty, health, and fitness—as by the ashram in Malsar. For this reason it can be said that Western healers and exercise instructors are every much the forerunners of the hatha yoga teacher as the guru, and Western natural health cure and exercise venues are every much the forerunners of the hatha yoga studio as the ashram.

3

SHRI YOGENDRA

Making Yoga into Calisthenics

Gymnastics and Calisthenics

In 1786, upon becoming the gymnastics teacher at the Schnepfenthal Educational Institute in Prussia, twenty-seven-year-old Johann Christoph Friedrich Guts Muths taught a variety of exercises "intended more for the improvement of the body, than for social diversion."[1] These practices included leaping, running, throwing, wrestling, vaulting, climbing, balancing, and lifting. The field of modern gymnastics formally began with the publication in 1793 of what would become its foundational text, *Gymnastik fur die Jugend* (*Gymnastics for Youth*), Guts Muths's writings about his teachings.

Another Prussian schoolteacher, though, became the great popularizer of modern gymnastics. In the spring of 1810 Friedrich Ludwig Jahn, who taught history, German, and mathematics at Plamann's School for Boys in Berlin, took his boys to Hasenheide, a nearby wooded area, for simple exercises. The *turner* (gymnast) movement was born. (Rejecting the Greek-derived word *gymnastics,* Jahn used *turnen* as his root word, believing it to be of German origin.)

The next year, in the spring of 1811, Jahn and his boys enclosed a stretch of the land for a *turnplatz* (grounds for gymnastic exercise). They set up apparatus such as vaulting horses (the first ones constructed out of tree trunks), a climbing rope (attached to a pole resting on the limbs of two trees), and a horizontal balance beam. By the end of the summer about two hundred boys (including students from a nearby school and an orphanage) were regularly taking part in activities there. In the next few years, as these gymnastic activities grew in popularity (adults were allowed to participate in them on Sundays), Hasenheide

Turnplatz took its place in the history of physical education alongside the grounds at Olympia in Greece (where sports were performed) and the Campus Martius outside Rome (where the art of combat was taught).

Turnvereins (gymnastic societies) quickly spread throughout Germany, sparking a vogue for gymnastics. By initiating an urgent impulse toward speedy, forceful, audacious, gravity-defying athletic movement to promote fitness among the populace, Jahn, building on the work of Guts Muths, had made physical exercise modern. But whereas Guts Muths advocated gymnastics as a means of improving the poor physical condition of children attending a school based on Rousseau's principles of education, Jahn enveloped his system in nationalistic ideology (used to serve the cause of making Germany free and united). He saw the *turner* (gymnast) system as a preparation for battle: "When all men, able to bear arms, have become valiant by warlike exercises, have become ready for fighting by warlike plays, belligerent and watchful by a patriotic spirit, then will a people be able to defend its frontier."[2]

Despite or because of this nationalist ideology, a gymnastics boom swept the West, especially in Germany, Sweden, Denmark, Great Britain, and America (where a far less nationalistic version of the *turner* system took hold).

By the mid-1800s the advocates of this fitness craze commonly argued that physical exercise, especially gymnastics, should be used to redress the deterioration of manhood, which, they thought, was endemic to each of their countries alone.

Typical in this regard was Thomas Wentworth Higginson, author of "Saints, and Their Bodies," published in *Atlantic Monthly* in 1858, which introduced Americans to Muscular Christianity, a Christian commitment to health and manliness imported from England, to which America still looked for ideas about health, fitness, and beauty.* Higginson sang the praises of gymnastics—"the invigorated life in every limb will give a perpetual charm to those seemingly aimless leaps and somersets"[3]—as a solution to the decline in men's health caused by (what he took to be) a peculiarly American set of historical circumstances: After the American Revolution, "a state of almost constant Indian warfare then created an obvious demand for muscle and agility. At present there is no such immediate necessity.† And it has been supposed that a race of shopkeepers, brokers, and lawyers could live without bodies. Now that the terrible records of dyspepsia and paralysis are disproving this, one may hope for a reaction in favor of bodily exercises."[4]

Inspired by Higginson and others, sedentary

---

*Over the course of his life Higginson was a Unitarian minister, a prominent abolitionist, a Civil War soldier (he commanded the South Carolina Volunteers, the first Union regiment recruited from former slaves), Emily Dickinson's mentor, and the author of numerous books, including *Army Life in a Black Regiment, Common Sense about Women,* and *Life of Margaret Fuller Ossoli.* In the early 1870s Higginson took an interest in Asian religions. He was an admirer of clergyman Samuel Johnson's volume on India in his *Oriental Religions and Their Relation to Universal Religion* series, which expressed the view that there is one universal religion.

†As Higginson himself would've surely acknowledged, one should be careful what one laments. Three years later men from the North and South would go off to fight each other in the American Civil War. More than 600,000 soldiers would lose their lives (a horrific toll equivalent to six million of today's population).

American men set about regaining their health and manhood through ardent devotion to the vigorous movements of gymnastics: darting, leaping, tumbling, and springing on the floor and, with the use of apparatus (such as the pommel horse, still rings, and parallel bars), balancing, folding, twisting, twirling, and swinging in the air.

The *turner* gymnastics system was soon rivaled by another gymnastics system, which eventually came to be called calisthenics, first developed by Per Henrik Ling in 1814 at the Royal Gymnastic Central Institute in Stockholm. Although it originally had a strong military component (the majority of the first students were young military officers; King Charles XIII had supported Ling's institute because he was anxious to prepare his country militarily), Ling's system became famous for its therapeutic component. Ling's "Swedish Movement Cure" was conceived as a system of medical treatment used to bring about recovery from chronic disease. "It is perhaps not readily understood," Ling wrote, "that a movement, or a mechanical action, is competent to affect interior portions of the organism. It is necessary first to understand that the human system is a *unit, complete* and *indivisible*."[5]

In general calisthenics is performed on the ground, without the use of apparatus, making its movements far more restricted than those of gymnastics. In contrast to gymnastics teachers, "Ling laid great stress on positions as distinguished from movements," Edward M. Hartwell wrote in a 1903 report on physical training for the U.S. government, "and also emphasized the necessity of making all move-

ments with ease and precision at the word of command."[6] "An exercise, in effect, consisted of movements from position to position, done on command," explains physical education historian Ellen W. Gerber. "The precision of the performance was thus the precision of the body position in each successive position. He divided all movements into trunk, head, arm, and leg movements and each position specified the exact location of each segment of the body."[7] This strict attention to form at the expense of movement was problematic. Students had to maintain strained positions while standing, kneeling, sitting, lying, or hanging for the length of time it took the teacher to correct the faults of each student. "The more conscientious the teacher," writes Gerber, "the less beneficial the exercise (in modern terms which stress dynamic strength and flexibility) and the more boring the class. As a result, Swedish gymnastics [in its original form] never became really popular even in Sweden."[8]

Müller's Calisthenics System

Born so small that he "could be placed in an ordinary cigar-box" and sick throughout his early childhood, J. P. Müller (1866–1938) grew up to become celebrated in his native Denmark for his amateur sports victories, robust health, and splendid figure.[9] In 1904 the thirty-eight-year-old Müller published a home exercise book, *My System: 15 Minutes' Work a Day for Health's Sake!* Originally composed for his comrades at the Copenhagen Rowing Club to keep them fit during the off-season, the book was an instant success. Five editions were printed in less than seven months. Subsequent demand led to

Swedish, English, German, American English, French, Finnish, Czech, and Dutch editions the following year. Eventually translated into twenty-four languages, the book would go on to sell millions of copies. In the early 20th century, Müller became "as famous as that other Danish export, [the father of the modern fairy tale] Hans Christian Andersen," writes journalist Sarah Wildman. "Maybe more."[10]

Müller's system is far simpler and livelier than the one created by Father Ling (as Müller reverently called him). In its emphasis on dynamic stretching, it resembles current warm-up routines for reducing muscle stiffness in preparation for sports competition and resembles some physical therapy routines for rehabilitating injuries. Believing that "suppleness and mobility in every joint being the primary condition essential to carrying one's youthful buoyancy into old age," Müller claimed that he had devised a system with more than a dozen exercises that "thoroughly exercise the joints."[11] They don't. However, they do make for a fairly comprehensive limbering-up set of exercises that can be performed in a short period of time without apparatus. They're easy, convenient, and cost-free. "Do not let a day pass without every muscle and every organ in your body being set in brisk motion, even if only for a short time," Müller advised his readers. "Stagnation in this case as everywhere else in Nature, is abnormal and leads to drooping and untimely death."[12]

Müller designed his home exercise routine as an antidote to the "mixture of exclusively intellectual culture, physical decadence, and mental morbidity" fashionable in Denmark. "There are people of both sexes," he wrote, "who actually make a parade of their ailments and what they consider to be their 'pale and interesting' appearance, under the impression that pallid, sickly looks are an infallible index of an aesthetic and soulful nature. Other signs of ill health and weakness, such as premature baldness or corpulency, are regarded by many as marks of dignity and distinction."[13] Müller sought to enhance the health and fitness of all kinds of people, including infants, the elderly, women, "literary and scientific men and artists," and the "town-office type," who is "prematurely bent, with shoulders and hips awry from his dislocating position on the office-stool, pale, with pimply face and pomatumed head."[14]

Müller well understood the transformative effect of daily exercise—not only on one's fitness and health but also on one's aspect and (by implication) outlook on life: "The entire body is strengthened, and grows flexible, mobile, and efficient. . . . As a matter of course you are healthy as well, and if healthy, at the same time—but only then—really beautiful. . . . A fresh complexion, clear eyes and a free carriage of the head—all of which are the outcome of a rational care of the body—lend a certain beauty to the most irregular features."[15]

In his manual *Yoga Asanas Simplified,* Shri Yogendra emphasized the differences between his hatha yoga system and the traditional hatha yoga system taught to him by his guru, Paramahamsa Madhavadasaji. The deviation in Yogendra's yogic exercise practice lies in elements that Yogendra appropriated from calisthenics— almost certainly from Müller's system, in particular. Although he dismissed Müller's course of home exercise (along with that of others) as "claptrap, charlatanry and pseudoscience," it seems that he wasn't above borrowing key concepts from it.[16] What Yogendra took from calisthenics enabled him to simplify and enliven the traditional hatha yoga exercise regimen.

Breaking with the Yoga Tradition

Short Routine

Yogendra selected only thirteen exercises to craft his routine, making it much less like the prevailing hatha yoga practice, with its eighty-four *asanas*, and much more like Müller's short calisthenics regime. Yogendra's routine—what he called "The Perfect Course"[17]—consists of the following *asanas* (the spelling and nomenclature are his):

1. *Sukhasana,* 2. *Talasana* and its Four Variations, 3. *Konasana* and its Three Variations, 4. A Variation of *Utkatasana,* 5. Antero-Posterior *Cakrasana,* 6. Simple *Bhadrasana,* 7. *Yogamudra* and its Two Variations, 8. *Pascimottanasana* and its Variation, 9. *Dhanurvakrasana,* 10. *Ardha-Matsyendrasana,* 11. Twofold *Pavanamuktasana,* 12. *Sarvangasana,* and 13. *Savasana.*[18]

Easy Routine

Modifying the original techniques of some *asanas* to create simpler versions had long been part of the hatha yoga tradition. Yogendra's systematic selection of largely easy *asanas* to comprise an entire yoga routine, however, was new (the spelling of the *asanas* is the author's, the main English translations are Yogendra's, and the parenthetical English translations are the author's).

Eleven of the thirteen exercises are conditioning *asanas*. Six of these are easy in their original form. Three—*Ardha-Matsyendrasana,*

Partial Matsyendra Pose (more commonly translated as Half Lord of the Fishes Pose), *Pavanamuktasana,* Antiflatus Pose (more commonly translated as Wind-Relieving Pose), and *Bhadrasana,* Throne Pose (also translated as Beneficial Pose)—are less difficult versions of more challenging poses. *Paschimottanasana,* Posterior-Stretching Pose (more commonly translated as Seated Forward Bend), has a simplified variation. And *Sarvangasana,* Semi-reverse Pose (more commonly called Shoulder Stand), is taught in graduated stages. So some form of all the conditioning exercises is easy to master, even for beginners.

Even the two nonconditioning *asanas* are easy. The routine begins with *Sukhasana,* Easy Pose, a preparatory meditation/relaxation exercise. Yogendra chose it over *Siddhasana,* Perfect Pose, and *Padmasana,* Lotus Pose, because "although unsuited to persons accustomed to sitting on a chair, to all others it may prove comparatively easy of practice."[19] And the routine ends with *Savasana,* Corpse Pose, a winding-down relaxation exercise.

Nothing if not keenly aware of the limitations of his middle-class clients, Yogendra created this routine to make yoga easier and more enjoyable for them to perform. "The perfect system of physical training, if it is to be popular," he maintained, "must not be so elaborate as to be prohibitive for daily practice, nor should it be so complicated and arduous as to offer much difficulty either in mastering its technique or in adapting it to the daily routine."[20]

Rodrigues defends Yogendra's innovations, arguing that his simplified yogic postures made yoga available to the general public while retaining its essence: "Yoga has become useful not just to the recluse but lay person and played its role in health, hygiene and therapy besides training of responsible individuals. Shri Yogendraji with his keen incisive mind has always preferred to get to the root of the practice taught and has applied himself with dedication to make some of the difficult practices of Yoga available for the modern man. He has simplified some of the *asanas*."[21]

In making hatha yoga more appealing to his middle-class constituents, Yogendra was taking his cue from Western physical culturists, probably, in particular, Müller, who promoted his system—a simplified and enlivened version of Ling's system—as "attractive and accessible to all."[22]

Dynamic Variations

All yogic conditioning postures involve stasis and movement. One must move one's body from its original neutral position in order to configure it into a yogic posture. While common to calisthenics, brisk, repetitive movements to and fro (backward and forward, side to side, and upward and downward) are antithetical to the essence of traditional hatha yoga *asana* practice, in which the controlled movement ends in a static, stretched-out position, which is then held. Yogendra, however, presented dynamic variations of yoga postures for ten of the eleven conditioning *asanas* in his yoga routine (the exception is *Sarvangasana,* an inversion pose, which is taught in stages and completed "only after a few weeks of initial training").[23]

Yogendra included the dynamic movements, he frankly admitted, as a means of retaining his followers. Students asked to perform traditional yoga postures right off gave up because they couldn't tolerate the strain of holding static stretches. Yogendra incorporated ballistic stretching into his routine in order to gradually introduce his students to the yoga postures:

> The series of rhythmic exercises . . . forming a part of yoga physical education herein set forth is based upon the less complicated yoga postures and their dynamic variations. The necessity for such a dynamic system . . . arose from the realization that the apparent rigidity of the static poses, when applied to the untrained ordinary people, called for much discomfort, strain and endurance. Consequently the disinclined and the sick, more often than not, dropped the very study of the yoga postures altogether. A graded physical training course that is to lightly lead the earnest to the successful practice of yoga poses, thus, became imperative both in the interest of the individual as well as the masses.[24]

Yogendra maintained that these variations barely diluted the benefits of the traditional yoga postures: "What with the scientific technique . . . employed in formulating these dynamic variations, nothing much has been actually detracted from the special hygienic virtues of the original *asanas*."[25] An example of a dynamic variation that functions as a warm-up or temporary substitution for a yoga pose is the variation for *Paschimottanasana,* which resembles the back-and-forth movements of rowing. "For the maximum stretching of the spine, however, genuine *pascimottanasana* may now [after the variation has been performed] be tried."[26] Performed quickly and repeatedly, some yoga postures themselves provide the same warm-up/temporary substitution functions. For example, the variation for *ardha-matsyendrasana* is repetitions of the original yoga posture held for a short period of time. "Repeat alternatively six turns to both sides in two minutes, as a dynamic exercise; or as a static pose, one minute to each side."[27]

Yogendra also argued that some of the dynamic variations improve the yoga poses. As an example, all four variations for *Talasana*, Palmae Pose (more commonly translated as Palm Tree Pose and more commonly called *Tadasana*, Mountain Pose), which involve a toe raise, are advanced exercises that "offer the very best means for increasing height."[28]

Yogendra insisted that he had generated all the dynamic variations from the yoga poses. Some of the variations, he claimed, were "suggested [to him] as an alternative consequent on the abstract descriptions in the Sanskrit texts which left enough margin for all possible variations."[29] The others, he claimed, were adapted from clearly defined yoga poses. In actuality, though, Yogendra cagily framed calisthenics exercises as dynamic variations of the yoga poses, and he almost certainly took these calisthenics exercises directly from Müller's system.

All of Müller's exercises are performed in rounds. Some involve a wide range of motion for opposing movements. For example, Exercise No. 11 is bending the body well back, with the stomach distended as much as possible, then, without stopping, bending the body forward as low as possible, with the stomach drawn in, and then, without stopping, swinging the body back again. These movements are repeated sixteen times. Yogendra's Antero-Posterior *Cakrasana*, Wheel Pose, is raising the arms overhead, inter-

lacing the fingers, leaning backward while pushing out the abdomen, and holding for six seconds, and then bending forward, touching the ground, and holding for three seconds. A modification of the forward bend involves bringing the arms up behind the back to a vertical position (fig. 3.1). Five rounds are completed in a minute.

Yogendra was so enamored of Antero-Posterior *Cakrasana* that he replaced traditional *Cakrasana* with it. This calisthenics exercise is superior, he maintained, because its vigorous movement develops anterior and posterior trunk muscles and, more critically, stimulates the intestines through stretching deep abdominal muscles. "As such, it acts as a remedial and a preventive measure in hepatic torpor and constipation by rousing the sluggish liver and colon to activity."[30]

Standing Postures

According to the 15th- to 16th-century *Hatha Yoga Pradipika*, the classic hatha yoga manual by Svatmarama, Siva taught eighty-four postures. "The number eighty-four traditionally signifies completeness, and in some cases, sacredness," writes Gudrun Bühnemann, scholar of South Asian religions.[31] But the *Hatha Yoga Pradipika* lists only fifteen *asanas*, and nine of them are seated poses for meditation. The 17th- to 18th-century *Gheranda Samhita* lists only thirty-two *asanas*. Over the subsequent centuries, the number of postures gradually expanded. Several illustrated manuscripts bridge the gap between the earliest hatha yoga texts and modern practice. Bühnemann identifies three sets of 19th-century drawings of eighty-four *asanas*: colored drawings illustrating a section

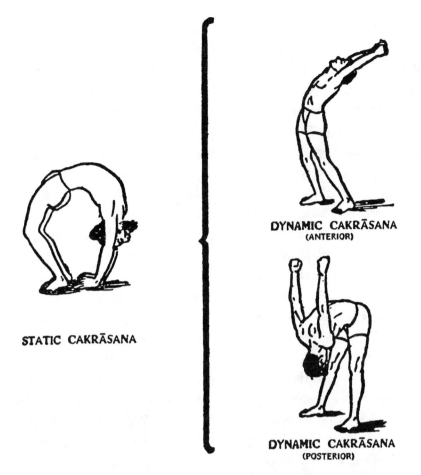

Figure 3.1. Static *Cakrasana* and dynamic *Cakrasana*
(From *Yoga Asanas Simplified*, by Shri Yogendra)

of Jayatarama's 1737 text *Jogapradipaka*, kept in the British Library; line drawings from Nepal, part of a manuscript preserved in a library in Kathmandu; and line drawings that are copies of older line drawings in the Jodhpur tradition, reproduced in a book published in 1968. Yoga scholar Norman E. Sjoman uncovered the *Sritattvanidhi* in the Sarasvati Bhandar Library, the private library of the Mysore Palace. Compiled between 1811 and 1868 by the maharajah of Mysore, Mummadi Krishnaraja Wadiyar, the manuscript contains a section with illustrations of 122 *asanas*.

In all of these pre-20th-century manuals, there are only two standing postures that involve bending the trunk: a forward bend with the arms wrapped around the calves shown in the Nepalese drawings and a backward bend with the hands squeezed between the legs shown in the Jodhpur drawings. Standing postures that involve twisting the trunk and/or bending to the side are completely absent. Conspicuously missing to modern-day practitioners are poses such as *Uttihita Trikonasana*, Extended Triangle Pose, and *Parivrtta Trikonasana*, Revolved Triangle Pose. Clearly these and many other standing poses are of recent origin. They were incorporated into yoga from calisthenics.

Yogendra appears to have been the first to incorporate standing exercises with bending and twisting movements into a hatha yoga exercise routine. If so, he probably adapted them from Müller's system. "Stand well up," Müller instructs his readers for Exercise No. 16, "with heels together and arms straight down by the sides. Quickly flinging the body (from the waist) over to the left, the left hand rubs down the left hip and outer side of the left thigh while the right hand is drawn up the right side of the body" (fig. 3.2).[32] The flinging is performed on the right side in the same manner. The movements are repeated a total of twenty times. Yogendra's version of this exercise is called *Konasana,* Angle Pose. For the first variation, Yogendra instructs his readers to place their feet apart and their arms at their sides. "Keeping the legs fixed, bend only the upper part of the body above the waist to either side . . . till the arm (of the side towards which the body is bent) slides below the respective knee. Also bring . . . the head to a right angle with the base, simultaneously sliding the other hand up to the armpit" (fig. 3.3).[33] The full movement is repeated three times in one minute.

In the second variation of *Konasana,* the pose is extended: one arm is lowered to the foot while the other arm is stretched upward. This pose is what's commonly called *Uttihita Trikonasana.*

Müller's instructions for his Exercise No. 4 are to stand with the feet about two feet apart, stretch the arms out to the side, twist to the left, bring the right arm down until the hand touches the floor between the feet, and extend the left hand overhead. Yogendra's instructions for the third variation of *Konasana* are to stand with the feet about two feet apart, hold the arms out to the side, and swing the arms "like the paddles of windmill, simultaneously rotating on the waist and turning the upper part of the body towards the right side. . . . Keep turning, thus, giving the body a half-twist, and bend downward till the left hand touches the right toe."[34] The right arm is stretched upward. This pose is what's commonly called *Parivrtta Trikonasana.*

Rhythmic Breathing

In 1918 Yogendra applied a method of breath control to yogic conditioning exercises, calling it the "Yogendra rhythm." Traditional *pranayama,* a series of breathing practices involving respiratory movement alone, is inadequate as physical exercise, Yogendra contended, because it doesn't mobilize the major body parts through exertion to ready them to receive oxygen. "One can go on expanding his chest and taking in deep breaths, yet he will find at the end that there are certain parts of his body still remaining inactive and undernourished. What is physiologically indicated . . . is either specified breathing with exercise or specified exercise with breathing. For this, the incorporation of [the] Yogendra rhythm of breathing with all forms for home exercises is the only corrective."[35]

In the *Jogapradipaka,* the oldest known text to actually describe eighty-four *asanas* (previously all eighty-four had only been named), "some *asanas* are combined with *pranayama* practices and are held for a long time," writes Bühnemann. "Thus Pachimatana/Pascimatana asana is recommended for a period of three to

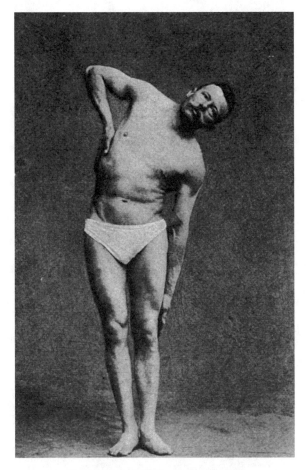

Figure 3.2. J. P. Müller demonstrating
Exercise No. 16, 1904

(From *My System*, by J. P. Müller)

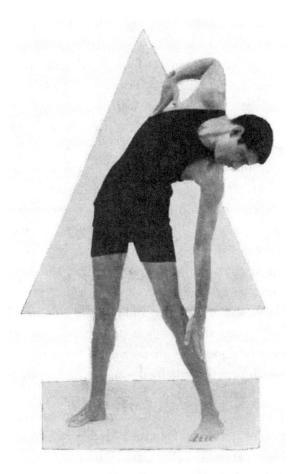

Figure 3.3. Shri Yogendra demonstrating the first variation
of *Konasana*, circa 1930

(From *Yoga Asanas Simplified*)

six hours."[36] This use of what we consider a conditioning posture as a meditative posture— with the body steady, the breath deep and even, the gaze fixed either on the tip of the nose or in between the eyebrows, and attention turned inward, leading to a state of tranquillity—is hardly what Yogendra had in mind when he recommended harmonizing *pranayama* with *asana*. What mattered to him was that deep breathing is enhanced by physical exercise, and physical exercise, in turn, is enhanced by deep breathing. "Unity and harmony between these two physiologic factors is what must be always desired in any muscular exercise."[37]

Yogendra recommended coordinating one inhalation or exhalation to one movement. His followers could easily achieve this rhythm because Yogendra's system involved continual movement interrupted by brief stasis. For example, during his alternate side-bending exercise, the first variation of *Konasana,* his instructions are to inhale while bending the upper body to one side, retain the breath for four seconds, exhale while returning to the standing position, pause for two seconds, and bend to the other side, using the same breathing pattern. Repeat the exercise for several rounds. Almost surely Yogendra adapted this practice of coordinating exercise movements with breathing from Müller's system, which Yogendra read about when he was a teenager.

Müller held that respiratory exercises should be accompanied by movement of the body. "To stand up and without any previous physical exertion take long breaths,—as often recommended, especially in German books—is unnatural and absurd, in fact may positively cause derangement in the relative pressure of the vessels of the body, and produce giddiness." He argued that taking a deep breath should only be done when there's a need for more air, which occurs naturally during strenuous physical effort. Respiratory exercises "are in their proper place only after a corresponding exertion of the body." He urged "drawing as deep a breath as possible, through the nose."[38]*

For the performance of his exercises proper, Müller advocated inhaling and exhaling on the beat of the movement, breathing evenly through the nose. For example, in his Exercise No. 12, he instructed his readers: "Bend 10 times to each side alternately, making 20 side bendings in all. Inhale briskly each time the body is straightened (from either side) and exhale evenly the rest of the time."[39]

While Yogendra picked up his breathing method from Müller (who may very well have copied it from someone else), it appears, however, that Yogendra was the first to apply it to the performance of conditioning (nonmeditative) yoga postures—the first, in his words, to have "prolonged, deep, and rhythmic breathing associated with each [postural] movement."[40] Previously, *pranayama* had (in general) been taught separately from conditioning *asanas*. In assessing Yogendra's achievements, his biographer Santan Rodrigues writes, "He has simplified some of the *asanas* and correlated them with a special breathing rhythm which derives the name from him—the Yogendra breathing rhythm. This has become such an accepted part of the *asanas* that we tend to forget that they were not there in the beginning but are a part of Shri Yogendraji's contribution."[41]

Benefits to the Internal Organs

Yogendra maintained that his system benefited the body's internal structures as well as the muscles. Each of his exercises had separate (although sometimes overlapping) physiologi-

---

*It would be a satisfying irony if Müller, in turn, had been influenced by traditional yogic breathing, which is practiced as an aid to seated meditation. Alas, he rejected what he called "Hindu-Yogi breathing," as Swami Kuvalayananda, the first great popularizer of modern hatha yoga practice, pointed out in 1926, because of his mistaken notion that it's performed with the mouth open.

"An author like J. P. Muller takes the writings of Yogi Ramacharaka [the pseudonym of William Walker Atkinson, the American author who helped popularize yoga as philosophy and Oriental occultism in America in the first decade of the 20th century] as the authoritative teachings of Yoga and starts condemning Yogic breathing," Kuvalayananda writes. As evidence he presents Müller's misdirected criticism: "In most of the Yogi breaths instruction is given to exhale vigorously through the mouth. Sometimes there is even added: 'in one great breath through the wide opened mouth.' That this method is wrong, and even in the long run dangerous, I [Müller] have proved in the foregoing chapters" (Kuvalayananda, "Rationale of Yogic Poses" [October 1926], 263).

cal benefits. For example, the spinal twisting of *Ardha-Matsyendrasana* relieves "the spinal nerves from the pressure consequent upon faulty habits of carriage and daily work."[42] In making his assertions, Yogendra was mirroring the claims of physical culturists. Müller, for example, contended that his method of exercising the spine through a variety of movements benefits the nervous system as well as the musculature:

> The chief advantage of rational physical exercise is thus not so much that the muscles and sinews grow stronger as that all the internal organs, including even the brain, heart and spinal cord are daily cleansed in a rejuvenating bath. Do you think that a vertebral column, for instance, which is daily submitted to as many stretchings, bendings, and twistings to its utmost capacity, as is the case in "My System," can get stiff and calcinated and possible impede the efficiency of the chief nerve fibres which pass through it?[43]

Assessment of Yogendra's System

One can't help but wonder why Yogendra didn't simply fess up to—or even boast about!—adapting elements of Müller's calisthenics system for use in fashioning his course of daily yoga practice. Granted, he would've had to admit borrowing much from Müller: the outline of an exercise format, a set of dynamic exercises, standing exercises, a breathing method coordinated to exercises, and a rationale for exercises. Perhaps his vainglory couldn't allow for such generosity. But if he was filled with excessive pride, then wouldn't this fierce, declared heretic who stridently set about subverting the centuries-old

hermetic hatha yoga tradition of transmission of knowledge from guru to *chela* by making yogic health practices available to the masses want to tout his yoga system for what it was—an innovative mix of East and West—and be hailed as a modernist syncretist? Alas, it seems that he and the members of the Hindu middle-class Indian milieu of which he was a part were so intoxicated with their nationalism—born of their humiliation and resentment over being subjugated by the British—that they couldn't acknowledge a debt to any Westerner.

It would've been easy for Yogendra to give Müller all the credit in the world; after all, Yogendra's "hatha yoga simplified" is clearly superior to Müller's calisthenics system. Needless to say, the two systems are very similar. Both are convenient for daily home use. Unlike gymnastics, they can be carried out without special apparatus. Comprising about a dozen and a half easy stretching exercises (when the variations are taken into consideration), they can be performed in a short period of time.

But the differences in the two systems are pointed. Müller famously promoted the brevity of his workout: exactly fifteen minutes. "A quarter of an hour daily is a very limited time," he conceded, "but when it is used to the best advantage it is, nevertheless, sufficient to prevent illness and preserve health, indeed in many cases regain it, so that the body is little by little transformed from a fidgety, hypochondriacal master, to an efficient and obedient servant."[44] "Most authors of home exercises regard fifteen minutes of [a] daily dose of vigorous gymnastics as a safe standard for persons of average capacity," Yogendra remarked, setting up his critique of Müller's exercises in order to make the case for his own exercises. "But, because of their static character in the case of the original poses and very slow movements in the case of their dynamic variations, the standard dose of daily yoga exercises may have to be varied between twenty-five to thirty minutes."[45] (If time is spent on the preparatory activities that Yogendra recommends—"Before beginning the exercise, it is advisable to evacuate the bladder and bowels, clean the nose and throat of all mucus, and drink a glassful of water neither too hot nor too cold"—then his routine is even longer.[46])

Müller's routine is performed with jerking and flinging (ballistic) movements and is restricted almost entirely to standing exercises, while Yogendra's routine consists of dynamic variations performed with slow movement and a brief stasis (not with "jerks and hasty or strenuous pulls"), along with traditional yogic floor poses, as well as new standing poses, that focus on static stretching.[47] The deliberation and control with which the poses are performed reduce the risk of injury. The variety of poses allows for joint movement through many planes of motion. The relatively wide range of motion of the poses, which are held in their extended position, promotes permanent elongation of muscles. All these factors make Yogendra's system safer, more comprehensive, and more effective than Müller's system, whether for practitioners pursuing yoga in isolation at home or in a group in a classroom setting.

Incorporating calisthenics into yoga, Yogendra's yoga routine is highly innovative. And eminently sensible. Its simplified *asanas* make it accessible, and their dynamic variations give it zest. It's perfect for those for whom it was created: the sedentary and infirm of the Indian professional class of the early 20th century. And it would be perfect for the inactive of today and, ramped up, for those yoga students of today who crave vigorous movement. But this visionary system never caught on. It was probably perceived by subsequent generations of yoga practitioners as derivative and impure or simply as insufficiently challenging. Even Yogendra himself apparently abandoned it. Currently, the Yoga Institute, which he founded, teaches solely static stretching. Students enter a pose slowly and steadily and then hold the stretch at their limit. This conventional style of yoga has a critical advantage over Yogendra's original mashup system: It's more conducive to looking within. It facilitates introspection.

Feminine Exercise

The controversy over which was the more effective system, gymnastics or calisthenics, raged from the early 1800s into the early 1900s. To an important degree, this was an argument over the appropriate behavior and physical capabilities of women. In his 1860 article "Gymnastics," published in *Atlantic Monthly* two years after "Saints, and Their Bodies," Higginson conceded that calisthenics, while ugly, was a useful warm-up exercise for the graceful and vigorous activity of gymnastics: "You will notice, however, that a part of the gymnastic class are exercising without apparatus, in a series of rather grotesque movements which supple and prepare the body for more muscular feats: these are calisthenic exercises."[48]

But Higginson dismissed "the favorite hobby of the day,—Dr. [Dio] Lewis, and his system of gymnastics, or, more properly, of calisthenics" as a stand-alone exercise. He well understood—and sniffed at—its raison d'être. There already existed apostles (such as William Bentley Fowle, the educator who introduced gymnastics exercises in New England, and George Barker Windship, the most well-known spokesman for lifting heavy weights to make the body as strong as possible) of what Higginson called "severe" exercises.[49] "There was wanting some man with a milder hobby, perfectly safe for a lady to drive," he reasoned. "The Fates provided that man, also, in Dr. Lewis. . . . [His method] is just what is wanted for multitudes of persons who find or fancy the real gymnasium to be unsuited to them. It will especially render service to female pupils, so far as they practise it; for the accustomed gymnastic exercises seem never yet to have been rendered attractive to them, on any large scale, and with any permanency."[50]

"Though Fowle, [John G.] Coffin, and many of their peers believed women to be capable of more than light exercise, domestic work, and dancing, there remained a strong bias against the sorts of vigorous exercise Fowle advocated," writes Jan Todd, historian of purposive exercise in the lives of American women. "By the 1830s, the tide carrying the vigorous exercises recommended by . . . Fowle [and others] had ebbed for women. It was replaced by a building wave of enthusiasm for the lighter, and supposedly more feminine, exercise system known as calisthenics."[51] A comparable movement took place in Europe.

While stating in his *New Gymnastics for Men, Women, and Children,* published in 1864, that his exercises, "like air and food . . . are adapted to both sexes," Lewis acknowledges that his system of physical training, with its "beautiful games, graceful attitudes, and striking tableaux, possess[es] a peculiar fascination for girls."[52]

Even without hatha yoga incorporating elements of calisthenics, calisthenics and yoga (i.e., a yoga based on conditioning *asanas*) inherently resemble each other. Their exercise principles are similar: unlike gymnastics, both use the human body without apparatus to perform exercises on the ground. Although these exercises work against gravity, they don't defy gravity: there's none of the bounding, leaping, and somersaulting that are essential to gymnastics. Although calisthenics movements tend to be quick, and yoga movements (in some styles) may be flowing, calisthenics and yoga don't have the speedy movements through space that are common to gymnastics (and dance). They're more related to the floor, the ground, and Earth than to the rafters, the sky, and the heavens. (Calisthenics and yoga are also alike when compared to sports. They're not competitive, governed by rules, and championed for instilling manly virtues, such as fair play, as sports were in England in the 1800s.) The similarities between yoga and calisthenics go a long way in explaining why modern yogins, in transforming traditional hatha yoga into an indigenous exercise system for Indians, used calisthenics as their primary model, and in explaining why, in the mid-20th century, hatha yoga would be largely categorized by all—and dismissed by men—as an exercise for women.

Lewis himself positioned his system not in contrast to a vigorous gymnastics but as the medium between the extremes of weight lifting and yoga contortionism. "The lifter and the India-rubber man," he warned, "constitute the two mischievous extremes." "Men, women and children should be strong, but . . . it should not be the strength of a great lifter." Instead, it should be "the strength of grace, flexibility, agility and endurance."[53] Nor should the flexibility be that of the yogin street performer, who configures his trunk and limbs in a way that twists the body out of its natural shape. The model exercisers "can neither lift great weights nor tie themselves into knots, but they occupy a point between these two extremes."[54] Lewis championed a "light" physical training system that developed elasticity, harmony, and grace—which is why, had he come across one of Yogendra's classes in Versova in 1918, he would've largely approved of the new exercise system that had been formed from hatha yoga.

The heart of Lewis's system is what he called "free gymnastics," consisting of standing exercises. They included "Rolling Head Movement," "Sinking and Raising the Body," "Bending the Body Forward and Backward," "Twisting the Body," "Raising the Knee," "Circular Arm Movement" (whirling the arms around), "Trotting Movement" (hopping on one foot), "Hands Upward" (stretching the arms overhead and pulling them down to the chest), "Legs Out and Back Sidewise," and "Deep Breathing with Body Bent Sidewise."[55] Each exercise was performed slowly but "with spirit and force" and repeated ten, fifteen, or twenty times.[56] The exercises were accompanied by music. (Lewis considered music to be a "delightful stimulus" to exercise. "Feeble and apathetic people, who have little courage to undertake gymnastic

[i.e., calisthenics] training, accomplish wonders under the inspiration of music."[57] He deemed the hand organ to be the best accompanying instrument.)

Higginson, ever the gymnastics proselytizer, heaped the kind of ridicule you'd think he'd reserve only for the habits of the slothful on a Lewis-style calisthenics class in a school gymnasium:

At the word of command, as swiftly as a conjurer twists his puzzle-paper, these living forms are shifted from one odd resemblance to another, at which it is quite lawful to laugh, especially if those laugh who win. A series of wind-mills,—a group of inflated balloons,—a flock of geese all asleep on one leg,—a circle of ballet-dancers, just poised to begin,—a band of patriots just kneeling to take an oath upon their country's altar,—a senate of tailors,—a file of soldiers,—a whole parish of Shaker worshippers,—a Japanese embassy performing *Ko-tow:* these all in turn come like shadows,—so depart. This complicated attitudinizing forms the preliminary to the gymnastic hour.[58]

Higginson's clever putdown of the calisthenics drill is such wicked fun that we ourselves may laugh. But ultimately the joke is on Higginson (and us, if we are complicit). If we ignore the sarcasm, his riff is revealed as a vivid and insightful description of calisthenics—and, even more, of its sister exercise, hatha yoga, and not just of hatha yoga's aesthetics but also its deeper meaning. The shape shifting in *asana* practice (even more than in calisthenics) richly evokes the movements of man-made objects, animals, and especially humans engaged in cultural activities (dance, social conventions, skilled and unskilled manual labor, and religious ritual). In so doing, *asana* practice illuminates both how the body bears a tradition of movements inherited or handed down from generation to generation, suggestive of life's timelessness, and how these movements, whether of nature or of civilization, are fleeting ("these all in turn come like shadows,—so depart"), suggestive of life's evanescence.

To think about yoga postures in this way is to explore our experience of our body in *asana* unencumbered by traditional ideology, something that we can do today, in part, because Yogendra—in his insistence on making yoga modern—helped strip hatha yoga of its (what he called) "mysticism and inertia."[59]

4

SHRI YOGENDRA

Taking Practical Yoga to the New World

Hatha Yoga in America

A Wonderful Dream

As word spread about Shri Yogendra's class on the beach at Versova, student enrollment swelled. After a month women were allowed to participate. There were no fees because Yogendra's patron Homi Dadina supported Yogendra and paid for all of the Yoga Institute expenses. (At future incarnations of the institute, Yogendra would initiate a payment policy based on a member's income.)

Within four weeks, after hearing about the health benefits of Yogendra's teachings, men began to arrive at the institute seeking treatment for debilitating medical conditions. Previously only a school offering *asana* classes to prevent disease, the Yoga Institute now also became a clinic to treat disease. The patients ate breakfast and participated in light activities (including a stroll on the beach) collectively, and they received individual instructions from Yogendra according to their needs. He set them up with an *asana* routine supplemented with purificatory and breathing exercises and a dietary program.

The first patient, registered on January 22, 1919, was Dadina himself. The yoga treatment Yogendra designed for Dadina's obesity, indigestion, and related conditions consisted of a regimen of physical exercises (*asanas*), purificatory techniques (*neti*, inserting a thread into the nostrils one at a time and pulling it out through the mouth as a means of removing phlegm, and *brahma datan*,

44

cleaning the throat with a long brush), breathing exercises (*pranayama*), and a prescribed diet. As a result of this treatment, Dadina's health improved considerably. He lost thirty pounds. His "heavy dull dyspeptic feeling" disappeared. "And on the whole [he felt] quite alert and cheerful."[1]

That Dadina and other Indians were eager to receive treatment at the Yoga Institute isn't totally a surprise. There was a vanguard of middle-class Indians who didn't have to overcome a repugnance of yoga, who didn't have to be convinced that it wasn't sorcery and self-penance. This group was receptive to yoga treatment because it had been primed by a Western current in health that had begun in the early 1800s in response to an antipathy toward conventional medicine: self-healing based on natural practices, such as hydrotherapy, fasting, and exercise. A patient writing appreciatively to the Yoga Institute on March 3, 1919, reveals how the congruence of this Western trend and hatha yoga was recognized by some in the Indian middle class.

I was suffering from Hemicrania [an unremitting headache on one side of the head] and the pain was so acute, so exacting that I was reduced from 122 pounds to 108 pounds which means a reduction of 14 pounds within a fortnight.

Having read some literature on physical culture and nature cure and myself being a believer in the same, I proceeded to Versova for a change and to try some method of nature cure. There I fortunately happened to encounter Swamiji [Yogendra], the founder of the Yoga ashram. I was charmed by his kind and sympathetic treatment of myself and at once placed my case under his care and now I am very much pleased to say that from the fifth day of my undergoing the treatment my headache has not recurred.

My confidence in nature cure has been doubly confirmed by this wonderful cure on myself within such a short period and I feel sure that the profound study of Swamiji Mani in the science of nature cure and Yoga, combined with his disinterestedness and his kind and sympathetic feelings towards the patient who being guided on the path of nature will not fail to regain his natural health and vitality.

In these hard times of epidemics and physical deterioration, India very badly stands in need of a number of such Yoga ashrams and health sanitariums. The more the knowledge of Yoga and Nature [*sic*] cure is defused, the better.[2]

The patient considered Yogendra's yoga treatment to be a complement to or a form of Nature Cure.

Nature Cure (or Natural Therapeutics) was developed by Vincenz Priessnitz (1799–1851), a farmer in Gräfenberg, a small village in the Silesian mountains of Austria, where Priessnitz opened the first hydrotherapeutic sanitarium in 1822. "His pharmacopeia consisted not in poisonous pills and potions," writes Henry Lindlahr in *Philosophy of Natural Therapeutics,* published in 1918, "but in plenty of exercise, fresh mountain air, water treatments in the cool, sparkling brooks, and simple, wholesome country fare, consisting largely of black bread, vegetables, and milk fresh from cows fed on nutritious mountain grasses." Among those who made the pilgrimage to Priessnitz's sanatorium were "wealthy merchants, princes and doctors from all parts of the world."[3]

"Rapidly the idea of drugless healing spread over the civilized world,"[4] Lindlahr, who was admired by Yogendra as an "authority on Natural Therapeutics,"[5] continues. Among those who "became enthusiastic pupils and followers of Priessnitz"[6]—along with such founders of disciplines as Friedrich Ludwig Jahn (modern physical culture), Phineas Parkhurst Quimby (New Thought), Andrew T. Still (osteopathy), and Daniel David Palmer (chiropractic)—was Louis Kuhne, "the German pioneer of Nature Cure, [who] claimed that 'disease is a unit', that it consists in the accumulation of waste and morbid matter in the system."[7] In rejecting modern medicine's view that disease is primarily caused by various germs (bacteria and viruses), Kuhne had created a theory that appealed to those with a nostalgia for a holistic conception of disease to replace the recently discredited humoral theory—which posits that disease is caused by an imbalance of four bodily fluids (humors)—held throughout much of Europe since it was systemized in ancient Greece.

Kuhne's book *The New Science of Healing or the Doctrine of the Unity of Diseases Forming the Basis of a Uniform Method of Cure, without Medicines and without Operations,* published in German in 1891 and translated from an early English translation into Telegu, Hindi, and Urdu at the turn of the century, "had a phenomenal impact . . . among those [Indians] who were seeking healthier, less invasive, and more natural alternatives to both allopathy

and Ayurveda," writes medical anthropologist Joseph S. Alter. "It is as though his book gave rise, almost overnight, to a whole school of Indian naturopaths."[8] Among those Indians who advocated self-purification as a means of ridding the body of toxins in order to maintain and restore health was Yogendra.

Unlike the Indian naturopaths who advocated Kuhne's method of hydrotherapy, Yogendra's treatment consisted of traditional hatha yoga practices for care of the mouth, ears, nose, eyes, stomach, small intestine, liver, and colon. And whereas "Kuhne [and other naturopaths], in advancing the uniformity of causes in disease, specifically rely on the data that the digestive organs are largely to be blamed for all kinds of constitutional diseases and pathogenic conditions,"[9] Yogendra, believing that "intestinal toxemia is the most universal of all maladies," primarily focused on "the most despised and neglected organ of the body—the colon."[10]

To facilitate the process of elimination, Yogendra recommended a dietary code (combinations of grains, dairy products, vegetables, fruits, nuts, and honey); antiflatulence postures (especially *pavanamuktasana,* anti-flatus pose); postures for abating constipation (*sirasana,* topsy-turvy pose, and *sarvangasana,* semi-reverse pose); postures for stretching the abdominal muscles (*dhanurvakrasana,* bow-curve pose); air irrigation (*sthula, suska,* or *vayu basti*) and water irrigation (*jalabasti*) of the colon; and internal massage (*mudras* and *bandhas,* practices that knead and massage the intestines through abdominal movements). (The spellings of the practices and their translations are Yogendra's.)

In Yogendra's view, Kuhne and the other naturopaths who believed that diseases, no matter how dissimilar, are all caused by toxicity were only now discovering what the ancient *rishis* had espoused: "It is now generally admitted by the practitioners of the various systems of medicine that, in fact, we almost always do die of poisons. Poisons, therefore, are the main factors not only in causing old age but also death not directly due to injury. Practical Yoga recognized this physiological fact 5000 years ago, and has accordingly provided for a large variety of purificatory processes (*malasuddhi*) for thorough and prompt elimination of all poisons from the body."[11]

While it's true that hatha yoga's implied theoretical underpinnings about natural healing preceded Nature Cure's zealous proselytization of natural healing by centuries, nevertheless it took the Nature Cure movement to prompt Yogendra and other yogins to bring the natural healing element of hatha yoga, practiced only by yogin ascetics, to the fore, creating yoga therapy as India's indigenous natural health treatment for improving public health. By presenting yoga as a practice of "perfect health, renewed youth and long life" (not as a spiritual discipline served by health practices)—that is, by integrating yoga into the Nature Cure movement—Yogendra was making yoga modern.[12]

In the first few months patients at the Yoga Institute were treated for heart trouble, obesity, asthma, prostate enlargement, gout, headache, diabetes, and other disorders. "The skeptics abounded and the *haute couture* of the neo-rich at Versova hardly allowed for anything serious," observes Yogendra's biographer, Santan

Rodrigues. "But with each success, doubts were replaced with beliefs."[13]

It seems, however, that Yogendra wasn't content with this modest success. After all, in his telling, "before his *mahasamadhi* (trance absolute [that is, his death]), Yogisara Paramahamsa Madhavadasaji, having imparted all the traditional secrets, finally *blessed and entrusted* [me] *in writing* with the Herculean task of [inaugurating a] practical Yoga Renaissance."[14] (While boasting about subverting the ancient *guru-chela* relationship with its hermetic tradition of knowledge transmission, here Yogendra is declaring that he was assigned by Madhavadasaji to spread yoga to the populace. Was Yogendra a heretic or a devotee? Apparently he wanted to claim the mantle of both.)

After a year of teaching students and treating patients day in and day out in Versova, Yogendra, in Rodrigues's account of events, had a realization: somebody needed to get the practical yoga renaissance "a foothold in the great continent," the New World (to where, after World War I, "all the endeavours, the events, the happenings took a flight"), particularly in America, where "the centre of the world had shifted from Britain."[15] Rodrigues describes the reasoning that undergirded Yogendra's thinking:

> Ideas and fashions accepted in America found a blind adherent in almost all the corners of the world. America had the best scientific talents and the most powerful mass media. It was essential for the advancement of Yoga, to get this ancient lore accepted by the best medical brains and then propagated by the omnipresent mass media. It was a wonderful dream.[16]

Who was more capable of carrying out this quixotic mission, Yogendra thought, than himself?

Vivekananda in America

Swami Vivekananda (1863–1902) had already introduced yoga in America as an exotic yet normative spiritual path during his arduous six-month lecture tour following his six addresses (including an electrifying speech on opening day) at the more than two-week-long World's Parliament of Religions in Chicago in September 1893. Vivekananda promulgated four yogic paths for manifesting divinity within: raja yoga (the path of meditation), karma yoga (the path of good works), bhakti yoga (the path of worship, what he called "the yoga of love and devotion"), and jnana yoga (the path of knowledge). Yogendra wanted to establish hatha yoga—the practical yoga—in America.

Vivekananda held a mélange of notions—some common and half-accurate, and others quite idiosyncratic and fanciful—about hatha yogins. "Thought-reading and the foretelling of events are successfully practiced by the Hatha Yogis."[17] In order to try to "overcome gravitation and rise by will into the air, . . . some of them in their efforts nearly starve themselves and become so thin that if one presses his finger upon their stomachs he can actually feel the spine."[18] "Twelve years training! And they begin with little children, otherwise it is impossible." "One thing [is] very curious about the Hatha Yogi: When he first becomes a disciple, he goes into the wilderness and lives alone forty days exactly. All they have they learn within those forty days."[19]

But Vivekananda's primary assessment of hatha yogins centered on their fitness and health goals. The aim of hatha yoga, he said in one of his early American lectures, "is to make the physical body very strong."[20] It "establish[es] a perfect control" over the muscles. (Making a mistake common to his times, he attributed gains in strength, not flexibility, to *asana* practice.) He also maintained that "health is the chief idea, the one goal of the Hatha Yogi. He is determined not to fall sick, and he never does."[21] But in his seeming praise for hatha yoga, Vivekananda was actually dismissing it. Hatha yoga provides fitness, health, and long life, he granted. "But that is all."[22] "From this body," he insisted in a later talk, "we have to separate the soul."[23]

"Vivekananda makes an emphatic distinction between the *merely physical* exercises of *hatha* yoga, and the *spiritual* ones of 'raja yoga,'" remarks yoga scholar Mark Singleton in *Yoga Body,* his groundbreaking book about the origins of modern yogic postural practice, "a dichotomy that obtains in modern yoga up to the present day." But making this distinction doesn't mean, as Singleton advances, that "Vivekananda uncompromisingly rejects the 'entirely' physical practices of *hatha* yoga."[24]

The Vedanta Society

After his lecture tour ended in early April 1894, an exhausted Vivekananda settled in New York. Amid a number of private talks in the homes of the rich—his "parlor lectures"—he delivered two public lectures, the first on India and Hinduism at the Waldorf Hotel on April 24, and the second on India and Reincarnation at the residence of Mary Phillips, on May 2. Most of his lectures, no matter what the topic, were on various aspects of Vedanta, the Hindu philosophy found in portions of the Vedas (ancient Hindu scriptures, especially the Upanishads, but also including the *Bhagavad Gita* and other texts). He considered the basic teaching of Vedanta to be the ultimate identity of the individual soul with God (the term for the Supreme Being that he frequently used when addressing Western audiences). When the Vedantist realizes his divine nature, Vivekananda explained, the world of misery vanishes for him and he finds absolute bliss.

One of the people who attended these lectures was Leon Landsberg, a Russian-born Jew, a journalist, and a member of the Theosophical Society. Vivekananda and Landsberg hit it off. After givings talks and lectures for the next six months, primarily in New England,* Vivekananda returned to New York on November 4, when he began to gather followers together, including Landsberg, into an informal group. (Some consider the formation of this group, which had officers but no headquarters or even registration, to be the beginning of the Vedanta Society.)

On January 27, 1895, Vivekananda moved into a room rented by Landsberg on the second floor of a rooming house at 54 West 33rd Street, one of a row of seedy rooming houses on the street. There, the very next day, Vivekananda started holding classes on yoga and Vedanta.

Thus, although its nucleus had been formed the previous November, the Vedanta Society may be said to have officially been founded by Vivekananda with Landsberg's assistance on Monday, January 28, 1895, in its first headquarters in this small room in New York.

Although finances were dire (classes were free, and donations, dropped in a basket hanging near the front door, didn't even cover basic expenses) and living conditions difficult (the twenty-foot-long, sparsely furnished room had no bathroom or kitchen), Vivekananda was contented in the period following the establishment of his headquarters. He welcomed the rest from the strain of touring. He greatly enjoyed Landsberg's companionship. ("He is a brave and noble soul, Lord bless him," he wrote to his close friend Mary Hale on February 1.[25] After classes they sometimes ate a light supper together at a cheap restaurant. They also cooked in the room, using a donated stove.) And he felt that he was of use to those who sought comfort in his words. He wrote to the socialite Sara Bull, who was among his most dedicated disciples, on February 14: "I am very happy now. Between Mr. Landsberg and me, we cook some rice and lentils or barley and quietly eat it, and write something or read or receive visits from poor people who want to learn something, and thus I feel I am more a Sannyasin now than I ever was in America."[26]

---

*One of Vivekananda's speaking engagements took place on the evening of August 13, 1894, before the Free Religious Association (of which Ralph Waldo Emerson was one of the founders) at the Davis Opera House in Plymouth, Massachusetts. Vivekananda had been invited by the president of the group, former Unitarian Minister Thomas Wentworth Higginson, who had introduced Muscular Christianity to America. Higginson and Vivekananda had met the previous year at the World's Parliament of Religions, where Higginson, a delegate, delivered a lecture, "The Sympathy of Religions," expressing his creed, shared by Vivekananda, that there is only one religion, which takes many forms.

Vivekananda gave philosophical talks on the four yogas and Vedanta to small gatherings of people at the society from 11:00 a.m. to 1:00 p.m. (though often the talks lasted longer). A follower, Josephine MacLeod, remembered arriving "in his sitting room [actually his room for working, cooking, eating, sleeping, and meditating] where were assembled fifteen or twenty ladies and two or three gentlemen. The room was crowded."[27] Sara Ellen Waldo, a follower who became Vivekananda's amanuensis, recalled: "The little room filled to overflowing, became very picturesque. The Swami himself always sat on the floor, and most of his audience likewise. The marble topped dresser, the arms of the sofa, and even the corner washstand helped to furnish seats for the constantly increasing numbers. The door was left open, and the overflow filled the hall and sat on the stairs."[28]

Another follower, Laura Glenn, recollected: "He began to speak; and memory, time, place, people, all melted away. Nothing was left but a voice ringing through the void. It was as if a gate had swung open and I had passed out on a road leading to limitless attainment."[29]

Vivekananda presented his more formal teachings at public forums in auditoriums and halls (e.g., a lecture on Hindu religion at the Brooklyn Ethical Association). While his talks and lectures to groups at the Vedanta Society and elsewhere had a deep impact on the public perception of Eastern spirituality, perhaps his most significant teachings were the meditation sessions that took place in the parlors of New York's fashionable set. In these intimate surroundings, he transmitted knowledge of yoga through practice.

Hatha Yoga to Facilitate Meditation

Vivekananda's meditation demonstrations had a powerful effect—not least of all on himself (fig. 4.1). He seemed as susceptible to slipping into *samadhi* as some people are to being seduced at first flirtation or to confessing to crimes they didn't commit. His method of achieving *samadhi,* in fact, seems more like precipitously falling into a trance than achieving the highest state of meditation through the patient, successive implementation of yoga techniques. Vivekananda biographer Marie Louise Burke writes: "Often times, he was lost in meditation, his unconsciousness of the external betraying his complete absorption within. Even while holding a class he would plunge into profound contemplation. When the Swami emerged from such states . . . he would feel impatient with himself, for he desired that the Teacher should be uppermost in him, rather than the Yogi. In order to avoid repetitions of such occurrences, he instructed one or two how to bring him back by uttering a word or a Name, should he be carried by the force of meditation into Samadhi."[30]

Vivekananda provided detailed instructions for sitting in meditation. Finding "a posture in which we can remain long," he said, is critical for accommodating the lengthy process of reaching higher states of consciousness.[31] He advocated for a meditative pose with "the spinal column free, sitting erect, holding the three parts—the chest, neck, and head—in a straight line [so that] you have an easy natural posture, with the spine straight. You will naturally see that you cannot think very high thoughts with the chest in."[32]

Vivekananda also provided detailed instruc-

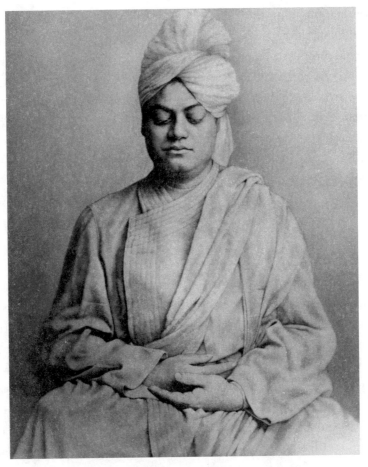

Figure 4.1. Swami Vivekananda sitting in meditation, 1896
(With the kind permission of the Vedanta Society of St. Louis)

tions for *pranayama,* yogic breathing exercises, which he considered an integral part of meditation. "After one has learned to have a firm erect seat," he said, "one has to perform, according to certain schools, a practice called the purifying of the nerves." Although this practice "has been rejected by some as not belonging to Raja-Yoga," he continued, the great teacher and philosopher Shankaracharya advises its use.[33]* Vivekananda quoted from Shankaracharya's commentary on the *Shvetashvatara Upanishad:*

The mind whose dross has been cleared away by Pranayama, becomes fixed in Brahman; therefore Pranayama is declared. First the nerves are to be purified, then comes the power

---

*Actually, Shankaracharya regarded *Nadi Suddhi,* Alternate Nostril Breath, the *pranayama* practice commonly considered to purify the nerves, to be preparation for *pranayama,* by which he meant either *Deerga Swasam,* Three-Part Breath, which involves breathing deeply into the lower, mid, and upper lungs, or *Antara/Bahya Kumbhaka,* Breath Retention on (respectively) the Inhalation or Exhalation, which involves stopping the breath.

to practice Pranayama. Stopping the right nostril with the thumb, through the left nostril fill in air, according to capacity; then, without any interval, throw the air out through the right nostril, closing the left one. Again inhaling through the right nostril eject through the left, according to capacity; practicing this three or five times at four hours of the day, before dawn, during midday, in the evening, and at midnight, in fifteen days or a month purity of the nerves is attained; then begins Pranayama.[34]

Vivekananda held that just as critical to meditation as *pranayama,* performed "after one has learned to have a firm erect seat,"[35] is the initial step in the "series of exercises, physical and mental, [that] is to be gone through every day, until certain higher states are reached":[36] conditioning *asanas,* performed to aid the removal of obstacles (fidgetiness and fatigue) to spiritual progress by providing steadiness and ease in a seated position.

An account of Vivekananda's hands-on teaching of conditioning *asanas* to the small groups of followers in his "parlor lectures" can be found in "Balm of the Orient Is Bliss-Inspiring Yoga," a snide article published on March 27, 1898, in the *New York Herald,* after Vivekananda had returned to India (he left New York in April 1896 and, after traveling in Europe, arrived in Calcutta in February 1897). "He explained to [his followers] various strange postures which they must assume illustrating his teaching with his own supple body, long trained to such acrobatic feats," wrote the uncredited reporter. "He described 'viparitakarani,' which consists of raising the body in the air by resting the crown

of the head and the shoulders upon the ground and supporting the loins with the hands. And 'paschimasana,' in which you stretch out both legs, and, having taken hold of the toes with the hands, place your forehead upon your knees. And 'gomukhasana,' in which you put the right ankle on the left side of the chest, and similarly the left ankle on the right side."[37]

These postures (*Viparitakarani Mudra,* Half Shoulder Stand, *Paschimottanasana,* Seated Forward Bend, and *Gomukhasana,* Cow Face Pose, along with several others that Vivekananda described and modeled) were performed in accordance with the hatha yoga tradition—that is, in preparation for seated meditation practices, including regulating the breath, shutting out external impressions, and concentrating on a single object as a means of seeking union with Being. But the author of the article treated Vivekananda's *asana* teaching with derision: "These and many more postures the Swami illustrated to his converts, telling them of the delightful results to be obtained from each. And the converts went home and tried to do likewise, to their great discomfort and the threatened dislocation of many joints."[38]

The primary source for the *Herald*'s scathing story of "how the Hindoo cult has captured New York society" was a certain Swami Kripananda, who witnessed the events, lent his expertise in yoga to the detailed descriptions of the poses, and modeled for the illustrative sketches that portray upper class New Yorkers as out-of-shape, clueless dupes struggling in vain to practice yogic poses in their homes.[39] Kripananda also wrote an accompanying article, "Just What Yoga Is," with even snarkier comments: "[Vivekananda] was a success from the start. Handsome, eloquent, charming in manner and convincing in his sophistries, this tawny beggar Prince soon had scores of our intelligent, practical, nineteenth century men and women sitting cross-legged in the privacy of their bedroom, gazing for hours at the tips of their noses, or, if not too plump, staring at their navels, and breathing by set rule with patient gravity and a decorous sense of their growing spirituality."[40]

Who was this swami who heaped ridicule and scorn on Vivekananda and his followers for what took place at "the séances of Swami Vivekananda" in the apartments of the upper crust?[41] It was none other than Leon Landsberg, given the name Swami Kripananda when he became the second of the two American swamis initiated into *sannyasa,* the stage in which worldly pursuits are renounced, by Vivekananda at Thousand Island Park in the summer of 1895. The apostate Landsberg—who once had been Vivekananda's intimate and shining disciple, tended to the practical details of establishing the Vedanta Society, and escorted Vivekananda around New York for his talks—evidently had soured on Vivekananda and his followers and was ready to dish the dirt.

According to Burke, Vivekananda's biographer, Landsberg's betrayal was due to his jealousy of other students who received Vivekananda's affection and attention. At first Landsberg had been smitten. "When I met the Swami [in April 1894] and realized the greatness of his soul," he wrote Bull, "all the love of which my heart was capable, and which was only waiting for an opportunity to escape its prison built up by prejudice and bad experience, blazed forth with all its intensity like a flame

that at last had found its way through the thick cover of ashes to the open air, and focused in his person."[42] But after Vivekananda's classes had grown and increasing numbers of students gathered around him in early 1895, Landsberg, resenting their presence, criticized them, sulked, quarreled with Vivekananda, and then, in April, promising to "break once for all my relations to [Vivekananda]," fled to another rooming house.[43]

After a reconciliation brokered by Bull, Landsberg received his final monastic vows from Vivekananda in the summer, and in December Vivekananda set up new quarters in Landsberg's rooming house. Since they had last lived in the same building, Vivekananda's following had greatly increased, necessitating much more help than Landsberg alone could supply. A devoted staff of students (who arranged scheduling, took dictation, kept accounts, cooked, and attended to other tasks) formed around Vivekananda. The brooding Landsberg withdrew to a small room in the attic, where he "sank deeper and deeper into a state of resentment and bitterness."[44] "Hypersensitive, self-centered to an extreme degree," Burke tells us, "he was subject to fits of black depression and violent temper, open to torments of jealousy, inclined to self-pity and delusions of persecution."[45] His dark nature, it might be said, blazed forth.

The last time Vivekananda and Landsberg saw each other was in March 1986, just before Vivekananda left America for England, the first stop on his journey back to India. Despite Vivekananda's reassurances of his love, expressed in a letter sent from Switzerland in August, and an invitation, made about a year later, to visit him in India, Landsberg deserted the fold, this time for good.

To ensure the continuity of not only his philosophical teachings but his yoga practice in America, Vivekananda anointed Swami Abhedananda, whom he had come to admire as one of his sixteen fellow disciples (some consider them as apostles) of Shri Ramakrishna in India, to be his successor at the Vedanta Society in New York in 1897. Abhedananda didn't disappoint. As well as vigorously popularizing Vedanta,* he faithfully carried on the hatha yoga meditation techniques taught by Vivekananda. In his *How to Be a Yogi,* published by the Vedanta Society in 1902, Abhedananda succinctly defined the place of *asanas* in aiding meditation: "Tremor of the body and restlessness of the limbs, which are such frequent obstacles in the way of gaining control over the mind, may easily be removed by the practice of *Asana.*"[46] Adhering closely to the *Hatha Yoga Pradipika,* the classic hatha yoga text, he presented instructions for several meditative and conditioning *asanas* (the names of the poses are added):

1. *Padmasana,* Lotus Pose. "Sit cross-legged on the floor, placing the left foot on the right thigh and the right foot on the left thigh, and keeping the body, neck, and head in a straight line."

2. *Baddha Padmasana,* Bound Lotus Pose. "After sitting in this posture, hold the right great toe with the right hand and the left great toe with the left hand (the hands coming from behind the back and crossing each other)."

3. *Virasana,* Hero Pose. "Sit straight on a level place, firmly inserting both insteps between the thighs and the calves of the legs."

4. *Kukkutasana,* Cock Pose. "Assuming posture No. 1, insert the hands between the thighs and the calves, and, planting the palms firmly on the ground, lift the body above the seat."

5. *Paschimottanasana* I, Seated Forward Bend, holding the toes. "Sitting on the floor, stretch the legs straight in front, hold the great toes with the hands without bending the knees."

6. *Paschimottanasana* II, Seated Forward Bend, holding the toes and touching the forehead to the knees. "Having accomplished this posture, touch the knees with the forehead."

7. *Akarna Dhanurasana,* Archer Pose. "Holding the toes as in posture 5, keep one arm extended and with the other draw the other toe towards your ear as you would do with the string of a bow."

8. *Mayurasana,* Peacock Pose. "Plant hands firmly on the ground and support the weight of the body upon the elbows, pressing them against the sides of the loins. Then raise the feet above the ground, keeping them stiff and straight on a level with the head."

9. *Savasana,* Corpse Pose. "Lie upon the back on the floor at full length like a corpse, keeping the head on a level with the body."[47]

---

*Like Vivekananda, Abhedananda was an active lecturer and prolific author who, by 1902, had published fifteen lectures, including "The Relation of Soul to God," "The Motherhood of God," "Religion of the Hindus," and "Why a Hindu Accepts Christ and Rejects Christianity," and four books, including *Spiritual Unfoldment* and *Reincarnation.*

Abhedananda taught these *asanas,* which are "familiar to many yoga students today," writes Stefanie Syman, who chronicled the history of yoga in America, to "several hundred students" at the Vedanta Society in order to facilitate their meditation.[48]

The positions of Abhedananda and Vivekananda on *asana* were virtually the same. With one critical difference: Abhedananda strongly believed in the ability of *asana* to eliminate two conditions that interfere with meditation: lethargy and sickness. He noted, "Another object in practicing *Asana* is to remove the *Tamas* element which causes heaviness of the body, and to free the system from the effects of cold, catarrh, phlegm, rheumatism, and many other diseases. Some of the exercises increase the action of the stomach and liver, while others regulate the activities of the other organs."[49]

Abhedananda recognized the temptation to practice *asana* as an end in itself. He sternly cautioned: "Thus we see that perfect health and longevity are the immediate results of the Hatha Yoga practices. To the real seeker after Absolute Truth, however, they have small value except as they become a means of attaining superconscious realization. . . . Raja Yoga . . . alone will lead the soul to God-consciousness and perfect freedom."[50] But he acknowledged that hatha yoga itself "does not claim that physical health is the same as spirituality. On the contrary, it tells us that if a healthy body were a sign of spirituality, then wild animals and savages who enjoy perfect health would be exceedingly spiritual; yet they are not, as we know."[51]

Abhedananda enthusiastically endorsed the value of yogic postural, breathing, and dietary (but not purificatory) practices in contributing to spirituality: "The principal idea of these Yogis is that physical maladies are obstacles in the path of spiritual progress while a healthy body furnishes one of the most favorable conditions for the realization of the highest spiritual truths in this life. Those who do not possess good health should, therefore, begin to practice Hatha Yoga."[52]

Vivekananda, in contrast, had a visceral abhorrence of hatha yoga as a fitness and therapeutic program (while favoring conditioning *asanas* as preparation for assuming a seated *asana,* and *pranayama* as a technique for facilitating meditation), decrying its practices as an impediment to salvation. Oddly enough, though, earlier in his life he had expressed an interest in learning hatha yoga to improve his own strength and health.

Vivekananda in India

Hatha Yoga to Improve Health

On January 18, 1890, about four and a half years after the death of his guru, Ramakrishna Paramahamsa, a major figure in the Bengali Renaissance from whom he was taught that all religions are true, and just a few years before beginning his lecture tour in America, Vivekananda arrived in Ghazipur to seek out the wisdom of Pavhari Baba. Baba was a hermit who lived not in a mountain cave or forest hut but in a proper house, fashioned like a spaciously roomed English bungalow and enclosed by high walls. He reputedly lived, however, in a burrow adjacent to the house, "wherein he lays himself up in Samadhi," Vivekananda wrote to

Pramadadas Mitra, a noted Sanskrit scholar. "Nobody knows what he eats, and so they call him Pavhari [one living on air] Baba."[53] Most peculiar of all, "he allows nobody to enter," Vivekananda wrote to Balaram Bose, a prominent devotee of Ramakrishna. "If he is so inclined, he comes up to the door and speaks from inside—that is all."[54]

Soon after they first "met" (Vivekananda remained on the outside and Baba on the inside of the door) in early February, it occurred to Vivekananda that he could learn mastery of hatha yoga from Baba. Ramakrishna had been knowledgeable about hatha yoga as, it seems, a methodological discipline for developing strength and obtaining good health through practicing yogic postures, deep breathing techniques, purificatory techniques, and dietary regulation, but Vivekananda, whose constitution was weak and health was poor, had never asked to learn it. He didn't want to pass up another opportunity. "One day I thought that I did not learn any art for making this weak body strong, even though I lived with Shri Ramakrishna for so many years," he reminisced to a disciple in 1902. "I had heard that Pavhari Baba knew the science of Hatha-Yoga. So I thought I would learn the practices of Hatha-Yoga from him, and through them strengthen the body."[55]

Vivekananda asked Baba to teach him the yogic health practices. The guru agreed. (Evidently neither of them considered the door between them to be an obstacle to transmitting hatha yoga techniques.) But then Vivekananda got spooked by a series of wordless visitations from Ramakrishna (although silent and dead, to his credit it can be said that Ramakrishna at least showed his face), who reproached him for being disloyal. "Thus when for several nights in succession I had the vision of Shri Ramakrishna," Vivekananda reasoned, "I gave up the idea of initiation altogether, thinking that as every time I resolved on it, I was getting such a vision, then no good but harm would come of it."[56]

Vivekananda wavered on passing up his chance to learn hatha yoga as physical culture and therapy from Baba. He believed he wouldn't be able to find as good instruction anywhere else in Bengal ("What little there is, is but the queer breathing exercises of the Hatha-Yoga—which is nothing but a kind of gymnastics"[57]). But just less than four weeks after his first so-called meeting with Baba and his many subsequent "talk[s] with him *ab intra*"[58] (what a sly use of the Latin legal term "from within"!), in which Baba wouldn't reply to direct questions ("What does this servant know?" he would demur) but then would go on rants, Vivekananda faced the reality that any kind of relationship with Baba was untenable.[59] On March 3rd, he wrote to Mitra about his frustration and disillusionment: "But now I see the whole matter is inverted in its bearings! While I myself have come, a beggar, at his door, he turns round and wants to learn of me! This saint perhaps is not yet perfected—too much of rites, vows, observances, and too much of self-concealment."[60] In early May 1890, about three months after his arrival, Vivekananda departed Ghazipur to go to Bareilly.

Even if he had had permission from Ramakrishna's ghost to take up hatha yoga with Baba and had a long, fruitful relationship with Baba, it seems unlikely that Vivekananda would've pursued hatha yoga training. For him, the real obstacle to learning hatha yoga wasn't Ramakrishna's shadowy form reproaching him for his fickleness or the brevity of his time spent with Baba but his resistance to improving his health. It's not that Vivekananda totally ignored the importance of good health in meditation practice: "There are several obstructions to practice. The first obstruction is an unhealthy body: if the body is not in a fit state, the practice will be obstructed. Therefore we have to keep the body in good health; we have to take care of what we eat and drink, and what we do."[61] And it's not that he didn't take some measures to alleviate his own pain and discomfort. During the time he was in Ghazipur, he recalled in 1902, "I was suffering diarrhea, and there [was] no food [that] could be had except bread." So he'd go to a garden with many lemon trees (near the ashram where he was staying), where, "to increase the digestive powers, I used to take plenty of lemons."[62] It's just that he had no interest in dedicating himself to a daily, systematic, vigorous practice of yogic conditioning postures, breath control exercises, purificatory exercises, and dietary rules. And he strongly disapproved of anyone who did.

In his American lectures Vivekananda granted that there's some benefit to hatha yoga purificatory practices: "One or two ordinary lessons of the Hatha-Yogis are very useful. For instance, some of you will find it a good thing for headaches to drink cold water through the nose as soon as you get up in the morning; the whole day your brain will be nice and cool, and you will never catch cold. It is very easy to do; put your nose into the water, draw it up through the nostrils and make a pump action in the throat."[63]

But in general Vivekananda expressed a strong antipathy toward hatha yoga as a health cure. It's not merely that he saw no efficacy in its health practices; he outright condemned them as harmful. The very goal of yogic health cure, he warned, is dangerously misguided. Hatha yogins "say the greatest good is to keep the body from dying. . . . Their whole process is clinging to the body."[64] But why would he express such agitated indignation about a discipline that holds out the possibility of improving health, especially considering that he himself suffered from diabetes (he was afflicted with swollen feet, loss of appetite, failing vision in his right eye, diarrhea, and fatigue), as well as asthma and severe lower back pain?

In Indian society it has traditionally been believed that we don't determine our destiny—that, instead, our destiny is determined by such factors as our past lives, the mixture of *gunas* (the three fundamental qualities: clarity, passion, and dullness) given us at birth, or the stars. In a conversation with a disciple in 1901, Vivekananda expressed his belief that having a diseased body was ordained for him by his birthplace.

Disciple: How are you, Swamiji?

Swamiji: What shall I speak of my health, my son? The body is getting unfit for work day by day. It has been born in the soil of Bengal, and some disease or other is always overtaking it.[65]

Believing that we're powerless to make changes allows us to be detached observers of life's vicissitudes, especially in times of suffering, but it also inculcates fatalism. In a lecture given at Washington Hall in San Francisco in 1900, Vivekananda mocked a hatha yogin in Calcutta who claimed to have lived five hundred years. "The walls can keep their bodies thousands of years," he scoffed. "What of that? I would not want to live so long. 'Sufficient unto the day is the evil thereof.' One little body, with its delusions and limitations, is enough."[66]* His followers would've received this rousing sermon as impassioned testimony about finding serene detachment from the impermanent body. But we, knowing that Vivekananda sensed that he wouldn't live long, may recognize his emotional display for what it is: an irrational outburst against a yogin's patently bogus claim of longevity that unmasks (unintentionally and without his awareness) Vivekananda's apathy in the face of, as he would put it to the disciple concerned about his ill health, "the few days that the body lasts."[67]

Knowing that Vivekananda died in 1902 at the age of thirty-nine (blood in his nostrils, mouth, and eyes indicates that the cause was a cerebral hemorrhage), we might consider his passiveness—his refusal to participate actively in improving his deteriorated physical condition with hatha yoga health practices—as a poignant coming to terms with (what he perceived as) the foreordained brevity of his life. But when we consider that he projected his resignation as a common good, we must condemn his attack on hatha yoga health practices—his damning of them as harmful to everyone without exception—because it swayed those whom

he had spurred into taking up yoga to shun the use of yoga for improving their health.

To be fair, Vivekananda's denunciation of hatha yoga as a regime for fending off and ridding the body of disease took place about twenty-five years before Yogendra and other yogins in India, in response to the Nature Cure movement sweeping the world, reframed hatha yoga as an indigenous natural health cure regime based in medical science for the mass of people (not just renunciates), and before this new perspective found acceptance among the Indian middle class. Had he lived during the time of these developments (which he was instrumental in making possible by stripping yoga of its traditional rituals, texts, and dogma), Vivekananda might've turned to hatha yoga to improve his health.

And no matter what his limitations, we shouldn't forget his great achievements. In the late 1800s in America, as modern yoga scholar Elizabeth De Michelis establishes, Vivekananda advocated for his new form of Neo-Vedantic Hinduism: "a technologically interpreted 'science of yoga' aimed at 'reattuning' the practitioner to the cosmos"—a spirituality born out of "eagerly absorbing the new . . . ways of life, but inwardly feeling a heart-rending nostalgia and longing for the old traditional forms." The publication of these teachings in *Raja Yoga* (Vivekananda's lecture published as a book in 1896), De Michelis notes, "immediately started something of a 'yoga renaissance' both in India and in the

---

*In the Sermon on the Mount according to the Gospel of Matthew (6:34), this proverb appears in a different context, and consequently has a different meaning. Jesus is telling his followers that if they seek the kingdom of God, then God will provide them with the necessities of daily life, so they should "take therefore no thought for the morrow" but address only the tribulations of each day.

West."[68] In his later years in India, he dedicated himself to addressing India's most pressing social issues (he ardently lectured on the need to lift up the poor, eliminate the caste system, and end British rule) and practiced *sewa,* organized service to others in the community (he founded the Ramakrishna Math and Mission, a social service organization).

If hatha yoga is defined as a discipline that facilitates meditation through the practice of conditioning *asanas* (yogic physical exercises that prepare one for sitting in "a posture in which we can remain long"[69]) and *pranayama* (breathing exercises that result in a "mind whose dross has been cleared away"[70]), then Vivekananda embraced hatha yoga, although he didn't identify it as such. So journalist Ann Louise Bardach, who's been researching the sage since the mid-1990s, is incorrect in attributing to Vivekananda an "utter lack of interest in physical exertions beyond marathon sitting meditations and pilgrimages to holy sites."[71] If, however, hatha yoga is defined as a discipline that imparts good health and long life or that removes lethargy and prevents disease to facilitate meditation through the practice of conditioning *asanas* (postures), *pranayama* (breath control), purificatory techniques, *mudras* (seals), *bandhas* (locks), and diet, then she's correct. Both definitions, of course, are true.*

Yogendra's ambition to introduce hatha yoga to America was based on the same misunderstanding (which still persists today) that Vivekananda totally rejected hatha yoga, while in actuality he believed that the conditioning *asanas* were a valuable aid to meditation, the yoga technique for attaining what he called "Existence Absolute," "Knowledge Absolute," or "Bliss Absolute." Although holding that yoga is an eight-step path that culminates in "a state of uninterrupted joy, peace eternal, consciousness absolute, and concrete self-realization," Yogendra was primarily a proponent of hatha yoga's ability to provide fitness and good health—the part of hatha yoga that Vivekananda rejected.[72] As such, he would be the first yogin to teach hatha yoga as physical culture and health cure—what he called "practical yoga"—in America.

---

*Bardach uses Vivekananda's lofty notion of yoga (to him, yoga "meant just one thing: 'realizing God'") to sneer at the contemporary yoga scene made up of an "estimated 16 million supple, spandex-clad yoginis in the United States, who sustain an annual $6 billion industry." When Vivekananda "introduced 'yoga' into the national conversation [in 1893]," she cuttingly remarks, "an exercise cult with expensive accessories was hardly what he had in mind" (Bardach, "How Yoga Won the West," 4 [phrases reordered]).

Interestingly enough, the journalists writing on the front page of a section of the March 27, 1898, *New York Herald* had a similarly contemptuous attitude about the yoga fad of their day—the one inspired by Vivekananda! Their target was "New York's fashionables [who] now attain perfect happiness by becoming amateur contortionists" (*New York Herald,* "Balm of the Orient"). The banner headline sarcastically instructs: "If You Want to Be a Yogi and Have Heavenly Dreams, Study These Postures." The postures are illustrated beneath the splashy headline (and above two scathing articles about yoga) in seven satirical sketches mostly of prosperous, middle-aged New Yorkers alone on the floor of their bedroom or living room, shoeless, looking pathetic or ridiculous or bewildered as they awkwardly struggle to assume the *asanas* taught to them by Vivekananda. Whereas Bardach implies that contemporary yoga followers in America have corrupted the spiritual yoga tradition introduced to America by Vivekananda, the *New York Herald* journalists implied that the late 19th-century yoga followers in America, in taking up weird yogic postures, were dupes, rich fools taken in by the charlatan in ocher robes and turban, Vivekananda.

Yogendra in America

In December 1919, accompanied by Dadina, Yogendra sailed to America, where he was enthusiastically welcomed by New York socialites entranced with both natural health cures and the supernatural (fig. 4.2). Accordingly, Yogendra put together for them a program consisting of yogic purificatory techniques, *asanas, pranayama,* and *siddhis* (yogic supernatural powers). He demonstrated *neti, dhouti* (various cleansing techniques, such as stimulating "fire" by repeatedly pushing the abdomen back toward the spine), and *basti* (the contraction and dilation of the sphincter muscle, sometimes performed with a tube inserted into the rectum—a form of yogic enema). He performed some difficult *asanas.* According to *World Magazine,* he "swell[ed] one lung to thrice the size of the other," controlled his bodily temperature, made "electricity stream from his fingers" in a darkened room, and stopped his watch through willing it.[73] The audience members, including many curious and skeptical medical practitioners, were astonished. Their wholehearted response gave Yogendra the opportunity to discuss his mission to bring yogic healing to America. He showed them case histories of patients in Versova.

A committee was immediately formed of three "reputed men of position" to find a suitable place for a yoga retreat.[74] In April 1920 a foreign branch of the Yoga Institute was established on an idle summer estate on Bear Mountain in Harriman, New York, in the Hudson Valley about forty-five miles north of New York City. Bear Mountain was an area of great natural beauty where wealthy businessmen made their summer homes and the middle class vacationed at resorts, inns, lodges, and campsites.

The Yoga Institute of America was formally opened to the public on June 30, 1920. Yogendra settled in, and over the next two years he treated a steady flow of patients and traveled to lecture on various Eastern spiritual topics, including yoga philosophy—the "philosophy of harmonious culture of body, mind and soul."[75]

In mid-1922 Yogendra received a letter from his aging father, Haribhai, saying that he was ailing and lonely. He requested that Yogendra return home to care for him. Yogendra was probably relieved. He had never felt at home in America. One of his first letters to his friend Popat in India shows his initial impression of America: "Here is a country of materialism and commerce, the vibrations are quite different; all seems to be superficial, they have no reality at the bottom. . . . To work in the midst of such people is undoubtedly trying and still more to convince them of any new philosophy."[76] A later letter to Popat confirmed this view: "Their reasoning is that battle of intellect which never can find its way within its own limits. They ought to be supplied with things and facts which their lower senses can comprehend, otherwise it has no meaning for them."[77] Yogendra sailed for India in the fall. He arrived in Bombay at the end of 1922 and continued on to Bulsar to join his father.

Yogendra Back in India

When Yogendra established his first ashram, the Yoga Institute, in Versova, a suburb of Bombay, in 1918, he had modest ambitions. But in 1923 he sought to open an international center—one that would "benefit not only the whole nation but also the world"—in Lonavla.[78] A philan-

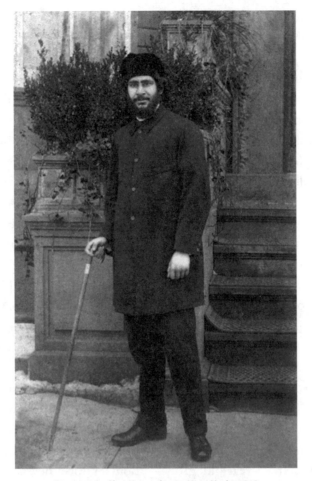

Figure 4.2. Shri Yogendra in New York, 1919

(With the kind permission of the Yoga Institute)

thropist had offered him a plot of land there "with a bungalow for his Yoga Ashram." But the project, alleges Rodrigues, acting as Yogendra's counsel, "fell into wrong hands"[79]—those of "another advocate of Yoga, claiming disciple-ship under Paramahamsa Madhavadasaji," who, after "dogging [Yogendra's] footsteps," cleverly stole his preparation.[80] The accused villain was Swami Kuvalayananda, the great popularizer of yoga as science-based health treatment.* Most

---

*Probably following Yogendra's quirk, Rodrigues never identifies Kuvalayananda by name but instead only makes (what some may consider comical) allusions to him. The references typically reveal Yogendra's lifelong grievance with Kuvalayananda for saying that he had been a disciple of Madhavadasaji. "The so-called rival rubbed salt in Shri Yogendra's wounds," Rodrigues asserts, surely reflecting Yogendra's simmering rage, "by claiming common teachership in Paramahamsa Madhavadasaji" (Rodrigues, *The Householder Yogi,* 174–75). What Yogendra really seemed to be accusing Kuvalayananda of was claiming to be not just another disciple of Madhavadasaji but his heir, a position Yogendra declined and yet believed to be his. How else to explain Yogendra's fixation with this groundless charge?

of Yogendra's groundwork, Rodrigues claims, was "usurped by the imposter" to open his own center.[81]

Putting his plans to found an international yoga center on hold, Yogendra moved on with his life. In 1927, after lecturing several times in Madras and Mysore, he delivered his discourse in Bangalore on the rightful place of yoga in the life of the householder. A group of admirers, including M. Ramachandra Rao Scindia, a well-known merchant and mill owner, asked Yogendra if he planned to become a *sannyasi* (a Hindu religious mendicant) or get married. Yogendra replied that "he planned to marry and bring up a family for he believed that by his own example he would make Yoga acceptable to modern men and women."[82] Upon hearing of Yogendra's plans, Scindia arranged for the tall, handsome young man to visit the house of a zamindar (a landowner who leases his vast property to tenant farmers) Venkataraman Rao, who had a marriageable daughter. Yogendra and the shy sixteen-year-old girl, Sita, got married the following year. They celebrated their marriage by witnessing the Dasara festival in nearby Mysore, led by the maharajah of Mysore, Shri Nalvadi Krishnaraja Wadiyar (see chapter 20), from the royal visitors' gallery, where they sat by invitation of an admirer of Yogendra's, Mirza Ismail, the diwan (prime minister) of the Kingdom of Mysore. After a few weeks, the newlyweds traveled to Bulsar, where they lived while looking after Yogendra's father.

During the next few years Yogendra studied, wrote, traveled, lectured, and started a family. Rodrigues portrays this time as idyllic: "The happy family spent its time in the verdant surroundings of a tranquil and unsophisticated town—Bulsar."[83] But it was a frustrating period for Yogendra in terms of advancing his career. The Yoga Institute that he established in Bulsar changed location from one rented house to another four times. Worse, the institute's out-of-the-way location discouraged admirers from visiting him. Even Rodrigues concedes that Yogendra "would have definitely preferred to be in a central [i.e., urban] location, where he could reach out to more people" and, no doubt, have a larger membership, greater recognition, and more financial security.[84]

Haribhai died in 1935 (nearly fifteen years after his entreaties to Yogendra to return from America to tend to him). He had asked his son to treat him "like a piece of wood" after his death.[85] Obeying his father's wishes, Yogendra cremated him without ceremonies. His only inheritance was a few cots and cooking utensils. Soon afterward, with "eyes cast to the city where things happened," Yogendra scouted Bombay for a new location for his institute.[86] In May 1936 he took his family to Chowpatty, even then Bombay's most famous beach, where they moved into a house that became the new headquarters of the Yoga Institute.

In the spring of 1938 Yogendra obtained a lease from the Bombay government for property in Kandivli, yet another suburb of Bombay. But "someone," Rodrigues contends, referring once again to Kuvalayananda, "wanted to have the Institute strangled just when it had started to grow and flourish."[87] In less than a day the acceptance of the lease was withdrawn—the result of "systematic interference from some interested quarters . . . a conspiracy that led to the cancellation of the Kandivli lease. . . . It

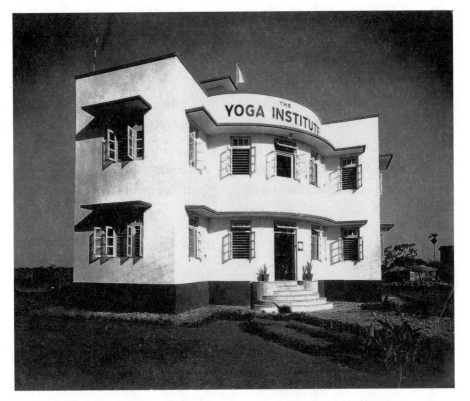

Figure 4.3. The Yoga Institute, 1948 (before landscaping was completed)

(With the kind permission of the Yoga Institute)

can only be a conspiracy hatched by one who did not cherish the progress of the Institute"—namely, "a so-called rival official yogi, having a close relationship with the Chief Minister, and thus [a] strong connection with the Government."[88] Making the final argument in Yogendra's case, Rodrigues even claims that a journalist, S. A. Brelvi, had "learnt about the foul play and wanted to expose the culprit" but, when told that the offender was Kuvalayananda, was afraid to continue his investigation because of Kuvalayananda's connection to the Indian Congress, one of the two major political parties in India.[89]

There's no evidence that Kuvalayananda had even heard of Yogendra in the 1920s and 1930s. But Kuvalayananda certainly loomed large in Yogendra's life during this period. Kuvalayananda, Yogendra believed, subverted Yogendra's greatest ambitions. Yogendra's paranoia is understandable. Not because Kuvalayananda was out to get him but because Kuvalayananda received the acclaim from the Indian elite that Yogendra sought and felt that he alone deserved. In the yoga world, Kuvalayananda was celebrated as *the* shaker of traditional beliefs. Yogendra's accomplishments went unnoticed.

Nevertheless, Yogendra persisted in his dream to establish a permanent internationally renowned yoga center (fig. 4.3). After buying property in Santa Cruz, a suburb of Bombay, he solicited loan money for construction of a building for a yoga center from past patients, some of whom were among Bombay's richest men. He either was turned down or found the interest rates exorbitant. Then, out of the blue, he was presented with an offer from Rustom J. Irani, a wealthy Parsi eccentric who had made his fortune in the café business.* Yogendra went to Irani's house and was led to the master bedroom, where he found Irani lying in a large bed. Instructing Yogendra to sit on the bed, Irani asked him how much money he needed. Yogendra said forty thousand rupees.† Irani quietly got up and returned with the money all bundled up, saying, "You may take it."[90] Using this loan, made on generous terms, Yogendra constructed the final incarnation of the Yoga Institute in 1948 (see fig. 4.3 on page 63).

---

*Representative of Bombay's cosmopolitanism, Irani's cafés were the first eating establishments in India to serve people from all walks of life, irrespective of class, religion, caste, or persuasion. Seated on bentwood chairs at marble tabletops, businessmen, migrant workers, artists, journalists, prostitutes, and lawyers rubbed shoulders.

†The rupee, a fixed-rate currency after independence, was pegged at 4.79 against the American dollar, so the amount Yogendra needed was about $8,300, which is about $83,300 dollars in today's money.

5

SHRI YOGENDRA

Making Yoga Gentle

Relaxation

"Modernity was experienced as a series of deprivations that invoked a fundamental sense of anxiety" in the new Indian middle class that emerged in colonial India in the nineteenth century, writes political scientist Leela Fernandes.[1] In the early 20th century Shri Yogendra pitched hatha yoga to members of the Indian middle class as a means of not only attaining good health but also finding relief from agitation. Yoga provides the kind of relaxation, he told them in *Hatha Yoga Simplified,* that "quickly recuperates or regalvanizes, as it were, the nerve centres, collects the scattered forces and thus reinvigorates the whole body. It is just as refreshing as a Turkish or a Russian bath, besides having many of the peculiar therapeutic advantages of a medical massage."[2]

Yogendra pointed to the yoga tradition of relaxation as the source of his practice and philosophy of yogic relaxation: "The ancient yogins, who are known for their self-mastery over the entire voluntary and involuntary organism, were fully alive to the many advantages of relaxation."[3] No doubt his initial, simple beliefs about bodily relaxation were acquired from his guru Madhavadasaji or Svatmarama's *Hatha Yoga Pradipika* and were therefore based in the yoga tradition; however, Yogendra's developed beliefs about bodily relaxation—both in their overarching arguments and most of their nuances—were derived from his readings in late 19th- and early 20th-century Western alternative medicine and physical culture, primarily Genevieve Stebbins's popular *Dynamic Breathing and Harmonic Gymnastics: A Complete*

System of Psychical, Aesthetic and Physical Culture, published in 1893. In fact, what Yogendra wrote about relaxation in his main text, *Yoga Asanas Simplified,* is purloined, with a bit of fussy touching up, from Stebbins, whom he also strategically quotes—what audacity!—in support of "his" theories. (In *Hatha Yoga Simplified,* Yogendra chose a more straightforward rhetorical strategy: he simply presented the supporting passage as if he'd written it.)

The American Stebbins promoted a spiritually infused physical culture system consisting of relaxing and energizing exercises based on the system created by Frenchman François Delsarte. Her American Delsartism "gave middle and upper-class women [a] means of celebrating the health and versatility of the human body," writes dance historian Laura Williams Iverson. "Focused on physical and spiritual transcendence, Delsartism was an exciting tool for women just starting to assert their rights in industrial America."[4]

Adopting wholesale Stebbins's polemics of relaxation (and using her wording with minor changes), Yogendra lamented in his section on *Savasana,* Corpse Pose, in *Yoga Asanas Simplified:* "Unfortunately, nothing perhaps has been so thoroughly misunderstood as the art of relaxation. For one thing, relaxation should not be mistaken for inertia; it also does not mean lying in a lazy manner or doing nothing."[5] "The object," he argued, "is to establish muscular equilibrium as soon as possible through the medium of relaxation—more truly, by conscious rest after conscious effort. It means that the more perfect the effort, the more perfect is the relaxation."[6]

Quoting Stebbins, Yogendra maintained

that completely relaxing the voluntary muscles allows for the transfer of energy to the involuntary muscles, producing "the necessary equilibrium for the renewal of strength."[7] To achieve this rejuvenation, Stebbins instructed her practitioners to "relax at once as completely as possible, so that the body or part shall be practically limp and lifeless, as though it was no part of you." This physical relaxation, she maintained, should be accompanied by mental withdrawal from the everyday world: "The mental idea to be used is a calm and perfect consciousness of your separate existence apart from and superior to the body or part undergoing the exercise. This must also be accompanied with the normal rhythmic breathing, while the imagination seeks unaided a pleasing but dreamy kind of rapport with the natural surroundings."[8]

Following Stebbins, Yogendra advocated separating the mind from the body: "What is important is that the consciousness of physical body should be necessarily and entirely forgotten."[9] And he, too, recommended normal rhythmic breathing: "Close the eyes as in peaceful slumber and follow normal rhythmic breathing."[10] But whereas Stebbins recommended fostering an ethereal connection to nature, Yogendra suggested making a connection to one's essential nature: "Keep watching the movements of the breath until at last the mind synchronises with the hazy sense of your being."[11]

In response to a claim that the American actor Steele MacKaye originated the concept of relaxation exercise, Stebbins attributed its first use in artistic expression to German philosopher

M. (Johann Jakob) Engel.* In his book on acting, *Practical Illustrations of Rhetorical Gesture and Action,* published in 1774 (and adapted for English drama by Henry Siddons in 1807), "the pupil is taught to lie upon the floor," wrote Stebbins, "and to withdraw all voluntary nerve-force from the extremities and thinking part of the brain, and to simulate death. This is strongly recommended as *the beginning of all control of the body,* and is illustrated by a picture of a man lying limp and helpless."[12] In the 15th- to 16th-century *Hatha Yoga Pradipika,* the first hatha yoga manual, Svatmarama wrote about *Savasana:* "Lying down on the ground, like a corpse, is called Sava-asana. It removes fatigue and gives rest to the mind."[13] The resemblance of Engel's exercise to *Savasana* is so strong that we can't help but wonder if Engel picked up his relaxation technique from hatha yoga. It's unlikely, though. The *Hatha Yoga Pradipika* wasn't translated into German until 1893. It's more likely he was influenced by accounts, common in his day, of travel to the Orient, which described the exploits of fakirs and the customs of nomadic Arabs, caravan merchants, and others who would lie down on the ground in a semilifeless state to recuperate from physical exhaustion.

In the late 19th century Stebbins held that along with restoring muscle-bound "congestion" to elasticity and enabling quick recuperation from physical exhaustion, a relaxation exercise "subdues over-excitement of the nerve-centres and stimulates calm self-control."[14] Believing that nervous disorders were the main cause of unhappiness in the early 20th century ("From what we now know of this world, it cannot be denied that the curse of modern civilization is nervous strain"), Yogendra incorporated Stebbins's relaxation techniques into his yoga system primarily to alleviate the anxiety of his Parsi and upper-caste Hindu middle-class students; in so doing, Yogendra introduced intricate, structured calming exercises into yoga.[15]

Relaxation Exercises

The preparatory posture in Yogendra's system is *Sukhasana,* Easy Pose, in which one sits with the legs crossed at the ankles and the hands placed palms downward on the knees (see fig. 5.1 on page 68). While taking this posture, "mentally watch the breath going in and out just for one full minute," Yogendra advised.[16] Similar to the usefulness of Stebbins's "perfect relaxation" exercise, which prepares for "energizing exercises," the value of *Sukhasana* "lies in establishing inner harmony with oneself, elation through poise and composure through elimination of muscular and nervous agitation, thus, providing the most favourable condition for the practice of other exercises to follow."[17] "Only after you are fully self-possessed 'like patience on a monument smiling at grief,' begin the other yoga exercises in perfect peace."[18]

The consummation of the subsequent routine of conditioning *asanas* is *Savasana.* In Yogendra's system, the final pose couldn't be

*After having studied under Delsarte for a year in Paris, MacKaye introduced the Delsarte system of expression to America in a lecture at the St. James Hotel in Boston on March 21, 1871. Over the next few years, while becoming a popular teacher and lecturer, he transformed Delsartism into an occult philosophy of emotion, pseudo-science of expression, and aesthetic exercise system for Americans.

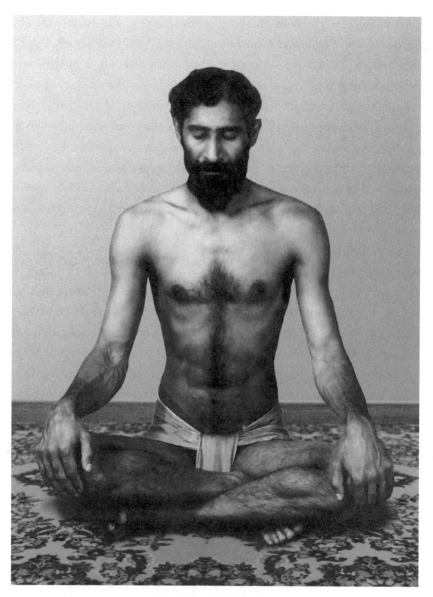

Figure 5.1. Shri Yogendra
demonstrating *Sukhasana,* Easy Pose, circa 1930

(With the kind permission of the Yoga Institute)

Padmasana, Lotus Pose, the most well-known seated position, or any other pose suitable for meditation because, from beginning to end, Yogendra's regime is structured for relief of stress, not preparation for meditation. *Sava-* *sana* completes the relaxation process with a thorough and systematic relaxation of body and mind. "Whenever physical or mental fatigue is experienced or the mind is agitated," he wrote, "the practice of *savasana* or the

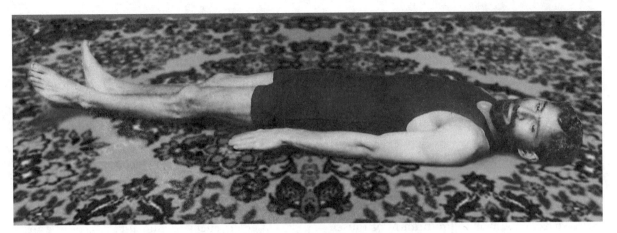

Figure 5.2. Shri Yogendra
demonstrating *Savasana,* Corpse Pose, circa 1930
(With the kind permission of the Yoga Institute)

corpse-pose is recommended by yoga authorities. The technique consists in simply lying supine with the face towards the sky and the arms and the legs extended passively to their full length. With that palsied sinking feeling as it is experienced during an early stage of collapse or the basal anaesthesia, keep motionless like a corpse and relax gradually, every muscle of the body"[19] (fig. 5.2).

No more than they had tolerance for the strain of holding poses, Yogendra's students had no interest in total renunciation of ordinary life, despite its difficulties and confusions. They turned to yoga not to reject the ordinary world of family, community, and work—considered by ascetics to be the cause of suffering—but to help them better cope with it. Keenly aware of their nervous state of mind, they turned to yoga for relaxation, not enlightenment. Yogendra's final exercise, *Savasana,* provides not only respite from the everyday world but preparation for returning to the everyday world: when we're

in a state of repose, we're better able to cope with life's challenges.

Yogendra also recommended relaxation exercises (in particular, *Savasana,* Corpse Pose; *Dradhasana,* Firm Pose, lying on the right side with the arm under the head "as if, for a pillow"; and *Makarasana,* Crocodile Pose, lying prostrate with the head resting on folded arms) for immediate relief of fatigue or stress: "Whenever physical or mental fatigue or strain is experienced, or the mind is agitated, the practice of certain postures which contribute greatly to muscle-relaxation is recommended by the yoga authorities."[20]

Conditioning Exercises

In Yogendra's system it's not only the first and last exercises that promote relaxation; it's also the conditioning exercises themselves. "The most characteristic feature of the yoga physical exercises is their non-violent and non-fatiguing disposition," Yogendra wrote. "For pure health, Yoga precludes exercises involving violence, strain or fatigue." In excluding any exercise that might involve strenuous exertion, which gives rise to such physiological reactions as an increase in blood pressure, pulse rate, and respiration—in other words, any exercise that is sweat producing—Yogendra created a gentle yoga, or in his words, "a system of non-fatiguing and non-violent physical training."[21] True yoga is "sedative, i.e., involving minimum of muscular and nervous agitation."[22]

Yogendra maintained that gentleness should be applied not only to one's method of performing yoga physical exercises (the technique) but also to one's state of mind. The *asanas* should be performed with a "fixation . . . undisturbed by any extraneous influences,"[23] with "ease and quietude."[24] By performing *asanas* in a placid manner, as well as slowly and rhythmically, students aren't subject to fatigue—to feeling tired or losing strength. More importantly, they won't get agitated. They won't be spurred on to violence against others. "The central objective of the yoga physical education is the cultivation of and habituation to the spirit of non-violence. Any system of physical training which is likely to breed militant spirit is, in terms of true Yoga, amoral."[25] In short, the nonviolent and nonfatiguing characteristic of the yoga physical exercises is "a special ennobling feature."[26]

This injection of pacifism into yoga seems like a lofty sentiment. And it would be, if it were espoused by a karma yogin, "a devotee," in Mahatma Gandhi's words, "who is jealous of none, who is a fount of mercy, who is without egotism, who is selfless."[27] But there's no outpouring of compassion in Yogendra's beliefs.

There are only rants—rants largely directed not toward hotheads crying out for rebellion against their British overlords but toward physical culturists advocating strength training, exercise drills, *surya namaskar,* and vigorous forms of hatha yoga:

Divorced from mental and moral purity, what are all systems of physical education, if not mere sources of biologic and mechanical enlargement of animality? According to [true] Yoga, physical education which metamorphoses man into a robot is vulgar, antihuman and perversive.[28]

[Physical training systems in educational institutions are a] very vile design of adding to man's bestial power without the compensating moral elevation.[29]

At the bottom of all aggressive outbursts in this world lie chiefly the ribald influences of bestial physical training which succeed in changing the chemistry of the brain.[30]

What needs emphasis in regard to yoga physical education is the fact that the objective of good health in the yoga sense is not the bestial urge for physical strength, bulging muscles and robust physique since brute force leads to violence.[31]

Yogendra was clearly worked up about how heated exercise can inflame passions. And he would know.

To make himself into a powerful wrestler, the teenaged Mani (as Yogendra was called in his youth) beefed himself up, combining indigenous Indian exercises with weight resistance exercises using fancy mail-order equipment (such as single and double chest expanders and dumbbells with five springs). In just two years Mani emerged as a skillful combatant with bulging muscles and prodigious strength. (Decades later, villagers in his hometown still recounted his superhuman feats. One time he bore the weight of a fully loaded bullock cart on his shoulders while villagers repaired the axle.) As his reputation as a wrestler spread, he began to receive challenges. One was from Arjun Bhim, a prominent local wrestler. In the spring of 1915, seventeen-year-old Mani agreed to the match.

When the imposing-looking Bhim arrived at Mani's home, Mani's father told Mani not to take him on. "I ignored father's caution, went outside near the well, rubbed my hands in the mud and went on the wrestling 'pad' made of yellow earth. The game started." After about a half hour, Mani sensed that Bhim wanted not just to defeat him but to make him submit to pain and humiliation. Mani went berserk. "I became violent and turned over and held him down with all my strength. Anytime he would try to get up I would make my grip stronger and rub his head hard to the ground."[32] Finally Bhim collapsed. Two days later he died.

Yogendra's revulsion to vigorous exertion was probably connected to this unbearably distressing violent event—he had killed someone!—in his youth. Memories of severely upsetting experiences remain buried in our minds forever. Although we may never bring them to consciousness, they nevertheless haunt our lives. They're usually brought to the surface not as memories but as behavior, say, a fit of inexplicable rage or sorrow—responses attached to a past experience sparked by a (sometimes trivial) present experience. In this way, unconscious feelings make us feel things we don't understand and act in ways out of our control.

Taking a man's life, like impregnating a woman, may be a heady experience for a man, especially a young man. If you can smite a mighty foe, you can do anything. It makes you bold. Yet killing someone out of pride, the great transgression, may lead to your becoming so overwhelmed with remorse that you feel disgraced and unworthy. And when you kill someone through losing your temper, you may always fear that your anger will get the better of you again, that you'll lose your head again. It makes you overly cautious.

Yogendra seems to have displayed elements of all of these behaviors throughout his life, but we don't know enough about him to say with certainty. All that we know for sure is that he responded to any hint of (what he perceived as) agitation in exercise with an angry outburst.

In Hindu psychology, our troubled emotions are called *prarabdha karma,* the portion of our total *karma* accumulated from past lives (*sanchita karma*) that is given to us at birth. *Karmas* are stored in a receptacle called a *karmasaya,* or womb of *karmas* (the unconscious), where, unless they're destroyed (often by changing our perspective), they give birth to new *karmas* (*agami karma*). Totally stripped of its allegorical meaning (i.e., its link to the doctrine of rebirth or cycles of existence), *karma* is strictly an expression of the unbreakable sequence of cause and effect. In Yogendra's case, *karmas* of his teen years (his displaced rage against his wrestling opponent and his depression upon leaving home), set off by childhood events, themselves brought forth still more unconscious reactions, which, in turn, became the primary determinants in his development as an adult. What's revelatory about Yogendra's unfolding *karmas,* however, isn't how they created and deepened his psychopathologies but how they helped give birth to his astonishing accomplishments—the innovations, such as his emphasis on gentleness in practicing yoga, that helped shape the course of modern hatha yoga.

Finding Peace

There's a yoga tradition in which yogins not only remain in but also make use of the quotidian world to practice yoga. Called kriya yoga, this tradition was defined by Patanjali, the fourth- to fifth-century author of the *Yoga Sutra,* considered by modern yogins to be the foundational philosophical text of yoga, as comprising *tapas* (bodily discipline or austerity), *svadhyaya* (study of self), and *ishvara-pranidhana* (surrender to God). Governed by these principles, the conduct of everyday life becomes a means of sensing the presence of God in all things through weakening the causes of our suffering, defined by Patanjali as the sense of "I," attachment, aversion, and clinging to life. Yogendra considered aversion to pain to be the primary cause of our afflictions, so he saw the paramount task of the kriya yogin as experiencing, facing, and accepting the pain of everyday life. In a letter

to his guru, Paramahamsa Madhavadasaji, sent in late 1920 to explain the differences in their approach to yoga practice, he wrote:

No doubt, [running away] is easy [*sic*] than to face experience because it is often bitter; but, after you once get used to it, it becomes a sort of pleasure. That is his past-time, the collecting of pebbles on the sand and throwing them back in the vast ocean. How pleasing it is when you lose yourself into it the realization of the Infinite through those manifold diversities. It is just like a diver. It is only the first thrilling sensation that you have to pass and then the ocean becomes your friend.

And what joy to realize that fathomless deep "Yato vacho nivartanta aprapya manasasaha" that Gnosis from which the mind and speech turn back baffled.[33]

Yogendra was quoting a famous saying from the *Taittiriya Upanishad,* "Upon trying to reach the Ultimate Reality, the mind, along with speech, are turned back disappointed," in apparent support of his belief that knowledge of the absolute nature of things cannot be comprehended by study or prayer but only by experience. Yogendra continued: "To me the joy of [my] senses is my joy of soul, filtered through myriad objects of his [*sic*] own. Then why should I renounce; why should I fear them?"[34] In the thrall, it appears, of Ralph Waldo Emerson and other American transcendentalists, Yogendra was proclaiming to Madhavadasaji that he believed that the union of one's divine spark within and the Divine is not attained through flight from everyday life but through opening oneself up to the sensory input of everyday life, through seeing, as Emerson put it, "the miraculous in the common"—the presence of God in the phenomenal world.[35]

Yogendra's great contribution to modern yogic spirituality, though, isn't his articulation of a provocative, heterodox defense of kriya yoga but his shaping of two aspects of hatha yoga, *asana* and *pranayama,* into what he called "yoga physical education." By stripping hatha yoga of its traditional ideology, methodology, and community in the early 20th century, he helped make possible (but, needless to say, didn't envision) the development of embodied yogic meditation—the integration of meditation right into one's conditioning *asana* practice—in the late 20th century.

One of those yogins who would later create a spiritually infused *asana* practice was Yogendra's kind, self-effacing, scholarly son, Jayadeva, who took over the directorship of the Yoga Institute in 1980, nine years before his father's death. (Even when his son was married and a father, Yogendra affectionately referred to him as "little Jayadeva" because of his gentle, childlike nature. Once, while watching his son climb the stairs in his home, the hot-tempered Yogendra was occasioned to remark, candidly and accurately, "He is the real yogi—he never gets angry."[36])

According to Jayadeva, yoga practice consists of four types of *asanas,* categorized by their configurations, and four corresponding *bhavas,* the complex of character traits, feelings, attitudes, and behaviors generated by the configurations. Practiced in sequence, the meditative postures (e.g., *Padmasana,* Lotus Pose) are experienced as *dharma* (self-direction, inner directedness, and quietude); the lateral, twisting, upward-reaching, and balancing postures (e.g., *Vrksasana,* Tree Pose) are experienced as *jnana* (concentration and body awareness); the forward-bending postures (e.g., *Yoga Mudra,* Yoga Seal Pose) are experienced as *vairagya* (humility, passivity, and detachment); and the backward-bending postures (e.g., *Bhujangasana,* Cobra Pose) are experienced as *aishwarya* (confidence and activeness).

Jayadeva holds that performing *asanas* as *bhavas* "automatically leads to spiritual states" that "cannot be described."[37] But his detailed descriptions of the four stages of *bhavas* indicate a spiritual path composed of four corresponding numinous states of mind: receptivity to an exploration of the individual self and an openness to the Universal Self; concentration on the individual self; surrender to the Universal Self; and identification of the individual self with the Universal Self.

This yoga practice isn't to be mistaken for a stress management technique, Jayadeva argues, which achieves merely "a peephole view of reality,"[38] but is a method for achieving the highest state of consciousness, *samadhi,* in which one "apprehends all objects of the world simultaneously."[39] As Armaiti N. Desai, dean of the Yoga Institute, says, "Thus at no point [when practicing yoga according to Jayadeva's precepts] do we end with the body beautiful only, but we follow the *Yoga Sutras* of Patanjali and the eight-fold path."[40]

But it was Yogendra père, through his foregrounding of *asana* in hatha yoga practice, who helped make it possible for his son and other later-generation yogins to realize the infinite through the experience of the movements of the *asanas* themselves. What he wrote about experiencing life in all its multiplicity, including pain, would be applied (not, needless to say, at his suggestion) to experiencing yoga: doing *asanas* is painful, but after a while you get used to the pain. It becomes "a sort of pleasure." You "lose yourself into it." In this way, *asana* practice becomes, as he aptly described everyday experience perceived with pure awareness, an "exercise of the soul."

6

SWAMI KUVALAYANANDA

Claiming Yoga Is Science

The Endocrine System in Popular Culture

Working into the night in the stifling summer heat in his temporary lab under the eaves of a medical building at the University of Toronto, Frederick Banting, a young doctor and researcher, and his lab assistant, Charles Best, a medical student, removed the islets of Langerhans (clusters of cells found in the pancreas) from several test dogs. The two men ground up the tissue, extracted a substance, and placed it in a vial left floating in a bowl of ice water. At 12:15 a.m., they injected five cubic centimeters of this substance into a dog that they had made diabetic by removing its pancreas, which caused excessive amounts of sugar to build up in the blood. Then they took urine and blood samples from the dog and tested them. The results showed that now the urine contained no sugar and the blood sugar levels were lowered by half. With this experiment, performed on July 30, 1921, Banting and Best isolated the pancreatic secretion that reduces blood glucose levels—soon named insulin—which had eluded physiologists for thirty years. This discovery was momentous. Not only had a treatment for diabetes (a disease so dangerous that those afflicted with it often died within a year) been found; henceforth, the existence and importance of internal secretions—hormones—released by glands to be set whirling through the bloodstream to affect distant tissues could no longer be in doubt.

Banting and Best delivered a preliminary report of their research to the Journal Club of the University of Toronto's Department of Physiology on November 14, 1921. Between late December 1921 and February 1922, newspapers around the world spread the story of the discovery of insulin on their front pages. In February 1922, a twelve-year-old boy, near death from diabetes, was administered insulin made from cattle pancreas and recovered. In early 1922, Eli Lilly & Company began to manufacture and sell insulin. In December 1923, Banting was awarded a Nobel Prize for his work.

Spurred by these events, the public imagination in the 1920s and 1930s became captivated by the ongoing wave of scientific discoveries about the endocrine system. People were enthralled by scientific revelations showing that every aspect of their lives from birth to death had a material cause within the body. Thus the workings of the body were found to be both more regulated, orderly, and integrated than previously thought and yet more astonishing and mysterious: hormones, in their awesome power to influence disease, determine sexual characteristics, and affect growth and mental capacity, seemed to be a miracle of nature, if not the handiwork of God made manifest in the body.

"There are many endocrine glands and they all work in perfect unison and harmony with each other" to regulate "our entire life, energy, and mental and physical activity," explained Swami Sivananda in the late 1930s. Sivananda, who had been a medical doctor in Malaysia for many years before becoming a renunciate in the early 1920s, considered this discovery about the workings of the endocrine system to be the "most important advance in Medical Science made during recent years." Yet he also believed that the "marvelous intelligence" of the cells of these glands was the latest proof that "the human body [is] the moving temple of God." "If you seriously ponder over [sic] for a while over the structure and working of this wonderful machine that is our body," he asserted, "you will be struck with awe and wonder. . . . This sort of balancing work in the harmony of nature is done by the intelligent [Mother] Prakriti [or Mother Nature, the avatar of *prakriti,* the ordinary material world manifested to our senses] under the direct guidance of the Lord of all nature."[1]

Scientific Exercise for Internal Organ Health

In the 1920s and 1930s, prominent Indian physical culturists made the claim that their exercise systems prevented and cured disease by, respectively, maintaining and restoring the proper working of the internal organs. In this, they took their cue from Western physical culturists who earlier had made the same claims for the favorable effect of their exercise systems on the internal organs. For example, Eugen Sandow, the renowned bodybuilder, asserted in 1897: "The benefits [of my system] are not, of course, confined to the visible muscular development. The inner organs of the body also share them. The liver and kidneys are kept in good order, the heart and nerves are strengthened, the brain and energy are braced up."[2]

J. P. Müller, the enormously successful purveyor of a home calisthenics system that influenced pioneer yogin Shri Yogendra, took aim at Sandow's system in 1904, saying that "the system is a good one for producing strong arm muscles; but verily the body's vital force does not reside in the arms."[3] Müller claimed that his system, in contrast, benefited the internal organs (as well as the skin), especially the lungs and the digestive tract: "No less than 11 [out of eighteen] of the exercises in 'My System' act directly on the internal organs and vigorously stimulate the muscles enclosing them which are hardly ever called into use by every-day occupations."[4]

Like Müller, the Indian physical culturists asserted that their exercise systems provided a harmony between the body's exterior (muscles and other soft tissue) and interior (inner organs) that was absent in bodybuilding/strength training. They characterized their harmonic systems as scientific.

The early part of the 20th century was an era when people had great faith in science (a faith that may be impossible for us to comprehend in our post-atomic-bomb age of profound ambiguity over many scientific endeavors). Almost any discipline—from painting, philosophy, psychoanalysis, and socialism to crime detection—could be given validity and respectability if it could be shown to be scientific in some way: if it could be proven by scientific procedures (tested, measured, compared, and recorded), if it used the scientific method (formulated and tested a hypothesis), or if it simply had scientific underpinnings (conformed to the latest scientific theories).

If Indian physical culture were to gain validity and respectability in educated circles (especially within India) in the 1920s and 1930s, when science had great cachet, it had to be shown—or at least asserted—by its exponents (especially those who championed hatha yoga, which had long been perceived as mysticism, magic, and self-penitence) to be a scientific system of treatment for disease. So the chief promoters of *surya namaskar* (sun salutations) and yoga—rival exercise systems during this period—forcefully stated that their disciplines were a science. Not a pure science but a body of systematically organized knowledge carried out according to a developed method, or, more specifically, an applied science, similar to medicine, which applies basic sciences, such as anatomy, biochemistry, and nutrition.

Bhavanarao Pant Pratinidhi, the rajah of Aundh, who refined and codified modern *surya namaskar,* contrasted the benefits of his scientific system to Sandow's bodybuilding/strength training: "The scientific and fundamental principles involved in our method of doing Surya Namaskars, Sun-Adoration, were at once recognized as enabling most of the vital organs to function normally, and to ensure robust health, rather than merely developing muscular strength."[5]

The pioneer Indian bodybuilder/strength trainer K. V. Iyer, who combined bodybuilding/strength training and hatha yoga practices, contrasted the scientific nature of his conjoined system to that of bodybuilding/strength training alone: "My ideally developed man whilst having both the symmetry and strength of a Sandow shall be immune to disease through his devout following of the dictates of Hata-Yoga. . . . [The reason is that] Hata-Yoga is a rational scientific course of human Mental and Physical discipline, based on a rationale [of physiological efficacy] as cogent and convincing as any proven truth in modern Western science."[6]

Yogendra contrasted hatha yoga, "a scientific course of daily exercises and coordinated breathing" for restoring, developing, and maintaining "the natural organic harmony and proportion between the outer muscular development—really, the growth and elasticity—and the development and functioning of the vital organs within,"[7] to bodybuilding/strength training, an "abnormal muscle-building" exercise routine for building an "orgastic physique associated with a brutish mind."[8] It's this "natural organic harmony," present at yoga's very inception, he argued, that makes yoga scientific. "For every part of the body and for every important physiological organ within, Yoga had to devise methods of exercise, purification and control which are to keep the body in uniform good health both *within* and *without*. . . . The practices, thus, effecting all parts of the body within and without . . . constitute, what may be rightly termed, the art and science of yoga health and hygiene."[9]

In "Raja Yoga," published in his collection of lectures on Vedanta philosophy in 1896, Swami Vivekananda declared raja yoga to be a science like any other.* If you want to be a chemist, "you must go to the laboratory, take the different substances, mix them up, compound them, experiment with them, and out of that will come a knowledge of chemistry. If you want to be an astronomer you must go to the observatory, take a telescope, study the stars and planets, and then you will become an astronomer. Each science must have its own methods."[10] The science of raja yoga, he reasoned, has a method for accessing the divine: meditation (the systematic application of the eight-step path expli-

cated by Patanjali in the *Yoga Sutra*). "The science of Raja Yoga . . . proposes to give men . . . a means of observing the internal states, and the instrument is the mind itself."[11] "So we see," comments modern yoga historian Elizabeth De Michelis, "that Vivekananda recommends yoga, and in particular (what he calls) *rajayoga* [the yoga of meditation] as the best, at times even the only, technique or rather 'science' apt to lead us to a self-validating 'realization' experience, the only locus where true religion may be found."[12]

In *How to Be a Yogi,* published in 1902, Swami Abhedananda, the successor to Swami Vivekananda at the Vedanta Society of New York, explained that hatha yoga, too, is a science:

Hatha Yoga is that branch of the Science of Yoga which teaches how to conquer hunger, thirst, and sleep; how to overcome the effects of heat and cold; how to gain perfect health and cure disease without using drugs; how to arrest the untimely decay of the body resulting from the waste of vital energy; how to preserve youth even at the age of one hundred without having a single hair turn grey, and how thus to prolong life in this body for an indefinite period. Anyone who practices it will in the course of time acquire marvellous powers; powers indeed, which must dumbfound a psychologist or anatomist.[13]

Abhedananda and others at the turn of the century believed that hatha yogins acquired

*In addition to being published in his 1896 collection of letters, Vivekananda's lecture on raja yoga was published as a book, *Raja Yoga: Conquering the Internal Nature,* also in 1896.

these powers through using *asana* and *pranayama* "to gain control over the involuntary muscles [especially cardiac muscle and the smooth muscle of the respiratory tract] of the body, which is impossible to the ordinary man. We all possess this power latent within us, but the Hatha Yogis were the first to discover a scientific method by which it could be developed."[14]

Defining hatha yoga as the science of preserving good health through maintaining the well-being of (not supernatural control over) the vital organs began in the 1920s—the yogic fantasy of suprapowers reduced to the practice of hygienics, and the yogic yearning for a correspondence between microcosm and macrocosm reduced to a prescription for harmony between musculature and viscera.

Benefiting the Endocrine Glands

For those in the medical field, knowledge of the workings of the endocrine system didn't exist merely to be understood, appreciated, or marveled at: it was to be used and acted upon. In an age of great medical optimism, researchers and doctors believed that scientific discoveries could be used to perfect nature. As Ernest Henry Starling, the British physiologist who coined the term *hormone,* wrote in *Lancet* in August 1905: "If a mutual control, and therefore coördination, of the different functions of the body be largely determined by the production of definite chemical substances in the body, the discovery of the nature of these substances will enable us to interpose at any desired phase in these functions, and so to acquire an absolute control over the workings of the human body. Such a control is the goal of medical science."[15]

By the 1920s and '30s, as Sheila M. Rothman and David J. Rothman, authors of *The Pursuit of Perfection: The Promise and Perils of Medical Enhancement,* document:

Students learned that [by manipulating hormones] medicine now had the ability to make the short taller and to prevent the already tall from becoming giants, establishing the idea that bodies could be shaped and reshaped.

No sooner was this idea glimpsed than a fascinating transition occurred in which cure moved into enhancement. Once the texts explained that endocrinology could redesign the body, it did not require a great leap of imagination to ask whether, if the short person could be made normal, could the normal person be made taller.[16]

Unlike some proponents of traditional medicine, Indian physical culturists—like their Western counterparts—neither had nor wanted the ability of the Creator to redesign or enhance the body (at least by unnatural means). They were far more modest. They simply made impassioned claims for the efficacy of their exercise systems on the endocrine system.

Shri Sundaram, who wrote the first modern hatha yoga manual, recognized that "the endocrinous system is very important. By intemperance, debauchery, abnormal work or sufferings from any chronic disease this system gets disarranged."[17] "[Yoga-Asana] benefits the endocrinous system most," he declared, "as no other exercise could do."[18] In contrasting hatha yoga to the calisthenics exercises recommended by that

American upstart (as Sundaram thought of him) Bernarr Macfadden, the self-proclaimed "father of physical culture," Sundaram exalted the contributions of the *rishis* (sages) of ancient India:

> [Yoga-Asana] is based on an expert knowledge of the endocrine organs. . . . To the lay mind, the subject might appear mysterious. Yet, the Physical Culturists of the West (notably Mr. Bernarr MacFadden [*sic*]) have commenced to take advantage of the endocrinous system and are racking their brains to invent suitable exercises. But thousands of years ago in their forest seclusion, the sages [of India] had discovered all that had been desirable. The proof lies in their Asanas. Whether the West would discover the equals of these remains to be seen. But any-way it is a desperate chance,—it may never be.[19]

No Indian physical culturist made—or had a right to make—stronger claims for the efficacy of yogic exercise for treating diseases of the endocrine glands than Swami Kuvalayananda.

Kuvalayananda

Jagannath Ganesh Gune (1883–1966), later known as Swami Kuvalayananda, was born into a middle-class family in Dabhoi in the state of Gujarat in 1883. (Swami Kuvalayananda wasn't a *sannyasi* [renunciate] name, as one might easily assume, but a pen name he took up for writing poetry when he was in his mid-thirties.) In 1897, when he was fourteen, Gune was orphaned, abruptly finding himself, in the description of his biographers Manohar

L. and Manmath M. Gharote, "deprived of all love and affection."[20] He was sent by relatives (who were probably too poor to take him in) to attend high school in Pune, considered India's center of learning, where he subsisted on *madhukari,* food provided in alms by Brahmin families. Despite being forlorn and destitute, he completed high school. After briefly attending Baroda College in 1904, he dropped out to devote himself to the cause of awakening the Marathi cosmopolitan elite to *swaraj* (self-rule). Inspired by Bal Gangadhar Tilak, "The Father of Indian Unrest," he performed a nationalist form of *kirtan* (Indian folk music that praises the divine), combined with a spoken discourse, in temples and on the streets. In June 1907, finding himself directionless, he returned to Baroda (also known as Vadodara) to attend college. But his real interest lay in studying *shastar vidya* ("the art of weapons"— a 17th-century Sikh martial art) from the master Rajratna Rajpriya Professor Manikrao.

Gune had first learned about Manikrao in 1906 from a newspaper account of his dazzling performance with weapons at the All India Exhibition held in concert with the National Congress at Calcutta. "In the very moment I thought of obtaining some light from such a resplendent person," recalled Kuvalayananda. On July 7, 1907, he presented himself before Manikrao at the Jummadada Vyayam Mandir (Jummadada Temple of Physical Education; Jummadada had been Manikrao's master). "Prof. Manikrao accepted me as his disciple and as a token he put 'pedha' [a delicacy primarily made of milk and sugar] in my mouth."[21] In Manikrao, Gune found the parental affection that he'd been missing for ten years, a period, he recalled, when "the entire world around me seemed to stare at me as if it was a Sahara desert, devoid of sympathy and compassion."[22]

During college and even afterward, Gune spent a great deal of time at the Vyayam Mandir. When he was ill, he stayed there day and night. "During such periods of illness, Bhau ["Brother," Manikrao's nickname] frequently came to me, sat on the bed, examined my fever and massaged my head," Kuvalayananda reminisced. "His loving hand [on my head] soothed my body. When the illness was of a more serious nature, he would place my head upon his lap, and pat me with love."[23]

Almost twenty years later, Kuvalayananda would pay tribute to Manikrao as the one "at whose feet I had the proud privilege of sitting for my lessons in non-Yogic physical culture, and to whose parental care I owe much that has made me what I am now."[24] Fifty years later, Kuvalayananda would say, "For such a love, at least in this life, I will never be able to pay back the debt."[25]

Gune studied with Manikrao for three years. Eventually he was forced to stop training because the intensity of the work required for the mastery of *shastar vidya* was too exhausting for him. After receiving a bachelor's degree from Bombay University in 1910 and working as a high school teacher and social worker from 1913 to 1915, he left Baroda to live in Amalner, Khandesh, where he got another job as a high school teacher. Dedicated to the nationalist agenda, he aimed to generate patriotism and a yearning for freedom in his students. "He introduced in the school physical exercises of various types both indigenous and foreign," the Gharotes write. "He took great personal interest in training the youths on

military lines infusing them at the same time [the] spirit of nationalism. With this end in view he composed several patriotic songs and poems. It was a sight to see the youths marching in tune with these songs in a spirit of utmost discipline and emotional fervour."[26]

In his private life, though, Gune was increasingly turning his attention to *yogabhyas* (the practice of yoga). He lived like a yogin, immersing himself in yoga practice and studies. He built a hut in an open field surrounded by a small garden, with a deer (named Venu) and a *mayuran* (an Indian blue peacock, named Uddhav) as pets. The hut served as the hub for local yoga enthusiasts (see fig. 6.1 on page 82). Among them were members of the influential Indian Institute of Philosophy, established in July 1916, which brought together academic philosophers and traditional scholars to promote nondualistic Vedanta. One of the members attracted to Gune was its founding patron and president, Pratap Seth, a wealthy industrialist and devotee of yoga.

As he became more involved in his *sadhana* (the practice of methods, such as the awakening of spiritual hunger, that enable one to pursue realization of Brahman), Gune realized that he needed formal guidance. "At the end of 1918," Kuvalayananda recalled, "my intensity about the practice of Yoga reached its climax. To receive initiation from Paramhamsa Maharaj was my intent desire."[27] (Kuvalayananda is referring to Paramahamsa Madhavadasaji of Malsar, Shri Yogendra's guru.) In their hagiographic portrayal of Madhavadasaji, the Gharotes write:

His Holiness Paramhamsa Madhavadasji Maharaj of Malsar was a spiritually perfect

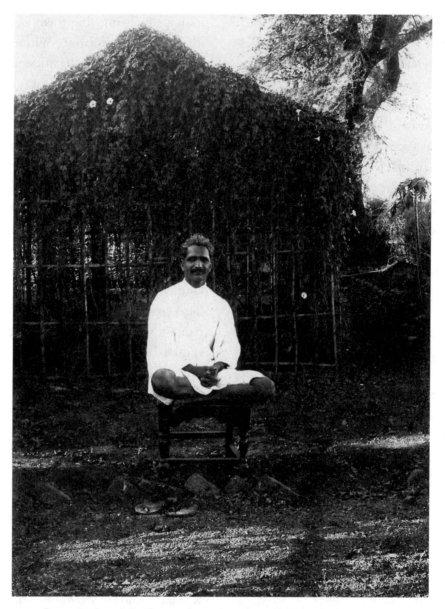

Figure 6.1. Swami Kuvalayananda sitting in front of the hut built at Amalner
during his *sadhana* period, 1915–1923

(With the kind permission of the Kaivalyadhama Yoga Institute)

and ideal Yogi who originally came from Bengal, lived in various parts of India for his spiritual development, stayed for twelve years on the sacred Kanakeshwar Hill, a few kilometers away from Bombay for his Tapasya [an endeavor involving great self-discipline, for which one must endure hardship and suffering, undertaken as a means of strengthening one's devotion to Brahman, the Ultimate Reality, the Absolute Being] and at last settled on the banks of the Narmada at Malsar in Gujarat where he organized a centre of spiritual culture for the upliftment of the humanity. . . . He left his mortal coil in 1921 at the age of 121 years.[28]

"I became the disciple of Shri Paramhamsa," wrote Kuvalayananda. "I devoted myself completely to him."[29] Not exactly. Unlike Yogendra, who had escaped from the guru's control only a few months earlier, Gune kept his distance from Madhavadasaji. Over the next two years, Gune would stay for several months at nearby Baroda, from where he would frequently visit Madhavadasaji in Malsar. During these stays, he "was blessed by his Holiness and trained in the Yogas of which he himself was a master."[30]

It's certainly far easier to believe that Madhavadasaji lived to 121 years of age than to accept that he was a spiritually perfect and ideal yogin. Yet there's no getting around the fact that he was a source of inspiration for two of the key figures in the formation of modern hatha yoga to serve humanity in a groundbreaking way: by using the medical aspects of hatha yoga—*asanas* (postures), *pranayama* (breathing exercises), purificatory practices, and diet—to alleviate or cure the ailments and diseases of ordinary people, not just of the votaries of hatha yoga.

As Gune became increasingly proficient in yoga, an odd thing happened: he became increasingly dissatisfied with his practice. In his historic declaration of purpose, "Towards Foundation and After," issued in a pamphlet in 1924, he presented an account of what led to his dissatisfaction, referring to himself in the third person as the founder of his yoga ashram: "As the organizer was being trained in advanced Yogic practices, he began to have experiences which were quite abnormal. Phenomena, physical and mental, that an average man is not able to induce, came slowly under his control. Naturally they excited curiosity in him as to whether these phenomena were purely physiological or purely psychological or whether they were psycho-physiological having their counterparts both in physiology and psychology."[31]

Upon realizing that mastery over the elements interferes with attaining *samadhi,* which represents true mastery, ideally yogins victoriously struggle against the temptation to use their command over physical and mental phenomena. Gune, in contrast, never struggled to give up his (unidentified) occult powers—because he was never in danger of succumbing to using them. He was always more interested in pursuing his curiosity about them. He met with yogins and consulted yogic literature. He talked with eminent doctors and researchers and read books on psychology and physiology. But he never found a scientific explanation for his experiences. This curiosity about the nature of his recently gained magical powers, however, led him to become curious about the workings of another aspect of yoga: "The Yogic culture has also a therapeutical side which constitutes a system of Naturopathy."[32]

Gune soon learned that, as was the case for yogic suprapowers, the therapeutical side of yoga also lacked scientific underpinnings. But that didn't discourage him. To the contrary: it presented him with a goal and fueled his ambition. Here was a field in which research hadn't been conducted but could be carried out, possibly to great effect. "The scientific study of Yoga would not only give a scientific basis to this system but also would show how it compares with other systems working in the same field." Gune sensed that he'd found his life's work: conducting experiments to prove the scientific viability of hatha yoga. "All this seemed so full of possibilities and so inviting that the organizer began to be restless over the matter. The idea of scientific research in the field of Yoga kept haunting him night and day."[33]

In 1920 Gune was made the principal and rector of the nearby National College, another school with a pro-independence agenda. Two years later, the college was shut down for its agitation against British rule, leaving Gune out of work—a misfortune that led him to realize his real mission in life. What he had yearned for was not to remain a teacher for the rest of his life but to become a *shankaracharya,* the head of an ashram. But not an ashram like any other—not a monastic retreat for practicing yoga as spiritual liberation but a place where he could give the therapeutic and physical culture side of hatha yoga a scientific underpinning and provide yogic treatment to those seeking a natural cure. The initial expenses for its foundation were met through a substantial donation (five thousand rupees) from the industrialist and yoga enthusiast Pratap Seth.

On October 8, 1924, the forty-year-old Swami Kuvalayananda, as Gune was now known, founded the Kaivalyadhama Ashram (*kaivalya* means "the solitariness or aloneness of liberation, the state of sheer presence," which is the highest achievement of the path of yoga, and *dhama* means "abode") in Lonavla, a city on a mountain-ous plateau on the rail line between Pune and Bombay in the state of Maharashtra. Lonavla was a hill station, where the well-off vacationed at a resort to escape the heat. (Because temperatures at the ashram were generally cool, Kuvalayananda advised visitors to bring sufficiently warm clothing with them even in summer.) The allure of its setting and climate, Kuvalayananda knew, was critical for appealing to the stressed urban professionals who would attend a health resort. "Situated at the foot of a hill on the heights of the Sahya mountains, the As'rama is cut off from the bustle and din of the modern society," he told them, "and a serene atmosphere characteristic of spiritual evolution perpetually settles over the whole of the Kaivalyadhama."[34]

The ashram included well-equipped laboratories for conducting original experiments on the different physical aspects of yoga (fig. 6.2). The results of the first experiments appeared in the initial issue of *Yoga-Mimansa*—a quarterly journal, written under Kuvalayananda's guidance, with "Scientific," "Semi-Scientific," and "Popular" sections—published on the day of the official opening of the ashram.

Kuvalayananda wasn't fully confident he'd succeed in bringing off his endeavor. Writing about himself in the third person, he expressed his doubts, which were in proportion to his wild ambition: "None can be more conscious of his weaknesses and short-comings than the organiser himself! The mere thought of the stupendous character of his work simply alarms him!" Perhaps he should take another path. "But he is helpless in the matter! He is called on to start the work by powers which he has not yet been able to fathom completely and he has answered the call!"[35]

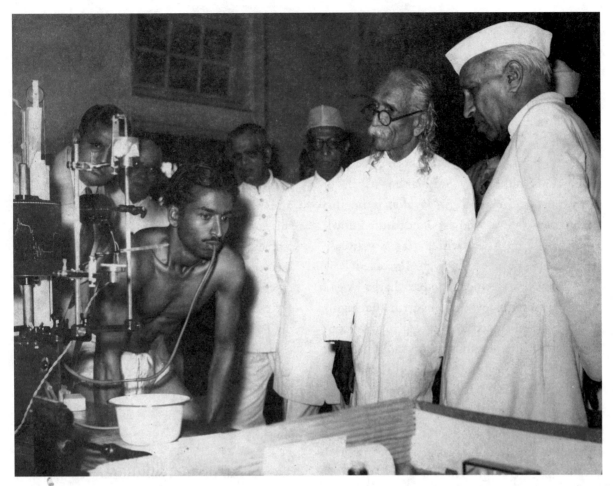

Figure 6.2. Swami Kuvalayananda and Jawaharlal Nehru observing a scientific experiment, 1958
(With the kind permission of the Kaivalyadhama Yoga Institute)

Needless to say, Kuvalayananda couldn't have even attempted to pull off this venture without having learned yoga therapeutics—the kernel of the entire enterprise—from Madhavadasaji. For which he was grateful. But Kuvalayananda's deeper gratitude was rightly for Professor Manikrao. Kuvalayananda "had had the privilege of being a humble disciple of Prof. Manikrao, the far-famed physical culturist of India. The fatherly love with which the organiser was trained in physical culture by the saintly Pro-fessor had created in him an undying interest in this field of human activity." It's difficult to determine which aspect of Kuvalayananda's relationship with Manikrao was more critical to his formation: Manikrao's parental love or his passion for physical culture. But Mani-krao was just as influential in shaping Kuva-layananda's identity for another reason, one decidedly prosaic: as the director of the Jumma-dada Vyayam Mandir, he was a role model for running a research institute. From Manikrao,

Kuvalayananda learned organizational skills ("Virtues necessary for ably conducting an institute . . . were all re-eminently present in Prof. Manikrao") and picked up his interest in research ("The very inspiration for research came through his example").[36]

Since its origin, hatha yoga had been considered a religion or philosophy. Svatmarama's 15th- to 16th-century *Hatha Yoga Pradipika* begins: "Salutation to Siva, who expounded the knowledge of Hatha Yoga, which like a staircase leads the aspirant to the high pinnacled Raja Yoga."[37] While giving a nod to hatha yoga's essence as soteriology, the pioneer hatha yogins of the early 20th century were primarily concerned with developing and promoting hatha yoga's ability to heal the body. To this end, they strenuously argued that hatha yoga wasn't mere exercise but was medical treatment—a kind of medical treatment that prevents and cures disease not by medication or surgery but by natural means: *kriyas, mudras,* and *bandhas* (respectively, cleansing techniques, seals, and locks, the three purificatory techniques); *pranayama* (deep breathing techniques); diet; and, chiefly, *asanas* (postures).

Beginning as a search for a scientific explanation of his own experiences, Kuvalayananda's ambitious and far-reaching project sought not only to make an indigenous natural health cure, yoga therapeutics, available to Indians but to investigate "the Yogic phenomena" and demonstrate their scientific basis to the world. The hypothesis of the research project, one might say, was that the benefits of hatha yoga weren't merely anecdotal but were verifiable by science. Just as traditional medicine is based on proven scientific

truths—which, we now know all too well, aren't always truths for all times (how quickly today's truths can turn into tomorrow's fallacies!)—Kuvalayananda wanted to show the world that the efficacy of yogic health cure could be proven by investigation of its practices through observation, experimentation, and explanation.

For the next forty years or so, Kuvalayananda, as characterized by William J. Broad, author of a book about the science of yoga, "worked with missionary zeal" to marshal scores of researchers to conduct experiments on the efficacy of various yoga practices in order "to recast the ancient discipline as a boon for health and fitness."[38] He largely succeeded, making him the key figure in changing the face of yoga. But was his research—although used by most 20th-century yogins (from S. Sundaram to B. K. S. Iyengar) to support their claims for yoga's scientific soundness, and recognized and honored among India's elite—valid?

To establish the intrinsic scientific character of yoga, nothing was more important than proving the efficacy of yoga on the health of the endocrine glands. In an article titled "A Note on the Ductless Glands" in the April 1926 *Yoga-Mimansa,* Kuvalayananda expressed his belief that the endocrine organs are of "supreme importance in the economy of human well-being."[39] The endocrine organs, he explained, secrete hormones into the blood or lymph to influence the functional activity, growth, or development of other distant organs. The hormones may work indirectly through the autonomic nervous system (comprising the sympathetic and parasympathetic nervous systems), which maintains homeostasis in the body, or directly through the endocrine organs. According to the latter method:

The endocrine secretions directly [without the intervention of the autonomic nervous system] affect the [distant] cells. Without discussing how this is done, we shall only exemplify it. The action of the thyroid secretion is the best example. As soon as this secretion suffers, the cells of the most distant parts of the human body slowly begin to undergo a change. The hair begin to grow grey, the nails have a tendency to be brittle, fatty degeneration starts in the arteries, the face tends to be wrinkled, weakness creeps over the brain, in fact, many senile symptoms begin to be apparent![40]

"Yogic Therapeutics," Kuvalayananda held, "aims at restoring the internal secretions to their normality by securing the health of the endocrine organs through Yogic practices."[41] But exactly which yogic practices? How do they work? And how can it be proven that they work? At the least, Kuvalayananda's case for yoga therapeutics' capability for maintaining or restoring the health of the endocrine organs ("Yogic exercises can restore to health many degenerated endocrine organs. Functional disorders can be very largely helped"[42]) succeeds or fails with the answers to these questions. At the most, his claims for the validity of yogic therapeutics itself—that is, for yoga as a cure for any disorder—are at stake.

7

SWAMI KUVALAYANANDA

Promoting Yoga as Health Cure

A Yoga Journal and Yoga Institute

Exercise for Healing

Like other founders of modern physical culture (the late 19th- and early 20th-century exercise-based practices considered to be part of the heterogeneous mixture of alternative practices to conventional medicine),* Swami Kuvalayananda held that his yogic exercise system could prevent and cure disease. Cures were effected, he maintained, through *asana* practice, aided by purificatory techniques, breath control, and diet.

In India, making claims for *asana* practice as health cure was nothing new. The assertions made by Svatmarama in his 15th- to 16th-century *Hatha Yoga Pradipika,* the first hatha yoga manual, for the healing powers of *asanas* are extravagant and unrestrained. *Matsyasana,* Fish Pose, "is an instrument for destroying the group of the most deadly diseases."[1] *Paschimottanasana,* Seated Forward Bend, "cures all diseases of men."[2] *Mayurasana,* Peacock Pose, "soon destroys all diseases."[3] *Padmasana,* Lotus Pose, is "the destroyer of the diseases."[4] Although these declarations have a shamanic character, they stop well short of

---

*Among them: Eugen Sandow (the showman bodybuilder who toured the world), J. P. Müller (the Danish athlete who championed "fifteen minutes' [calisthenics] work a day for health's sake"), Bhavanarao Pant Pratinidhi (the rajah of Aundh, who revived, modified, codified, and popularized *surya namaskar,* sun salutation exercises), and K. V. Iyer (the Indian bodybuilder who taught strength-training exercises complemented with *asanas* at his gymnasium in Bangalore).

making claims about restoring the dead to life or attaining immortality through absolute mastery of the body. Thought to destroy diseases by correcting humeral imbalances, *asanas,* in conjunction with the purifying and breathing exercises, were traditionally practiced by yoga votaries simply to achieve good health.

But these traditional practices were decidedly not a therapeutic system for the general public; they weren't prescribed to outsiders to guard against or cure disease. In a seismic departure in the 1920s, yogins began to promote yoga as an organized measure (whether public or private) to prevent disease, in particular, and promote good health, in general. As yoga scholar Joseph S. Alter observes: "Before about 1900 there were countless *sants* [those who have united with Brahman], *swamis* [religious teachers] and *sannyasis* [religious mendicants] who practiced yoga and used their powers to heal, but they did not prescribe yoga to heal, and the techniques of yoga they employed to enhance their power, to whatever end, were defined as esoteric, arcane, and a matter of great secrecy. Yoga, in this sense, was distinctly metaphysical, transcendental, and otherworldly. It was in no sense viewed as a practical aid to recovery or self-improvement for the masses."[5]

The early 20th-century yogins who prescribed hatha yogic exercises as medical treatment for the populace—as, in effect, a public health measure that could benefit anyone, including those who weren't devotees of yoga philosophy—had many models in the Western physical culture movement to emulate, notably the American Bernarr Macfadden (1868–1955), the self-proclaimed "father of physical culture," whose voluminous published works included a wildly popular magazine and over sixty books from 1900 to 1930 alone.

Macfadden

The brash, satyric Macfadden fasted on raw foods (especially carrots), abstained from alcohol and tobacco, railed against white bread, exposed his skin to sunshine whenever possible, rejected medicines, thoroughly chewed his food ("Masticate every morsel of your food until it is practically a liquid"[6]), favored a randy sex life, took cold baths, practiced deep breathing, denounced corsets (he claimed that by decreasing sexual desire, they were a primary cause of divorce), got plenty of hard exercise, and kept "a hopeful mental attitude."[7] And if you wanted "the joy of that superb, abounding radiant health which is the privilege of every human being to enjoy,"[8] then you, he felt, should do the same (see fig. 7.1 on page 90).

Macfadden promoted physical culture in his magazine *Physical Culture.* The first issue, entirely written by Macfadden, appeared in March 1899. The magazine was an instant success. By late 1900, Macfadden was the most famous promoter of natural healing in America. His motto could be found in the intimidating legend on the cover of his magazine: "Weakness [is] a Crime. Don't Be a Criminal" (a secular—and perhaps typically male and American—twist on the basic tenet of Muscular Christianity that weakness is a sin).

Macfadden preached the glorious redemption of the human body from decline and corruption. The body, he maintained, is naturally healthy. Allowing it to become run down and undernourished makes it susceptible to disease.

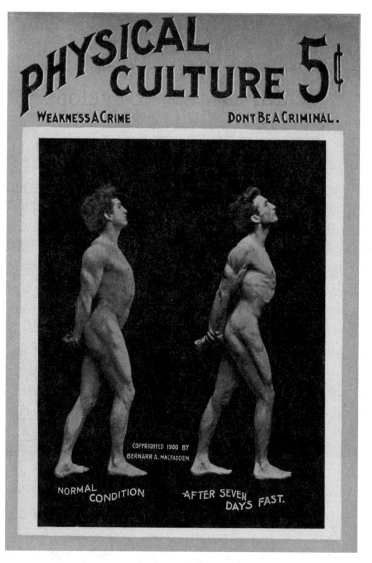

Figure 7.1. Cover of *Physical Culture,* showing Bernarr Macfadden, 1900
(With the kind permission of David L. Chapman)

Physical culture provides vigorous health by restoring "vital power" through "enabling all the organs of the body to perform their individual functions in that orderly fashion that Nature intended that they should when she designed them."[9]

As was the case for most people of the time who embraced physical culture, exercise was just one component of Macfadden's regimen; he believed that a complete system of natural healing could be found only in his entire regimen (with fasting as its keystone). Nevertheless, he considered the role of exercise in attaining good health to be critical: "No part of the body can be normal unless exercise is taken in some manner, in order to affect various physiological processes."[10] In the summers he walked barefoot twenty miles from his seasonal home to his Manhattan office in the Flatiron Building (although he decorously put on his hat, coat, and shoes before entering the city "in order to assume the articles of clothing that qualify one to become one of the conventional human sheep"[11]). He often stood on his head (occasionally while dictating editorials for his magazine). He regularly lifted weights. He published many exercise manuals, beginning in 1900, when he was thirty-two. (That first manual, *Macfadden's Physical Training,* was illustrated with nude photos of the bushy-haired and barrel-chested Macfadden.[12] And nude photos of him appeared in profusion in his magazine. What could be more fortuitous for an exhibitionist than to live in an age when the human body was being extolled as Nature's most beautiful handiwork?) His earliest interest in the healing powers of physical activity, though, was in treating disease by prescribing and/or assisting with body movements.* In the late 1880s he hung from his St. Louis apartment window a gold and black lettered sign advertising his credentials: Bernard McFadden/Kinistherapist/ Teacher of Higher Physical Culture.† (According to Macfadden biographer Robert Ernst, Macfadden had cleverly coined the term *kinistherapist*—which derives from *kinesis,* the Greek root for "motion"—because it "sounded impressive."[13])

In his 1904 book *Building of Vital Power,* Macfadden contended that not just daily exercise but particular exercises helped to prevent or cure particular diseases. In one example, he advised that for the treatment of Bright's disease (a form of kidney disease), "in addition to the massage, kneading and percussion as already described, exercises that call for the turning and twisting of the trunk and bending of the body, should be employed."[14]

In another example, Macfadden recommended an exercise that is the same as *Halasana,* Plow Pose, to combat symptoms of illnesses caused by poor digestion. The exercise was presented as one of a series of exercises that produce quick and vigorous movement of the abdominal muscles to "strengthen the involuntary [peristaltic] muscles and in so doing increase the digestive functional power." "Continue the exercise until slightly fatigued," he directed.[15]

About twenty years after Macfadden and other physical culturists first made claims for the effects of particular exercises on preventing and curing disease, proponents of hatha yoga followed suit: they claimed that particular *asanas* prevented or cured particular ailments and diseases—only they did a better job of it than Western exercises. *Asanas* more effectively acted upon organs, especially the endocrine glands, they asserted, by mechanical (i.e., natural) means—by pressing, moving, jostling, inverting, and massaging them. (Although he asserted that certain *asanas* remove digestive

---

*The first modern doctrine of exercise as a method of therapeutics was developed by Per Henrik Ling. In his principal work on gymnastics, *General Principles of Gymnastics,* published by two of his pupils in 1840, after his death, Ling wrote that his "medical gymnastics" is the means by which "one seeks, either by his own proper postures or with the help of another person and by helpful movements, to diminish or overcome an ailment which has arisen in his body through its abnormal relations" (Ling, *General Principles of Gymnastics,* quoted in Hartwell, "On Physical Training," 743).

†Macfadden's birth name was Bernard Adolphus McFadden. He was still using his given name and the original spelling of his family name during this period.

disorders, such as indigestion and loss of appetite, Svatmarama emphasized the more generalized claim that certain *asanas* cure disease, not that they have specific therapeutic effects.)

In 1931 Kuvalayananda published *Asanas,* a kind of medical handbook for treating specific diseases and disorders with yoga postures. The instructions for performing the yoga exercises and the descriptions of their therapeutic effects were strikingly similar to Macfadden's exercise prescriptions: for example, six turns of *Halasana* repeated in four minutes' time, Kuvalayananda advised, "is useful in combating dyspepsia and constipation, especially when they are due to the degeneration of the abdominal muscles or the nervous mechanism of digestion."[16]

The information in this book was based on articles previously published in Kuvalayananda's journal, *Yoga-Mimansa,* which touted specific yogic conditioning postures as the cure for specific diseases in each issue.

Yoga-Mimansa

First published in October 1924, the quarterly journal *Yoga-Mimansa*—a more restrained version of Macfadden's combative, sensationalist *Physical Culture*—was Kuvalayananda's chief vehicle for popularizing his system of yogic exercise and therapeutics (fig. 7.2). Kuvalayananda knew that in order to have hatha yoga accepted as physical culture and health cure, he had to overcome the attitude of the majority of middle- and upper-class Indians (those who owned property, were well educated, and held a professional post), who either dismissed yoga as being irrelevant to their lives or looked down their noses at yoga as weird spiritual practice or

street theater. What could make yoga relevant and respectable to them, he understood, was for it to be considered indigenous physical culture and naturopathy whose efficacy could be scientifically proven. The contents of the magazine were therefore intended not only to inform but also to impress: they were divided into "Editorial Notes," "Scientific," "Semi-Scientific," "Popular," and "Miscellaneous" sections.

When *Yoga-Mimansa* was launched, Indian newspapers and journals wholeheartedly adopted Kuvalayananda's strategy to get the middle class to support his endeavor. "Physical culture is being subjected to experimentation in America, and the periodicals of that country publish scientific criticism on the results. *Yoga-Mimansa* is the first journal in India publishing scientific and experimental criticism on Yoga," the *Maharashtra* informed its readers. "The scientific character of [Shrimat Kuvalayananda's] work is placed beyond all doubts, as he makes no concession for blind faith." This "experimental evidence shows that Yoga is not a mystical nonsense," and therefore, the newspaper forcefully concluded, "it is the duty of every educated and monied Maharashtriya to help this scientific study of Yoga."[17] The *Kesari* concurred: "Yogic culture is looked upon as something mysterious and secret. This endeavour to bring it before the popular gaze and interpret it in the light of modern sciences . . . deserves patronage in every respect."[18]

Tatvajnana Mandira, the quarterly organ of the Indian Institute of Philosophy, reported:

Yogic culture has been encouraged in India since very old days. Even to-day perfect Yogins are reported to be present in the caves

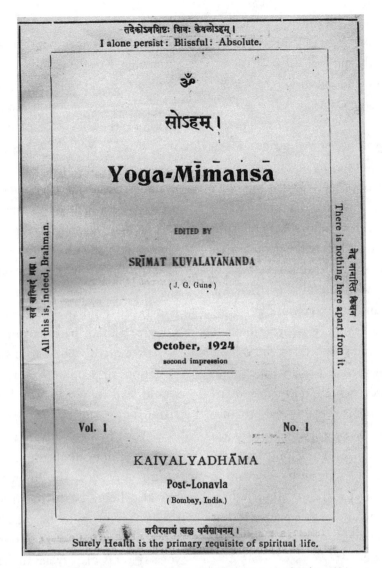

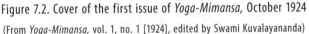

Figure 7.2. Cover of the first issue of *Yoga-Mimansa*, October 1924
(From *Yoga-Mimansa*, vol. 1, no. 1 [1924], edited by Swami Kuvalayananda)

of the Himalayas. There is extensive literature available on this subject. The aphorisms of the divine Patanjali are too well known to require a mention. Swami Vivekananda and Swami Ramatirtha have also added to the original stock. . . . Very often pseudo-Yogins are seen imposing upon the credulous public and giving performances in the streets of a town. Perhaps it is due to the baleful influence of this class of people, that latterly Yoga is being looked upon with some disfavour in our land.

So it is a matter for congratulations that Srimat Kuvalayananda has founded an institution for a critical study of Yogic culture. His researches in the path of Yoga . . . from the viewpoint of the present day sciences, are altogether a new activity in this country. Even if we ignore the spiritual aspect of Yoga, its physical culture side and therapeutics are, in themselves, of great importance.[19]

Nava-Sangha wrote about the inaugural issue of *Yoga-Mimansa:* "One of its main features lies in its copious illustrations, representing yogic details about asana, nervous chakras etc.—a subject hitherto confined to mystical literature, which has been brought before the popular gaze as a highly instructive and exhaustive field of study and placed under careful scientific treatment, experiment and interpretation."[20]

Prabuddha Bharata, a Calcutta journal, expressed its praise and support: "In the volume before us are given various poses with copious illustrating pictures, which may cure many chronic diseases. This is properly the province of Hat Yoga [*sic*]—a science which has got a bad reputation as encouraging only mystery and miracle-mongering. The author's scientific treatment of the subject will clear all prejudices from the public mind and enable people to test it for themselves. We wish success to this altogether new enterprise."[21]*

Bolstered by newspapers and journals, the campaign Kuvalayananda carried out in *Yoga-Mimansa* to get middle-class Indians to take up hatha yoga was met with success. Although promoting hatha yoga as health cure with a scientific basis was his primary strategy in winning them over—countering their view of yoga as an irrelevant or déclassé, even shameful and repulsive, activity—he also used two supplemental strategies.

The first was touting yoga's ancient origin as emblematic of India's glorious precolonial past. In a time of rising indignation among the middle class over British rule, a nationalistic fervor had taken hold in India. One aspect of this surge of Indian nationalism (which was actually part of the worldwide fanatical devotion to nations or peoples that, among other things, would lead to World War II) was the endless flaunting of India's great and superior antiquity. Yoga had the advantage, Kuvalayananda argued, of not only being up to date (a natural health cure with the imprimatur of science) but also being based in an ancient and pure tradition. In fact, hatha yoga isn't ancient; it's a few centuries old. More importantly, the hatha yoga systems of Kuvalayananda and the other

---

*None of these articles in Indian newspapers, no matter how disparaging of yoga practices, accuse yogins of unsavory sexual acts. So there's no evidence here that would give credence to William J. Broad's sensationalizing, unsupported assertion in *The Science of Yoga* that "no small part of the disrepute" in which mendicant yogins were held by educated Indians in the early 20th century "centered on sex" (Broad, *Science of Yoga,* 15). In fact, as scholar of South Asian religions David Gordon White shows in his account of the tantric sexual practices employed by yogins for the realization of *siddhis* (supernatural powers) in *Sinister Yogis,* debauchery among wandering ascetic yogins in modern times, while persistent, wasn't pervasive or even thought to be pervasive.

A Western critique of mendicant yogins can be found in a remark made by American Christian missionary Reverend W. M. Zumbro in a 1913 *National Geographic* article: India "has kept alive for centuries an army of five million idlers, who, though able-bodied men, produce nothing and live on the charity of those who work" (Zumbro, "Religious Penances," 1291). This view was evidently shared by India's British colonizers. White notes that in the 1891 British imperial census, Nath yogins (a religious order founded in the late 12th or early 13th century) were listed under the category of "Miscellaneous and Disreputable Vagrants" (White, *Sinister Yogis,* 240).

founders of modern yoga were hardly pure.

The transformation of traditional hatha yoga into modern hatha yoga was achieved by privileging the means, *asanas* (the various yogic conditioning postures, which, according to the *Hatha Yoga Pradipika* should be "practiced for gaining steady posture, health and lightness of body"[22]), over the ends, *samadhi* (defined by the *Hatha Yoga Pradipika* as the attainment of "oneness of the self and the ultra self"[23]), in response to the physical culture movement sweeping the world. In applying Western physical culture tenets to the conditioning *asanas* of hatha yoga, the yogins created a syncretic blend of Eastern and Western exercise: modern postural yoga.

But for the most part, Indian physical culturists couldn't bring themselves to admit that they were influenced by the West. Whereas liberal constitutionalists in early 19th-century India acknowledged their debt to the political ideologies of Locke, Mill, and Bentham and the movements for self-government and against absolutism in Europe, yogins in early 20th-century India refused to acknowledge that their transmutation of yoga into an exercise system for fitness and health was inspired by Sandow, Müller, Macfadden, and other leaders of the physical culture movement in Europe and America. Instead, they dismissed Western exercise systems as recent, inferior versions of this centuries-old, indigenous Indian practice.

While boldly remaking yoga in the image of Western physical culture, Kuvalayananda and the other yoga innovators—instead of expressing gratitude toward the Western physical culturists who influenced them, taking pride in having combined seemingly contradictory exercise systems, or even framing their achievements as an absorption of the new into India's enduring identity—insisted on pointing solely to the ancient and pure Indian lineage of their yoga systems.

What accounts for the yogins' promotion of Hindu India's cultural (as well as religious and racial) supremacy? Almost surely it was a matter of their having embraced the strident chauvinism that had arisen among upper-caste middle-class Hindus to shore themselves up against the West—a reaction to their sense of inferiority to, even victimization by, the West.

Kuvalayananda's second supplemental strategy was expunging spirituality—the essence of yoga—from his writings. While his own *sadhana* (spiritual practice) involved daily yogic meditation, Kuvalayananda omitted (to a great extent) the topic of yoga as salvation in part because it was irrelevant to and beyond the reach of the yogic physical culture and therapeutics he was developing and in part because it was largely associated by his targeted middle-class audience with the extreme practices of nomads who utterly rejected middle-class aspirations.*

---

*There's no evidence to support Broad's assertion that Kuvalayananda (and the other yogins who forged modern hatha yoga) censored information about the influence the medieval form of Tantra that emphasized sexual ecstasy as the path to transcendent consciousness had on the formation of hatha yoga in the 10th and 11th centuries. There are no grounds for believing that Kuvalayananda even knew about the influence of Tantra on yoga, or that he "maintained a virtual taboo on the word 'Tantra'" (Broad, *Science of Yoga,* 26). Hence, there's no evidence that, in order to "giv[e] yoga a bright new face that radiated with science and hygiene, health and fitness," Kuvalayananda "shed the old emphasis" on "eroticism" that lingered in current-day yoga practice (ibid., 26, 37) by concealing—indeed, by not extolling!—yoga's "tips about extended lovemaking" and "thrills similar to the bliss experienced in sexual orgasm" (ibid., 26). All of these assertions by Broad are unsubstantiated, defamatory, and silly.

The shift in thinking in the Indian middle class that resulted from Kuvalayananda providing hatha yoga with a scientific underpinning allowed its members to engage in some yoga practices—once they were made easy, palatable, and convenient enough—and ignore the rest. We know that they took up yoga as health cure with alacrity in part because of the large number of people from all over India who flocked to Kuvalayananda's clinic.

Clinic

Kuvalayananda offered yoga therapeutics at his ashram, Kaivalyadhama, from the time of its opening in October 1924 in Lonavla. Not only effective for disseminating the results of the scientific research, *Yoga-Mimansa* also spread word throughout the provinces of the availability of treatment at the ashram. "Therapeutic advice is given gratis at the As'rama to patients that come for consultation," the first issue announced. "As soon as it becomes economically possible, a regular Yogic hospital will be managed by the Institute."[24] In this way, Kuvalayananda proselytized hatha yoga and made it available to all comers (not only as health cure but also as classroom exercise with free instruction)—marketplace practices that gurus (throughout the millennia sought out by postulants, whom they accepted or turned away) surely would have found abhorrent.

The ashram attracted so many patients from all parts of India that in January 1927 Kuvalayananda was obligated to open a clinic, Rugna Seva Mandir, in a new separate bungalow, where all therapeutic activities (examination and treatment) were transferred.* In the three and a half years after the opening of this medical facility, about 1,300 patients were examined there free of charge. Many were treated with yoga therapy. (Some were sent to different medical institutions, such as the Government Hospital at Khandala.) Doctors devised the yogic treatment plans based on the information learned about yogic techniques from the scientific investigations conducted in the ashram's Rana Natavarsingh clinical laboratory, which had opened in October 1926. Trained yoga teachers (males for the male patients, females for the female patients) carried out the plans. When medical complications existed, the yogic treatment consisted of many practices, which sometimes required days for the patients to learn. During the course of all treatments, the doctors regularly reexamined the patients and the yoga teachers regularly carried out assessments in order to introduce more effective results into the program.

Most patients stayed in nearby lodgings, but the new bungalow allowed for inpatient treatment. It had only nine beds (although in the summers as many as twenty-five patients were accommodated inside the building). Only men

---

*In 1932 Swami Kuvalayananda opened a two-part branch of Kaivalyadhama in the suburbs of Bombay. Called Pranavakunja, its headquarters were in Borivali (where the *Yoga-Mimansa* office was relocated) and its health center was in Santa Cruz. The next year the health center was moved to a rented building in the heart of Bombay (across from the Charni Road railway station) to make it more accessible to the public. The health center was moved again two years later to Marine Drive, where the British government donated a plot of land and Sir Chunilal Mehta, a wealthy patron and council member (and later governor) of the Bombay Presidency, donated money toward construction of a building.

were admitted. They received free boarding and lodging for the first two days. They were required to bring their own bedding. Patients with contagious or infectious diseases were not admitted. (They did receive treatment, though; those with venereal diseases, however, were turned away altogether.) Rules and regulations were strictly enforced: "No unholy act or word should disturb the peace."[25]

Kuvalayananda reported in a review of Kaivalyadhama's activities from October 1924 to March 1930 that "nearly two thousand people have been treated either as indoor or outdoor patients." "People suffering from constipation, dyspepsia, auto-intoxication, nervous debility, asthma, piles, seminal weaknesses, heart troubles and a variety of other diseases," he wrote, "found great relief from Yogic Therapy."[26]

Treatment

A typical yoga therapy treatment designed by Kuvalayananda was the prescription, dated May 5, 1927, for the preeminent leader in the struggle for Indian independence, Mahatma Gandhi, who was afflicted with poor circulation (perhaps caused by diabetes), high blood pressure, and nervous tension (Kuvalayananda feared that recent political setbacks had put him on the verge of a nervous breakdown): saline (at 5 a.m.); diluted milk; enema ("to be dropped after a fortnight"); *ujjayi* (a breathing technique); *Savasana,* Corpse Pose (ten minutes); *Sarvangasana,* Shoulder Stand (five minutes at a fifteen-degree angle the first week and gradually increased over several weeks to twelve minutes at a thirty-degree angle); and massage ("of the spine, abdomen and heart at bed time").[27]

Gandhi, who was taking time off from his heavy schedule to recuperate in Nandi Hills, an ancient hill fortress near Bangalore, had written to Kuvalayananda on April 17th expressing interest in taking up *asanas* and other yogic measures to aid in his recovery. "The growing self abuse among the students has as you know attracted me to the Yogic Asanas as a possible cure of that evil habit," he wrote. "In the course of my reading I saw that Asanas were recommended as a remedy for the cure of many other ills."[28] In late April Kuvalayananda traveled to Nandi Hills, where, over the course of about two weeks, he examined Gandhi, made a diagnosis, designed a suitable holistic protocol, and showed him how it should be carried out. After Kuvalayananda returned to Lonavla, the treatment continued by mail.

In early June Kuvalayananda reassured Gandhi: "Shavasana should have a soothing effect upon the nerves; you should come out of it as from sleep quite refreshed. . . . Sarvangasana . . . should leave you in possession of doubled energy."[29] Gandhi replied: "I did not notice the effect you ascribed to Shavasana. May it not be that the prescribed period is too short, that is two minutes. I did feel refreshed when I used to lie flat on my back for nearly 15 minutes. Nor do I notice any positive effect of Sarvangasana. Would you advise increasing the angle or increasing the period of the pose at the present angle?"[30] Kuvalayananda recommended performing both exercises for fifteen minutes and increasing the angle of *Sarvangasana* to thirty degrees. Gandhi took this advice but admitted that he might not be practicing *Sarvangasana* at the correct angle because he had no measuring device.

Kuvalayananda suggested to the Mahatma that he "get a big protractor in the local market [in Bangalore] such as is used in the school room either by the teachers of geometry or drawing. This will enable you to measure the angle accurately."[31]

Gandhi remained especially interested in the *asanas*: "I want to give the practice of these yogic exercises a full trial, if only because I regard them of all the methods of medical treatment to be the freest from danger."[32] But all along he worried that *Sarvangasana* might cause his blood pressure to rise. About six weeks after beginning his regime, he wrote to Kuvalayananda that he'd stopped practicing *Sarvangasana* and *Halasana* (which he'd taken up on his own) on the advice of his doctors, who'd found that his blood pressure had risen, and announced that he was returning to his normal activities.

Writing back on July 4, 1927, Kuvalayananda pleaded with Gandhi not to resume his sociopolitical actions: "I have been reading with considerable alarm about your preparation to start your tour. I intended writing to you in the matter even a week ago. But refrained from doing it, as up to now I had already repeatedly requested you to take *complete rest* to the end of July or even August. It was clear that you were acting under advice of local doctors and I did not think it desirable to once more call your attention to my advice which was already there."[33] Kuvalayananda's alarm sprang from more than concern for Gandhi's health: "I am anxious to see that you regain your lost vitality, as much for your own sake as for the sake of our nation. But my greatest anxiety," Kuvalayananda candidly admitted, "is to see that the results of your single case are counted as the result of one case only and that no one tries to jump at any general conclusions on the strength of these results which are being affected by the peculiar circumstances of your life."[34]

"Already the [Yoga-]Shastra [the science of yoga, based on observation and experiment, in contrast to the yoga of belief] stands condemned at the hands of the educated people who do not want to give it even a hearing in its defence," Kuvalayananda continued, "which is allowed even to the worst of criminals!" He warned Gandhi of the danger "to which the Shastra is likely to be exposed either for my miscalculations or yours. So for God's sake do not do anything that will lead to your own trouble or to the trouble of Yoga-Shastra. I should request you with all the earnestness I can command not to begin your work or *even to think* of beginning it earlier than the middle of August."[35]

Kuvalayananda was in a panic, it seems, over the prospect of his prized patient either telling people that he'd just wasted his time with a course of yoga therapeutics or dropping dead, which people would blame on his course of yoga therapeutics—either way, with the calamitous result that Kuvalayananda's entire mission to elevate hatha yoga to physical culture and therapeutics would be discredited. In closing, he strongly tried to impress on Gandhi that his faith in the efficacy of *Sarvangasana* was unshaken. "N. B. [the abbreviation for nota bene, Latin for "note well"]," he concluded, "the note of warning I have sounded in the above letter has little reference to the present disturbance.

It is aimed at avoiding future trouble."[36]*

Earlier in the letter, Kuvalayananda had insisted that *Sarvangasana* doesn't raise blood pressure: *Sarvangasana* is "a remedy against high blood pressure. . . . In your case when the pose is passively practiced [i.e., with the assistance of somebody to lift Gandhi into the pose] according to prescription, [it] should certainly help to reduce blood pressure as it had done previous to the recent disturbance." While granting that "it is very difficult from at a distance to apportion the blame among the different factors suspected rightly or wrongly to be responsible for the rise," Kuvalayananda attributed the setback to Gandhi having overworked himself in promoting a *khadi* exhibition† and arranging for a subsequent tour and "not at all Sarvangasana, unless it was taken without due regard to the prescribed technique," by which he meant "the angle at which it was taken was in the neighbourhood of 50°." Kuvalayananda conceded, however, that he himself might be to blame. "It was only the glow which you felt all over the body," he wrote by way of explanation, referring to Gandhi's reaction to performing the pose at a broad angle in Kuvalayananda's presence at Nandi, "that made me advise you to take a pose at an angle more acute."[37]

It's easy to understand how Kuvalayananda was blinded by Gandhi's *Sarvangasana* glow into suggesting a more challenging form of the exercise. He was, in general, bedazzled by *Sarvangasana*. It was the central posture—the queen (or mother) of all *asanas*—in his system.

*Kuvalayananda had no cause for concern. Gandhi didn't speak ill of yoga therapy (in fact, he reported in January 1928 that he was continuing his *asana* and *pranayama* exercises), and he went on to live a long life (he was assassinated in 1948 at the age of seventy-nine).

†*Khadi*, a coarse homespun cotton cloth, was the icon of *swadeshi*, the economic strategy of encouraging domestic production and boycotting the purchase of foreign goods as a means of achieving Indian independence.

8

SWAMI KUVALAYANANDA

Investigating the Yogic Phenomena
Yoga Research

Articles on *Sarvangasana*

Each issue of Swami Kuvalayananda's periodical, *Yoga-Mimansa,* featured at least one article on an *asana.* Presented in the "Popular" section, the *asana* articles were divided into four parts: name, technique, points of study, and note. Illustrated with photos of yogins (most commonly intense, sometimes fierce and scary, long-haired, bearded men) modeling the *asanas,* the technique part contained instructions for doing the *asanas.* Previously, the *asanas* performed, by yogins in city squares, on beaches, or on the grounds of ashrams must've seemed mysterious to onlookers. By making available detailed, step-by-step instructions for assuming *asanas,* Kuvalayananda, like a magician revealing the secret of how magic tricks are done, took the mystery out of hatha yoga. Destroying the perception that performing *asanas* is an esoteric skill was one of the critical acts in making yoga modern.*

---

*The impulse to disclose centuries-held secrets was also a key ingredient in the formation of modern wrestling in India. In the mid-1920s, just as *asana,* separated from its spiritual path practiced in ashrams, began to be practiced in *vyayamshalas* (gymnasiums) solely to maintain and acquire good health and vigor, Indian wrestling, severed from its ancient ethos, ritual, and tutelage in *akharas* (training halls), also came to be practiced in *vyayamshalas* as stripped-down sport.

The 1927 manifesto of the English-language *Vyayam* (*The Body Builder*), the magazine of the *vyayamshalas,* states: "There are some who know the science [of wrestling] but they are anxious to

But perhaps even more instrumental in the demystification of *asana* was the clinical presentation of the fitness and health benefits of *asana* to the muscles, vertebrae, blood vessels, and nerves in the points of study part of the articles. In describing these effects, Kuvalayananda was showing his readers that the physical aspect of hatha yoga is nothing less than India's indigenous form of physical culture and natural health cure. So you'd be foolish to reject yoga, he was saying, out of a belief that it's a repellent practice, some sort of self-torture or black magic that you want nothing to do with.

The central place of *Sarvangasana* in Kuvalayananda's yogic system—and hence in early modern hatha yoga—is underscored by it being the subject of the first (in the inaugural October 1924 issue) and longest ever (continuing in the July 1925, October 1925, and January 1926 issues) article on an *asana* in *Yoga-Mimansa*. In that article, titled "Sarvangasana or the Pan-Physical Pose (more commonly translated as Shoulder Stand)," Kuvalayananda stated that the featured *asana* (the expansive discussion of *Sarvangasana* is accompanied by a brief discussion of its complementary exercise, *Matsyasana,* Fish Pose) "holds a very conspicuous place in the field of Yogic physical culture because it is one of the most powerful agencies that ensure and improve the health of the thyroid; and the health of the thyroid means for the most part the health of the whole body."[†]

Sarvangasana achieves this miraculous health of the thyroid, the two-lobed endocrine gland located in front of and on either side of the windpipe, naturally, Kuvalayananda maintained—that is, by mechanical (not pharmaceutical) means (see figs. 8.1 and 8.2 on page 103).

The first means is by inversion of the body. In the upright position, blood has to rise against gravity when it flows from the heart to the thyroid. But the upside-down position of the trunk in *Sarvangasana* obviates the struggle to force the blood upward. "Then the law of gravitation operates and attracts far more blood" from the heart and "sends it to the thyroid gland."[2]

The second means is by the chin lock.

The sharp angle of the neck and the consequent pressure of the hyoid bone [the horseshoe-shaped bone in the front of the neck between the chin and the thyroid] exert a considerable check on the blood circulation of the two carotids [the paired arteries that supply oxygenated blood to the neck and head], at a point which is situated just above the root of the superior thyroid arteries. Thus the blood stream running through the common carotids gathers volume and is largely driven through the superior thyroids considerably increasing their normal supply.[3]

---

guard it as a secret. Under these circumstances, there is no wonder that wrestling is seen in its roughness and unrefined boorish nature. We, therefore, will try our best to explain to our readers the tricks and counters thereon with as many explanatory notes and exact illustrations as possible" (Dadape, "Wrestling," 124).

[†]*Sarva* means "whole, all, entire or complete"; *anga* means "body or limb"; *asana* means "pose." Contemporary texts sometimes include the literal translation of *Sarvangasana* as "Whole Body Pose" along with the more familiar appellation "Shoulder Stand." Kuvalayananda and other early 20th-century yogins gave "Pan-Physical Pose" as the literal translation.

Turning the body upside down increases blood circulation to the thyroid gland. Pressing the chin against the thyroid gland impedes the outward flow of blood, thus damming up the blood. This blood overflow supplies the gland with such an abundance of nutrients, Kuvalayananda argued, that the thyroid's ability to manufacture its secretions is increased.

Influence of the Articles on *Sarvangasana*

The influence of the publication of "Sarvangasana or the Pan-Physical Pose" in the mid-1920s on how hatha yoga was perceived and presented was immediate, long lasting, and far-reaching. More than any other pose, *Sarvangasana*—through its beneficial effects on the endocrine glands—came to embody the notion that through yoga practice one could attain not magical powers but radiant health. The great influence of Kuvalayananda's writings on *Sarvangasana* can be attested to in the teachings of three esteemed yoga teachers over the course of the rest of the 20th century.

S. Sundaram: "Messrs. Muller and MacFadden [*sic*] have developed exercises for the health of the thyroid," S. Sundaram explains in his 1929 *Yogic Physical Culture or the Secret of Happiness,* the first modern hatha yoga manual, published only five years after Kuvalayananda's article. "The exercises invented by them chiefly consist of resistance movements of the neck. By way of example, the hands are clasped over the occipital region (behind the head) and they are made to press the head down, while the neck muscles resist the movement; then vice-versa; and then

from side to side, etc. Obviously the object of these movements is to draw extra blood-supply to the thyroid gland." Sundaram finds these exercises wanting: "The benefit to the thyroid thereby is very small."[4]

But Macfadden, at least, never claimed that his neck exercises benefited the thyroid. He recommended the exercises to strengthen the muscles of the cervical spine, and decidedly not for reasons of health or even fitness: "Well-developed muscles are desirable not merely because of the added strength, but because they make the body more beautiful. . . . A well-developed body is, to our eyes at least, a thing of beauty."[5]

What is the yogic alternative to Macfadden's supposed attempt to increase the blood supply to the thyroid gland? "It is Sarvangasana," pronounces Sundaram. "Many have been doing Sarvangasana blindly and reaping its benefits nevertheless. The first to notice its physiology and scientifically discuss its mechanical advantages has been the Yoga-Mimamsa [*sic*] journal. And its three or four articles on this pose are very valuable and convincing."[6]

B. K. S. Iyengar: "The importance of Sarvangasana cannot be over-emphasised," writes B. K. S. Iyengar in his groundbreaking, encyclopedic *Light on Yoga,* published in 1966, more than forty years after Kuvalayananda's article. "It is one of the greatest boons conferred on humanity by our ancient sages. Sarvangasana is the Mother of Asanas. As a mother strives for harmony and happiness in the home, so this asana strives for the harmony and happiness of the human system. It is a panacea for the most common ailments."[7]

Having adopted Kuvalayananda's claims wholesale (probably after reading them in Kuv-

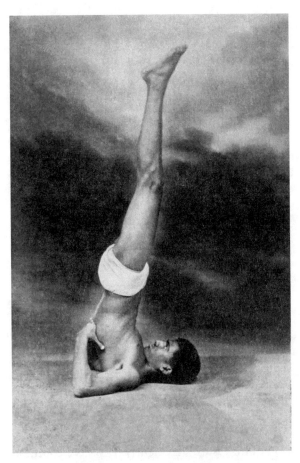

Figure 8.1. "Sarvangasana or the Pan-Physical Pose (Side View)"

(From *Yoga-Mimansa,* vol. 1, no. 1 [1924])

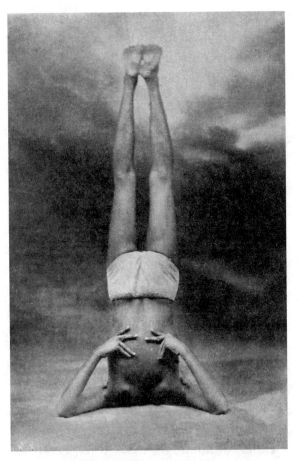

Figure 8.2. "Sarvangasana or the Pan-Physical Pose (Back View)"

(From *Yoga-Mimansa,* vol. 1, no. 1 [1924])

alayananda's *Asanas* and/or S. Sundaram's *Yogic Physical Culture*), Iyengar explains how *Sarvangasana* works:

> There are several endocrine organs or duct-less glands in the human system which bathe in blood, absorb the nutriments from the blood and secrete hormones for the proper functioning of a balanced and well developed body and brain. If the glands fail to function properly, the hormones are not produced as they should be and the body starts to deterio-rate. Amazingly enough many of the asanas have a direct effect on the glands and help them to function properly. Sarvangasana does this for the thyroid and parathyroid glands which are situated in the neck region, since due to the firm chinlock their blood supply is increased.[8]

Gary Kraftsow: In *Yoga for Wellness: Healing with the Timeless Teachings of Viniyoga,* published in 1999, over seventy-five years after Kuvalayananda's article, Gary Kraftsow, who teaches yoga using a methodology developed by T. Krishnamacharya (Iyengar's teacher) that emphasizes individual needs and capacities, presents two sequences of *asanas* to enhance the workings of the endocrine system. The first sequence, for hypothyroid conditions, is designed to stimulate the area around the thyroid (located at the base of the neck), parathyroid (attached to the back of the thyroid), and thymus (situated behind the top of the breastbone) with the "intention of balancing the function of these glands." The second sequence, for type 2 diabetes, is designed to stimulate the area around the adrenal gland (sitting atop the kidneys) and pancreas (lying behind the stomach) with the "intention to stimulate and nourish these glands and to restore balanced functioning." Both sequences feature *Sarvangasana*.[9]

Sundaram, Iyengar, and Kraftsow didn't carry out their own research on *Sarvangasana* to establish or bolster their claims for its efficacy in treating endocrine disease or other ailments. Nor did they base their claims for the benefits of *Sarvangasana* on their experience with patients (or, at least, they don't provide anecdotal evidence). They relied on Kuvalayananda's original research from 1924. In fact, almost all claims about the benefits of *Sarvangasana* can be directly or indirectly traced back to Kuvalayananda's series of articles. But what was the actual evidence presented in those articles?

Benefits of *Sarvangasana*

Kuvalayananda proved his claims for the benefits of *Sarvangasana* with case studies that are less like qualitative descriptive research and

analysis and more like absurdist tales found in contemporary flash (sometimes called nano, *micro,* very short, or short, short) fiction or offbeat stand-up comedy acts: almost all of the studies have morbidly compelling beginnings and oddly comical endings. The first study is about a leper patient who, under the care of a yogin at an ashram, had been making progress (the "gaping ulcers between his toes and fingers that discharged loathsome fluids" healed) by following the *Sarvangasana* treatment supplemented by a milk diet. But "there was a fearful relapse when the patient preferred to be in a leper asylum where he died of this disease some three years later."[10] "Notwithstanding the tragic end," Kuvalayananda concluded that *Sarvangasana* treatment "is capable of largely controlling leprosy, although it may not eradicate it."[11]

The second study is about "a young man in his thirties [who] developed a mode of life which was calculated to lead to the degeneration of his testes." (Evidently this was a common problem among young Indian males: "A number of young men suffer from testicular degeneration for various crimes committed against themselves and the society," Kuvalayananda reported.) After three months of *Sarvangasana* practice, readers must've been relieved to learn, "the testes [of the young man] reverted to their original size and weight." "The Sarvangasana treatment," Kuvalayananda concluded, "is one of the best remedies [the young men] can adopt to repair their losses."[12]

Kuvalayananda informed his readers that the effect of *Sarvangasana* on the thyroid can further be demonstrated by the clinical facts gathered from treatment of the ovaries, spleen, appendix, and liver. He gave, as an example, his third study about a sixteen-year-old boy who had a degenerated spleen and, as a consequence, was susceptible to attacks of malaria. The boy "took to Sarvangasana and in something like six months became permanently free from his spleen trouble." This promising result, Kuvalayananda hopefully concluded, "could save the boy against malarial infection."[13] Kuvalayananda also briefly explained how in aiding the parathyroid glands, *Sarvangasana* aids in maintaining muscle tone.

The portion of the article published in the July 1925 issue is devoted to the beneficial effects of *Sarvangasana* treatment on the parathyroids, the four small glands (each about the size of a grain of rice) located on the posterior surface of the thyroid gland. Healthy parathyroids prevent convulsions, Kuvalayananda asserted. "One of the forms these convulsions take is *epilepsy,* popularly known as *falling sickness.*"[14] As reported in the fourth case study, a young man who suffered from epilepsy "followed [his treatment] half-heartedly; and yet, within a six months' time, the patient reported to us that he was fast improving. We had no occasion to hear from the patient any more, nor had we any occasion to try this treatment in any other case." Kuvalayananda admitted, "The clinical evidence adduced here is too meagre to authorise any generalisation." So why bother even including this case? "It has been introduced here solely with a view to encourage epileptics to take to Sarvangasana treatment."[15]

The continuation of the article, in the October 1925 issue, is solely dedicated to *Sarvangasana* treatment's ability to increase venous circulation in order to alleviate the symptoms of varicose veins, swollen and often painful veins,

commonly on the leg, that have filled with an abnormal collection of blood. "The whole column of venous blood stands inverted in this pose," Kuvalayananda stated. "At once the force of gravity begins to help the circulation, instead of going against it; and the valves are relieved of their pressure and begin to get complete rest. The veins start draining under the pressure of their own contents and the whole work becomes very smooth."[16]

The conclusion to the series, published in January 1926, is entirely devoted to the scourge of sexual dysfunction—what Kuvalayananda calls "seminal weakness"—that was afflicting young, urban middle-class Indian males: "Premature ejaculations and feeble erections are the ailments that we would notice here," he announced.[17] "In what follows we shall try to study the effects of Sarvangasana on these defects."[18] In the manner of the fire-and-brimstone sermons, pulp fiction, yellow journalism, and melodramas of the times, Kuvalayananda's description of the plight of these young men is sensationalistic: "These two disorders have become so common that they . . . are tormenting the souls of youths."[19] "Darkness, unending darkness, hangs over not only their present life but threatens to cloud the future also!"[20]

Kuvalayananda elaborated on the "darkness, unending darkness": "The unmarried section of these unfortunate youths tries to forget his weakness by drowning his anxieties in the din and dash of the busy city life by day, and sleeping over his worries at night!"[21] But these young men "are perpetually haunted by a sense of unworthiness which does not leave them even in their dreams!"[22] (With whom these young single men are having sex, we're curious to know. And what were the exact circumstances under which they confessed their torment to Kuvalayananda?) "But the married—they have a partner before whom it is worse than death to confess their weakness; and from whom there can be no hiding, at least, in this regard! . . . Even the idea of meeting the wife chills their heart!"[23]

The salvation for these doomed young men is, of course, according to Kuvalayananda, *Sarvangasana*. *Sarvangasana* is beneficial for treating premature ejaculation, he explained, because "the engorged vessels of the reproductive apparatus are elevated in this pose and are bound to be drained of their extra blood, if the pose is maintained for a sufficiently long time and the practice is daily kept up for a considerable period."[24]

"The muscle responsible for feeble erection can . . . be strengthened [by practicing] Asvini-Mudra," a seal that is basically the contraction of the anus but involves contraction of not only the sphincter but also the perineum and pelvic floor muscles.[25] "Asvini-Mudra can be advantageously practiced during Sarvangasana," Kuvalayananda relayed to his readers, "but only in the latter half of the time devoted to the pose daily."[26]

After granting that "we have been trying Yogic Therapeutics only of late and that its unlimited possibilities have not yet been fully fathomed," Kuvalayananda stated: "By our personal experience, we can say that Yogic remedies are by far the best that we have ever seen, and that they are capable of making up *much* of the damage done to sexual powers, though they may not be able to effect a complete cure."[27]

Conclusions for Claims for *Sarvangasana* Treatment

"The clinical evidence produced here when taken collectively," Kuvalayananda declared with certainty, "irresistibly leads to one conclusion only. It clearly proves that the Pan-Physical Pose very effectively helps the thyroid to regain its health and strength" (fig. 8.3).[28] Although stated by a man who by all accounts was without pomposity, this claim is claptrap. The case studies aren't in-depth, longitudinal, and systematic. Their analysis and results don't provide objective information about the physiological effects of *Sarvangasana* treatment. As a result, the studies hardly provide a sharpened understanding of how *Sarvangasana* treatment works, or whether it actually works at all. (Besides, although having their place in medical research, case studies—even when they're rigorous— aren't nearly as valuable as well-conducted, long-term, randomized controlled studies.)

In fact, these case studies are so flimsy that they don't even lend themselves to generating or testing hypotheses. As evidence for *Sarvangasana* treatment curing leprosy, testicular degeneration, epilepsy, poor venous circulation, premature ejaculation, and erectile dysfunction, they're more like a collection of old wives' tales than case studies.

How could it be otherwise? The cause of leprosy is a bacteria believed to be spread from person to person through infection (respiratory droplets). The cause of epilepsy is some sort of injury to the brain. Psychological factors are commonly the major contributor to erectile dysfunction and premature ejaculation. (Performing an exercise—similar to what

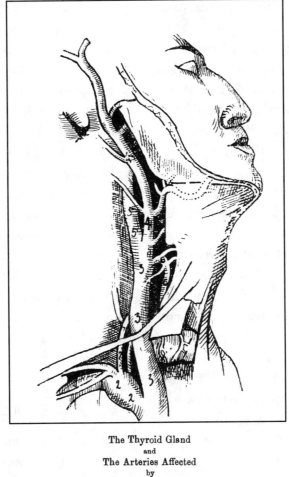

The Thyroid Gland
and
The Arteries Affected
by
The Pan·Physical Pose.
1 The Thyroid Gland.

2 The Subclavian, Ist Part.	5 The Internal Carotid.
3 The Common Carotid.	6 The Superior Thyroid.
4 The External Carotid.	7 The Inferior Thyroid.

Figure 8.3. Illustration, "The Thyroid Gland and the Arteries Affected by the Pan-Physical Pose"
(From *Yoga-Mimansa*, vol. 1, no. 1 [1924])

Kuvalayananda advocates—for contracting the pubococcygeus muscle does, however, aid in gaining control over ejaculation.) The causes of varicose veins are congenitally defective venous valves and conditions such as pregnancy (when the growing uterus puts pressure on the inferior vena cava, which in turn increases pressure on the leg veins) and standing for long periods of time (when blood tends to pool in the lower extremities, causing sluggish venous blood flow). (*Sarvangasana,* like other inversions, does relieve pressure in varicose veins, especially at the end of a long day on one's feet, by improving drainage of blood in the veins, but it isn't nearly as effective as simply walking, which uses the muscle action of the legs to pump venous blood through the veins.) None of these disorders are caused by the poor functioning of the thyroid or parathyroids. And even if they were, they couldn't be cured by applying pressure to the thyroid gland with a chin lock. "There is no medical evidence to support the common yogic point of view that applying external pressure to an endocrine gland will stimulate it to release its hormonal load," writes Mel Robin, author of *A Physiological Handbook for Teachers of* Yogasana, "unless the pressure is so extreme that the glandular cells are ruptured."[29]

Positing yoga as rational health cure, "Sarvangasana or the Pan-Physical Pose" is the most important and influential article about the health benefits of hatha yoga ever written—and perhaps the silliest. Kuvalayananda promised to examine clinical evidence, but what he delivered is nothing more than flimsy and bizarre anecdotal evidence. He provided no evidence whatsoever that practicing *Sarvangasana* maintains a healthy thyroid or restores a debilitated or diseased thyroid to health.

But then, Kuvalayananda was up against an obstacle that's difficult to overcome: yoga practices—*kriyas, mudras, bandhas, pranayama,* and *asanas*—don't maintain or improve health. Or, at least, they haven't been proven to do so. This is borne out by the fact that there's no substantiated (science-based) evidence for the therapeutic effects of *asanas* and the other yogic practices on health—for their facilitating the workings of the internal organs, boosting the immune system, cleansing the body of toxins, improving lipid profiles, increasing insulin sensitivity, lowering blood pressure, or the like. To tout the health benefits of yoga, William J. Broad, author of *The Science of Yoga,* relies heavily on the evidence found in "Risk Indices Associated with the Insulin Resistance Syndrome, Cardiovascular Disease, and Possible Protection with Yoga: A Systematic Review," an assessment of all the relevant literature (seventy original clinical research studies) published from 1970 to 2004 on the effects of yoga on cardiovascular risk factors. Broad reasons: "The studies range from anecdotal to rigorous. But their large number . . . argue persuasively that yoga works remarkable well."[30] His conclusion (and its specious rationale) flies in the face of the evidence. As the reviewers themselves sensibly conclude, while yoga may improve cardiovascular disease and other insulin resistance syndrome conditions, "the methodologic and other limitations characterizing most of these studies preclude drawing firm conclusions."[31]

A Grand Folly

Kuvalayananda's ambitious endeavor to put yoga cure on a scientific footing—his claim that specific yoga practices were devised in a way to rehabilitate specific organs, including the endocrine glands—was a grand folly. Individual *asanas* cannot be assigned a therapeutic value. (They have no physiological mechanism that stimulates internal organs.) And hatha yoga practice doesn't work holistically to maintain or improve health.

Not that the outcome of Kuvalayananda's undertaking was ruinous. The conversion of the Indian middle class to hatha yoga practice, made under the mistaken belief that the health benefits of yoga have scientific underpinnings, helped Indians cope with their anxieties. Through its vaunted relaxation techniques (controlling the breath and resting the body after exertion), hatha yoga does promote a shift in the autonomic nervous system balance from primarily sympathetic to parasympathetic, thus temporarily reducing the physiological effects of stress (stress hormones return to normal levels). But then, so apparently do many other activities, such as puttering in the garden, sitting on a boardwalk bench at the sea, watching television, and brisk walking.

The efficacy of a course of hatha yoga *asanas* for lowering disease risk or treating disease remains unproven against such rival protocols as lifestyle modifications (primarily, a largely whole-foods vegetarian diet, aerobic exercise, discontinuation of smoking, some sort of group support, and stress management), pharmaceuticals, and even herbal remedies. There is, however, something of clear and unique value about *asana* practice: its ability to benefit musculoskeletal fitness.

Physical health may be said to be the absence of disease or infirmity but is perhaps better described as physical wellness or vigilant and active resistance to illness. Fitness, in contrast, is the capacity to meet the demands of some physical task, such as running a long distance, holding a heavy object, or reaching down to tie one's shoes. One can be fit without being healthy (well-conditioned runners can have undiagnosed cardiovascular disease) and healthy without being fit (the disabled can be free of disease). The three primary components of fitness are cardiovascular endurance (the ability of the heart, blood vessels, and lungs to deliver oxygen to working muscles), strength (the ability of muscles to exert force), and flexibility (the ability of joints to move through their full range of motion).* Commonly leading lives that don't naturally keep them physically fit, in modern times people usually turn to exercise to maintain the primary components of fitness.

During the same period in which he was attempting to prove the benefits of yoga as health cure, Kuvalayananda was establishing the viability of yoga as flexibility exercise par excellence—especially as manifested by its exercises for conditioning (enhancing the mobility and stability of) the spine.

---

*Other components of fitness are local muscle endurance, power, speed, reaction time, agility, balance, and coordination.

9

SWAMI KUVALAYANANDA

Standing Up Straight

Yoga and Good Posture

Correctives to Poor Posture

Looking at people walking along a busy downtown street, we see that ideal (i.e., standard) posture is rare. Most of us—whether young or old—are bent over, at least to some degree. Poor posture is damaging to more than appearance. Ideal skeletal alignment—the mechanically efficient placement of the joints while standing—allows muscles and other connective tissue to remain at their optimal resting length (neither shortened nor elongated) and affords optimal positions for the internal organs. If even slight deviations from standard aren't regularly adjusted, over time they become habitual and progressively worsen, until one day we find ourselves having a myriad of musculoskeletal tissue and organ system problems such as lower back pain, proneness to injuries, poor digestion, increased susceptibility to respiratory ailments, and hypertension.

Alarm over the deleterious effects of poor posture has been expressed in the West since the formation of industrial societies in the early 19th century, when people's lives were reordered around long hours of arduous work in factories and offices. In 1833 Peter Gaskell, chronicler of the destruction of the harmonious family by the urban factory system, stood near the single, narrow doorway of a large cotton mill in England to witness the workers exiting the building. "An uglier set of men and women, of boys and girls, taking them in the mass," he concluded, "would be impossible to congregate in a smaller compass." They were made ugly by their work conditions: a long day cooped up in stifling heat, remaining in one position for hours, and forbidden any exercise. "Their complexion is sallow and pallid—with a peculiar flatness of feature. . . . Their stature low. . . . Their limbs slender, and playing badly and ungracefully. A very general bowing of the legs. Great numbers of girls and women walking lamely or awkwardly. . . . Nearly all have flat feet, accompanied with a down-tread. . . . A spiritless and dejected air, a sprawling and wide action of the legs. . . . Beauty of face and form are both lost in angularity."[1]*

While social reformers and laborers themselves took steps to alleviate the horrendous working conditions in factories and offices that caused deformed bodies, shambling gait, and slumped posture, physical culturalists took up the cause of fixing the resultant bad posture. Early on, the military posture—standing "at attention," chin tucked in, chest puffed up, shoulders wrenched back, lumbar curve exaggerated, front thighs vigorously contracted and outwardly rotated, knees tightly locked, and feet angled outward—was commonly promoted as the corrective. But over time, its value was increasingly questioned.

In the late 1880s, in an effort to understand the resistive forces that German soldiers, draped with equipment, must overcome during movement, University of Leipzig professor of topographical anatomy Christian Wilhelm Braune, aided by his student Otto Fischer, set out to sci-entifically determine the efficacy of the military posture by locating the body's center of gravity, which, in turn, would enable them to locate the places where the line of gravity falls in relationship to the weight-bearing joints. (The line of gravity connects the body's center of gravity with the center of Earth. Upright posture is most stable when we stand in accord with the line of gravity.) The two men conducted their experiment on corpses. "Altogether we had four fresh, normally built cadavers (suicides) at our disposal."[2] The researchers found an ingenious solution to the tricky problem of dissecting an upright corpse: they froze the cadavers with an artificial freezing mixture to make the bodies hard and nailed them to a wall with "a pointed iron rod, as slender as possible, but still strong enough and hard enough to prevent it from being bent by the weight of the body," supplemented by steel rods.[3] In effect, they crucified the dead. (Surely, no matter how grisly, scientifically lofty, or filled with practical consequences for the German military this experiment was, the quest to find the very center of the body, an undiscovered geographic location, which even no skilled surgeon had knowingly excavated, must've held out the same romantic allure that compelled 19th- and early 20th-century explorers to attempt to reach the North Pole.)

Dissecting the bodies with "a broad, fine-edged saw, much in the same way two workmen

*The Lumière brothers' historic film *La sortie de l'usine Lumière à Lyon* (commonly titled in English as *Workers Leaving the Lumière Factory*) presents an entirely different picture of industrial workers after a day's work in the 19th century. Made in 1895, the film shows a spirited, mostly female workforce briskly exiting a factory (built by the brothers' father for his photographic equipment manufacturing business) and walking off-screen. Most of the men and women move with their torsos quite erect. But this scene of laborers leaving their factory, it turns out, isn't an actual documentary. It's a reenactment. So we don't know if the ebullience of the workers is typical. Yet the film is persuasive evidence that the posture of at least some Victorian factory workers was far superior to our own.

would saw the trunk of a tree," to locate the points of intersection of the anteroposterior, lateral, and transverse planes, Braune and Fischer established the center of gravity of the body as 4 cm (1.57 inches) anterior to the first to the third vertebrae of the sacrum.[4] (Inserted like a wedge between the two hip bones at the base of the spine just above the tailbone, the sacrum—a curved, forward-tilting, triangular bone—is composed in adults of five fused vertebrae.) The position of an upright man with this center of gravity was plotted on a life-size drawing. (Not all four corpses proved equally useful: one couldn't be dissected because Braune lacked permission to cut it, and another started "to break up during the measurement"—that is, it began decomposing.)

The results of the study were published in 1889 by the Royal Academy of Sciences of Saxony in a treatise titled "The Center of Gravity of the Human Body as Related to the Equipment of the German Infantry."[5] When Braune and Fischer compared the "corpse" position to the military position, they concluded that the "unsatisfactory placement of the gravity line in the military position causes severe muscular strain, that leads to great fatigue on being held for any length of time. It is, therefore, a very undesirable position."[6] The more a soldier (especially one loaded down with gear) assumed this unnatural perpendicular position, the more likely he was to become (in World War II slang) a sad sack.

As a result of their systematic and extensive work on the body's geography, Braune and Fischer helped discredit the military posture. This was a good thing. But they had done it

with incorrect findings. They were off the mark in their location of the body's center of gravity, placing it behind the actual center of gravity, which is correctly placed midway between the hip joints, approximately 5 cm (1.96 inches) anterior to the second sacral vertebra (the precise location depends on a person's proportions).

(The design of Braune and Fischer's experiment was flawed. The corpses were frozen when they were supine. The curve of the lumbar spine is much less when we're lying on our back—especially when we're dead—than when we're standing, a position that shifts the center of gravity forward. Furthermore, a corpse suspended by rods or even merely propped up—especially one that's frozen—has a different center of gravity from an upright living person. That's because the distribution of fluids and positions of organs change in a dead body.)

As an apparent consequence of their inaccurate mapmaking, a harmful corrective to both the stooping posture, with its abnormal protrusion of the shoulder blades, and the distorted, stiff military posture gained popularity: the flattened back position. Instead of carrying out the order to "stand up straight" by throwing the shoulders back and up, expanding and elevating the chest, narrowing the upper back, and arching the lower spine, one merely drew in the abdomen, tilted the pelvis backward, and flattened the back and neck.

And as a consequence of Braune and Fischer's use of what they called *normalstellung,* the reference position, another harmful corrective gained popularity: the on-center position. In their reference position, a plumb line falls (when the body is viewed from the side) directly through the centers of the hip, knee, and ankle joints (the weight-bearing joints), as well as through the tips of the ear and shoulder. "This position offers great advantages for making measurements and calculations," Braune and Fischer explained, "because it presents a definite point of origin, due to the fact that it makes the centers of gravity of the separate sections of the body all lie one above the other in one vertical plane."[7]

Mistaking this reference line (which passes through the centers of weight-bearing joints) for the line of gravity, doctors, physical therapists, and physical education teachers began to exhort those under their sway to take this on-center position—an unstable position that can be held only momentarily because it calls for intense, constant muscular effort in the presence of normal external stresses.* The true line of gravity, anatomists would later discover, passes through the lobe of the ear, just in front of the shoulder joint (midway between the front and back of the chest), through the highest portion of the sacrum (midway between the back and abdomen), through the leg slightly behind the center of the hip joint, slightly in front the center of the knee joint, and slightly in front of the bony prominence on the outside of the ankle.

Maintaining an unnatural posture—whether slack (drooping from exhaustion, loss of enthusiasm, a habitual slouch over a desk, and the like) or rigid (mimicking soldiers at attention or taking the on-center position)—requires perceptibly strained muscular activity; maintaining a relaxed erect posture, in contrast, requires only the largely untended minimal contraction of a few muscles. Equipped with knowledge gained from neurology, biomechanics, kinesiology, and other fields or based on their own keen observations of bodily movements and experience gained in therapeutic practice, physical culturists of all stripes came to recognize that ideal postural alignment is attained chiefly by relaxing muscles, not tensing them. As a result, they placed emphasis on "not trying so hard" and "letting go" to avoid tension.

Some physical culturists further realized that a regular physical fitness program that balances and coordinates the antigravity postural muscles (the muscle groups that stabilize joints to oppose the effects of gravity in standing) is a necessary prerequisite to relaxed standing. Concerned with good posture as an element not of aesthetic or ethical refinement but of physical functionality—of fitness and health—they began to configure physical conditioning programs that would make relaxed standing effortless. One of Swami Kuvalayananda's greatest insights was his recognition of the suitability of yogic exercise for achieving and maintaining ideal upright posture, which allows for relaxed standing and graceful carriage.

Postural Alignment Introduced into Yoga

In "Some Practices for Increasing Stature," a sincere bit of quackery published in the April 1926 *Yoga-Mimansa,* Kuvalayananda promoted

---

*Perhaps the misunderstanding took place because, as Swedish pioneer physical therapist, teacher, and researcher Signe Brunnström believed, *normalstellung* was mistranslated as "normal posture" (Brunnström, *Brunnström's Clinical Kinesiology,* 368). Or perhaps it took place because the plate that illustrates the reference line (which may have been many people's primary source of information about the research) appears to be illustrating the line of gravity.

yoga poses as a natural means (as opposed to faddish mechanical devices invented by physical culturist hucksters) of stimulating bone growth in adults to gain height. He shilled his yoga treatment with a decidedly nonyogic scare tactic based on a popular misconception of Darwin's theories: "In these days of keen competition, only the fittest can survive. A tall figure has immense advantage over a stunted frame."[8]

To give his pitch the authority of science, Kuvalayananda based yoga's efficacy in stimulating bone growth in its conformity to Meyer's law, which states that while a bone's structure—its basic architecture—was determined over millions of years by the mechanical forces imposed upon it, a bone's formation takes place during an animal's lifetime when the stresses of pressure and tension are placed on it (i.e., bone adapts to an altered load).* Kuvalayananda gave examples of seven yogic practices that operate according to the law.

After describing four yogic practices (two postural and two cleansing exercises) that increase pressure on the vertebrae, Kuvalayananda concluded, "Ancient Yoga teaches scientific exercises for the longitudinal growth of the trunk by pressure stimulus and thus helps human beings to increase their stature."[9] And after describing three postural exercises for increasing tension, which is produced by muscles groups pulling in opposite directions on bones at their joints, he similarly concluded, "All these stretching exercises increase the muscular tension on the bones and thus stimulate them to growth."[10]

Kuvalayananda made clear that he wasn't referring to bone growth in early age. "The exercises noted here . . . are, in every way, capable of increasing human height. They should, however, be begun just after puberty, because at that age the bone-building activity is unusually great. . . . As the skeleton reaches maturity in the fifth decade, these practices may be available *at least* up to the fiftieth year."[11]

Perhaps out of a mixture of ignorance and wishful thinking, Kuvalayananda misunderstood how bone growth works. Bones are alive and do respond to stress: they adapt to the loads they're placed under. When the loading is increased, the bones remodel themselves to become stronger to resist that amount of loading; when the loading is decreased, the bones become weaker. But bones grow in length only in our childhood, adolescence, and early adulthood. The stimulation of weight-bearing exercises (which, to a limited degree, yoga postures are) maintains and increases bone density, but preserving the integrity of bones as we age doesn't make them longer.

Kuvalayananda well understood, however, that "the erect posture which the man has assumed" flattens out intervertebral disks and that yogic stretching exercises are even more effective than sleep in "disburden[ing]" the "greatly taxed" disks.[12] The stimulation of fluid-circulating flexibility exercises (which, in their special attention to lengthening the spine, yoga postures amply are) helps prevent intervertebral disks (which account for approximately 25 percent of the length of the

---

*Georg Hermann von Meyer proposed his theory in 1867, but Julius Wolff—who, in 1892, presented the first evidence that bone remodels in response to mechanical forces—advocated, defended, and popularized the theory. For this reason, it came to be known as Wolff's law.

spine) from losing their elasticity and height.

Preventing the deterioration of intervertebral disks was hardly the only valid and compelling reason that Kuvalayananda gave for practicing yoga. Amid his misguided discussion of increasing bone growth through tension stimulus, he offhandedly introduced an even more powerful rationale for practicing yoga: attaining ideal postural alignment.

In support of the yogic principles for attaining ideal aligned posture, Kuvalayananda quoted an unidentified passage from an unnamed "learned author."[13] The passage is from *Adolescence: Its Psychology and Its Relations to Physiology,* by Granville Stanley Hall (1844–1924), which was published in 1904, and in which the term for the extended hiatus between childhood and adulthood was coined.* Instead of ecumenically granting that this modern Western source brings new insights to the subject of aligned posture, Kuvalayananda praised Hall's writing because, despite "bear[ing] on a system different from Yoga," it "beautifully describes some of the fundamental laws of the ancient Yogins in evolving their system . . . of physical culture."[14]†

Kuvalayananda could've declared the supreme adaptability of hatha yoga's centuries-old stretching exercises to this new field of postural training being explored by Hall and others in the West. His failure to do so wasn't singular. It was the wont of all prominent Indian physical culturists of the period, in the thrall of Indian nationalism, to boldly borrow practices from Westerners, claim primacy for the practices in the distant yoga tradition, and, to top it off, hold up the Western practices as confirmation of the validity of the supposedly ancient yogic practices. (Needless to say, in the period between World War I and World War II, this rhetoric of grandeur of national heritage wasn't restricted to India.) Yet in Hall, Kuvalayananda recognized a unique and sagacious proponent of relaxed standing whom he could not "withstand the temptation" to quote at length.[15]

Hall grasped that in order to stand comfortably, we first have to remove all lethargy and ungainliness from our habitual way of standing and moving. For this, we need to systematically rearrange our bone structure. Only when skeletal bones are properly aligned can muscles be unburdened of the strain of holding up the parts of the body that are out of place. Methodically addressing the postural defects of slouching, Hall suggested prescriptive

---

*Hall, it would seem, was a very unlikely source of information for a swami: Founder and first president of the American Psychological Association and president of Clark University, he was an acclaimed American psychologist and educator. Finding a kindred spirit in Sigmund Freud (both emphasized the importance of sexuality in children and adolescents), Hall became the United States' most ardent proselytizer of psychoanalysis. In 1909 he hosted Freud, his most eminent disciples (including Carl Jung), and about twenty other participants at a conference at the university, in which Freud, the star attraction, gave five lectures in German on the origin and development of psychoanalysis and received an honorary degree. Whereas Hall was enthralled by Freud, the doctor who had forged the talking cure to treat neurotics in Vienna, Kuvalayananda, in contrast, was inspired by Paramahamsa Madhavadasaji, the guru who had trained disciples to shut up along the banks of the Narmada River at Malsar in Gujarat.

†In a less generous description, Kuvalayananda wrote that Hall's passage "very adequately expresses some of [ancient yoga's] basic ideas" (Kuvalayananda, "Some Practices for Increasing Stature," 149).

movements to correct them: "The head must balance on the cervical vertebrae and not call upon the muscles of the neck to keep it from rolling off; the weight of the shoulders must be thrown back off the thorax; the spine be erect to allow the abdomen free action; the joints of the thigh extended; the hand and arm supinated etc."[16]

When the parts of the body are rearranged in vertical alignment, Hall realized, muscles are relieved of their extraneous work. Unlike the slouching posture or equally enervating military posture, in which the chest is thrust out and the lower back is markedly arched, the aligned posture can be held effortlessly (at least for a short while; even relaxed standing in place isn't comfortable for any length of time).

Hall was aware of the effects of posture on the internal organs: "the interests of the viscera are never lost sight of."[17] A lengthened spine keeps the chest from collapsing on the abdominal region. As a result, the lungs can fully expand (which facilitates effortless breathing and combats respiratory ailments) and the intestines are unconstricted (which facilitates good digestion).

Hall also brought keen psychological insight (commonplace to us now) to his analysis of posture. "Extensor action goes with expansive, flexor with depressive states of mind; hence courage, buoyancy, hope, are favoured and handicaps removed," he declared.[18] The folded-up posture of bent ankles, knees, hips, and spinal column "goes with" (which can mean "is a sign of" and "gives rise to," as well as "is associated with") being filled with doubt, while the straightened up posture "goes with" being upbeat.

What especially interested Kuvalayananda, though, was the exercise principle Hall advocated to achieve "erect, self-respecting carriage": "relax the flexor and tone up the extensor muscles and . . . open the human form into postures as opposite as possible to those of the embryo which it tends persistently to approximate in sitting, and in fatigue and collapse attitudes generally."[19] This protocol was developed (according to Hall but not universally agreed on) in the early 1800s by the Swedish originator of medical gymnastics, Per Henrik (in English sources, "Peter Henry") Ling, and his immediate pupils to correct the "ill-shapen bodies of most men about them."[20]*

Although endorsing all of Hall's insights by the very fact of quoting them, Kuvalayananda elaborated on only this one aspect of Hall's analysis. The bones of the human skeleton are kept in position by muscle groups—flexors and extensors—that perpetually exert opposing pulls on the bones. The flexor muscles bring bony parts together at their joints. "Their action is counteracted by the extensors," Kuvalayananda explained, "which keep these parts from closing upon themselves."[21] In order that the tension exerted by opposing muscles (flexors and extensors) to keep bones in position be balanced—in particular, to prevent the loss of

---

*Brunnström implies that at least the popularization of the military posture can be attributed to Ling. "It is impossible to tell whether this conception of desirable posture originated with . . . Ling," she speculated in 1940, "or whether it was accepted by him and his followers from an already existing army conception of posture. However this may be, the 'military' type of posture soon was accepted everywhere" (Brunnström, "Changing Conception of Posture," 79).

balance caused by tight (shortened) muscles—muscles must be kept flexible. This ability is "secured in Yoga by various postures which stretch all the different muscles of the body and keep them perfectly elastic," he maintained. "A scientific study of the different poses shows very clearly, however," he continued, introducing a critical qualifier, "that Yogic Physical Culture aims at making the flexors more elastic than the extensors, so that the whole frame may easily stand erect."[22]

On the face of it, Kuvalayananda's favoring flexor muscles over extensor muscles for stretching is puzzling. Why would he (following Hall) advocate stretching that seems to promote muscle imbalance in order to achieve standard posture? The answer is that Kuvalayananda recognized the natural disproportion of pull in (i.e., force between) the flexors and extensors: the body has a tendency toward flexion due to the downward pull of gravity on the bony structures at the ankle, knee, hip, and spinal column joints. For example, the pectoralis muscles of the chest, serving as flexors, exert a greater pull than the opposing back muscles, resulting in the thorax collapsing upon itself. Through conscious effort, however, "the latissimus dorsi and the trapezius keep the thorax and the head from curving forward and serve as it were as extensors."[23] Therefore, an effective yogic protocol calls for stretching the chest more than the upper back. *Bhujangasana,* Cobra Pose, is more important for good posture than *Paschimottanasana,* Seated Forward Bend—at least as far as the upper trunk is concerned.

But while adopting Hall's advice to perform exercises that relax—*stretch*—the flexor muscles, Kuvalayananda ignored the other equally critical part of Hall's paradoxical formulation: performing strengthening exercises to tone up—*strengthen*—the extensor muscles. The tendency to fold in on ourselves when standing is opposed by the lower limb and trunk extensor muscles, as well as the muscles that retract, depress, and downwardly rotate the shoulder girdle.

In order for us to stand up straight, we must not only stretch the flexor muscles, which tend to become tight and short through slouching, but we must also strengthen the extensor muscles, which tend to become slack and elongated through slouching. (Poor postural habits only exacerbate the natural tendency of our bony skeleton to bow to the constant, wearying pull of gravity toward the center of Earth.)

Kuvalayananda advocated (or at least didn't disapprove of) mixing strength training with flexibility training: "There is no harm in undergoing the Yogic exercises and strenuous muscular exercises side by side." His only caveat was to practice the two disciplines twenty minutes apart; he advised that those who want to finish their exercises "with a balance introduced into their system" take yogic exercises last, and that those who want to have "a spirit of exhilaration at the end" take their muscular exercises last. (He also suggested guidelines for walking as the cardiovascular component of a fitness routine, cautioning that "walk when taken as an exercise must be brisk" and, like strenuous muscular exercise, should be performed twenty minutes before or after yogic exercises.[24] For his ecumenicism in providing protocols for practicing strength training and brisk walking, Kuvalayananda would probably be scorned by today's yoga teacher purists, whose careers wouldn't exist without his pioneering efforts.) But he never articulated—probably even for himself—a regime of strengthening exercises that would complement stretching exercises to attain vertebral alignment. That would be left to one of his most unlikely adherents.

Indian bodybuilder K. V. Iyer was a close observer of "the posture usually adopted by the town-dweller, the students, the office going folk and the business-men who have not taken any pains whatsoever with the welfare of their bodies. The head is carried in the peering position forward of the chest; [the] chest [is] sunk deep by contraction, due to the forward droop of the shoulders and to depression of the sternum (breast-bone); the abdomen [is] thoroughly relaxed and protuberant."[25] Iyer well understood the ill effects of this poor posture. When habitual, these postural faults strain the neck, causing headaches; elongate the middle and lower fibers of the trapezius (the parts of this mighty muscle that keep the shoulder blades back and down), diminishing their ability to assist arm elevation; reduce the mobility of the thoracic cavity, restricting the lungs and making breathing difficult; displace the digestive organs (causing, as Iyer points out, "digestive trouble and every sort of bowel complaint"); strain the lower back muscles, resulting in lumbar back pain; and tighten the legs, causing cramps.[26]

Iyer had a remedy for poor posture: "Cultivate straightness, and you prolong and intensify your youth. Bodily erectness depends upon maintaining the straightness of the spine. If you drift into careless habits of sitting, standing and walking, the body's weight is thrown on the bones of the body and the spine. The sign of infirmity and old age is made more and more pronounced, with the result that the body itself gets actually warped into a round-back, flat-chested, distended-abdomen type" (fig. 9.1).[27]

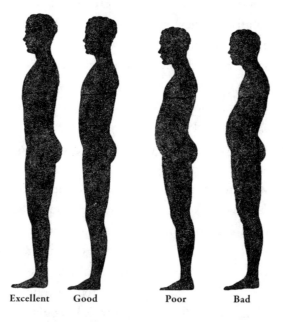

Excellent   Good   Poor   Bad

Figure 9.1. "Illustrations of Posture Standards"
(From *Physical Training through Correspondence,* by K. V. Iyer)

But exactly how is straightness cultivated? Unlike Kuvalayananda, Iyer recognized the need for practicing strengthening exercises as well as *asanas* to foster aligned posture. In "The Correct Carriage of the Body," a chapter in his major work, *Physical Training through Correspondence,* Iyer—whose hatha yoga teachings were enormously influenced by the articles published by Kuvalayananda, "to whom India owes gratitude for having revived the 'Hata-Yoga'"[28]—suggested innovative correctives that combined *asanas* and Western strengthening exercises.*

For example, for the "drooping shoulders and a cramped chest" aspect of poor posture, Iyer recommended an *asana* to open up the chest (whose muscles originate on the breastbone and collarbones) and a strengthening exercise for developing the upper back (whose muscles originate on the shoulder blades) in order to "keep the shoulders in position."[29] For stretching the chest, he recommended *Dhanurasana,* Bow Pose, in which you lie prone, bend the knees, grab the ankles, and pull on the legs while "raising the chest as high as possible and throwing the head well back" (see figs. 9.2 and 9.3 on page 120).[30] He suggested repeating the *asana* "two or three times, —successively, maintaining the posture some 15, 20 or 30 seconds each time according to your ability."[31] For strengthening the upper back, he recommended a basically isometric exercise in which you clasp the hands on top of the head, raise the shoulders, and "start pulling your arms strongly apart" while moving "the arms straight above the head" (see figs. 9.4 and 9.5 on page 121).[32] This movement is repeated eight to twelve times.

For those of us who tend to increasingly slouch during the day, performing exercises on a daily basis in this manner—balancing our bony structure through strengthening the anti-gravity muscles and stretching the muscles that oppose them—enables us to cope with gravity's constant pull.

The Cause of Poor Posture

When our muscles, tendons, ligaments, and fascia don't align our bones at their contacting surfaces (the joints), our bony skeleton bows to the constant, wearying pull of gravity toward the center of Earth. But which is the cause and which the effect? Are we bent over from poor postural habits or from the pull of gravity?

Iyer saw postural deficiencies as a cultural issue. They were the plight of modern man who sits slouched over his desk for long hours: "Young men in class-rooms and in private studies, officials and clerks in their offices, work with spines bent, throwing all the weight of their body on the table or the desk before them. I have seen them with their pens or pencils almost poking into their eyes. They work on in this posture, four or five hours per day; the curve in their spine becomes more and more pronounced. Devitalisation and old age set in before their time, when they ought to be in the prime of their lives."[33]

In contrast, American physical educators Gene A. Logan and Wayne C. McKinney,

---

Physical Training through Correspondence is still the only manual on combining yogic postures and Western strengthening exercises for fitness and health (depending on whether the strengthening exercises in Richard Hittleman's 1964 *Yoga for Physical Fitness* are considered to be yogic or Western).

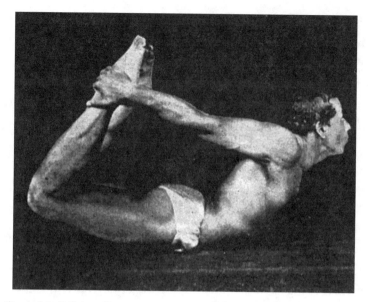

Figure 9.2. K. V. Iyer demonstrating *Dhanurasana,* Bow Pose, photo study for
the illustration in *Physical Training through Correspondence,* circa 1940

(With the kind permission of Shashidhar Tokanahalli Nagabhushan Rao)

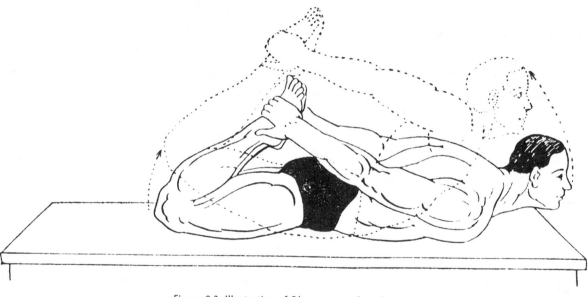

Figure 9.3. Illustration of *Dhanurasana,* Bow Pose

(From *Physical Training through Correspondence*)

experts in the theory and practice of anatomic kinesiology, posit two altogether different reasons for the tendency toward flexion in man: the "(1) anatomic or bony structure of the joints at the ankle, knee, hip, and spinal column, and (2) effect of the downward pull of gravity on these joints."[34]

Like Iyer, Hall recognized the cultural

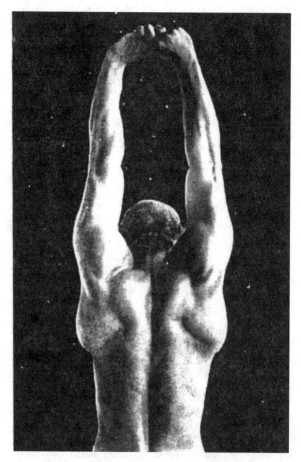

Figure 9.4. K. V. Iyer demonstrating an exercise for strengthening the upper back, photo study for the illustration in *Physical Training through Correspondence,* circa 1940

(With the kind permission of Shashidhar Tokanahalli Nagabhushan Rao)

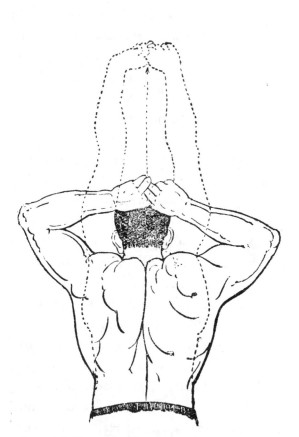

Figure 9.5. Illustration of an exercise for strengthening the upper back

(From *Physical Training through Correspondence*)

aspects of poor posture: "The great majority of city bred men, as well as all students, are prone to deleterious effects from too much sitting."[35] But, more psychologically attuned to human behavior than Iyer, Hall also recognized that not only sitting and fatigue but also some mental states (what he called "collapse attitudes," such as defeat, grief, and despair) increase the natural tendency toward giving in to the pull of gravity. (To these three causes of poor posture,

he might've added a fourth: the purposeful slouching of adolescence, a rejection not only of adulthood but of membership in the community of humankind, for it's our upright posture that distinguishes the human genus from all other living creatures.)

Like Logan and McKinney, Hall also recognized the body's natural tendency toward flexion, which is why he argued for strengthening the body's antigravity musculature to maintain upright posture. But, possessing an existential bent absent in Logan and McKinney, he fully understood the melancholy nature of standing erect—that is to say, of what it means to be human. He recognized that the body's inherent structure and a law of nature (gravity) conspire to doom us to a lifetime of surrendering to defective posture. Hence his cri de coeur to resist: we must, he insisted, constantly "open the human form into postures as opposite as possible to those of the embryo which it tends persistently to approximate."[36] But over time the struggle wears us down. Postural alignment in the elderly commonly exhibits a more flexed posture than in the young, due to sedentary living and the aging process itself—a gradual return to the fetal position.

Kuvalayananda not only incorporated into hatha yoga Hall's admonition to stretch the flexors more than the extensors in order to improve posture but also, in giving over an entire page to Hall's observations, endorsed Hall's sophisticated analysis of the causes of poor posture. While he didn't expand on Hall's astute observations about the social context and psychological states of poor posture, Kuvalayananda did embrace Hall's observation that most of us give in to the natural inclination to revert to curling up in the fetal position, especially as we age. We know this not from anything Kuvalayananda wrote but from the peculiar image that he used to illustrate the passage from Hall.

The Yogic Body

Kuvalayananda illustrated Hall's discussion of posture—in particular, how the human form "tends persistently to approximate" an embryo—with "The Embryo," a startling etching of a floating figure with the body of a

fetus and the face of an adult man (fig. 9.6). Lost in contemplation, Fetus-Man seems to define humans in their inception—in their very essence—as the thinking animal, *Homo sapiens*. Being unborn—being still inside the womb—is not too early to turn one's thoughts inward.

Fetus-Man's strange aspect—the head of an adult is affixed to the body of a fetus (or is it the other way around?)—brings up a myriad of questions. Is he a regressed adult returned to his amniotic surroundings, or is he a prodigy fetus? Is his adult destiny already determined? Is he in a state of accelerated or decelerated aging? What's he contemplating—his past or his future?

Some may find it hard not to simply see the figure as some freak of nature displayed in a formaldehyde-filled jar on some dusty shelf. Is his grotesquely strange appearance the result of a rare disease or a scientific experiment gone disastrously awry? If the latter, we wonder, where is the conjoined adult body and fetus head? In some parallel universe? Others, however, may find this image less weirdly disturbing than deeply dolorous in its portrayal of the human condition. Rather than showing a worn-out, corseted factory worker leaning on her machine, a pale clerk bent over his desk, or a downcast rejected lover in a park, this depiction of Fetus-Man simultaneously reveals life's beginning and end. That our fate is determined by biology is far sadder (it seems to me) than that our fate is determined by culture. We can oppose our culture. We can't escape our biology.

Fetus-Man is, most of all, a portrait of our biological fate (at least for those of us who live a long time): as we approach our ending, incre-

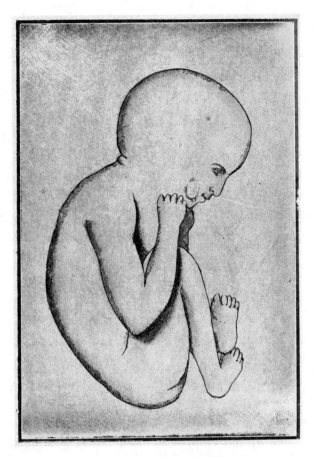

Figure 9.6. Illustration, "The Embryo"
(From *Yoga-Mimansa*, vol. 2, no. 2 [1926])

mentally bent over, we recapitulate our beginning, curled up in the womb. Just as the fetus has recently emerged from nothing, we, weary to the bone from resisting gravity year after year on Earth, will someday tip over just a bit more and pitch ourselves back into nothing.

But is it inevitable that we turn in on ourselves?

In the course of making an argument for the capability of yogic stretching to alleviate the flattening out of spinal disks (which get compressed through sitting and standing, bending and lifting) more effectively than sleep,

Kuvalayananda referred to "the erect position which . . . man has assumed" in opposition to animals, none of whom fully stand erect on two legs.[37] In this allusion to the evolutionary status of humankind, he showed that he recognized standing erect as a key aspect of the human condition. Which, of course, is why he incorporated a regime for perfecting our standing posture—attaining postural alignment—into his yogic physical fitness program. He felt compelled to assert—with clumsy and obvious legerdemain—that this concern for postural alignment is part of the yoga physical culture tradition. At the same time, he failed to grasp (what we decades later and worlds apart can grasp) that a concern for standing tall fits right in with the yoga tradition of contemplation.

As historian of religion Mircea Eliade points out, the immediate purpose of yogic techniques "is to abolish (or to transcend) the human condition by a refusal to conform to the most elementary human inclinations."[38] Some amount of slouching is a natural human tendency. Even if we didn't hunch over our desks or sink into depression, we'd still overly tighten our flexors and curl up (to some degree) like a fetus due to our bony structure and the pull of gravity. Standing erect in perfect alignment, as we do when we assume *Tadasana,* Mountain Pose, during our classroom or home yoga practice—like the traditional meditative practices of sitting still in a relaxed, stable position (commonly, *Padmasana,* the Lotus Pose), breathing rhythmically, concentrating on a single point, and emptying the mind by stopping the mental flux—is unnatural. In other words, standing in aligned posture—like the series of traditional yogic meditative refusals to move, to breathe non-rhythmically, and to be distracted—is an act of repudiation, a rejection of or a means of dissociating ourselves from our customary behavior in the world and outlook on life, which are expressed by the way we usually stand.

To attain *Tadasana,* we don't draw ourselves up; we harmoniously arrange our bones. As a result, we're not holding our body stiffly erect.

We're letting our body relax. With the body's line of gravity the reference point around which our skeleton organizes itself, and its center of gravity over our base of support, we're securely planted on Earth. Which is why this pose is so calmly exhilarating. And so conducive to contemplation. We stand responsive to the Divine alone. This experience may be transferred to our everyday life.

During quotidian activities, having our skeleton in alignment allows us to stand with our arms, once forelimbs, fully free for use in performing motor tasks or gesturing—acts that help define us as humans. When we move, we have a lilt in our walk. Our head is stabilized with respect to the vertical so our gaze takes in the environment. (Humankind's erect posture is closely related to its well-developed eyesight. Creatures who walk on all fours have excellent powers of smell, enabling them to follow a scent on the ground. We, who have good vision, stand tall and hold our heads high, enabling us to take in an expanse of land, sea, or sky or, for that matter, cityscape.) As a result, we go about our lives both fully involved in the world and removed from the world. In response to situations that would ordinarily disturb us, we take in what's around us as a land surveyor does: by gathering information through observation and instantly analyzing it. Which means to say, we remain calm and undisturbed, receptive and humble. We welcome the Divine spirit flowing into us.

10

SWAMI KUVALAYANANDA

Youthifying the Spine

Yoga and Chiropractic

Inanimate and Human Machines

We tend to associate the plight of workers in the industrial age with machines in factories. Beginning with the mechanization of the textile industry in Great Britain in the late 18th century and continuing over the course of the 19th century, home-based artisans were largely replaced by unskilled laborers brought together in factories to mass-produce high volumes of products by operating spinning jennies and other machines in return for wages.

But the rise of large-scale, mechanized factory production, we sometimes forget, greatly expanded ancillary industries, such as banking, insurance, transportation, and retailing. Clerks, accountants, secretaries, managers, lawyers, agents, and other employees were needed to process orders, keep records, file documents, and so on. This booming population of workers who assisted in the transactions of the manufacturing industry was often brought together in that other critical workplace of the industrial age: the intricate and complex office, located in multistory buildings in cities. There, workers sat at desks. (As the number of office employees grew, desks themselves became mass-produced in factories, where they were manually assembled from parts churned out by machines.) Just as much as factory workers, who performed physically repetitive or demanding activities at machines, office workers—hunched over papers at their desks for long hours—became victims of a plague of back problems.

In Herman Melville's story "Bartleby, the Scrivener," published in 1853, the narrator, who runs a Wall Street law practice that deals in rich men's bonds, mortgages, and title deeds, clinically observes how Nippers, one of his scriveners (a scrivener makes handwritten copies of documents), is tormented by his work-table: "Though of a very ingenious mechanical turn, Nippers could never get this table to suit him. He put chips under it, blocks of various sorts, bits of pasteboard, and at last went so far as to attempt an exquisite adjustment by final pieces of folded blotting-paper. But no invention would answer."[1]

Getting the table adjusted to the right height was hardly an idle matter. "If, for the sake of easing his back, [Nippers] brought the table lid at a sharp angle well up towards his chin, and wrote there like a man using the steep roof of a Dutch house for his desk:—then he declared that it stopped the circulation in his arms. If now he lowered the table to his waistbands, and stooped over it in writing, then there was a sore aching in his back."[2] (At his wit's end, Nippers, if he was certain of anything at all, knew he wanted "to be rid of a scrivener's table altogether.")

Although back pain didn't originate with the industrial revolution (as paleontological evidence shows, prehistoric humans suffered from degeneration of the spine; as the 550 BCE medical writings of Hippocrates recorded, Greeks were afflicted with back pain; and, as 18th- and early 19th-century studies reported, millers, quarrymen, tailors, and other traditional tradesmen were subject to backache), the back distress suffered by Nippers was a virulent modern version of occupational back pain incubated in factories and spread to offices. Some of those with back, neck, and shoulder pain turned for relief

to so-called bonesetters, practitioners of joint manipulation, a folk remedy. Although popular among the common people, bonesetters were denigrated for their lack of study (even of anatomy) and formal training (they were self- or family-trained) or ridiculed as charlatans (for their seemingly miraculous cures) by members of the medical profession. Largely illiterate, they left no records of their training, treatment, or results. Ironically, the most detailed account of bonesetting is found in an 1871 four-part article, "On the So-Called 'Bone-Setting,' Its Nature and Results," in *Lancet* (the first medical literature on the subject) by a physician, Wharton Hood. His admiring profile of the famous bonesetter Richard Hutton describes case after case of successful treatments: "A joint, previously stiff, painful, and helpless, was almost instantly restored to freedom of action by his handling, and the change was often attended by an audible sound, which he regarded as an evidence of the return of a bone to its place."[3]

Bonesetters mostly treated patients for impaired mobility that remained after an injury. To restore the full range of motion to a joint, they applied a quick twisting movement to the stiffened body part (they typically had a strong grip). But for healing chronic back problems, they pressed hard with the thumb and forefinger about the spine, moving gradually over the entire problematic area until the pain was alleviated.

Manipulative therapies had been practiced in many parts of the world in ancient times and over the subsequent centuries. The first historical reference to manipulation (a patient with scoliosis was tied to a ladder and inverted) is found in Hippocrates's 400 BCE book on joints. But it wasn't until practitioners in the late 19th century began to ballyhoo the musculoskeletal system as essentially a mechanism with moving parts used to perform various tasks—in other words, as a machine, the very thing that was largely responsible (directly and indirectly) for the prevalence of back pain in the modern era in the first place!—that bone manipulation, because it seeks to place the body in harmony with its inherent mechanical principles, could be claimed to be scientific. In addition to having a concept with which to counter the common criticism that bone manipulation lacked scientific validation, practitioners now also had a metaphor (the body is a machine) so compelling and easily understood, so prosaic and yet poetic, that it could be used with great effect to explain and promote their system.

At 10:00 in the morning on June 22, 1874, forty-six-year-old Andrew Still, a brawny American physician who had become disillusioned with prevalent medical practices after his experience as a de facto surgeon in the Civil War and the death of three of his children from spinal meningitis in the spring of 1864, had an epiphany: disease "is effect only. Ninety-nine times out of one hundred" the cause of disease is that "the machine [the human body] has a wobbling saw; it has left the line."[4] Plainly put, disease is caused by a misaligned spine (the manifest mechanical cause that sets off the underlying physiological cause: the failure of the nerves to adequately regulate blood flow). Therefore, the cure for disease is spinal manipulation (which, by restoring the proper functioning of nerves, removes obstructions to blood flow).

Still began manipulating his patients' vertebrae to alleviate their medical conditions. In so doing, he created the first mechanical treatment for ill health: osteopathy, a new alternative medicine derived from the practice of bonesetting. In traditional medicine, in Hippocrates's formulation, the cure of disease lies within the body (where disease is caused by internal imbalances of the humors and bodily fluids), and methods of treatment include bloodletting, purges, and herbs. Over the course of the second half of the 19th century, when medicine entered the modern era with germ theory, the prevailing view became that most diseases, such as tuberculosis and influenza, are caused by the invasion of a host by outside agents (pathogens—bacteria, viruses, and other microorganisms) and can be prevented by vaccines or cured by medication. According to Still's alternative modality, based on the theory that health can be maintained (and, therefore, disease conquered) only by maintaining the normal functions of the musculoskeletal system, cures are found through manipulating bones (i.e., bringing them into conformity with the principles of mechanical balance). In fact, the patient isn't so much in need of a cure but a tune-up.

Still found that he could cure all the cases under his care. Eager to share the success of his work, he approached the "thinking people" of his hometown, Baldwin, Kansas. "But, alas! when I said, 'God has no use for drugs in disease, and I can prove it by his works'; when I said I could twist a man one way and cure flux, fever, colds, and the diseases of the climate; shake a child and stop scarlet fever, croup, diphtheria, and cure whooping-cough in three days by a wring of its neck, and so on, all my good character was at once gone." Ostracized by his fellow citizens (including some—evidently those who believed he'd committed blasphemy for emulating Jesus by the laying on of hands—who prayed "to save [his] soul from hell"), Still moved with his wife and six children to Kirksville, Missouri, where he opened an office on the town square in March 1875.[5] After a long period of study and practice during which he cured patients of illnesses such as palsy, asthma, pneumonia, consumption, gallstones, heart disorders, and rheumatism (or so he said), he founded a school of osteopathy in Kirksville on May 10, 1892, and published the first of his four books, *Autobiography of Andrew T. Still with a History of the Discovery and Development of the Science of Osteopathy* in 1897, thereby breaking with the long-standing custom of bonesetters of keeping their methods to themselves and their family members.

Chiropractic

In the mid-1890s, about twenty years after Still began developing osteopathy, Canadian-born Daniel David Palmer, who had been practicing magnetic healing in Iowa for nine years, developed chiropractics, a rival system for adjusting the skeleton, under (in Palmer's accounting) decidedly more amazing and auspicious circumstances. While attending a Mississippi Valley Spiritualist Association camp meeting held in Clinton, Iowa, he received his first messages on the principles of chiropractic from Dr. Jim Atkinson, a Davenport physician who had been dead for about fifty years. "The method by which I obtained an explanation of certain physical phenomena from an intelligence in the spiritual world," Palmer explained to doubters, "is known in biblical language as inspiration."[6]* Receiving knowledge of chiropractic from "an intelligent spiritual being" was a sign of Palmer's self-effacement and special authority.[7]

During the nine years he had practiced magnetic healing, Palmer had been obsessed with discovering the cause of disease in his patients. To him, this was life's great mystery. While it was commonly thought that disease was caused by bacteria, viruses, or other microorganisms from some outside source, he was convinced that the the cause was to be found in the body. But exactly where?

Under Atkinson's tutelage, Palmer gradually came to believe that all disease originates in the spinal column, caused by nerves being impinged in the intervertebral foramina (the openings between vertebrae through which nerves leave the spine and extend to other parts of the body). Since the nerves are occluded by the displacement of vertebrae misaligned due to tension or trauma, a chiropractor need only adjust the displaced vertebrae—by this means relieving the pressure on the pinched nerve—to cure the disease.

---

*This was an era when claiming to have received afflatus from otherworldly and divine sources wasn't unusual. Thousands, perhaps even millions (it's impossible to verify the estimates), of Americans participated in Spiritualism, talking with the dead. (Founded in upstate New York by three sisters in 1848, modern Spiritualism first gained wide popularity after the American Civil War when bereft family members yearned to contact soldiers killed in the conflict.) And religious cults were formed when prophets declared that they had received revelations through dreams, visions, and visitations of apparitions, angels, the Holy Spirit, or God.

"The cause of disease has been, and is yet, mysterious to humanity. Chiropractic has solved the mystery," Palmer declared at the beginning of the new century. "The old idea, that the cause of disease [originates] outside the patient [and enters into the patient's body], still prevails in most of the schools of healing, and the remedy consists in finding something which, by being introduced into the body of the sufferer, will drive the disease out." In contrast, "the Chiropractic idea is that the cause of disease is in the person afflicted, and the adjustment, in correcting the wrong that is producing it."[8] This model of disease is entirely based on the concept of man as machine, an idea which Palmer embraced.

"Man is a machine, one of the most wonderful ever created," Palmer marveled. But "like all other machines it is liable to have some portion displaced by wrenches."[9] In fact, "is not the human body much more liable to have its difficult parts racked out of their proper position, and resultant consequences are more severe and far reaching than that of an inanimate machine?"[10]

If you're convinced that man, a living machine, is more susceptible to malfunction than a nonliving machine, why not turn to "a human machinist who understands the cause of disease, a man who can detect and adjust that which is out of alignment?" Unlike the doctor, Palmer pointed out, "the Chiropractor does not treat disease; he adjusts some part of the skeletal frame, replacing it in its normal position." Contrary to what many think, the chiropractor doesn't rub, stretch, slap, or press (and certainly doesn't magnetize, hypnotize, apply heat or electricity, perform surgery, prescribe drugs, or alleviate agitated mental states) to get his results. "He puts [the skeletal frame] into its natural position with his hands," Palmer noted. "There is nothing extraordinary about this; machinists use their hands when adjusting parts of a machine that is out of alignment."[11]

On September 18, 1895, Harvey Lillard, the janitor of the building where Palmer rented his office, visited Palmer. Lillard had lost his hearing seventeen years previously. He couldn't even hear the loud rumbling of a wagon on the street. He had become deaf, he recounted, when he was "in a cramped position, and felt something give in his back."[12] Upon examining him, Palmer found a displaced vertebra. Palmer made two adjustments, freeing nerves that had become paralyzed by pressure. Lillard's hearing returned. More than ten years later, Palmer provided an update in his first book: "Mr. Lillard can hear as well today as other men." And if anyone had any doubts, well, he or she could go ask Lillard himself. "He resides at 1031 Scott Street, Davenport, Iowa."[13]

Palmer opened the Palmer School of Chiropractic in 1897 in Davenport. The school graduated fifteen chiropractors in 1902—the beginning of Palmer's expansion of his form of alternative medicine. He explicated his principles in three books: *The Science of Chiropractic* (1906), *The Chiropractor's Adjuster: The Science, Art and Philosophy of Chiropractic* (1910), and *The Chiropractor* (1914).*

---

*Palmer died under controversial circumstances in 1913 at age sixty-eight. His son was accused of running him down with a car during a parade. Palmer probably wasn't even struck by the car (it appears that he merely stumbled to the street). And, according to Palmer's biographer, Vern Gielow, the official cause of death was typhoid fever (one of any number of diseases that chiropractic is helpless to treat), not injuries.

Yoga as Chiropractic

By the mid- to late 1920s, approximately thirty years after Palmer started his chiropractic school, the maintenance of a healthy spine had become a common mandate in many systems of physical culture. In 1929's *Yogic Physical Culture or the Secret of Happiness,* the first modern hatha yoga manual, S. Sundaram observed: "One who knows the a, b, c, of physical culture pays much attention to the spine. He recognises its importance. On its elasticity and health depend the vitality and youth of an individual. The stiffness of the back-bone means old age. This factor has come to be well-realised in the world of physical culture. Any modern treatise on this subject devotes some attention to this important member of the body."[14]

"The clarion call is therefore sounded by the Western physical culturists," Sundaram exclaimed, "to 'youthify the spine.' All honour to them and may they meet with success!" But they should know, he continued, that "the cry for youthifying the spine was started thousands of years ago, when as civilized countries their lands had no existance [*sic*]"—the cry uttered by "bookless sages experimenting without laboratories and vivisection." The scientifically derived spinal exercises developed by Westerners could never equal the instinctual exercises "left by the Indian sages to posterity for the benefit of humanity."[15]

This assessment is ahistorical. Though most *asanas* involve movement of the spine, they were not designed by the Indian sages—not even instinctively—to "youthify the spine." These poses were developed, and probably haphazardly performed, as preparatory limbering-up exercises for holding a seated posture with steadiness and ease during a long meditation. This modern purpose—youthifying the spine—was first assigned to *asana* practice in the mid-1920s when Kuvalayananda brought hatha yoga into the Western mechanical healing tradition.

At the forefront of the ambitious early 20th-century project to transform the soteriological discipline of hatha yoga into physical culture, Kuvalayananda shrewdly branded yoga as the exercise par excellence for the health of the spine. In his four-part article "The Rationale of Yogic Poses"—the founding document of modern hatha yoga (i.e., modern postural yoga)—published in the July and October 1926 and January and April 1928 issues of *Yoga-Mimansa,* he described the aims of the ideal system of physical culture and then proceeded "to see whether these features are present in the system of Yogic Physical Culture, incidentally introducing comparisons between the Yogic and non-Yogic systems."[16] An ideal system of physical culture ensures the health of the endocrine, circulatory, muscular, and nervous systems, Kuvalayananda pronounced. He singled out the nervous system—which "mainly consists of the brain, twelve pairs of the cranial nerves, the spinal cord and thirty-one pairs of the spinal nerves"—because, he felt, it was under stress as never before.[17]

"Nerve culture," Kuvalayananda contended, "should be the most important feature of an ideal system of body-building" because "nerve culture has become perhaps the most imperative thing for every human being. It is the forward march of our civilization and the consequent changes which have come over our life that are making nerve culture extremely urgent." What are those changes? "The most striking change that has dominated our civilized life is the concentration in big cities. The conditions of city life are almost entirely different from the conditions of village life. The din and bustle of the city . . . [and] the tediously long hours for which the majority of business men are kept to their desks . . . put such a strain upon the human nerves, that nervous diseases are as rapidly developing as the civilization itself!" "The industrial evolution that has revolutionized our life," he bemoaned, places great nervous strain on urban dwellers working in factories and offices and living in "unhealthy and inadequate housing accommodations."[18] Even its touted technological advances, which seem to improve the lot of modern men and women, increase stress on the nerves. For example, the advance in communication (telegraph, telephone, trains, and planes) "that has enabled man to annihilate time and space, has [merely] shifted the strain from the muscle to the nerve!"[19]

"Hence," Kuvalayananda argued, "an ideal system of Physical Culture must make special provision for nerve-building."[20] Yoga is that ideal system. Yoga benefits the nerves—the "fine thread-like or wire-like structures connecting the brain and the spinal cord with the different parts of the body"—through mechanical means: a set of yogic exercises.[21] "Yogic Physical Culture gives exercises principally for the roots of the nerves. It does not, however, neglect their branches. Yoga promotes the health of the nerves by bringing to them a liberal supply of fresh blood and also by automatic message done either by stretching or by the rapid vibrations of the tissues."[22]

In the nerve-building regime that Kuvalayananda proposed, the *asanas* that supply blood are *Sirsasana,* Headstand (to the brain); *Sarvangasana,* Shoulder Stand or what Kuvalayananda called Pan-Physical Pose (to the cervical region of the spine); *Halasana,* Plow Pose, and *Mayurasana,* Peacock Pose (to the thoracic and lumbar regions of the spine); and *Padmasana,* Lotus Pose, and *Paschimottanasana,* Seated Forward Bend (to the lumbar and sacral regions of the spine). The *asanas* that "stretch and bend the spine in different ways and thus give it a sort of massage" are *Halasana* (anterior bending); *Bhujangasana,* Cobra Pose, *Dhanurasana,* Bow Pose, and *Matsyasana,* Fish Pose (posterior bending); and *Ardha-Matsyendrasana,* Half Spinal Twist Pose (left and right twisting).[23]

This regime for the health of the spine is nearly identical to what Kuvalayananda called "A Course of Yogic Physical Culture for the Average Man of Health," consisting of ten *asanas* (as well as two purificatory exercises), which Kuvalayananda had presented one year earlier in the October 1925 *Yoga-Mimansa.* The set of *asanas* in that course of yogic physical culture became the hatha yoga canon (with variations) in the mid-20th century. (This compact *asana* routine was primarily spread by Swami Sivananda—who based his regime on that of S. Sundaram, who, in turn, based his regime on that of Kuvalayananda—and was upended by B. K. S. Iyengar, who promoted a variety of far more expansive routines.)

That the ten yogic postures chosen as the most effective for the course of yogic physical culture are nearly identical to the ten yogic postures that make up the regime for spinal health indicates that the course was specifically designed for maintaining the health of the spine.* Instead of promoting the full panoply of *asanas*—the dozens of available yogic postures—developed through the previous four or five centuries, Kuvalayananda sharply customized the yoga regimen to address a prevalent modern concern: alleviating or preventing back pain. Thusly, modern hatha yoga practice was shaped into a set of exercises for systematically maintaining the integrity of the spine.

Yoga as Preventive Chiropractic

Understanding the tendency for slight spinal misalignments to occur, Kuvalayananda presented *asana* practice as the best means of keeping the spine aligned. But he didn't use this belief to make a critical assessment of chiropractic. It would be the famed Indian bodybuilder K. V. Iyer who, in the early 1940s, would make explicit a yogic critique of chiropractic. First, Iyer expounded the principles of chiropractic: "Many ailments, physical and mental, are caused by interference with nerve impulse."[24] Even heart and other organ diseases are the result of impinged nerves, Iyer contended. Rather than prescribing drugs to cure the organ disease, "the Chiropractic way is to start at the other end; remove the cause of the trouble by removing the impingement on the controlling nerve or nerves" by adjusting displaced vertebrae and spinal deformities.[25]

In his description of chiropractic, Iyer, following Palmer, wildly overstated the effects of impinged nerves on the body and hence the reach of chiropractic. Chiropractic isn't capable of curing disease because diseases aren't caused by dislocated vertebrae. (To be sure, misalignment of vertebrae, with consequent pressure on nerves, does have some far-flung effects, from headaches to fatigue, indigestion, and cold feet. Largely limiting its treatment to repairing various back injuries, contemporary chiropractic has greatly reduced the claims of its scope as medical treatment. And so, it must be said, has contemporary yoga.) Iyer also didn't understand that nerve impingement has many causes, not just misalignment of vertebrae or spinal deformity. But he then rightly pointed out a critical limitation of chiropractic in permanently restoring the health of the spine: "Mechanical adjustment alone is not sufficient in itself." To prevent a reoccurrence of a dislocation of vertebrae, Iyer recommended routinely practicing yoga postures: "When there is marked tendency to spinal curvature and displacement of vertebra [*sic*], many of the simple spine-stretching, spine-bending, spine-twisting exercises . . . will be of immense value."[26]

In giving this advice, Iyer was following Kuvalayananda's teachings from 1931. "If the spinal column is to be maintained in the best of health," Kuvalayananda asserted, "it must be trained to execute all the movements through which it is capable of going. The natural movements of the spine may be of six varieties; forward and backward bents [*sic*], side bents [*sic*] to the right and left, the left twist and the right twist."[27] But Iyer also recognized the critical limitation in Kuvalayananda's protocol for spinal health: yogic stretching exercise alone isn't sufficient in restoring the health of the spine.

---

*Both the course for the average man and the spinal regime were slightly modified in Kuvalayananda's book *Asanas,* published in 1931.

"The adjusted vertebra has always a tendency to slip into its old faulty position," Iyer pointed out, "partly because of going back to the bad old posture of the body, and partly because of the weakness of the muscles of the spine and the back." What's the remedy for weak muscles? "There are many cases of seriously displaced-vertebra and spinal-deformity which need . . . special exercises to strengthen the back and the erector-spinae muscles not to let it subluxate (Slip) [sic] again."[28] To reestablish adequate and permanent health of the spine, Iyer knew, one needs to take up yogic stretching postures supplemented by strengthening exercises. Once the spine is aligned through stretching and strengthening exercises, the alignment must be vigilantly maintained with good posture.

Then Iyer took his criticism of chiropractic one step further: the regular practice of yogic stretching exercises and Western strengthening exercises isn't only remedial; it prevents the occurrence of most back problems. While chiropractic treats the cause of ailments (although not nearly to the extent that Iyer believed), it doesn't prevent them from occurring again and, needless to say, doesn't (wasn't created to) prevent them from occurring in the first place. "One who possesses a normal healthy spine," Iyer asserted, setting his preventive system in contrast to chiropractic, "can maintain it the same way throughout, by the cultivation of proper carriage of the body, and good exercises for the spine and the back."[29]

Order of Postures

"Yoga has reaped the harvest of thousands of years' experience, and nothing is left to chance—the *sequence* of asanas is subject to the most precise ruling," writes André Van Lysebeth, a follower of Sivananda, about Sivananda's renowned "Rishikesh series" (the spelling and nomenclature, but not the italics, are Van Lysebeth's): *Sarvangasana,* Candle; *Halasana,* Plough; *Matsyasana,* Fish; *Pashchimottanasana,* Forward Bend; *Bhujangasana,* Cobra; *Shalabhasana,* Locust; *Dhanurasana,* Bow; *Ardha-Matsyendrasana,* Spinal Twist; and *Shirsasana,* Headstand (see fig. 10.1 on page 134).[30]

This order of *asanas* in a session was discerned, in Van Lysebeth's telling, by "the intuitive genius of the Rishis of former days" and has the same truth as "the conclusions of one of Einstein's equations."[31] Although it can be argued that the order of postures in Sivananda's system is based on a discovery of a law of biomechanics (the principle of reciprocal innervation) already present in nature, the application of this knowledge to yoga (and the discovery itself) certainly wasn't made thousands of years ago; the notion of following a set order of *asanas* was first formulated by Kuvalayananda in 1925.

In his 1931 book *Asanas,* Kuvalayananda presents "A Full Course of Yogic Physical Culture for an Average Man of Health," which presents eleven *asanas* in the same order recommended in the nearly identical original version of the regime in the October 1925 *Yoga-Mimansa.* "In practicing Asanas students will do well to preserve the sequence of the various poses that has been followed . . . here."[32] Those who are starting their training "may pick up the different Asanas in any order he likes, the easiest being taken up first and the more difficult being taken up later on."[33] Any prescription for

CANDLE **SARVĀNGĀSANA**	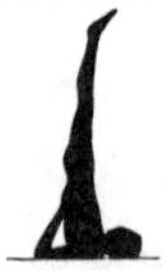	1 MIN.
PLOUGH **HALĀSANA**	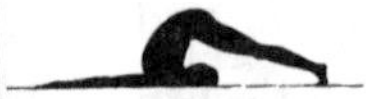	2 MIN. INCLUDING THE DYNAMIC STAGE
FISH **MATSYĀSANA,**	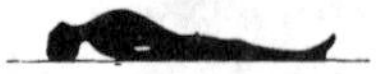	1 MIN.
FORWARD BEND **PASHCHIMOTTĀNĀSANA**	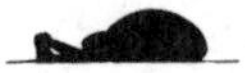	2 MIN. INCLUDING THE DYNAMIC STAGE
COBRA **BHUJANGĀSANA**	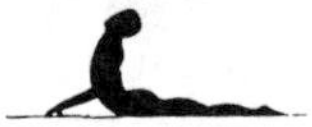	1 MIN. INCLUDING THE DYNAMIC STAGE
LOCUST **SHALABHĀSANA**		1 MIN. INCLUDING THE HALF LOCUST
BOW **DHANURĀSANA**	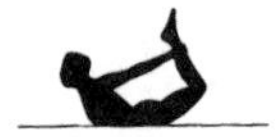	½ MIN.
SPINAL TWIST **ARDHA-MATSYENDRĀSANA**	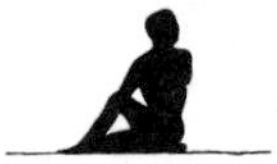	1 MIN.
HEADSTAND **SHĪRSĀSANA**	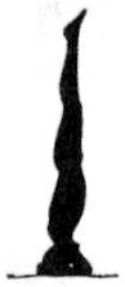	1 to 10 MINS. OR MORE.
UDDIYANA AND/OR NAULI		1 MIN. or 2 MINS.
BREATHING		3 MINS.
SHAVĀSANA RELAXATION		3 MINS.

Figure 10.1. Illustration, "Session of Asanas" (Rishikesh series)

(From *Yoga Self-Taught,* by André Van Lysebeth)

practicing conditioning *asanas* in a particular order is totally absent in all previous hatha yoga texts.

Although Kuvalayananda didn't spell out the principle that underlies his order, a rationale may be discerned in his instructions for *Matsyasana,* Fish Pose, which immediately follow those for *Sarvangasana,* Shoulder Stand (what he called Pan-Physical Pose), found in the very first issue of *Yoga-Mimansa.* In discussing *Matsyasana,* Kuvalayananda argued that "the practice of this pose cannot be neglected if one wants to reap the full benefits of the Sarvangasana." "The pose is antagonistic to [which means to say, "cooperates with"!] the Pan-Physical Pose," he explained, "at least as far as the cervical and upper dorsal regions are concerned." He advised that when *Matsyasana* is "undertaken as a complement of the Pan-Physical Pose," it should be held for

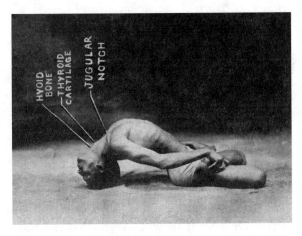

Figure 10.2. "Matsyasana or the Fish-Pose (Side View)"
(From *Yoga-Mimansa*, vol. 1, no. 1 [1924])

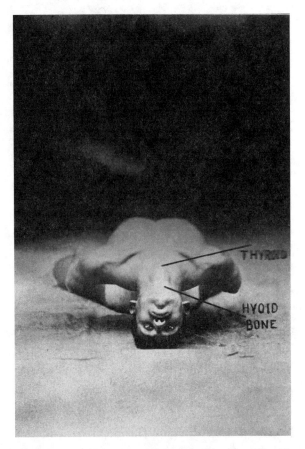

Figure 10.3. "Matsyasana or The Fish-Pose (Front View)"
(From *Yoga-Mimansa*, vol. 1, no. 1 [1924])

about a third of the length of time devoted to the main pose.[34]

This protocol of engaging muscles on opposite sides of the cervical and thoracic joints with complementary poses is implicitly based on the principle of reciprocal innervation: when muscles (called agonists) shorten, or contract, the muscles located on the opposite side of the joint (called antagonists) elongate, or relax. In pairing up yogic postures with opposing (agonist and antagonist) muscle groups, Kuvalayananda recognized the need for maintaining the proper resting length (neither too short nor too long) of the opposing muscle groups. The shortening of the cervical and thoracic muscles caused by the Shoulder Stand is alleviated by the lengthening of these muscles through the Fish Pose, thereby ensuring a balanced musculature (figs. 10.2 and 10.3).

Sundaram greatly expanded on this implicit rationale by describing the biomechanical reasons for performing *Matsyasana* immediately after *Sarvangasana:* "to relieve a certain crampiness and stiffness in the neck and shoulders,"

to open up the chest, and to tone the posterior muscles of the neck and shoulders. He singled out the reason for performing these two opposing postures in their effect on the neck: "The bending of the neck in opposite directions by a practice of these poses, gives an unexampled tone to the nerves and muscles of the neck."[35] (He also added two physiological reasons for balancing these two postures: to increase blood circulation to the thyroid and parathyroid glands and to facilitate "very deep breathing."[36])

About twenty years later, Sivananda, in the Rishikesh series (his adaptation of Sundaram's routine), would make explicit Kuvalayananda's rationale for performing the Fish Pose after performing the Shoulder Stand and its application to the order of the entire yoga regime. Van Lysebeth explains: "Within a series each posture falls into place, completing or accentuating the previous one, preparing for the next one or acting as a counter-posture to balance another."[37] This is an ingenious order, pleasing in its logic and largely and soundly based on the principle of reciprocal innervation. As one posture unfolds from the other, the muscles of the skeleton—especially those of the spine—are alternately compressed and released, leaving them at their optimal resting length.

Thus the necessity for practicing *asanas* in a particular order (basically defined by a measured unfolding of complementary pairs of *asanas*)—and, hence, the very rhythm of the popular hatha yoga class in mid-20th century—was firmly established (until it was subverted later in the century by the popularity of the arrhythmic system of Iyengar and the dynamically rhythmic system of Pattabhi Jois).

Kuvalayananda-Style Class

"One of the most sacred duties that the As'rama has to perform is giving free instruction in Yogic culture to outsiders," Kuvalayananda announced. "There are a number of people anxious to develop along Yogic lines, if they could do so without being required to give up their vocation." All people, he said, were welcome to attend classes at Kaivalyadhama "whenever they find spare time."[38] Almost all of the visitors to Kuvalayananda's ashram came from afar and so had to make arrangements for boarding and lodging in the neighborhood. They were

screened by Kuvalayananda, who, always hard pressed for time, limited interviews to fifteen minutes. One of these early visitors was the Russian-born wife of the commercial attaché to the Czechoslovak Consulate in Bombay, Indra Devi, who would become instrumental in popularizing yoga in America in the 1950s and 1960s.

At the suggestion of Prince Mussoorie, the brother of Devi's friend Princess Bhuban of Nepal, Devi went to what she called the Kaivalyadhama Yogic Health Center in 1937 (or possibly 1936) to learn yoga. After her interview with Kuvalayananda, she was examined by a doctor. He suggested to her that she attend the women's class the next day one hour after breakfast or in the afternoon two or three hours after lunch. (Evidently there were no set times for classes.) The class was held in a medium-sized room with a matted floor. At the doctor's suggestion, Devi wore a sari (but later switched to shorts, which were more comfortable).

The actual classroom instruction—seemingly in defiance of the structured regime (in which a sequence of *asanas* is maintained) described in Kuvalayananda's articles and book—was, from appearances alone, desultory but perhaps was undergirded by the principle that each student should be allowed to master the poses at her own pace. When Devi arrived the first day, several women were already present, each doing a different yogic posture. The female instructor invited Devi to sit on the floor next to her and showed Devi how to do deep rhythmic breathing. Then the instructor showed Devi a chart with illustrations of yogic exercises. She asked Devi to assume three of the poses (the spelling and nomenclature are Devi's): the Stretching, the Reverse, and the Plough (respectively, *Paschimottanasana*, Seated Forward Bend, *Sarvangasana*, Shoulder Stand, and *Halasana*, Plow Pose). Devi couldn't correctly perform the poses because she was too stiff. The next class she asked a fellow student to press against her back so she could reach her toes in *Paschimottanasana*. The teacher forbid this, cautioning Devi that forcing the pose might result in an injury. She assured Devi that she would be able to do all the poses in time. "Which will probably be in my next incarnation!" a disheartened Devi exclaimed.[39] Devi was just beginning to make progress when she had to leave Lonavla in order to return with her husband to Prague.

Although the yoga sessions taught by Kuvalayananda teachers in the 1920s and 1930s would certainly be recognizable to us today, they would seem fussy, cramped, and pinched. Focusing on the internal organs, the selected *asanas* weren't expansive and dynamic; they didn't allow for easeful or free movement. Students in Kuvalayananda's classes performed *asanas* that were thought to mechanically affect internal organs, either by applying pressure (forward bends, side bends, twists, chin locks, and abdominal contractions) or by relieving pressure (backbends and inversions). These yogic postures, it was said, massage, stimulate, reposition, or relax internal organs to provide good health. This new take on hatha yoga—yoga as health cure—was epitomized by *Sarvangasana*, Shoulder Stand, exalted as the Queen of Exercises because it was said to stimulate the thyroid gland through reversed blood flow and the chin lock.

Whereas Kuvalayananda teachers told students to literally turn their attention inward—to the physiological workings of the body—contemporary yoga teachers, in contrast, instruct their students to be attentive to the shape and structure of the body—to the bones, muscles, and joints. They place emphasis on extending, or "opening," joints, on expansiveness and movement. A class might be typified by *Virabhadrasana* II, Warrior II, which is performed by standing in *Tadasana*, Mountain Pose, jumping the feet apart, extending the arms, turning the feet as in *Trikonasana*, Triangle Pose, bending the right knee, moving the left shoulder slightly back, opening the chest, tucking the buttocks under, keeping the left groin moving back, and keeping the left leg straight—the posture of a warrior dancer.

Awakening the Spine

Kuvalayananda introduced into the centuries-old practice of yogic conditioning *asanas* a modern rationale: maintaining the flexibility of the spine to prevent disease. In so doing, he reframed yoga as a system of mechanical maintenance based on the principle that the body is made up of an interrelated system of tangible parts—bones, aided by connective tissue, acting as pulleys, levers, hinges, and plates—that may become stiff through insufficient use or misaligned by stress and tension and, therefore, require daily upkeep. In this way, Kuvalayananda made hatha yoga into a teacher-taught or self-applied preventive chiropractic.

Kuvalayananda's emphasis on yoga's capacity for comprehensive spinal movement to provide health for the nerves led to the touting of yoga as the exercise par excellence for the fitness of the spine—defined as the ability to satisfactorily perform common muscle and joint work of the spine. If we don't put effort into maintaining the flexibility of the spine as we get older, yoga teachers came to correctly point out, its joints, like all synovial joints, become more rigid: the less a synovial joint is moved, the more its joint capsule shrinks and stiffens, reducing range of motion.

Defining yoga as the definitive exercise for conditioning the spine led to the focus of some contemporary yoga classes on creating balance, lightness, extension, and spaciousness of the trunk and limbs (often while retaining special attention on the alignment, stability, and mobility of the spine). This aesthetic element was first added to yoga by T. Krishnamacharya and was further developed by his students Iyengar and Jois. Iyengar's manual *Light on Yoga* (published in 1966) and his demonstrations "created in the Western public an awareness of the . . . artistic potential of postural practice," observes modern yoga scholar Elizabeth De Michelis. "These developments opened up spaces for the aesthetic appreciation of *asanas,* something quite novel in the field of yoga."[40] An Iyengar-style class showcases the elegance, verve, and drama of assuming *asanas,* and a Pattabhi Jois *vinyasa*-style class showcases the grace, flow, and exhilaration of performing *asanas* mixed with *surya namaskar.*

This emphasis on pleasing and dynamic yogic postures, in turn, has led some yoga practitioners to inhabit their body as a means of accessing the spiritual. Rather than viewing their yoga practice as utilitarian (Practice yoga to ensure good health and a long life) or aesthetic (Practice yoga to achieve beauty), they use their *asana* practice as a vehicle for transcendence.

In her book *Awakening the Spine,* Vanda Scaravelli advocates accompanying each pose with rhythmic breathing and, during the exhalation, elongating the spine without effort. "We learn to elongate and extend, rather than to pull and push." As a result, "an unexpected opening follows, an opening from within us, giving life to the spine, as though the body had to reverse and awaken into another dimension."[41] Today we yogins can engage in this transcendent act—channeling the energy of the spine in order to experience the universe as the concrete manifestation of divine energy (from which the universe was formed)—during moving *asanas* because Kuvalayananda incorporated a concern for the health of the spine into the practice of yogic conditioning postures in the 1920s.

Coda

Kuvalayananda meditated every day after his morning bath. Seated in a quiet corner, he withdrew his senses from the objects of the world by closing his eyes, which facilitated the arousal of an internal visual sensation, a blue light, on which he concentrated (fig. 10.4). The rest of his day, though, wasn't spent perfecting his spiritual practice—or, at least, perfecting it in isolation from the world. The overarching goal of his life was to instigate and ensure the success of India's revival by making yoga modern: "The As'rama is trying to bring Yoga in correlation with the present-day culture by attempting a scientific interpretation of its truths."[42]

Toward this end, Kuvalayananda conducted research on the therapeutical (health) aspects of hatha yoga. Under his supervision, *asanas, bandhas, mudras, kriyas,* and *pranayamas* were

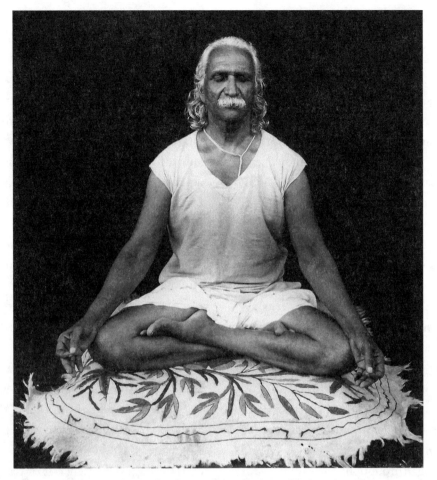

Figure 10.4. Swami Kuvalayananda sitting in meditation, circa 1960
(With the kind permission of Kaivalyadhama Yoga Institute)

subjected to laboratory experiments, using chemicals, microscopes, X-rays, and other means. He planned and conducted these experiments, analyzed the resultant data, and made scientific connections previously unproven or unobserved. Or so it appeared. His claims for the beneficial effects of yoga on health were largely inflated. But his prescriptions for yoga as fitness were inspired.

Although yoga practices don't have a rehabilitative effect on the body's physiological systems (or, at least, the practices haven't been convincingly shown to prevent, alleviate, or cure diseases that don't have neuromuscular involvement), and they don't have an ability to develop strength (through resisting progressively greater weight loads at a high intensity) or improve aerobic capacity (through controlling heart rate, respiration, or metabolism), hatha yoga's capacity to make the musculoskeletal system more flexible and aligned excels. In taking up yoga, people around the world have discovered a way to alleviate lower back pain and joint stiffness and facilitate standing tall. The first to recognize yoga's matchless salutary effect in these areas, Kuvalayananda customized the hatha yoga routine to maximize its effectiveness in providing critical elements of musculoskeletal fitness.

Although his claims for yoga were a mixed bag, Kuvalayananda's dream of transforming hatha yoga into a widely practiced physical exercise in India was an unambiguous success. Kuvalayananda strongly advocated making physical education an integral part of general education and making yogic physical culture the center of physical education. He dedicated himself to this cause out of a motivation to render public service to the nation, but the impetus also arose from a strong conviction that he owed a dept of gratitude to Professor Manikrao, whom he revered as his guru in physical education and as his caring father figure. Kuvalayananda was convinced that the only way to discharge this debt was through promoting his mentor's cause. Through *Yoga-Mimansa,* Kuvalayananda popularized yoga throughout the provinces. As a result, various educational institutions sought his help in organizing physical culture courses based on yoga.

Kuvalayananda's most lasting influence, though, was on making yoga acceptable as exercise for middle-class adults, and then to all Indians. They took up yoga in small groups in commercial settings and individually in their homes. In spreading yogic physical culture and therapeutics in India, Kuvalayananda succeeded in uplifting his people and in gaining respect from the West for India's ancient achievements made modern. And he helped make yoga available to all peoples around the world.

❦

In early December 1965, the eighty-two-year-old Kuvalayananda had a heart attack. While recuperating in bed at his own Ishwardas Chunilal Yogic Health Centre Kaivalyadhama in Mumbai, he wrote an upbeat and chatty letter to his anxious *shishya* and proud subject of many of the scientific experiments at the ashram, Manohar L. Gharote, to put him at ease. "There should be no worry about me. I feel confident that I shall have no more heart-attacks hereafter. Please accept my congratulations for the highest scored marks that you have secured in your last examination. . . . It pleased me very much to see that you will be coming to Lonavla during the next X'mas holidays."[43]

After his bed rest, Kuvalayananda was allowed by his doctor to move about but not to exert himself. He was ordered to walk slowly and climb stairs step by step. He wrote Gharote to reassure him once again. "One thing is certain. I am definitely out of danger and making satisfactory progress in my health. So there should be no worry about me."[44] On April 18, 1966, after a second heart attack, Swami Kuvalayananda, in the words of his biographers, Gharote and his son Manmath, made his "journey to the great beyond."[45]

Kuvalayananda considered the needs of others until the end. But he couldn't have built Kaivalyadhama and his other institutions without being firm of purpose. He made it clear to his workers that he didn't consider his unflagging activities to be a sacrifice for the sake of the mission of propagating yoga but simply a duty that he had chosen—and that he wished them to feel the same. "His manner was modest and unassuming," remarked Arthur Koestler, the writer best known for his novel *Darkness at Noon*, "yet impressive in its gentle authority—a particular mixture shared by so many Indians, from Gandhi downward."[46]

Reflecting on Kuvalayananda's character, Manmath M. Gharote holds that "those who are selected by Almighty for the Noble cause [of dedicating their lives to others] had to suffer in their lives." While the experience of suffering may be a precondition to dedicating one's life to others, having endured suffering doesn't inevitably lead to benevolent behavior. In the case of Yogendra, the despondency of his troubled early years (which he never examined and overcame or had soothed by a mentor) led, in part, to his delusional resentment directed at Kuvalayananda—an assigning of blame to Kuvalayananda for Yogendra's failures. Although he would get married and have a loving family, he remained ill-tempered and self-centered his entire life. In contrast, out of the loneliness and distress that Kuvalayananda suffered, as Gharote points out, "*karuna* (compassion) arose."[47] By becoming detached from—not slave to—his own suffering, the genial Kuvalayananda, a *brahmachari* (celibate), spent his life in service to others. His primary means of achieving union with the Supreme Universal Soul was through selfless action.

11

K. V. IYER

Mixing Bodybuilding and Yoga

Muscle Cult

In 1922 twenty-four-year-old Kolar Venkatesha Iyer (1898–1980) founded the Hercules Gymnasium in Bangalore, the first commercial Western-style gymnasium in India. It consisted of one small room, available after working hours, in the headquarters of the Mysore Troop of Boy Scouts (established by the maharajah of Mysore, Shri Nalvadi Krishnaraja Wadiyar, in 1909), attached to the rear of Tipu Sultan's summer palace (long owned by the state), an ornate, two-storied, Indo-Islamic structure made of wood, with pillars, arches, and balconies. At first there were only four students. They trained with Iyer not so they could boast of their great strength, enter competitive weight-lifting contests, or excel at sports; they sought, instead, to develop a harmonious, muscular physique, as well as to attain good health and more than adequate strength.

Classes were held six days a week at 5:30 p.m. Every Saturday evening, after finishing their exercises, Iyer and his students bathed and put on clean clothes in preparation for *puja* (a form of ritual worship). Iyer conducted *bhakti* (devotion) to invite the blessings of Hanuman, the deity whose portrait sat on a table covered with an altar cloth. (Hanuman, the mighty Monkey God, is revered by gym enthusiasts, including bodybuilders and wrestlers, not so much for his traditional role as faithful servant to Rama but as the giver of strength.) Accompanied by Iyer's harmonium playing, the worshippers sang *bhajans* (devotional songs, especially those of Tiger Varadachar, a composer and singer). Afterward, they offered food and incense to Hanuman, passed their hands three times through a camphor flame, and lightly touched their eyes with sanctified water cupped in their right hands, drank the water, distributed *prasad* (the offered food that had become sanctified), and sat for meditation.

Unlike the discus thrower's or blacksmith's bodily makeup, Iyer's muscular physique wasn't formed as a by-product of some physical task; it was an artificial physique that Iyer designed, as if he were chiseling a stone sculpture, to be pleasing in appearance. Although bodybuilding as an aesthetic endeavor—the urge to transform the human body, the very size and shape of it, into (something like) a work of art—didn't begin until the 19th century (the term "bodybuilding" was coined by Robert Jeffries Roberts in 1881 to describe the workout that he'd devised as director of the Boston YMCA), Iyer validated his pursuit of physical beauty as a continuation of "the ideals of perfect beauty of figure" formulated by ancient Greeks and embodied in their statues, made familiar to people of the early 20th century, including Iyer, mostly through photos of the Greek statues, or, more accurately, photos of Roman copies of the Greek statues. "These ancient classical statues," he declared in "The Beauties of a Symmetrical Body," an article he published in the June 1927 issue of *Vyayam,* an Indian physical culture magazine, "have given us models to admire, learn from and even to imitate."[1] Following the fashion of the times created by Western bodybuilders, Iyer posed as an actual or seeming Greek statue for many of his publicity and illustration photos (see fig. 11.1 on page 144). For the first photo caption in his gallery of self-portraits in his 1936 pamphlet *Perfect Physique,* he selected these words of praise to burnish his reputation and, in effect, define his essence: "'The living ideal of ancient Grecian Manhood,' writes Carl Easton Williams, Editor of Physical Culture, a Bernard Mc Fadden [*sic*] Publication."[2]

Iyer also positioned his pursuit of beauty in the context of ancient India. During the Gupta period (3rd to 6th centuries), considered the classical artistic and scientific peak of Indian culture, instructional manuals, called *Shilpa Shastra* or *Vastu Shastra,* were created by Brahmin priests and *shilpin* (master sculptors) for holy pictures, carvings, and statues. Iconometric rules for the presentation of the major gods included, for example, exact measurements for the width of the shoulders and waist and the depth of the chest. For six years, "through sheer physical culture," Iyer recollected, he sculpted his body to bring it into accord with "the ideal proportions of the *Silpi Shastra,*" producing a body "identical, limb to limb and inch to inch, with the same."[3]

In the October 1927 issue of *Strength,* a magazine devoted to weightlifting, bodybuilding, and fitness, editor-in-chief Mark Berry, who would become Iyer's biggest booster over the next six years, introduced his readers to Iyer with a photo of Iyer displaying his broad back muscles ("One of the finest poses we have ever had the pleasure to present to our readers").[4] Berry described Iyer as an "example of the ambitious youth who worked hard with his mind set on physical perfection; that he has achieved it, can hardly be denied, though he may not consider such to be the case, being an Indian idealist."[5] Berry was mistaken about Iyer's modesty. Just a few months earlier Iyer had proclaimed (as perhaps only a young man could or would)

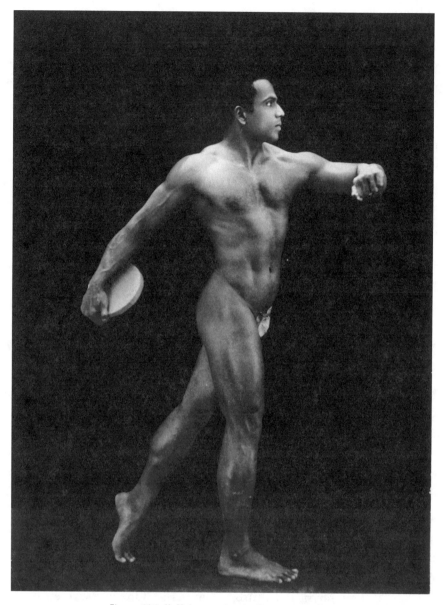

Figure 11.1. K. V. Iyer posing in the manner of a
Greek statue of a discus thrower, 1930s
(With the kind permission of Michael Murphy)

his pride in possessing "a body which Gods covet."[6] Although the desire of the gods cannot be affirmed, from all accounts it can be said with some certainty that Iyer was entirely justified in his claim to the title of "India's most perfectly developed man."[7]

What made Iyer "perfectly developed" was his muscular symmetry and its effect on his carriage. Only a muscular body with pleasing proportions, he argued, could radiate "ease, grace and poise."[8] For this reason, he abhorred the kind of body developed by the *vyayam,* the centuries-old Indian system of physical training practiced in the service of wrestling (and feats of strength). As in Japan, wrestling is a way of life in India. It's been practiced since ancient times, probably then, as now, as more of a dueling art than a military combat art. Anthropologist Joseph S. Alter fruitfully explains *vyayam* through its relationship to yoga: "As with yoga, a key concept in vyayam is the holistic, regulated control of the body. In yoga, however, the body is manipulated through the practice of relatively static postures. Vyayam disciplines the body through strenuous, patterned, repetitive movement."[9]

Vyayam exercises fall into two categories. The first is exercises to develop explosive movement, agility, and stamina. These include *dands* (something like push-ups) and *bethaks* (squats), which are performed together. The second is exercises to build strength and muscle bulk. These include swinging *sumtolas* ("Indian barbells") and *korelas, joris,* and *gadas* (types of heavy clubs) and lifting *nals* (stone weights) and *gar nals* (stone wheels). The body that's formed from the strengthening exercises is hardly like that of a Greek statue or a god. "It pains me awfully to look at a modern wrestler," Iyer lamented. "One in fifty does not possess a symmetrical build. These wrestlers devote themselves *only* to increase the bulk of their flesh."[10] While they aid wrestling, *vyayam* strengthening exercises, he realized, aren't effective for bodybuilding because they aren't based on scientific principles.

To achieve symmetry, Iyer turned to Western means of muscle development, primarily bell exercises practiced according to Sandow's three principles of bodybuilding: selectivity, progression, and high intensity.* Selectivity is choosing particular resistance exercises to target muscle groups. For example, straightening bent arms to target the triceps; pulling the arms down and/or back to target the latissimus dorsi (lats); and curling the trunk up to target the abdominals (abs). Progression is increasing muscle growth by gradually adding more weight resistance. High intensity is lifting an amount of overload much heavier than we're used to.

Iyer well recognized that these scientific principles could be misapplied. He found repugnant not only wrestlers who ignore the scientific principles of muscle development but also bodybuilders who use heavy weight lifting to develop a massive musculature: "While exercising one should bear in his mind that he is performing [the exercises] to acquire a good build, a sound and healthy body with ample strength. The desire for only big bulging biceps might mar the symmetry of the body and make him knotty and abnormal."[11] Even worse, "heavy weight lifting . . . when applied unscientifically . . . often results in rupture, heart strain, [and] nervous break down, [as well as] in an ugly unsymmetrical body."[12]

Through introducing and promoting bodybuilding to the average man in the 1920s and 1930s, Iyer helped popularize the Sandowian image of modern male beauty in India, nurturing an avidity for transforming the body among Indians to match the zeal of the ancient Greeks. How thrilling it must've been to be a part of

---

*Iyer also practiced and taught Maxalding, the muscle control system developed by Maxick and Monte Saldo based on the isometric contraction of muscles in isolation. Practitioners will a muscle to contract (without moving a bony segment), hold the contraction, and then relax the muscle.

the gathering of men in the various incarnations of Iyer's gymnasiums (from the early 1920s to the mid-1930s, Iyer moved to bigger spaces to accommodate his growing membership) who were involved in this new project to perfect their bodies!

Reconciliation of Muscle Cult and Hata-Yoga Cult

Along with his fervor for conferring physical perfection on his countrymen, Iyer was equally dedicated to improving their fitness and health. He was concerned with imparting not just the ability to do daily physical activities with a minimum of fatigue but also the capacity to ward off chronic disease, "to remain active to a ripe old age."[13] He bemoaned the then current concept of wellness:

> The attitude of the physician towards health seems to be to classify all people under two heads—the sick and the well. If actual disease is not present, the individual is classed as well. But there are degrees of health, just as there are degrees of humidity and temperature. One person may have excellent health, another fair health, and still another poor health, yet none of these would be classified as sick from the view-point of the physician. One may be organically sound, in that, no defect could be found in any organ or tissue of the body: and yet he may not be a robust healthy individual.[14]

Iyer described the manifestations of robust health by comparing it to the symptoms of poor health:

> A person in poor physical condition is easily exhausted by mental and physical exertion; he is irritable, likely to have morbid thoughts, petty ailments, and low morale; he may have a sallow complexion and dull eyes; and he frequently complains of constipation, head-ache, nervousness and insomnia. On the other hand, it is equally common to observe in a man of good physical condition, evidences of mental and bodily vigour such as alertness, cheerfulness, high morale, bright eyes, elastic step, healthy complexion, and capacity for arduous mental and physical work.[15]

How is one to obtain this "mental and bodily vigour"? According to Iyer, it could only be accomplished by complementing bodybuilding with the health-building aspects of hatha yoga: *asana* (consisting of conditioning postures, as opposed to the postures suitable for prolonged immobility), *pranayama* (consisting of breathing exercises), *kriya* (consisting of cleansing techniques), *mudra* (consisting of seals), *bandha* (consisting of locks), and diet. He proclaimed:

> The dissimilarity between Hata-yoga Cult and the Western Cult of Body-building lies in the very goal that these two systems aim to achieve. Longevity of life—a life healthy and free from ailments functional and organic, to fit the individual human unit to fulfil his obligations to himself, his home and the society he is a part of, succinctly sums up what Hata-yoga imparts to the worldly man.
>
> Europe—ancient, mediéval and modern—in her Cult of the human body, has ever been aiming at the symmetry, bulk and strength in the developed man.[16]

Iyer was the first practitioner of physical culture to combine the "Cult of Body-building" and the "Hata-yoga Cult." "My aim in My System," he declared in 1930 in his manifesto *Muscle Cult—A Pro-em to My System,* "is to reconcile these two great systems to assure the future Culturist of robustness of health and beauty of limb and trunk."[17]

Iyer brokered this reconciliation in a period of great agitation, recollected in a kaleidoscopic rush of words: "Born of early motherhood, puny boyhood, Sandow's pictures, earnest emulation, unguided headlong rush into spring-bells and cold-baths, small reward of sprouting muscles and stern reprisals of recurring colds and fevers, a depressing period of no gain in bulk or strength,—a baffled mind steeped in Western Physical Culture turns to Hata-yoga, India's heritage—blending of the two systems."[18] The result of this febrile revelation was newfound good health and a fine physique. Having created his own system (although he modestly wrote, "I have invented no system of my own" but just made an "experience-guided selection" from other systems), Iyer would then turn to initiating others into it.

"It is absolutely necessary," he advised prospective bodybuilders, "that all those who are ambitious of a beautiful and symmetrical body, combined with the highest efficiency of strength and endurance, should tone up their everlasting health, by developing the internal muscular organs of the body, and their functionings, through proper Yogic Asanas first, and thus overcome once and for all times, all functional defects, to restore the body in every part."[19]

It turns out that Iyer was largely mistaken about the benefits of hatha yoga. While providing a degree of good health, hatha yoga practices don't promote the abundant good health that he believed. However, *asana* practice does provide superb flexibility, as well as grace. Which is why *asana* imparts just as much beauty of limb and trunk as does bodybuilding. He was largely correct, though, about the benefits and limitations of bodybuilding. Bodybuilding provides "symmetry, bulk and strength." It doesn't impart "longevity of life," although it does have some health benefits.

Around 1940, after he'd become India's most famous bodybuilder and the owner of India's largest and most successful gymnasium, Iyer came to feel that he'd overemphasized the value of attaining "the beauties of a symmetrical body." In his 1943 book *Chemical Changes in Physical Exercise,* he not only warned again against developing large muscles for a showy physique, with the attendant "pitfall of overstrain," but seems to have abandoned bodybuilding (weight-resistance training with the goal of developing a well-proportioned musculature with large, well-defined muscles) altogether. Instead, he promoted strength training (he used the term "physical training") as a means of providing good health to the internal organs, especially those of the circulatory and respiratory systems.[20] In actuality, strength training, like yogasana (the practice of yogic postures to maintain or improve fitness and health), has little effect on maintaining good health or improving poor health. It primarily provides a key aspect of fitness: the strength to perform everyday activities involving lifting, lowering, pulling, and pushing with ease

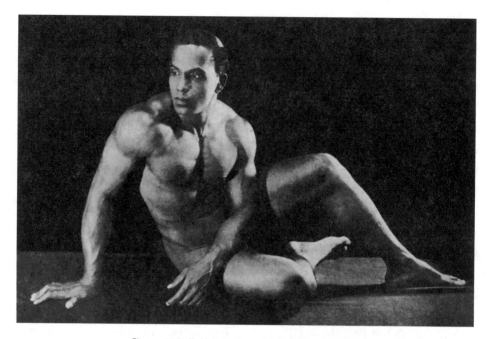

Figure 11.2. K. V. Iyer, "In a Pensive Mood," 1936
(From *Perfect Physique,* by K. V. Iyer)

(yogasana provides the flexibility to perform everyday activities involving bending forward, backward, and sideways and twisting with ease).

Not that Iyer didn't recognize the fitness benefits of strength training. It makes us "fit enough to accomplish each day's work with minimum fatigue and to remain active to a ripe old age," he wrote.[21] He provided training guidelines accordingly. "Hence, it is advisable to exercise each muscle or group of muscles separately."[22] "For "strenuous exercise, . . . exercise the extremeties [*sic*] of the body one day and the torso the next day." "If graded exercise is taken day after day, the load of work may be gradually increased and, finally, that which formerly was a heavy load is comfortably carried."[23] Fatigue is determined in part by "habits of muscular use. . . . And so, exercises that have rhythm of movement, tempo of breathing, and harmony of co-operation of the

motor nervous system are a potent factor in preventing fatigue."[24]

Like Sandow, Iyer drew heavily on photography to promote his system. As art historian Tamar Garb observes in *Bodies of Modernity,* her exploration of the representation of masculinity and feminity in the late 19th century, photography was an especially felicitous medium for making the connection between modern and ancient Greek muscle cult: "It was the newest of pictorial media, photography, which became an important vehicle through which modern endeavours could establish their links with an ancient and noble past. The modern body-building or 'physical culture' movement, as it was then called, depended on photography for its publicity and for propagating an image of ideal masculinity based on ancient prototypes."[25]

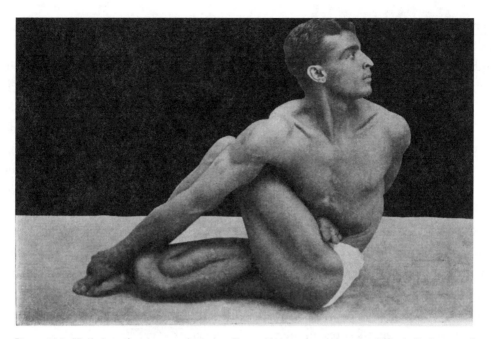

Figure 11.3. "T. K. Ananthanarayana depicting 'Purna Matsyendrasan,' a very difficult Yogic pose of great chiropractic value. He is now an adept and a finished pupil of Yogic School of Physical Culture," 1936

(From *Perfect Physique*)

To promote the three-month correspondence course for his Correspondence School of Physical Culture, founded in 1928, Iyer created a booklet, *Muscle Cult—A Pro-em to My System,* in 1930, which was replaced in 1936 by a more polished version, *Perfect Physique—A Proem to My System*. The booklets contain a plenitude of photographs of men (some beefed up, but others quite trim, even slight) showing off their muscular development. (None of them are doing exercises; they're all posing.) The front of the booklets contains a gallery of photographs of Iyer (taken by Iyer, who was an avid photographer). He's naked, or nearly so, dramatically lit to emphasize the chiaroscuro of his musculature, and often posed like a Greek statue of an athlete. But it's the casual poses, the ones with Iyer in repose, that catch our eye: they both startle us and draw us in with their seeming intimacy and candidness. On of them, entitled "In a Pensive Mood," shows Iyer sitting on the floor, looking off contemplatively (fig. 11.2).

Iyer used photographs to link not only modern and ancient muscle cult but also bodybuilding and yogasana, two disciplines ordinarily opposed in people's minds. Included in *Perfect Physique* is a photograph of a student performing a seated twisting yoga pose cited in the *Hatha Yoga Pradipika*. The caption reads: "T. K. Ananthanarayana depicting 'Purna Matsyendrasan,' a very difficult Yogic pose of great chiropractic value" (fig. 11.3).[26] *Muscle Cult* contains photographs of a student demonstrating yogic purificatory exercises of the abdominal region. A single caption reads: "S. Sundaram. An exponent of Hata-Yoga performing '*Uddiyana* and *Nauli*.'"[27] Although he includes many more muscle cult than hatha yoga cult photographs, by placing the photographs from the two disciplines side by side—or, perhaps better said, by dropping the hatha yoga cult photographs into the middle of the muscle cult photographs—Iyer was showing that they make up one capacious exercise system.

Legacy

When he was a teenager in the early 1930s, Jack La Lanne (or LaLanne, as his name is often spelled), who would become a famous American fitness expert and bodybuilder best known for his prodigious feats of strength and his long-running (1953–1985) television show, "began to see stories and pictures in magazines about a Hindu physical culturist named K. V. Iyer. He was not a 'strong man' in the classic sense of being able to perform great feats of strength," La Lanne recalled in 1973. "But he was a perfect physical specimen, with a muscular and fully developed body that I, skinny Jack La Lanne, envied."[28] After realizing that he and Iyer had the same slight build (their height and bone structure were nearly the same), La Lanne made Iyer his model for changing his body, which means to say, for changing his life. Although Iyer "lived on the opposite of the world," La Lanne wrote, "he became my inspiration."[29] Following Iyer's recommendations for weight-resistance exercises, La Lanne worked out, "taking my own measurements, always aiming toward the dimensions of K. V. Iyer," until a few years later he finally achieved a physique like Iyer's.[30]

But more compelling praise for Iyer came from an unsolicited testimonial made by a correspondence school student, Ooi Tiang Guan, from Penang, Malaysia, on June 6, 1929, published in *Muscle Cult:* "I have now come to the last lesson. I can honestly say that your course is the best, because it is not mere muscle culture. The internal organs too are strengthened and nerves are toned up. It unfolds to me the precious and vital secrets of life 'The Yogic Culture' which accounts for the long and healthy lives of the Indian Sages."[31] Ooi understood what La Lanne didn't: that Iyer's full teachings were groundbreaking, and what made them so was that Iyer wasn't merely a bodybuilder but, in Berry's words, "a professional physical culturist, teaching modern methods of progressive [weight-resistance] exercise, combined with the science of yoga."[32]

Iyer was the ideal person to implement this merger of Western and Eastern physical culture. By upbringing and inclination, he was cosmopolitan (without ever having left India), yet steeped in his own traditions. Moreover, he had a conciliatory temperament: for him, there was no conflict between muscle cult and hatha yoga cult. They simply complemented each other.

In this conviction, Iyer was far more sensible and ecumenical than the oft-intolerant contemporary hatha yogins who feel that they're upholding the purity of the yoga tradition when they reject other forms of exercise. They're ignorant of their own history. Two of the yogins who created modern hatha yoga, Kuvalayananda and Sundaram, approved performing both yogasana and strength training. Kuvalayananda recommended waiting twenty minutes between the exercises: "Those that want to finish their exercises with a balance introduced into their system, should take the Yogic exercises last. But those that want to have a spirit of exhilaration at the end, should finish with the muscular exercises."[33] Sundaram recommended doing the exercises at opposite times of the day: "If the Yogic system is practiced in the mornings, the Muscular exercises ought to be done in the evenings and vice versa. The former works up the internal organs and attracts greater blood to them: while the latter do the same thing for the superficial body."[34] But Kuvalayananda and Sundaram didn't integrate the two disciplines into one system.

Iyer's legacy is in having brought muscle cult and hatha yoga cult together into one workout: the understated muscularity and strength of intense strength training complemented by the graceful suppleness and flexibility of a dedicated yogasana practice. An Indian enthralled with the bodybuilding systems of Europeans, yet proud of and indebted to the centuries-old Indian practice of hatha yoga, Iyer forged a dynamic West-meets-East physical exercise system, in which movements to resist opposing forces are coupled with movements to surrender to opposing forces.

12

S. SUNDARAM

Publishing a Yoga Manual

Demonstrations and Lectures

When traveling to hold exhibitions of muscle cult for the Indian populace in the 1920s, famed bodybuilder K. V. Iyer brought along with him Seetharaman Sundaram (1901–1994) to perform yogasanas (yogic postures practiced to maintain or improve fitness and health). "I had to go with Professor K. V. Iyer on Physical Culture tours through the Mysore Province and Madras," recalled Sundaram, seeming to express some reluctance for what turned out to be an immensely rewarding experience. "Welcome opportunities came to me for delivering many lectures and demonstrations of Yoga-Asanas. The inventions of the Rishis were much appreciated by the public, consisting of elderly people and students of various ages."[1]

Sundaram's proficient displays of *asanas,* executed with "his nimble rubber-body," and eloquent and erudite talks about the health benefits of *asana* practice wowed his audiences, for whom being exposed to a yogin proselytizing about yoga physical culture was a novelty.[2] "Sir! Are you a medico?" shouted a member of the surging crowd that surrounded him after a discourse on yogic healing in a *pandal* (a temporary structure) put up for the Youth Congress, a "sideshow" to the 1927 Indian National Congress session held in Madras.* "What

---

*In 1888 the Indian National Congress became the first organized political body on a national level to be accepted by the British. Although the seventy-two representatives who met at the first session belonged solely to the English-educated Indian middle class (comprising technicians, doctors, lawyers, professors, journalists, managers, clerks, and others), they served all classes of India. (The 474 delegates who attended the second session came from a wide range of Indian society, including *zamindars,* shopkeepers, merchants, agricultural laborers, bankers, and miners, as well as members of the professional class.) At the forty-second session, held in Madras from December 26 to 28, 1927, an independence resolution was adopted for the first time.

a lucid exposition of the rationale of yoga asanas and pranayam [yogic breathing techniques for controlling the life force] you have given! A layman could not marshal this amount of physiology and anatomy!" "Sorry, friends!" replied Sundaram, extricating himself from the admiring crowd. "I am not what you imagine. Study, research and experience furnish a fund of knowledge!"[3]

There was another way in which Sundaram wasn't what he seemed to his admiring public: he'd been struggling to find rest, stability, and order in a life long filled with turmoil. Born into a poor Brahmin family in 1901 in Mathurai, Tamilnad, Sundaram lost his mother when he was eight. His self-absorbed father quickly remarried to a callous woman, leaving Sundaram and his two sisters, according to his official biography, like "babes in the red wood forest, with no one to care for or comfort them."* Sundaram became withdrawn. "Timid, retired, morose, unknown to game and merry boyish life, he appeared as if dreaming even while walking." In 1915, when he was only fourteen, a marriage was arranged to a ten-year-old girl, Nagalakshmi. After a year, he felt "manacled for life."[4]

In 1917 sixteen-year-old Sundaram, who "had match-stick limbs, knock knees, dry skin, heated body, and roofy chest," turned to physical culture.[5] Over the next three years, he developed a strong and shapely (although still slender) body through practicing *dands, bethaks,* club swinging, and parallel bar exercises. It was during this period that he first took up hatha yoga—*asanas, pranayama* (which he practiced four times a day, including once at midnight in solitude), and *shatkarma* (yogic cleansing techniques) (see fig. 12.1 on page 154).

His spiritual awakening also began during these years: "He frequented the local Theosophical Society; read books on mysticism, hypnotism and mesmerism, phrenology, palmistry and theory of numbers and in no time became an expert in their application." But his "fancy for the mystic sciences came to an abrupt end. . . . [when] Swami Vivekananda's Raja Yoga set his spiritual fire ablaze."[6] Thereafter, he longed to find a guru who would initiate him into the experience of *samadhi.*

At the same time, Sundaram's family life was falling apart. "With a step-mother in the house and a father whose thoughts seldom travelled beyond his skin and having little guidance," his marriage foundered. In 1919 Sundaram sent his wife back to her family. "The world appeared to him to be only misery and bondage."[7] His only solace, for all the wrong reasons, was escape in *vairagya,* nonattachment or dispassion.

Running away from his debts, Sundaram's father moved with his wife to Bangalore in 1919. In the following year, at his father's bequest, Sundaram joined them. He got a temporary job as a law clerk at the office of the British Resident of Mysore, where he spent his days pasting correction slips, taking shorthand,

---

*Sundaram's official biography was composed under his supervision for his sixty-first birthday, when the completion of his sixtieth year of life—the time, according to Indian tradition, when a man increasingly turns away from worldly matters and toward spiritual concerns—was celebrated.

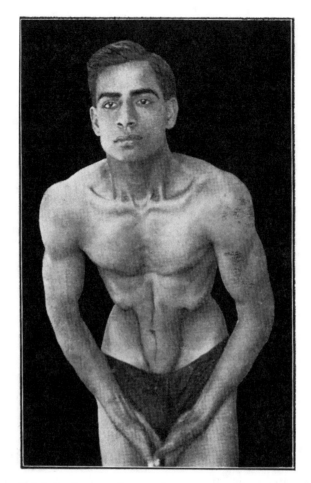

Figure 12.1. S. Sundaram performing "Nauli or the Rectus Isolation," 1929

(From *Yogic Physical Culture,* by S. Sundaram)

and typing letters.* (He hated being a law clerk. In fact, he hated courts and the law in general; he had wanted to be a doctor or a forest ranger.) After elders brought about a reconciliation, his wife rejoined him.

From 1920 to 1924 Sundaram studied for the series of law exams, while working as an account's clerk in the Mysore comptroller's office in Bangalore. Throughout this period, domestic life with his self-absorbed father and cold stepmother placed pressures on his marriage. "Many a day the young householder was on the point of running away and embracing sanyasa [the life of renunciation]." But "something prevented this":

---

*The Resident, a civil officer appointed by the central British government, administered the Assigned Tract of Bangalore (previously the Bangalore Cantonment), which contained the quarters for the British army and its family members. The jurisdiction of the Resident's court extended over the entire area, which consisted of "an agglomeration of people of different religions, castes, creeds and races, speaking different tongues—both Indian and European" (Hasan, *Bangalore through the Centuries,* 128). Located at the western end of the parade ground, the Residency was housed in a stately bungalow, in front of which, on a flagstaff, flew the Union Jack—surely a daily reminder to Sundaram, an ardent nationalist, that he was working for his rulers.

the birth of a child, his daughter Javalakshmi, early in 1924.* Even though his life was now a "trouble factory [that] started growing in right earnest," the young man who was neglected as a child couldn't abandon his own child.[8] After passing his last exam, he enrolled as a first-grade pleader (a lawyer who's entitled to practice civil law before the chief court) with the Bangalore Bar in October 1924. He soon became a junior in a law firm, which enabled him, on earnings of fifteen rupees a month, to get his own housing and support his wife and infant daughter.†

Within six months, although "he was in an adopted province with no God-father to help in the profession," through "energy and push" he set up his own law practice. "He had once vowed not to be a Legal Practitioner but destiny had made him one" (see fig. 12.2 on page 156).[9]

Magazine

During these difficult times, Sundaram continued his pursuit of yogasana. He began strength and *asana* training at Iyer's gymnasium in the early 1920s, which led to his touring with Iyer to lecture on and demonstrate yogasana. In 1927 he became associated with a "a group of dedicated souls" who "propagated the advantages of doing asans and pranayama. That was the nucleus and dynamic foyer of the Cult of

Psycho Physical Exercises contained in the Asanas."[10] Headed by the learned literary critic Brahmachari Ramachandra, the group lived at a *prem ashram* (spiritual community) near Lalbag (the 240-acre garden located in the south of Bangalore, started by Haider Ali in 1760 and completed by his son Tipu Sultan).

The group's mission to propagate yogasana included serving the poor. In the early 20th century, social service was being developed in India by an active citizenry. Social service associations proliferated. Blending newly introduced modern Western ideas of social service with traditional Indians ideas of *seva* (also *sewa*), selfless service, members of the urban elite promoted the welfare of the people living in slums. The appalling living conditions of the slums—the flimsy housing (clusters of mud huts with roofs and/or sides made of rags, scraps of wood, tin sheets, or other waste materials), crowded sleeping conditions, lack of sanitation, and poor nutrition—made them breeding grounds for disease. Many of the social service associations attempted to improve the health of the slum dwellers through teaching Indian practices of physical culture and therapeutics. Sundaram joined the "group of dedicated souls" who taught *asana* and *pranayama* in Seva Centres in the industrial slums of Bangalore, mostly in the old areas of Malleswaram and Basavangundi.

---

*There's contradictory evidence about the year in which Javalakshmi was born. In a list titled "Important Dates" in the authorized biography of Sundaram, the 1924 entry reads: "Enrolled as legal Practitioner/birth of a daughter—first child" (Members of the Committee, "Biographical Sketch," 36). But in the chronology of Sundaram's life in the main text, it appears that she was born in 1920. And a family record states that she was born on May 5, 1922.

†It might be argued that his father and stepmother, ground down by poverty and, as a result, preoccupied with survival, could hardly have been expected to be selfless and loving parents and that Sundaram never gained the objectivity to understand their plight. But Sundaram (implicitly) insisted that they should be seen not in economic, sociological, or political terms but in psychological terms—they were self-absorbed and uncaring—and that he needed to distance himself from them in order to establish his own life.

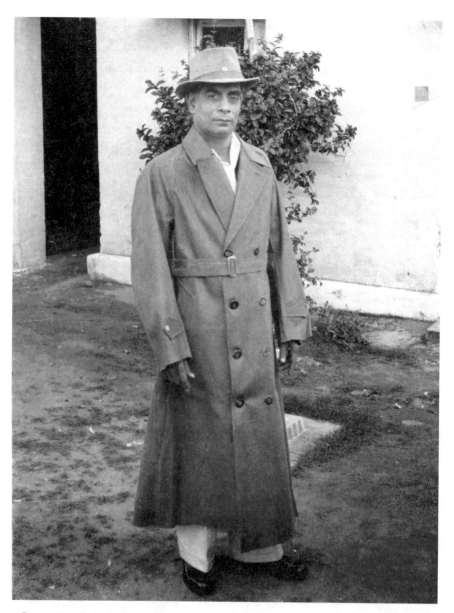

Figure 12.2. S. Sundaram, in front of his home, dressed for work at his law office, 1950s
(With the kind permission of Hari Shankar R.)

Under Ramachandra's leadership, the group extended their platform for widely promoting the benefits of yoga to journalism by publishing *Brahmacharya,* a monthly English-language magazine, for which Sundaram became the associate editor. His more significant work for the magazine, however, was writing articles about *asanas* and *pranayama* with a scientific rationale, illustrated with photos of him performing the exercises. In performing this task (as well as presenting his lectures), Sundaram found Swami Kuvalayananda's *Yoga-Mimansa* invaluable: the research published in the journal verified Sundaram's experiences and teachings, increased the depth of his knowledge, "and helped him against the destructive and scoffing criticisms of the unbelieving world."[11]

Although *Brahmacharya* had a thousand subscribers, it stopped publication after three years, in 1930, when Ramachandra became more involved in other endeavors.

The First Modern Hatha Yoga Manual

The most significant result of the lectures and demonstrations and magazine writing was that they produced the impetus for Sundaram to write a hatha yoga manual. "Wherever I went [on the tours with Iyer to promote *asana* practice]," he recounted, "persons asked for a book of instructions, a guide or text book on the subject."[12] "After the publication of my articles on 'Yoga in Physical Culture' in the Brahmacharya, the demand for a book increased. My profession and its dry-as-dust duties claimed most of the time and attention. My ambition to popularise Yogic Physical Culture and make the sons and daughters of India partners in the enjoyment of its benefits, remained unfulfilled. Then the indefatigable Editor of the Brahmacharya, Sjt. Ramachandra, found the ways and means for the publication of a work on this subject. All that remained for me was to write it up."[13]

A studious, accomplished writer who was an expert on yogic health cure, Sundaram worked on his manual in 1928, finishing in December. Published in English in 1929, *Yogic Physical Culture or the Secret of Happiness* was the first (or, at least, the first extant and ear- liest documented) modern hatha yoga manual. Fully illustrated with photos of Sundaram, this pioneering book places a course of hatha yoga bodily practices—*asanas, kriyas* (purifying techniques), and *pranayama*—at the center of hatha yoga, and health cure as its raison d'être.

At least two other claims have been made for prior publication of a modern hatha yoga manual. The Yoga Institute maintains that Shri Yogendra's *Yoga Asanas Simplified* was originally published in 1928; however, no copies of this original edition are extant. (The archivists at the institute say it's lost.) In any case, in all likelihood, it was a pamphlet.

Modern yoga scholar Mark Singleton places the publication date of *Practical Hatha Yoga, Science of Health: How to Keep Well and Cure Diseases by Hindu Yogic Practice* by R. S. Gherwal as 1923. Singleton writes: "The book, based on a lecture-demonstration tour of the previous year, is probably the earliest photographic manual of modern, populist *hatha* yoga—even predating by one year the launch of Kuvalayananda's *Yoga Mimamsa*."[14] But existing copies of *Practical Hatha Yoga* don't have information about the place of publication, publisher, date of publication, printer, and person who reserved the copyright. The book isn't chiefly a modern hatha yoga manual anyway. It's a compilation of three lectures, the first of which is a discussion in three parts of the "regeneration of the thyroid gland and the correction of constipation" through yogic physical culture and therapeutics.[15] (The other two lectures are the New Thought–influenced "The Power of Mind over Body," an argument for the application of willpower to achieve a muscular build, and the Vivekananda-influenced "The Way to

Nirvana," a guide to finding divinity within.*) What's more, this thirty-eight-page section on yogic health cure isn't even original: rather than predating Kuvalayananda's *Yoga-Mimansa,* it's mostly plagiarized from the first four issues (October 1924, February 1925, July 1925, and October 1925) of the magazine! For example, near the beginning of five pages of purloined text about constipation, Gherwal wrote:

> The aim in tonight's lecture is to study the effect of the fecal matter delaying in the ceacum, that is to say, of cæcal constipation, and to see how Yoga proposes to cure it. The modern world has devised various remedies against this disease. A reference to these will first be made with a view to see how the Yogic methods compare with the modern ones.[16]

The only difference between this text and Kuvalayananda's text is the substitution of the words "tonight's lecture" for "this article." Sometimes Gherwal's changes were more creative. For example, Kuvalayananda wrote, "Now in India Yogic tradition claims to cure lepers by the Sarvangasana treatment which requires a milk diet. A great yogin of the Deccan used to prescribe this practice to his leper patients. The Yogin has left the mortal coil long since."[17] Gherwal, in contrast, wrote, "My Master cured lepers by the Sarvang treatment. He always prescribed a milk diet."[18]

Gherwal, an Indian who had established an ashram in Southern California's San Marcos Pass in 1920, assumed (probably correctly)

that he could pass off Kuvalayananda's text as his own because no member of his American audiences would've read *Yoga-Mimansa.* Even if *Practical Hatha Yoga* was published before *Yogic Physical Culture,* Sundaram's book—with its single-minded focus on performing yogic exercises to maintain and improve health, its full course of yogic exercises, and its original authorship—can be said to be the first hatha yoga manual that mainly and comprehensively foregrounds yogic exercises and isn't stolen.

"There is a sort of psycho-physical balance in these Yoga-Asanas," Iyer wrote in the foreword to *Yogic Physical Culture.* "The author has taken a keen interest in depicting truly his personal experience and achievement in the field of Yogic-therapy and its application over the endocrine, nervous, and vascular systems which are the foremost factors in maintaining the correct working of all the internal organs of the human body."[19] Sundaram deferentially acknowledged his great debt not only to Iyer and Ramachandra but also to Kuvalayananda for his critical help in building a medical model of yoga: "But for [his research], my labours may have been neither convincing nor supported by scientific and clinical data." But Sundaram realized the personal nature of his book: "My intuition and experience guided me through the task more than anything else."[20]

Publishing a book about hatha yoga was just as critical to modernizing hatha yoga as was making it available as a class and testing

---

*New Thought originated in the early 19th century in the United States as the theory that sickness originates in the mind, and therefore can be overcome by willpower (see chapter 15). Over the course of the 19th century and the first decades of the 20th century, the tenets of New Thought became increasingly theological and the scope of its application expanded to such areas as finding financial success and achieving a muscular physique.

it in a laboratory. Previously, gurus, secretive and reclusive, had made yogic health practices (*asana, pranayama,* and purificatory techniques) available only to a select few. Sundaram believed that the yogic system of physical culture is the ideal "system of Physical Culture intended for masses." His mission in publishing *Yogic Physical Culture* was to make yogic physical culture indiscriminately available to anyone who cared to take it up. He ended the preface to his book with an invocation: "Our duty in this World is to work and leave the results in His hands. May He who is All-powerful infuse enthusiasm in the readers and enable them to reap the rewards of Yogic Physical Culture in benefits enduring and substantial! Om!"[21]

Impact of the Book

Sundaram's creation of *Yogic Physical Culture or the Secret of Happiness* in 1928 was attributed by the prolific renowned poet whose works proclaimed the universality of religion, Kavi Yogi Suddhananda Bharatiar, in his encomium to celebrate Sundaram's 60th birth year in 1962 to the felicitous matching of Sundaram's determination, skills, and knowledge of yoga with an opportune circumstance: the availability, for the first time, of research on the viability of yoga as health cure. "Sundaram was serious in gathering facts and figures for a standard work on Asans," remarks Bharatiar in the spirit of a colleague, not only as one yogin to another but as one writer to another. "Kuvalayananda of Lonavla was then publishing his wonderful Yoga Mimamsa [*sic*] journal. He wrote volumes on Asans. Sundaram brought out a neat handy book on Asans, clearly illustrated and his book

on Asans stands peerless even today. He was well qualified for this purpose with his refined English and deep plunge into the details of the subject and the noble object in view."[22]

Yogic Physical Culture is very much of the combative times of late colonial India: it's a kind of jingoistic tract. From the beginning to the unfortunately bellicose end, Sundaram's stance is ardent and polemical. As if at a lively dinner party that's gone late into the evening, he immensely enjoyed provoking controversy:

Of course people rush into a sea of medicines and bathe there profusely and in most of the cases drown themselves in the waters of drugs. Latest researches and doctors who do not pander to their patent drugs by inventing new diseases in their victims, conclusively prove that drugs are very harmful and oftentimes, ineffective. They advise restoring the harmony of the internal forces and a healthy regeneration of the organs, nerves and muscles through natural and therefore physical culture methods. But even there, could the modern physical culture exercises equal the therapeutic value of these yogic ones? One may say without hesitation "Never!"[23]

Here Sundaram is making an appeal to Indians to reject not only conventional Western medicine but also one of its popular alternative therapies, Western physical culture, and instead take up (what he considered to be) the only true natural therapy, Indian physical culture—specifically, India's ancient, indigenous exercise system ("the inventions of the Rishis"), the conditioning *asanas* of hatha yoga. Pointing out (in his book and at his lecture/demonstrations) yoga's link to a distant, singular, and superior cultural heritage was critical to Sundaram's political agenda: promoting yogasana not merely as a response to the Western physical culture movement but also as an assertion of India's worthiness to be free of British colonialism—to be, in other words, an equal among nations. What he refused to see (or admit) was that he and the other pioneer yogins, influenced by the West, had molded these exercises—created to serve a centuries-old religious discipline, hatha yoga—into physical culture, which means to say, had made them Western.

Later generations of authors of hatha yoga manuals no longer needed to stridently advocate for hatha yoga, and not only because they no longer needed to justify (to the world and to themselves) the reasons why India deserved to be an independent nation; yoga's wide popularity, due in no small measure to the efforts of Sundaram and the other pioneer yogins, made heated and prolonged arguments over its merits unnecessary.

While surpassed in achievement nearly forty years later by B. K. S. Iyengar's *Light on Yoga,* Sundaram's *Yogic Physical Culture* nevertheless remains the most significant modern hatha yoga manual—and not just because it was the first. According to Sundaram's biographers, it "attracted the intelligentia [*sic*] to the practice of Yogasanas in India and abroad. Very modest in size, unattractive in get up, this book priced low has converted many thousands to Yogic life and earned encomiums at home and abroad as top ranking in the subject."[24] Some of those inspired to take up yoga after reading the book were Englishmen in the top ranks of the Indian civil service. Among them was the last British Resident in Mysore, Sir Walter Fendall Campbell, who, before leaving India after Swaraj in 1948, personally expressed his thanks to Sundaram.

The readership abroad was scattered. Hundreds of copies of a foreign edition printed on high-quality paper (the paper in books published in India was often extremely thin, yet relatively opaque) were circulated in America, in England, and on the Continent. "This created a stir in the western world," write Sundaram's biographers, "and revolutionised its thinking in the field of Yoga Asanas, normally associated with Eastern 'physical torture and penance.'"[25]

Unfortunately, these larger claims are unsubstantiated. Although *Yogic Physical Culture* played some role in paving the way for the acceptance of hatha yoga in India and the West, there's no evidence that interest in it was far-reaching, long lasting, or intensely held. Even his biographers concede that the sales numbers for the book were low as Sundaram was too busy as a yogin, householder, and lawyer to find the time and means to promote it. A second (revised) edition wasn't published until 1971. And no coterie developed of followers devoted to the book. Nevertheless, there was a way in which the book had an impact out of proportion to its sales: its influence on subsequent books written by yogins, including Sivananda and Iyengar.

Modified Canon

A childhood friend of Sundaram recalled that after a few years apart, he and Sundaram met up again in Bangalore in 1928. "I saw him an adept in Hatha Yoga. . . . He taught me about 80 Asanas."[26] Part of what makes *Yogic Physical Culture* what Bharatiar accurately described as "a neat handy book on Asans," though, is that it calls for just a small number of conditioning *asanas*. Probably thinking that it would be unrealistic to expect most people of his times to practice eighty or so *asanas*, Sundaram adopted Kuvalayananda's 1926 canon (a slightly revised version of his original course devised in 1925) for "an average man of health," consisting of eleven *asanas* (as well as one *bandha*, one *mudra*, one *kriya*, and two *pranayamas*). To these, he added two more *asanas*. (The eleven *asanas* in Kuvalayananda's 1926 routine were *Sirsasana, Sarvangasana, Matsyasana, Halasana, Bhujangasana, Salabasana, Dhanurasana, Ardha-Matsyendrasana, Paschimottanasana, Mayurasana,* and *Savasana.* Sundaram added *Thrikonasana* and *Padhahastasana.*) The thirteen conditioning *asanas* in his routine, Sundaram asserted, gave the votary a systematic and complete workout.

> In discussing the physiology of the poses, so far, it has been seen, that when one set of muscles is contracted, another set is relaxed and stretched. The Asanas have covered the whole muscular system and have alternately and in turn relaxed almost all the sets of muscles, whose health and activity are important. The perfection of the poses themselves would be physically impossible if that which has to be relaxed remains contracted or vice versa. Therefore, if one practices these Asanas, it may be taken for granted, that he or she has contracted and relaxed the whole muscular system of the body.[27]

Sundaram's goal was to make available a manual that was handy, not encyclopedic, consisting of a series of exercises that were highly effective but not off-putting and imposing. His modification of Kuvalayananda's canon was later widely exported to the West through its adoption by Swami Sivananda in his *Yogic Home Exercises*. But there was another, subtler way in which Sundaram's book influenced subsequent hatha yoga: by its format.

Format

Heavily influenced by articles on *asanas* (postures), *bandhas* (locks), and *shatkarma* (purificatory practices) in *Yoga-Mimansa*, Sundaram's *Yogic Physical Culture* established the format for most hatha yoga manuals: a brief account of the name of the exercise; an explanation of the technique for performing the exercise; an accompanying photo illustration; and a description of the therapeutic benefits of the exercise. This format is the model for the two most influential hatha yoga manuals, Sivananda's *Yogic Home Exercises* and Iyengar's *Light on Yoga*.

Photographs

In the 1920s and 1930s, the role of photography was critical in the dissemination of hatha yoga through book and magazine illustrations. *Yogic Physical Culture* is illustrated with photos of Sundaram "taken under the supervision and direction of Professor K. V. Iyer, who is an artist in this respect."[28] At first look, the photos of Sundaram demonstrating the exercises are startling. There's absolutely no trace of everyday reality in them. The wiry and seemingly diminutive Sundaram, wearing skimpy shorts, appears to be a man vitally alive, yet an apparition. He appears to be atop a marble slab or stone sarcophagus situated on the edge of earth, over which loom the vast empty black heavens—a mix of the intimate and the immense, life and death, the temporal and the eternal. The various positions that he takes sometimes seem less ethereal than precarious: if he were to slip, he would tumble into the black nothingness.

Our common sense, however, tells us that Sundaram is demonstrating the poses on what is probably a small, light-colored platform in front of a black backdrop—the visual elements (the décor, props, costume, and lighting) chosen, no doubt, to make his body look sculptural, not sepulchral. The practice of illuminating a well-lit foreground figure and contrasting it against a dark background (the photos are touched up to increase the contrast) was common in the 1920s and 1930s, as evidenced by the photos of Iyer (which he also took) in his own books. The setting isn't an ashram or a yoga institute; a home (in a living room or a room set aside for exercise or meditation) or its environs (a garden or yard); an auditorium, arena, or lecture hall; a park; the woods or seaside or other natural settings; or a temple, shrine, or other holy locations—environments that evoke some aspect (such as finding respite, imparting knowledge, or feeling calm) of what is deemed the yoga spirit in our times. It's probably Iyer's studio.

Sundaram's demeanor in the photographs seems passive, if not submissive. The taking of the poses seems perfunctory, not at all dynamic. Perhaps the intention was to show him placid.

I suspect, though, that Sundaram, unlike Iyer, simply didn't take to the spotlight.

To appeal to the middle-class readership, it was important for the model to be ordinary—not like the wild-eyed yogins seen on the streets of India, who look as if the mortification of their flesh in life could only be fully consummated in death, the total annihilation of the body. Sundaram is slight, but not self-deprived; self-contained, but not antisocial; confident, but not imposing. He doesn't look deranged or threatening. His shape and aspect are pleasing. He doesn't wear a turban, large earrings, a sacred thread, or a loincloth. He doesn't have three horizontal stripes of ash across his forehead. He doesn't have a shaven head or long, matted hair and a beard. His hair is short and neatly combed. In sum, he doesn't have any of the distinctive marks of a renunciate yogin. Instead of connoting a life of austerity, marginality, or infirmity, his lithe, sprightly, unadorned, groomed, and toned body displays good health.

But what's most striking about the demonstration photographs in *Yogic Physical Culture* is something easily unnoticed: they are of the author. That the photos are of Sundaram lends a quality to—or, more accurately, reinforces a quality in—the book that's absent in Kuvalayananda's *Yoga-Mimansa* articles and his book derived from them: a sense of personal journey, or, at least, of personal statement. Whereas Eugen Sandow, Bernarr Macfadden, and J. P. Müller expressly presented their systems as their own creations and unflaggingly promoted them as such, Sundaram modestly presented the yogic system of physical culture as having been handed down to him from ancient sages; but, just as with the photos of the Western physical culturists in their books, the photos of Sundaram demonstrating exercises implicitly but emphatically declare the book's unique, idiosyncratic, and personal nature.

Stages

Sundaram's *Yogic Physical Culture* explains how to perform yoga postures using three kinds of stages, all picked up from Kuvalayananda's *Yoga-Mimansa*. (Kuvalayananda created the concept of stages in *asana* pedagogy. "These stages have not been prescribed in the Yogic texts," he wrote in an article in *Yoga-Mimansa* about performing *Halasana*, Plow Pose, "nor are they required by different Yogic traditions.[29])

Stages for Assuming *Asanas*

Sundaram's instructions for performing *Bhujangasana*, or Cobra Pose, consist of five stages. The student lies facedown on the ground, places both hands just beneath the shoulders, lifts his head up, bends his spine backward, and, lastly, bends his spine well back, with "the navel remaining as near to the ground as possible."[30] Sundaram illustrated the posture with only the completed pose, what he called "the perfected pose."

Explaining (and illustrating) the stages for assuming *asanas* was the most effective aid in helping readers learn how to perform *asanas,* but it had more than a practical effect. It turned *asanas* into mere exercises. It demystified them. Sundaram's description of the method for assuming *Bhujangasana* and other *asanas* stripped them of their appearance as penitential self-torture or a manifestation of superhuman powers. (It's practically impossible for us today to comprehend how difficult, weird, and mysterious *asanas* looked even to Indians, who were familiar with them—let alone to Westerners, who had never seen them before—in the 1920s.) The *asanas* didn't repulse. They didn't inspire awe. They were merely a means of improving one's health. They were physical exercises.

Stages for Varying the Final Position in *Asanas*

In Sundaram's instructions for performing *Halasana,* he directed the student to lie on his back with his hands palm-downward at his sides, lift his legs, lift his trunk, and then, while keeping his knees straight, lower his legs over his head until his toes touch the ground. Ignoring the preliminary steps, Sundaram identified the completion of these movements as the first stage (see fig. 12.3 on page 164). Pushing the toes further is the second stage. Pushing the toes as far beyond the head as possible without raising the arms is the third stage. Clasping the hands behind the head and pushing the toes to their extreme limit is the fourth stage (see fig. 12.4 on page 164).

What made these stages remarkable is their purpose: they're variations of the final position, each with an equal value. Sundaram elaborated on how "each different stage affects a particular region of the spine" and other parts of the body: in the first stage, "the lumbo sacral region of the spine is pulled" while the abdominal and quadriceps muscles are contracted; in the second and third stages, "the dorsal region of the vertebral column is affected" while the contraction of the abdominal and quadriceps muscles is lessened in the second stage and negligible in the third stage; in the fourth stage, the cervical

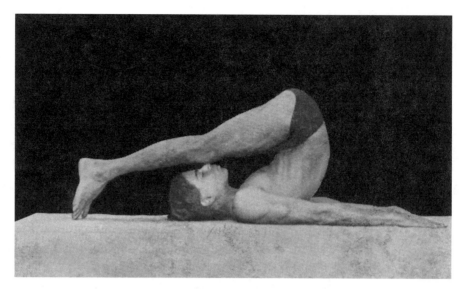

Figure 12.3. S. Sundaram demonstrating the first stage of *Halasana,* Plow Pose, 1929
(From *Yogic Physical Culture*)

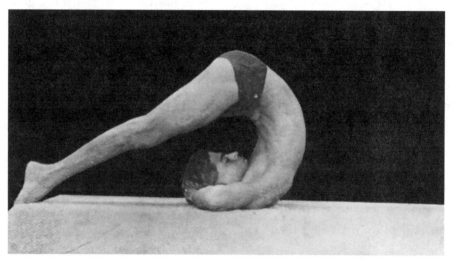

Figure 12.4. S. Sundaram demonstrating the last stage of *Halasana,* Plow Pose, 1929
(From *Yogic Physical Culture*)

region undergoes a "regeneration . . . unrivalled in any system of physical culture."[31]

The instructions for these slight variations would have been difficult to understand without illustrations. Thankfully, Sundaram (following Kuvalayananda) provided plates for each of the stages.

Stages for Extending the Final Position in *Asanas*

Sundaram also explained *asanas* using a third kind of stage, this one for increasing the difficulty of the pose. For example, he described four stages for *Paschimottanasana,* Seated Forward Bend or Posterior Stretching Pose. In the first stage, the student lies supine on the ground, extends his arms overhead, raises his trunk, and bends forward over his legs. He tries to reach his toes, and then goes back to the prone position. In the second stage, he catches his toes, and then returns to the supine position. In the third stage, he catches his toes and touches his forehead to his knees, and then goes back to the supine position. In the fourth stage, he buries his face between his knees.

The last three positions are extensions of the final position in *Paschimottanasana*. They increase the range of the final position by incrementally increasing the intensity. By describing these progressively difficult refinements of the final position, Sundaram enabled the willing and able student, through perseverance, to complete the pose to maximal effort (during a session or over time). Describing stages that increase in intensity also made *asanas* accessible to students of varying abilities and experience. The graduated stages imply beginning, intermediate, and advanced levels.

Presenting variations that increase in intensity also reinforced the need for safety. "Go slowly, cautiously and inch by inch," Sundaram advised in his instructions for *Paschimottanasana*. "Never strain beyond reasonable and comfortable endurance."[32] By explaining the incremental steps in extending the completed pose, he reinforced this caution.

Presenting stages with equal variations of *asanas* is quite rare in subsequent yoga manuals. Explaining and showing stages for assuming and extending *asanas*, though, became quite common. All these stages weren't used to their full advantage, however, until Iyengar systematically applied them to poses in his acclaimed encyclopedic *Light on Yoga* (1966). (While admitting that he'd read the manuals written by the early modern yogins, Iyengar stubbornly contended that his book is sui generis. In regard to Sundaram's book in particular, Iyengar flatly insisted to me: "The formats are not at all similar."[33])

The Nature of *Asana*

Scholar and popularizer of yoga history and philosophy Georg Feuerstein describes Patanjali's eight-limbed spiritual path—found in his *Yoga Sutra*, considered by modern yogins to be the foundational philosophical text of yoga—as "leading from the common life of self-involvement to the uncommon realization of the Self beyond the ego-personality."[34] The eight limbs (or steps or aspects) of this path are *yama* (external discipline), *niyama* (internal discipline), *asana* (posture), *pranayama* (breath regulation), *pratyahara* (withdrawal of senses), *dharana* (concentration), *dhyana* (absorption), and *samadhi* (contemplation). Most yoga practitioners today are most familiar with the third limb, *asana,* which they commonly consider to consist of the conditioning postures taught in yoga classes.

When Patanjali explicated *asanas,* though, in the *Yoga Sutra,* he was referring to the seated postures for meditation. In the three aphorisms on *asanas* (II.46, II.47, and II.48), he wrote (in Chip Hartranft's translation of what he calls *The Yoga-Sutra of Patanjali*): "The postures of meditation should embody steadiness and ease. This occurs as all effort relaxes and coalescence arises, revealing that the body and the infinite universe are indivisible. Then, one is no longer disturbed by the play of opposites."[35] The conditioning postures, in contrast, notes the out-of-fashion mid-20th-century author of books on Indian philosophy Ernest E. Wood (in his commentary on what he calls *Patanjali's Yoga Aphorisms*), "are regarded simply as health exercises, beneficial in general if properly selected and practiced and beneficial indirectly for yoga purposes inasmuch as they conduce to an obedient, quiet and healthy habit of body."[36]

In his first book, *The Yoga Tradition of the Mysore Palace*, published in 1996, yoga teacher and iconoclastic modern yoga scholar Norman E. Sjoman extends Patanjali's definition of seated meditative postures to conditioning postures. Based on his interpretation of Patanjali's *sutras* on *asanas*, Sjoman posits four stages in assuming conditioning *asanas:* effort, letting go, balance, and transcendence. In describing the last three stages, he writes that the *sutras* call for "loosening, relaxing or letting go, for stretching beyond the trammels of the mind until we find balance, . . . the state of unhindered perfect balance, Patanjali's . . . meditation on the endless. This is the only way that one can transcend the conditioning of past habits recorded in the unconscious or involuntary nervous system." Sjoman concludes by emphasizing the importance of the first stage: "The prerequisite for relaxation is effort, of course, as only a muscle that is worked is able to relax (that is, there is a distinction between dormancy and relaxation)."[37] He elaborates on this point in his second book, *Yoga Touchstone,* published in 2004: "The sutra indicates that effort is necessary to perform the asana; that one must let go of this effort and attain to a total stillness (meditate on the endless). This is a significant state-

ment. It tells us that each asana involves body mechanics, and at some point has to transcend body mechanics, right up to the very desire to move, in order to attain fullness, stillness."[38]

In the late 20th century, some yoga teachers, notably Iyengar, began to consider the conditioning postures as a suitable vehicle for systematically applying all eight limbs of Patanjali's path of liberation. Taking note of this trend, Gudrun Bühnemann, scholar of South Asian religions, observes, "Several contemporary teachers have begun to claim that all ancillary parts of Patanjali's eightfold Yoga are inherent in their *asana* practice. They assert that the ancillary parts either unfold naturally *after* or are even experienced *during* the practice of the postures."[39] All eight steps, in other words, can be condensed within the rhythm of performing the conditioning postures: effort, letting go, balance, and transcendence.

Sundaram's contribution to the developments in modern yoga that led to this contemporary discourse about using the conditioning *asanas* as a vehicle for attaining to Being is his book's unprecedented emphasis (inspired by Kuvalayananda's *Yoga-Mimansa* articles) on the conditioning *asanas* as yogic physical culture, not as an aid to the yogic spiritual practices that consummate in *samadhi*. He provided two rationales for this shift. First, the conditioning *asanas* can provide fitness as an end in itself; they are not limited to preparing the body for holding a seated *asana* with steadiness and ease because an uncomfortable position distracts from meditation. Second, the conditioning *asanas* can provide good health as an end in itself; they are not limited to preventing illness because the symptoms of illness interfere with meditation. But Sundaram's equally significant contribution to today's embodied yoga practice is his instructions, which can be seen not so much as commands but as detailed descriptions of the process of performing conditioning *asanas* (the first to be found in book form).

Sundaram's detailed instructions refined the performance of conditioning *asanas,* which in all likelihood had been being performed perfunctorily and haphazardly. He moved conditioning *asanas* away from habit and imprecision and toward the attentiveness and exactitude previously only approached in assuming the traditional meditation *asanas*. He showed that performing conditioning *asanas* involves mindful mechanical effort—specifically, the deliberate shortening and lengthening of muscles. In so doing, he helped initiate the evolution in hatha yoga practice that has led contemporary practitioners to pay close attention to the subtle tensions of their musculature when assuming conditioning *asanas*.

In exposing the process in detail, Sundaram also led the way for yoga practitioners to bring their attention to other equally important tasks involved in assuming a pose: moving slowly, steadily, and in a controlled manner to enter a pose; using the constant interplay between mind and body to make assessments (such as locating an imbalance or obstruction) for needed adjustments; correctly positioning the body according to the unique anatomical demands of the pose; and holding the pose at the limit of their ability. Attentive to these mind/body tasks, contemporary yoga practitioners become totally absorbed in performing *asanas* (there's no opportunity for the mind to wander; there's so much to attend to), thereby dissolving opposites (such as pain and pleasure), and then go beyond: discovering the absolute through the experience of their body in *asana*.

13

S. SUNDARAM

Meditating on the Body in Yoga

Relaxation

Born in Württemberg, Germany, in 1882, the great bodybuilder Maxick (his real name, suitable for a macabre cautionary tale for English-speaking children, was Max Sick) was a sickly child who "contracted diseases such as usually spell death to a child of tender years."[1] At five, he became afflicted with rickets. When he attended school for the first time at seven, it was brought home to him that he was a weakling among robust boys. He longed to be strong and healthy. When he was ten, he sold all his cherished belongings to schoolmates to buy a ticket to the circus so he could see a strongman named Hercules, whose crowning feat of strength was supporting twenty-five adults on a plank.

Inspired by Hercules's strength and muscular physique, Maxick (1882–1961) began to secretly exercise using a dumbbell fashioned from a stone slab. Upon discovering him exercising, his father (warned by doctors that the boy shouldn't exert himself) smashed the crude weight to bits. Undaunted, Maxick cleverly turned to a means of developing muscles without apparatus: isometric, or static, contraction, which occurs when there's tension on the muscle but no bony movement (the length of the muscle remains the same).* Throughout his school years he perfected his system. When he was a young adult earning a living as an engineer's apprentice, he joined a weight-lifting club. After winning contests in the light-, middle-, and heavyweight classes (despite weighing barely

---

*Raise your right arm out to the side at shoulder height with your palm facing upward. Bend your elbow until your forearm is perpendicular to the floor. Make a fist. Contract your biceps muscle simply through willing it (i.e., without moving your forearm). This is an isometric contraction.

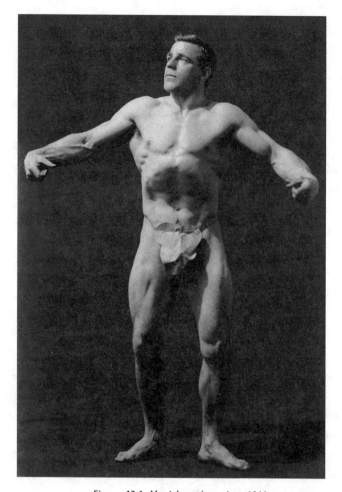

Figure 13.1. Maxick posing, circa 1910
(With the kind permission of David L. Chapman)

112 pounds), he became something of a local celebrity. At twenty-three, he moved to Munich, an art center, to become an artist's model (not surprisingly, he made a fair amount of money at it). His next few years, though, were almost exclusively occupied with teaching weight lifting and muscle control to pupils and perfecting his system.

In 1910 Maxick went to London to compete in a weight-lifting competition (only to learn upon his arrival that it had already taken place). While there he was discovered by a bodybuilder once apprenticed to Eugen Sandow, Monte Saldo (his real name was Alfred Montague Woollaston), who recognized a physical phenomenon when he saw one (fig. 13.1). Saldo arranged for Maxick to give a demonstration of his muscle-control skills—isolating one group of muscles at a time, including the left and right rectus abdominals—for Britain's weight-lifting elite. The physical culture magazine *Health & Strength* covered the event: "His will seemed to act as commander-in-chief, and at a signal from him, and without any forcing, the latissimus dorsi, the abdominals, the deltoids, etc., seemed to do whatever they were told. His body, in fact, was like a transformation scene. . . . It was really very wonderful indeed."[2]

The muscle control demonstration brought Maxick acclaim. Managed and promoted by Saldo, Maxick succeeded in building up a large clientele in England, where he made his home. *Muscle Control or Body Development by Will-Power*—his influential manual on "The Maxick-Saldo System of Physical Culture," which came to be called, for short, first Maxaldo and then Maxalding—was published in 1911.

In the book's second chapter, "How Muscle-Control Was Revealed to Me," Maxick gives an account of the key realization in developing his system: relaxing muscles is just as important for muscular development as contracting them. There are three reasons for this. First, relaxing muscles prevents muscle binding, thereby keeping muscles supple. Second, systematically relaxing the targeted muscle beforehand facilitates its subsequent contraction: "unless a muscle be supple enough to lie soft when relaxed, real control is out of the question."[3] Third, relaxing nontargeted muscles while contracting the targeted muscle allows for full contraction: "I learned that while one group of muscles is being employed, other muscles are involved. . . . When I had grasped this fact, the idea came to me that, to allow each muscle to put forth to the utmost the energy therein contained, it was absolutely necessary that other muscles must not be allowed to interfere—in a word, they must by the effort of will, be relaxed."[4]

The yogin Seetharaman Sundaram had learned Maxalding at K. V. Iyer's Hercules Gymnasium, where it was a regular part of the curriculum, along with bell lifting and yogasana, from the very start in 1922. Maxalding appealed to Indian physical culturists for an easily understandable reason: it shares much in common with modern hatha yoga. Performed without machines or even tools (dumbbells or barbells), Maxalding exercises, like yoga postures, are self-contained and self-sufficient. Furthermore, both Maxalding and hatha yoga demand great mental as well as physical control. And not just concentration. The near suprahuman control of the body exerted by Maxalding and yoga adepts is ultimately realized by a powerful force of will.

Maxick was considered by Swami Kuvalayananda, whom Sundaram revered for establishing a scientific rationale for hatha yoga, to be the only Western physical culturalist "to have approached the subject of muscle building with some scientific insight."[5] Not, according to Kuvalayananda, that there was anything to learn from Maxick. After all, his two key relaxation principles, which "Mr. Maxick claims to have discovered," had been "anticipated" in the practices of "ancient Yogic savants": the principle "of keeping a particular muscle contracted while others round-about it are thoroughly relaxed" is found most notably in *Nauli* but also in "a number of other Yogic exercises requiring perfect contraction of particular muscles," and the principle of "enjoin[ing] the most willful and complete relaxation of every muscle tissue" is found in *Savasana*.[6]

In his 1929 yoga manual *Yogic Physical Culture or the Secret of Happiness,* in the opening paragraph of his commentary on *Savasana,* Sundaram, too, acknowledges the validity of Maxick's principles about relaxation while claiming that they had long been known by yogic sages: "Relaxation is as important for muscular development as contraction. . . . [Maxick] claims this principle to be his discovery. . . . It may be a new discovery for him and the West. But the Yogic Savants of India had this knowledge many, many years ago, and incorporated it in the system of Yogasana."[7] Yet, despite his dismissal of any originality in Maxick's system, Sundaram wisely realized that Maxalding included a new and vital element that could be adapted with great benefit to yoga.

As spelled out in Exercise 1, "Relaxation," which is performed while standing, Maxick tells students that before they can embark on systematically contracting the major muscles of the body, they first have to systematically relax all their muscles:

> This is a most important exercise—the beginner must learn to relax all the muscles.
>
> Study the pose [displayed in a figure in the book], and it will be seen that not a single muscle suggests contraction.
>
> Think of each part of the body in turn, beginning at the head and working downwards.
>
> Allow each muscle to droop as you think of it; but care must be exercised that, while doing so, you do not contract other muscles which you have already relaxed. . . .
>
> The whole back, as the front, is in repose.[8]

Sundaram's systematic relaxation technique for *Savasana,* for which there's no precedent in yoga literature or practice, was adapted from this step-by-step method of total body relaxation adumbrated by Maxick. Sundaram simply fleshed out the instructions.

In *Yoga in Modern India,* sociocultural anthropologist Joseph Alter contrasts B. K. S. Iyengar's "incredibly detailed and exact" descriptions on how to perform *asanas* in *Light on Yoga,* the encyclopedic hatha yoga manual published in 1966, to the "rather vague and cryptic" descriptions in Svatmarama's 15th- to 16th-century hatha yoga manual, *Hatha Yoga Pradipika,* the first text that recommends conditioning *asanas* among its hatha yoga techniques: "With regard to savasana (corpse pose) Iyengar gives us almost two pages, with careful anatomical reference and measurements, phenomenal concern with the details of body-plane and ground-plane interface, and a complex calculus of geometric positioning that is virtually poetic."[9] But Sundaram's instructions for bodily relaxation in *Savasana* in his hatha yoga manual, written about forty years before Iyengar's book, are even more detailed and poetic than Iyengar's instructions. For example, whereas Iyengar directs students to "keep the heels together and the toes apart,"[10] Sundaram directs them to "let the heels remain together and the toes separated, permitting the thighs to roll outwards, in an absolutely relaxed condition."[11]

Alter further rhapsodizes about Iyengar's formulation of a hatha yoga that, while "devoted primarily to the physical dimension of practice rather than to metaphysics, meditation, and liberation,"[12] links to the original power of hatha yoga to bring about liberation through physical transubstantiation: "The *Hathayogapradipika* hardly says more than 'lie flat on your back like a corpse,' the homology with embodied death—and by extension enstasy—being rather obvious. In Iyengar's elaboration the homology is refined, and the corpse pose becomes both more physical and more metaphysical. His genius is in making the arcane nature of medieval practice explicit, clear, and unambiguous. In Iyengar Yoga, as in medieval Hatha Yoga, the body becomes the materialization of magic."[13]

In his commentary on *Savasana*, Iyengar largely relies on quotations from the *Hatha Yoga Pradipika* and the *Gheranda Samhita*, the late 18th-century hatha yoga manual, to make his case that the object of this corpse-like pose is not only to make the body motionless but to make the mind calm, thereby leading to liberation of the soul. But when all is said and done, he primarily considers *Savasana* to be a relaxation exercise: "By remaining motionless for some time and keeping the mind still while you are fully conscious, you learn to relax. This conscious relaxation invigorates and refreshes both body and mind."[14] "The stresses of modern civilization," he concludes, "are a strain on the nerves for which Savasana is the best antidote."[15]

Sundaram, as we've seen, also defines *Savasana* as relaxation exercise. "There is a pose, the very name of which indicates complete supineness and immobility. This is Savasana. And it relaxes the whole body. The muscular exertions are made to cease and complete rest and tranquility are afforded to this wonderful machine, the human body."[16] But Sundaram defines *Savasana* as something more than relaxation exercise to a much greater extent than Iyengar: Alter's impassioned praise of Iyengar's commentary on *Savasana* can be more accurately applied to Sundaram's commentary on *Savasana* because the latter is not

only far more detailed and poetic but also far more physical and metaphysical.

The Body as Vehicle for Transcendence

In *Yogic Physical Culture,* Sundaram intuitively places his instructions for *Savasana* within the framework of the eight-limbed path of transcendence, which was explicated in the *Yoga Sutra,* the text compiled by Patanjali between 325 and 425 CE, and espoused since the late 19th century by Easterners and Westerners alike as the "classical yoga" (fig. 13.2). Sundaram begins with the third through sixth limbs: posture, or *asana;* breath control, or *pranayama;* concentration, or *dharana;* and sense withdrawal, or *pratyahara.* First he tells his votaries to, "lie flat on your back on a soft spread," with the hands at the sides, the legs straight, the heels together, and the face looking up. Then, he instructs them to "breathe normally and steadily. Concentrate your thoughts and allow the mind to dwell within. Forget all outside emotions and sensations. Remember that you are relaxing the whole body and giving it absolute ease and relief."[17]

After this initial preparation, Sundaram guides yoga practitioners—frequently by urging them to use the New Thought practices of creative visualization and autosuggestion—through a sequence of relaxation exercises for bony segments and muscles, moving upward from the feet to the legs, trunk, hands, arms, and head:

Begin at the feet, loosen your calf-muscles, proceed up the knee joints, to the thighs and

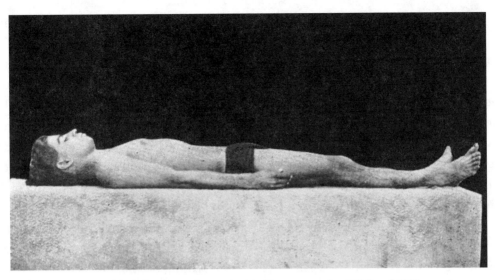

Figure 13.2. S. Sundaram demonstrating "Savasana or the Still Pose," 1929
(From *Yogic Physical Culture*)

then the hips. Repeat mentally at every place, "the muscles are relaxed; the body is relaxed; I am at ease." . . . From the hips and the gluteous [*sic*] muscles, come up the sides, the rectus muscles, and the loins, relaxing them perfectly. Rest and ease the back. . . . Then ascend the chest. While passing up the trunk . . . there should be corresponding relaxation of the fingers, the wrists, the elbows, the arms and the shoulders. . . . Pass up the throat. Relax the neck muscles, the chin, the mouth, the eyelids and the forehead.[18]

Toward the end of these instructions for the limbs, trunk, and head, Sundaram takes the practitioners in a surprising direction: literally inward. He directs them to relax their viscera: "Slowly in your mind carry the message of rest and peace through the bowels, the liver, the kidneys and then ascend to the chest."[19] At first this seems weird. After all, it requires visualizing the abdominal organs, which can't be seen or, for

that matter, directly touched, the way our toes or chest or belly can. To a great extent, internal organs have an implied existence: they're generally only palpable when swollen from disease. We usually know our inner organs through their effects (inhalations and exhalations of the lungs, flutterings of the heart, stirrings of the bowels, and the like).

Then the guided visualization gets downright goofy. Adherents are asked not just to relax the organs of the thoracic cavity but also to "circle round the heart in a stream of health and restful sensations and filter into the lungs, vitalizing the cells, carrying them the message of love, rest and peace."[20] Practitioners are being asked to comprehend their internal organs not through studying or observing or even considering their workings but through bathing them in love, rest, and peace. The internal organs are freed from exertion, absented any disturbance or agitation, and adored. Thusly, the seventh limb, meditation, or *dhyana,* is initiated. (On another level, this is a kind of lucid return—a going back that's different, needless to say, from an incoherent regression—to the first stage of infancy. Sundaram evokes this period of infancy when the infant is preoccupied with sensations inside its body. The infant imagines, it is posited, that the serenity and bliss that infuse its body, while actually emanating from the mother during feeding, are self-generated.)

The interior of their body suffused in bliss, votaries can complete the meditation by following Sundaram's next instruction: "All thoughts turned within, the mind following the calm and reposeful breath pronouncing the secret symbol of universal love and omnipotence 'OM!' in silence, remain as long as you can, from 5 to 10 minutes."[21]

Then the rapturous state is interrupted: "As the muscles relax, as the minutes pass, there would be the welcome feeling of a sort of deadening, cool and comfortable." This brief observation is terrifying, and not just because it describes an experience that's an anticipation of death: it reveals not our fear of death but our yearning for death. Death is welcoming. The total tranquillity brought about by yogic withdrawal from everyday life—enstasy—is the same as the tranquillity of death. *Savasana* becomes a ritualistic preparation for dying.

Seemingly with some alarm in his voice, Sundaram then urgently cautions devotees not to fall asleep, as if to scold them for seeking to escape a comprehension of death too unbearable to sustain. He is actually asking them to approach death in order to be reborn. By withdrawing from profane life, he's saying, they could find a deeper and truer life—one in tune

with the cosmos. For this transformation to take place, they must remain awake. "Keep the mind awake; awake to the sensations of rest and peace; awake to the thought that the organs are recuperating." And then comes the culmination of all that preceded it: the entry into ecstasy. "[Keep the mind] thrice awake to the music of the myriad worlds whirling in endless space, creating the perpetual vibration of 'OM!'"[22] The vibration of OM generated in their body unites with the cosmic vibration of Om. This is the eighth limb, union with the object of contemplation, or *samadhi*.

This final state is preverbal, which means to say, prethinking: it's a body/mind consciousness. Practitioners are liberated from their preoccupation with inner bodily sensations by a feeling of oneness with the outer world. (On another level, this is a kind of recapitulation of the second stage of infancy, in which the infant feels one with the mother—the stage, naturally enough, that is the source of our oceanic feeling of oneness and contentment with the world. But *samadhi* is not, it must be clearly understood, a regression to the stage of infancy in which we're at our mother's breast or held in her arms; it's a transcendence of the fragmented world.)

And then, after this transcendent journey, the transition back to the everyday world: "Fatigue is removed," Sundaram suddenly declares, his words sounding like a clap of the hands, snapping the practitioner back to ordinary life, as if the withdrawal from it had hardly been more than mere relief from physical effort and mental stress, as if the liberated state had been a dream.[23]

From where did Sundaram get this peculiar meditation?

Traditionally, we sit in a still, steady, and comfortable position during yogic meditation. Sundaram suggests lying down in *Savasana,* Corpse Pose, in a totally relaxed state. This spiritualized relaxation seems to derive, directly or indirectly, from Genevieve Stebbins's 1893 *Dynamic Breathing and Harmonic Gymnastics: A Complete System of Psychical, Aesthetic and Physical Culture,* in which Stebbins describes a spiritual consciousness that's accessed through relaxation while lying supine.

During meditation, all ordinary mental functions are arrested as we begin by concentrating on a single object, a point in space, an idea, or an image. Traditionally, the object of concentration includes features of the body, such as the navel or the space between the brows (locations of *chakras,* vital energy centers), but only for their symbolic value. The corporeal body is ignored. (We sit in a still, steady, and comfortable position in the first place so our consciousness won't be troubled by the presence of the body.) But Sundaram draws attention to the body! For him, the object of concentration *is* the body—the gross (not the subtle) body, the material and destructible body that stiffens inside and out, the pitiable body that makes us agitated and lonely, the body that lies lumpily on the ground (or floor) like a corpse.

Traditionally, the subject of the meditation is Vishnu or some other god (whom the yogin imagines being in the lotus of the heart). For Sundaram, the subject of the meditation—an extension of the object of meditation—is the body itself. Like the traditional meditation on fire (in which the meditation is begun by concentrating on glowing coals placed before the yogin), the meditation on the body expands to the universe.

This idiosyncratic meditation subject likely derives from three of Sundaram's strongest identities: physical culturist, parent who had suffered loss and neglect as a child, and yogin. The meditation mixes the physical culturist's fixation on the health of the internal organs, the mother's soothing love for her child, and the Hindu's spirituality. In addition, the meditation is infused with the quality that novelist W. Somerset Maugham, who met Sundaram in 1938, described as Sundaram's "poetic sensibility; landscape and rivers, flowers, the sky by day and the sky by night were a delight to him."[24] The sui generis end result is yogic meditation as poetic lullaby—a lullaby intended not to put children to sleep but to awaken yoga practitioners to an embodied spirituality.

In his article "Salvation through Relaxation: Proprioceptive Therapy and Its Relationship to Yoga," modern yoga scholar Mark Singleton traces the Western influences (the "amalgam of proprioceptive therapies, early humanistic psychology, and a variety of Western esoteric speculations") on yogic spiritualized relaxation. Singleton, who remains impartial about whether this "relatively new and composite phenomenon" is a corruption or merely a development of the yoga tradition, remarks, "Relinquishing tension during formalised relaxation sessions, it is said, leads to self-realisation or at the very least furnishes insights into one's fundamental, true, and eternal nature."[25] Sundaram would argue that these kinds of transformations are exactly what yoga facilitates, and yoga modernists would argue that in every age yogins create a version of yoga relevant to their times and that Sundaram's version of yogic meditation practiced during *Savasana*—despite, or perhaps because of, it being a composite of physical culture, Western esotericism, personal history, and traditional yogic philosophy—is relevant to our times, in which agitation commonly prevents us from comprehending underlying realities.

In his 1962 tribute to Sundaram, "Diamond Jubilee of the Yogacharya," Kavi Yogi Suddhananda Bharatiar praises Sundaram for having "carved a glorious destiny for himself through his impeccable service to humanity in the demonstration of Yogasanas." But "Sundaram is not a mere Asan-Vala," Bharatiar continues. "Even street jugglers do Asan and it has become very cheap and common today though the technique is very defective. . . . His psychic being measures the heaven of Yogic Realisation soaring higher and higher to unknown planes of divine consciousness."[26]

Bharatiar (as would Sundaram himself) attributed Sundaram's possession of "the deeper mysteries of knowledge far beyond mere bending and stretching of the body" to his initiation by Swami Sivaprakasa Ananda Giri into "Vedantic Yoga which perfects the whole being en-masse and brings real peace and bliss to human life."[27]

Sundaram had been smitten by Giri not when he was an impressionable youth but when he was a thirty-nine-year-old responsible husband and father and accomplished professional. While in court one day in 1940, he heard that a great *sadhu* who frequently experienced *bhava samadhi* (an ecstatic devotional state often translated as "trance") had come to an ashram in Bangalore. Sundaram rushed over to the ashram. When he walked into the hall and saw Giri sitting on the dais, Sundaram felt as if "the

Himalayas were sitting there in human form." He prostrated himself in a gesture of surrender. Giri stayed in Bangalore, and Sundaram became one of his disciples. Sundaram hailed Giri as "the Great One."[28]

Shortly before Giri died in late 1942, Sundaram went to Giri's Mallikarjunaswami Temple for his midday devotion. He retired to the *puja* room. A while later, Giri brought a disciple into the room, where they found Sundaram sitting before the shrine, absorbed in worship and unaware of them. "To test the dept [*sic*] of Sundaram's yoga," Giri commanded the disciple to strike Sundaram (presumably in the head) with all his might. The disciple dutifully punched Sundaram as hard as he could. "Nothing happened. Sri Sundaram was sitting there as [if] carved out of stone, insentient." Giri and the other disciple left the room. When Sundaram come out later, Giri asked him, "Do you feel bodily pain?" Although puzzled by the question, Sundaram simply answered, "No."[29] While the magical story element more suitable for a folk tale—Sundaram's imperviousness to a blow—is almost certainly apocryphal, Sundaram had finally achieved the *samadhi* that he had sought since he was seventeen.

But nearly fifteen years earlier in his *Savasana* meditation, Sundaram showed that we could comprehend deep mysteries not by blotting out the body but by being exquisitely attentive to the body—if not to the body as it bends and stretches, then at least to the body exhausted by bending and stretching. Not that the body assuming a yoga pose isn't a suitable subject of meditation—which we've come to learn, in part, because Sundaram, by meditating on the body in repose, opened the way for later yogins to meditate on the complexities of the movements of the *asanas* themselves.

Coda

Sundaram led an austere life. He got up at five each morning to meditate. He rigorously observed all the orthodox Hindu precepts concerning bathing and food. His chief nourishment was milk, fruit, and nuts. He went off to work at his law office. Unlike Iyer, who mounted plays on a stage in his gymnasium and regularly went to the movies, he never attended the theater or movies.

Sundaram taught yoga at his yoga center, Sri Sundara Yoga Shala, founded in the 1930s in the Payappa Garden area. Maugham observes that he was "extremely nice" to his students, without having any "cloying affectionateness. . . . He was natural and human."[30] Feeling obligated to relieve the suffering of others, in 1947 Sundaram opened an inpatient/outpatient section in the yoga center, where patients afflicted by chronic diseases not cured by drugs could find relief through yoga therapy.

In his work circle, Sundaram's activities as a yogin were largely unknown and therefore unheralded. We know this from an event that took place in 1949, toward the end of his legal career. At close to nine o'clock one evening at the Central Railway Station in Madras, as the train to Bangalore was about to depart, a retired high court judge of Mysore stood in the doorway of his first-class compartment to watch a large crowd of prominent people (which included a zamindar, a presidency magistrate, a number of businessmen, and several yogins) sweeping toward the train. Upon reaching his compartment, the members of the crowd stopped and prostrated themselves, one by one, before a bountifully garlanded figure revealed in their center. "Their dress braving the dust of the public platform, [they] touch[ed] his feet."[31] The ex-judge instantly recognized the adored man, his arms filled with presents, including fruits, as a lawyer who had argued many cases before him: Sundaram. The ex-judge ducked inside the car.

As the train whistle blew, Sundaram boarded the compartment, went to the lower berth, put down his presents, sat down, and, as the train moved out of the station, waved good-bye to his admirers.

A voice familiar to Sundaram rang out from the upper berth: "Mr. Sundaram, you seem to be something grand here. All these tributes and salutations! We in Bangalore never knew you were revered like this."

Sundaram rose to address his former colleague. "They believe I am a spiritual personality and guide," he explained in a modest tone.

"Well, Mr. Sundaram, we in Bangalore, have taken you as an ordinary lawyer with some knowledge of Yoga Asanas," the ex-judge replied. "This scene is an eye opener!"[32]

Not the least of Sundaram's virtues was his acceptance of his householder responsibilities. His wife's pregnancy in 1921 could've been the tipping point in a series of dispiriting events that propelled the twenty-year-old husband to enter the life of self-denial of an ascetic, donning a saffron cloth and becoming a *sannyasi* studying scriptures. However, instead of succumbing to the temptations of religious escapism, he became a dependable husband,

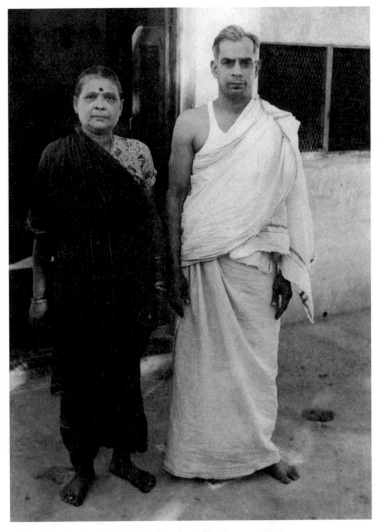

Figure 13.3. S. Sundaram and his wife, Nagalakshmi, 1940s

(With the kind permission of Hari Shankar R.)

father to his daughter, and lawyer. He went on to have eight more children. "He was evidently devoted to his wife and children and proud of them," Maugham notes (fig. 13.3).[33] Applying himself with "zest, intelligence and integrity," Sundaram maintained his modest law practice until 1952, when he retired.[34]

There's a grimness to a life defined by accepting responsibilities—caring for one's wife and children, waking and dressing and going to work, making the best of things. And there's a nobility. But then Sundaram, who led such a life, had something to rely on for support. "Not choosing to run away from the world and not caring to fortify himself by external renunciation," his biographers perceptively write, "he has been living in the midst of turmoil and distress, firmly rooted in Yoga and daringly beckoning all to taste its glorious fruits of inner peace and dedicated action."[35]

PART II

Making Yoga Dynamic
The Sun Salutations as Yogic Exercise

14

BHAVANARAO PANT PRATINIDHI

Reviving *Surya Namaskar*

Bodybuilding

"In 1897 we read about Sandow, the famous physical culturist," recalled Bhavanarao Pant Pratinidhi (1868–1951), the rajah of Aundh, "and purchased all his apparatus and books, and for full ten years practiced regularly and continuously according to his instruction."[1] In taking up bodybuilding at his palace in Aundh, a small princely state then under British authority but ruled by the rajah (and now a part of the state of Maharashtra), Bhavanarao was nothing if not up with the latest trend in physical culture. Eugen Sandow's *Strength and How to Obtain It* had just been published in 1897. A training manual, the book was illustrated with dumbbell exercises that could be performed at home. "Thus physical fitness," explains Sandow's biographer David L. Chapman, "was made available to large numbers of interested people who might never have tried it before."[2]

By "all his apparatus" Bhavanarao meant Sandow's patented Grip Dumbbells and Developer, which Sandow advertised in his books and promoted on world tours. The Grip Dumb-bell was separated into an upper and lower half connected by springs. The pupil (who was, until 1911, assumed by Sandow to be male) had to exert force to keep the two halves together. When using ordinary dumbbells, he might exercise in "a desultory and half-hearted manner"; squeezing the grip provided him with "a definite point upon which to concentrate his mind."[3] "Sandow's Own Combined Developer" was an Indian rubber strand device that was attached to a wall or closed door (one strand to the top, the other to the knob) and vigorously yanked. The handles were weighted with removable light dumbbells. Exercises for the developer complemented dumbbell exercises.

Sandow claimed to be a physical culturist promulgating a system for preventing and curing disease: "The body, in fact, like a child, wants to be educated, and only through a series of exercises can this education be given. By its aid the whole body is developed, and, as will be seen, pupils who have conscientiously worked at my system testify freely to the good results obtained, not only in the direction of vastly increasing their muscular strength, but of raising the standard of their vitality and general health."[4]

But Sandow's primary identity (in the eyes of others) was as bodybuilder, not physical culturist. He was the first showman bodybuilder. In the 1890s, under the management of Professor Attila (Louis Durlacher, Sandow's teacher as well as promoter) in Great Britain, and under the management of Florenz Ziegfield Jr. (who would later gain fame as a Broadway impresario, best known for his series of theatrical revues, the Ziegfield Follies) in America, the German-born Sandow traveled the variety theater circuit as Sandow the Magnificent, displaying to rapt audiences, as reported in the *New York Herald* in 1893, "such knots and bunches and layers of muscle that they had never before seen other than on the statue of an Achilles, a Discobolus, or the Fighting Gladiator."[5]

The history of male beauty in the modern (i.e., postmedieval) era may be said to have begun with the display in 1508 of the recently discovered marble statue of Apollo, a Roman copy of the bronze Greek original.* This stunningly graceful statue, which captures the Greek god midmoment slipping from tautness into repose just after he's shot an arrow and slain a foe, was the first of Pope Julius II's collection of ancient statues to be displayed in the Vatican's Belvedere Courtyard, the first public museum since antiquity, and was immediately considered to be the sculptural embodiment of ideal male beauty.[†]

The modern aestheticization of the male body evolved over the next four hundred years through such diverse developments as leisure travel (particularly the Grand Tours made by wealthy Britons) to Italy, where the ancient statues could be seen; the dissemination of images of the statues through prints; published reflections (particularly the works of Johann Joachim Winckelmann) on the ideal beauty of the statues; the celebration of anatomy based on dissection; scientific discoveries in biomechanics and kinesiology about muscle function (such as contraction and relaxation); the prescribing of corrective exercises by physicians for improving physical function and disability; the formation of northern European systems of gymnastics; technological innovations (such as plate-loaded barbells); the cult of beauty (a sensuous response to Victorian sedateness); the urge to refashion the body; and the sanctioning of self-love (in the guise of self-realization).

---

*A case can also be made for this history beginning with the depiction in early Renaissance paintings of hunky naked men as mythological or religious figures, including Christ, but perhaps most notably the martyred St. Sebastian.

†Its reputation would remain very much the same throughout subsequent centuries but would be most celebrated during the Enlightenment. In 1771 Johann Wolfgang von Goethe would chastise the statue: "Apollo of Belvedere, why do you show yourself to us in all your nakedness making us ashamed of our own?" (Goethe, quoted in Mosse, *Image of Man,* 32).

Recent historians (some swayed by contemporary observers in the 19th and early 20th centuries) generally depict the origin of modern physical culture in a particular region or country as a bellicose response by its peoples to a unique plight (e.g., by Germans to the defeat of the German states by Napoleon Bonaparte, by settled Americans to the competition from waves of immigrants, and by Indians to the oppression of British colonialists). Bodybuilding, the most flamboyant aspect of physical culture, is commonly considered to be a compensatory response by modern men to a blow to their masculinity dealt not only by adversaries but also by sedentary factory and office life—by, in effect, modernization. Bodybuilding deserves better than this facile reductionism. It should be treated in the same manner as other glorious phenomena of the 19th century, such as the train, the cinema, and impressionist painting.* The history of modern male beauty, sparked around 1500 by the classical idiom of male perfection found in the body and carriage of statues of nude male youths, culminated in the supreme bodybuilder, Eugen Sandow—an ancient Greek statue come alive. As such, in the popular imagination circa 1900, Sandow was the embodiment of perfect manhood.

In *Strength and How to Obtain It* Sandow proffered to his readers the same benefits that his pupils had received: "Pupils who have followed my system testify not only to their increased muscular strength but to their general health."[6] But his expressed concern for the strength and good health of his readers is belied by the book's illustrations: photos of Sandow displaying his heroic, godlike physique, an appeal to the reader's fantasies of becoming a pumped-up superman. In becoming an acolyte of Sandow, Bhavanarao was not merely seeking to achieve physical fitness; he was attempting to perfect his body by adorning it with bulging muscles as a means of attaining a new ideal of manhood—one that made it acceptable for men to display hard, sculpted, sexually charged bodies in physique contests and, just as for women in the bathing beauty pageants that became a regular part of summer beach life in the 1880s, to be gazed at and adored (fig. 14.1).

After ten years, Bhavanarao rejected Sandow's bodybuilding regimen (although not, as we shall see later, all that was implied by it). He did so because it didn't achieve the results he was seeking: a shapely figure. While the measurements of "the waist and abdomen showed a marked reduction," "the chest measurement remained the same."[7]

As practically anyone who lifts weights nowadays at the local gym could tell you, obtaining a symmetrical, muscular body by following Sandow's home exercise instructions was doomed to failure. Sandow achieved his Herculean physique by training for bulk and power according to the three principles taught to him by Professor Attila: selectivity (choosing resistance exercises for targeted muscles), progression

---

*A historical account of male beauty that sings the praises of bodybuilding has already begun with Kenneth R. Dutton's *The Perfectible Body: The Western Ideal of Male Physical Development,* supplemented by articles such as Charles Musser's "'A Personality So Marked': Eugen Sandow and Visual Culture," Mary M. Lane's "Why Naked Men Get Short Shrift," and Anne Hollander's "Men in Tights." These works are correctives to the typical late 20th- and early 21st-century cultural histories that trace discourses of masculinity in crisis, such as George L. Mosse's *The Image of Man: The Creation of Modern Masculinity* and Tamar Garb's *Bodies of Modernity: Figure and Flesh in Fin-de-Siècle France.*

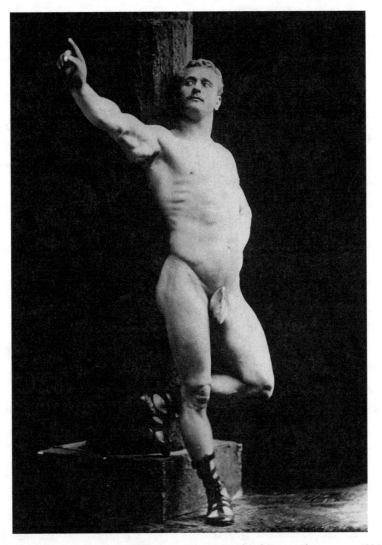

Figure 14.1. Eugen Sandow, pointing, oracle-like, in his famous column pose, 1894
(With the kind permission of David L. Chapman)

(gradually increasing the resistance against the targeted muscles), and high intensity (placing a high overload on the targeted muscles). The regimen Sandow advocated in his book not only couldn't develop a body with the massive musculature of a bodybuilder, it couldn't even develop a toned, sinuous body, which many prefer. In fact, it couldn't even provide the moderate amount of strength needed to carry out daily tasks with ease. The best that could be said for the strength-training methods found in Sandow's book is that they could supply a modicum of muscular development for "weaklings and invalids to improve their health," says Chapman, and might inspire others to join a gymnasium where they could progress to lifting heavier weights.[8]

It was lucky for those who practice hatha yoga, however, that Sandow's book, apparatus, and instructions were largely useless marketing gimmicks; otherwise, Bhavanarao might never have turned to reviving a centuries-old exercise that had apparently fallen into neglect.

Taking Up *Surya Namaskar*

In 1908, influenced by the example and advice of his "esteemed friend" Gangadharrao Patwardhan II, the rajah of Miraj Senior, a princely state, Bhavanarao took up *surya namaskar* (sun salutation exercise) with zeal. *Surya namaskar* is a series of positions (mistakenly thought to be adapted from yoga postures) performed at a fairly fast pace with fluid transitional movements accompanied by rhythmic breathing. The series is repeated for a length of time, say, ten minutes, becoming a form of vigorous yet graceful and seemingly relaxed cardiorespiratory exercise.

This was Bhavanarao's version of the exercise. (Although the positions of *surya namaskar* were not considered to be *asanas* at this time, for convenience's sake, they are anachronistically described here using B. K. S. Iyengar's nomenclature, which has become the lingua franca in yogasana.)

- First position: Stand in *Tadasana,* Mountain Pose, with the hands folded at the chest in prayer.
- Second position: Bend down into *Uttanasana,* Standing Forward Bend, with the arms straight and the hands flat on the floor.
- Third position: Raise the head, bring the right leg back, and bend the left leg (lunge). The arms remain straight.
- Intermediate position: Bring the left leg back along the right leg with the arms still straight (plank).

- Fourth position: Bend the arms, flick the toes under, and dip to the floor in a position that closely resembles *Chaturanga Dandasana,* Four-Limbed Staff Pose, but with the knees on the floor and the pelvis somewhat thrust upward.
- Fifth position: Straighten the arms, lift the torso and head up, and bend back into a position that closely resembles *Urdhva Mukha Svanasana,* Upward-Facing Dog. (This position also somewhat resembles *Bhujangasana,* Cobra Pose, because the knees and lower part of the front thighs are on the floor.)
- Intermediate position: Raise the hips, straighten the legs, and bring the trunk and head down with the arms still outstretched into *Adho Mukha Svanasana,* Downward-Facing Dog.
- Sixth position: Bring the left leg forward. Bring the right leg forward. Straighten the knees and rise to the first position.
- The sequence is repeated with all the single leg movements reversed.

Bhavanarao would go on to practice *surya namaskar* "continuously, regularly and systematically . . . with Vedic and Bija Mantras" in darkness between 3 and 4 o'clock in the morning, well before sunrise, every day for the rest of his life.[9]

When Bhavanarao began to practice *surya namaskar* in earnest, he had long been familiar with it: he'd learned it as a child, probably in the 1870s, from his father, who practiced it for fifty-five years. Rather than merely repeating what he'd learned from his father, though,

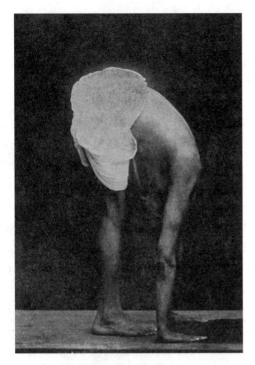

Figure 14.2. Bhavanarao Pant Pratinidhi, demonstrating the second position of *surya namaskar*, 1924

(From *Surya Namaskars [Sun-Adoration] for Health, Efficiency & Longevity*, by Bhavanarao Pant Pratinidhi)

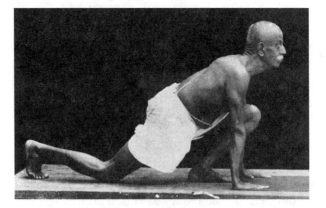

Figure 14.3. Bhavanarao Pant Pratinidhi, demonstrating the third position of *surya namaskar*, 1924

(From *Surya Namaskars [Sun-Adoration] for Health, Efficiency & Longevity*)

Bhavanarao experimented, making subtle modifications to some *surya namaskar* positions.

It was in 1908 that we first began to do Surya Namaskars in the old style. According to this the knees were not straightened while bending over, nor was the foot brought forward on a line with the palms, and it was not necessary to stand erect at the beginning of each Namaskar or to regulate the breathing in the way we have indicated.

After doing the Namaskars in this way for about a year, we tried one day to bring the toes of one leg forward on a line with the palms, and found that it put a greater strain on the abdomen and waist. This was the first improvement made on the old style.

On another occasion, while attempting to straighten the knees while bending over to place the palms on the ground, we experienced a still greater stretching sensation in the calves, thighs, waist, abdomen, and throughout the back. A material improvement resulted.[10]

In this account of his simple adjustments to the old style of *surya namaskar,* we find just as great an achievement as Bhavanarao's later indefatigable promotion of his new style of *surya namaskar,* through which it became popular in India and, later on, around the world (figs. 14.2 and 14.3).

History of *Surya Namaskar*

Surya namaskar is undoubtedly named for its resemblance to the sun worship ritual in which Brahmin priests kneel and lie prostrate in adoration of the sun—a ritual that seems to have been practiced continuously in India since Vedic times. Performed at sunrise while facing east, the sun worship ritual is the priest's expression of the community's gratefulness to Surya (the Sun God) after the night's seclusion and austerity. The ritual is part entreaty for Surya's continued beneficence and part giving thanks for Surya's light of life, without which we wouldn't exist, and, by extension, for all that comforts and nourishes us and helps us endure. A critical part of the worship is the chanting of the celebrated *gayatri* mantra: *Om tat savitur varenyam bhargo devasya dhimahi dhiyo yo nah pracodayat* (We meditate on the ineffable effulgence of the resplendent Sun; may That direct our understanding).

The sun worship ritual isn't practiced by the laity nor, for that matter, even found entrancing to the laity. "No one really pays close attention to the ritual," says Roxanne Gupta, a scholar of Indian dance. "They feel it will benefit them with or without their attention. When people go to the temple to worship in the morning, they go straight to the main altar (sanctum) and walk right past the Brahmins doing the sun worship ritual. It's their thing, not the public's, even though the public knows it will benefit them. Hindus don't have a fascination for [priestly] rituals. They take them for granted."[11]

The basic movements of the ancient sun worship ritual, still practiced in the sun temple in Andhra Pradesh, one of only seven Hindu temples dedicated to Surya remaining in India today, are austere: the priests stand, crouch over, put their weight on their hands, drop to their knees, fall forward supported by their hands, lie prostrate (in the position most deeply expressive of supplication) for a few seconds while chanting, resume kneeling, and get up again. These larger movements are accompanied by an elaborate pattern of smaller movements with symbolic meaning—movements that in another context would be seen as compulsive and debilitating rituals used to ward off some sort of danger or, perhaps, as a variation of a children's game, such as patty-cake, with its sometimes complex sequence of hand clapping. These smaller symbolic movements consist of the following: While standing, the priests cross their hands at their groin. After kneeling (and before kneeling again), they fleetingly place one hand over the other on the floor, tapping their closed hands together and to the floor. After lying prone, they cross and uncross their legs at the ankles three different times, and they bring their arms back and cup their hands at the small of the back, twice swivel their downward-facing head to the left and right, jutting the chin out to the floor, and then dramatically extend their arms in front with their elbows on the floor, bring their hands together in prayer position, pat the floor near their face, quickly touch their collarbone, and tuck their head in, with their forehead to the floor.[12]

Although this ritual, unlike Western prayer, involves rhythmic chanting and movement, the basic movements are performed awkwardly. They have a restricted range of motion. Despite being repeated 108 times, they don't demand a great deal of energy. All in all, it can be said that this ritual has none of the grace, complex whole-body movement (especially of the spine) and dynamism of *surya namaskar* (not to mention the theatrical panache when performed by Iyengar, who practically flung himself into the positions and then held them an extra moment as if pausing for applause).[13] As Gupta points out: "The sun worship movements aren't an exercise. They have nothing to do with fitness of the body."[14]*

The *surya namaskar* exercise appears to have been first developed—or, at least, can only be traced back—a few hundred years ago. In the July 1926 issue of *Yoga-Mimansa,* Kuvalayananda provides this tantalizing glimpse (without citing a source) of the colorful history of *surya namaskar:* "This system of exercise [*surya namaskar*] has been in vogue in Maharashtra at least for a few centuries and is very much favoured by the upper classes of the society. In the eighteenth century it was not unusual to find youths making as many as twelve hundred prostrations every morning. Among such youths were to be seen some of the Brahmana rulers of the land."[15]

In his *Encyclopedia of Indian Physical Culture* (a one-volume English condensation, published in 1950, of the ten-volume Marathi original published from 1935 to 1950), editor D. C. Mujumdar encapsulates the history of *surya namaskar* in the same sketchy manner (also without a citation), highlighting the efforts of Samartha Ramdas (1608–1681), the firebrand wise man who proselytized a militant Hindu revivalism primarily in Maharashtra, a large region in India that includes Mumbai (Bombay): "Samartha Ramdas, whose renowned disciple was Shiwaji, the founder of the Maratha Empire in the latter half of the seventeenth century, was the pioneer in reviving and spreading Namaskaras in every nook and corner of Maharashtra. He was a man of such a formidable strength that he used to practise 1200 Namaskaras daily. His disciples developed like him strong but supple bodies. The Hindus had immense respect for this great bachelor who successfully preached his doctrines with singular zeal and personal example, throughout his life."[16]

The original purpose of *surya namaskar* exercise isn't known. It was probably developed as preparation for strength exhibitions, sports (especially wrestling), or military training, not as an exercise solely for developing and maintaining fitness. At Ramdas's urging, Shiwaji established numerous *akharas* (wrestling gymnasiums) throughout Maharashtra, where in all likelihood he implemented *surya namaskar* as part of the wrestler's extensive exercise regimen.

While the general shape of *surya namaskar* exercise was derived from the ancient sun worship ceremony, the influences that formed the particular positions are also unknown. If *surya namaskar* preceded the birth of Ramdas (1608–1681) or even originated in his youth, then the positions that make up *surya namaskar* don't derive from hatha yoga. Of the three primarily hatha yoga texts—*Hatha Yoga Pradipika,* from the 15th to 16th centuries; *Gheranda Samhita,* possibly from the 17th or 18th century; and *Shiva Samhita,* apparently from the late 17th or early 18th century—only *Gheranda Samhita* describes a yoga posture, *Bhujangasana,* Cobra Pose, that even resembles a position found in

---

*In the late 1980s, after witnessing Brahmin priests performing their daily worship in the sun temple in Andhra Pradesh, Gupta, who was tutored in *surya namaskar* by Bhavanarao's son, Apa B. Pant, demonstrated *surya namaskar* for the priests. Never having seen this elaborate set of rhythmic exercises that somewhat resembles their ancient sun worship ritual, they were quite bemused.

surya namaskar—what is simply called the "the fifth position" by Bhavanarao. (And actually, *Urdhva Mukha Svanasana*, Upward-Facing Dog, more closely resembles this position.) So the rest of the *surya namaskar* positions (and perhaps even this one) must've been incorporated into the yoga canon from *surya namaskar,* perhaps as late as the mid-1800s. This sequence of events seems likely because the positions of *surya namaskar* were designed to facilitate what Bhavanarao described as "a large number of different springlike, quick and buoyant movements of the body" and don't (directly) lend themselves to enhancing the ability of sitting in repose, with steadiness and ease, for a long period of time in meditation, as do the original conditioning postures of traditional hatha yoga.[17]

The positions of *surya namaskar* exercise may have been influenced by *dands* (jackknifing push-ups) that, along with *bethaks* (deep squats), constitute the core wrestling *vyayam* regimen. The preliminary position for *dands* isn't standing up but lying prone on the ground with the palms directly below the shoulders. The two positions of the *dand* proper closely resemble two of the six basic *surya namaskar* positions. In the first *dand* position, one straightens the arms, bends at the knees, and thrusts the hips up and back into a position that resembles a slack *Adho Mukha Svanasana*, Downward-Facing Dog. In an intermediate position, one bends the arms and further bends the legs, pushes the torso down and forward, and brings the chest between the hands. In the second position, one pushes the torso up by straightening the arms (thus strengthening the arms, shoulders, and upper back), with only the palms and the toes on the ground, into a position resembling a droopy *Urdhva Mukha Svanasana,* Upward-Facing Dog.

But the questions remain: Did *surya namaskar* exercise evolve solely from the religious ceremony, and two of its positions were later appropriated by wrestlers as the *dand*? Or did *surya namaskar* exercise evolve from the religious ceremony by incorporating the *dand* from the wrestling tradition? At this point, the origin of *surya namaskar* exercise remains murky.

Surya namaskar was practiced both as worship of Surya and as exercise at the turn of the 20th century. Historian of Aryan medicine Bhagvat Sinh Jee observed in 1896 that in India "there are various kinds of physical exercise indoors and outdoors. But some of the Hindoos set aside a portion of their daily worship for making salutations to the Sun by prostrations. This method of adoration affords them so much muscular activity that it takes to some extent the place of physical exercise."[18] But it appears that practicing *surya namaskar* as exercise was in decline.

According to Mujumdar, "in the nineteenth century, zeal for Namaskaras gradually deteriorated and many people practically neglected it. Until at last [in the early twentieth century] Shrit. Bhavanrao Pant Pratinidhi Raja of Aundh, who got inspiration from Shrit. Balasaheb Mirajkar the late Raja of Miraj, systematized the science of Namaskaras, analysed it and put in a Book-let on the Namaskar-exercises with illustrations."[19]

15

BHAVANARAO PANT PRATINIDHI

Promoting *Surya Namaskar* as Health Cure and Strengthening Exercise

Worshipping the Sun Indoors

"There are [those] who seriously question why the Sun should be bowed to," Bhavanarao Pant Pratinidhi, the rajah of Aundh, provocatively declared in his 1928 illustrated exercise manual, *Surya Namaskars (Sun-Adoration) for Health, Efficiency & Longevity,* in seeming disbelief that anyone would not hold the sun as an object of worship, and therefore would not want to take up *surya namaskar* (what is now commonly translated as "sun salutations" rather than "sun adoration" but is perhaps more accurately translated as "salutations to the Sun God"), a rhythmic exercise composed of a sequence of ten or so positions performed in rounds.[1] Influenced by Auguste Rollier, the world-famous physician who popularized heliotherapy, sun cure, in the early 1900s, Bhavanarao held "that sun-light was just as necessary to the growing child, and to everybody else too for that matter, as it is to the growing plant, and in exactly the same way—that is, in *direct* contact with the skin." As proof, he referred skeptics to the expert testimony of Rollier and several Western physical culturists who had recently discovered the scientific value of treating illness by exposure to direct sunlight. One of them, quoted by Bhavanarao from Bernarr Macfadden's July 1926 issue of *Physical Culture,* advised: "Bathe your body in the Sun. The Sun is the greatest of healers. . . . Tuberculosis, pneumonia, [and other diseases

189

and illnesses] are being cured with regularity, speed and certainty by this new method called Heliotherapy."[2]

In actuality, though, practicing *surya namaskar* as a kind of sun bathing was of no importance to Bhavanarao. He performed his sun salutations from 4:00 to 5:00 a.m. in his mansion in Aundh, greeting the sun in worship without absorbing its healing rays. (In doing *surya namaskar* indoors, commonly in an austere room set aside for yoga classes, contemporary practitioners have followed in his footsteps, as well as his hand placements.) His great fervor for *surya namaskar* was based instead on the health and fitness benefits derived from practicing it as vigorous exercise, which, in fact, is how he primarily promoted it.

Bhavanarao advocated practicing a daily regime of *surya namaskar* cycles, with one cycle taking twelve seconds: 25 to 50 cycles for children from eight to twelve, 50 to 150 cycles for boys and girls from twelve to sixteen, and 300 cycles for everyone over sixteen.[*] "If this practice be religiously and constantly observed," he asserted, "one can defy all preventable disease and will keep oneself fit in mind and body as long as the exercises are persisted in."[3] But there was a proviso: the sequence of exercises must be performed with what he called "will power" (or sometimes "mind force," "will force," or "auto-suggestion"). "Long-continued Surya Namaskars done loosely or in a slovenly manner may give the body some benefit," he asserted,

"but the full development of every part, cure of disease, or removal of pain cannot be produced unless the whole will-power is brought to bear upon the particular part of the body while actually performing the Surya Namaskars."[4]

Although this conviction that exerting the will over parts of the body while performing *surya namaskar* develops muscles, cures disease, and removes pain may seem to come from the tradition of yogic magical thinking, it's actually derived from the New Thought movement that had sprung up in America in the 1890s and first decades of the 20th century, based on the mid-19th-century philosophy and practice of Phineas Parkhurst Quimby, who sat beside his patients to gently persuade them that disease is an error of the mind (a belief that he termed "the Truth") in order to effect a cure.[†]

Bhavanarao extolled the insights of the influential New Thought author Frank Channing Haddock: "Says he in his great book, *Power of Will* [published in 1907]—'Physical health is . . . reached through the resolute and persistent Will.'"[5] But his praise was given only to lend authority to his own statements about the need for applying willpower "in the performance of any bodily exercise and especially in doing Surya Namaskars"[6] (Haddock's "observation . . . will further elucidate our point"[7]).

Willpower (as well as mental control, positive thinking, and auto-suggestion), Bhavanarao argued, is an original Indian concept recently (re)discovered by Westerners. Because

---

[*]In the mid-1930s Bhavanarao drastically curtailed the daunting recommendation for adults, made in the late 1920s, to twenty-five *surya namaskar* cycles to be completed in five or six minutes. (Presumably, he reduced the recommendations for children proportionally.) He himself continued performing three hundred *surya namaskars* in an hour.

[†]Unlike mesmerists, Quimby never claimed to be a medium, went into a trance, or even maintained that he possessed any unusual healing powers.

the ancient Indian sages "were not able to make their teaching acceptable by presenting it in terms of modern medical science . . . we had . . . to wait till . . . a Haddock appeared to instruct us in the value of will-power [and other Western authors taught us similar constructs]. . . . Any one who reads the works of these authors even cursorily and compares their teachings with those of our 'rishis' will not fail to be struck with wonder at the deep wisdom of our ancient 'rishis' and to bow down his head in speechless adoration."[8] Bhavanarao, like his fellow Indian physical culturists who made similar claims for the rishis, didn't provide any textual evidence to support his assertion.

Exercise: Health Benefits

Moving the Body in Particular Configurations

Bhavanarao claimed that the particular arrangement of body parts in most of the *surya namaskar* positions provides benefits to the internal organs, and hence cure diseases and ailments related to the organs. For example, in the fifth position (which resembles *Urdhva Mukha Svanasana,* Upward-Facing Dog), "all internal derangements, such as liver and spleen disorders and bowel complaints, disappear. . . . All predisposition to tonsillitis, enhanced by wrong eating, gradually vanishes. And it is believed that even scrofula [tuberculosis of the lymph nodes, especially in the neck] might be cured by this exercise."[9]

Chanting Bija Mantras

Since as early as the Vedic period, *bija* mantras (primary or "seed" mantras, consisting of an elemental sound followed by a nasal aftersound), although meaningless, have been considered to be a magical vehicle of salvation. The power of producing these sounds has been accorded great value for harmonizing with the vibrations of the cosmos. While chanting is an integral part of the ancient sun ceremony, Bhavanarao harnessed mantras for a new purpose: to serve health.

In a section of *Surya Namaskars* aptly titled "Health through Speaking," Bhavanarao explained: "There must now be described the wonderfully healing and vitalizing powers—physiological as well as psychic—possessed by the apparently meaningless Bija Mantras—Om, hram, hrim, etc., and how they influence several organs, such as the heart, stomach, brain, etc., and how they serve not only as prophylactic (preventive) but as therapeutic (curative) as well." "The mantras have to be recited in the standing position with hands folded," he instructed. "During actual exertions, such as bending down, prostrating and rising, all efforts are concentrated on inhaling and exhaling through the nose only."[10]

The claim that a mere sound can have an effect on the internal organs wouldn't have been made before the late 19th or early 20th century. Chanting mantras had long been held to be a technique of mystical physiology used to awaken a divine manifestation through the *chakras,* centers in the body where aspects of spiritual consciousness and physiological functions merge. In the late 19th century, scientifically minded Indians began to associate the *chakras* with key nerve plexuses in the body. Mid-20th-century yoga scholar Ernest Wood notes:

> Some modern scholars have strongly associated these chakras with important nerve

plexuses in the body—notably Major B. D. Basu of the Indian Medical Service, who explained these in the Prize Essay published in the Guy's Hospital Gazette in 1889. This eminent doctor and scholar gave the list as follows: 1) the sacral plexus [at the base of the male genital organ], 2) the prostatic plexus [at the perineum, situated at the base of the spinal column], 3) the epigastric plexus [the lumbar region at the level of the navel], 4) the cardiac plexus [region of the heart], 5) the pharyngeal plexus [region of the throat], and 6) the cavernous plexus [between the eyebrows].[11]*

To mold *surya namaskar* into physical culture, Bhavanarao redefined it as a system for preventing and curing disease by aiding the internal organs. Once the *chakras* were defined as plexuses, it was a short jump for Bhavanarao to claim that mantras, long held to have a correspondence with the *chakras,* could affect the organs associated with those plexuses: "Bija Mantras produce stimulation and vibration in different vital parts of the system, such as the heart, abdomen, throat, palate, windpipe, brain etc., purify their blood, and consequently remove disorders, ailments and diseases in those regions."[12] Realizing full well that this mixture of yogic magical thinking and alternative medicine sounded like hokum, Bhavanarao had a ready response: "If this sounds absurd I can't help it. I am dealing with facts. The thing happens."[13]

Exercise: Fitness Benefits

Strength

Although iconometric rules for the presentation of the major gods exist in the *Shilpa Shastra* (Gupta-period instructional manuals with strict rules for presenting the physiques of Indian gods in holy pictures, carvings, and statues), there's no Indian exercise tradition for attaining the harmonious physique of the gods. It's not *vyayam,* the centuries-old Indian system of physical training practiced in the service of wrestling and feats of strength. And it's certainly not *surya namaskar.* Sociocultural anthropologist Joseph S. Alter argues that Bhavanarao nonetheless turned to *surya namaskar* to achieve a beautiful physique: "In Bhavanrao's conception *surya namaskar* was a form of body-building."[14] It's true that Bhavanarao rejected Sandow's home exercises because they failed to provide him with the shapely figure he desired. And he did indeed make claims for *surya namaskar* as a kind of body sculpting. He praised the position that resembles Upward-Facing Dog mixed with Cobra Pose because "the girth of the chest increases, whilst that of the abdomen decreases" (the primary aesthetic result he sought when he took up Sandow's methods using mail-order apparatus).[15] Even so, Bhavanarao's primary concern was with *surya namaskar* as strength training (building strength to provide functional benefits), not body sculpting (maximizing muscles for display). On page one of his manual, in his declaration of principles, "The Necessity and Essentials of Exercise," in support of his conception of *surya namaskar* as

---

*The word *plexus* has been added to items 2 through 5 of this extract.

strength training, he quotes Macfadden: "You cannot keep throbbingly alive unless you give your body the muscular activity essential to thoroughly develop it. And *all through life* a certain amount of exercise is needed to maintain super strength and vitality."[16]

In "The Best Exercise" chapter of *Surya Namaskars,* Bhavanarao enumerated in great detail which muscles are strengthened in each position. For example:

> You will find that in [the second] position [the Forward Bend] the muscles of the calves, the rear part of the thighs, the hips, the waist and almost all of the muscles of the back receive a severe strain, which means a gradual development of those parts, where the roots of premature decay and decline find lodgment. Special strain will be felt on big muscles joining the back and shoulders. The triceps are also brought into action. Considerable stress is brought upon the abdomen and stomach muscles while stooping forward.[17]

Here (and with all the other positions), Bhavanarao got the mechanics of this exercise almost entirely wrong (see fig. 15.1 on page 194).

The "severe strain" that he described in the posterior parts of the body results from elongating muscles, not contracting them: the posterior muscles are being stretched, not "developed" (i.e., strengthened). Of course, without realizing it, Bhavanarao was right in attributing some degree of strength gain to what is basically a flexibility exercise. A basic principle of kinesiology is that muscles are so designed that as the agonist elongates, the antagonist contracts. (Though in this case, it's the muscles on the anterior side of the body—that is, those muscles *opposed* to the ones that Bhavanarao indicated—that are being strengthened through contraction.) But *some degree of strength gain* doesn't make for an optimal amount of strengthening, which is what's necessary for maintaining ideal posture, easily performing routine physical activities, and preventing injury. What does is performing strengthening exercises that are taxing, selective, and progressive—principles most efficiently applied by using free weights or resistance machines.*

So Alter goes further astray when he posits that "the modern form of the exercise [*surya namaskar*] was inspired by a theory of bodybuilding developed by the world-renowned physical

---

*While all the major modern hatha yogins made strength claims for yoga, the current common belief among yoga teachers that yoga develops sufficient muscle tone to prevent "flabbiness and general fatigue," "preserve the good appearance . . . of the body," and keep the body from "appear[ing] old long before its time" can be traced back to Richard Hittleman's *Yoga for Physical Fitness,* published in 1964 (Hittleman, *Yoga for Physical Fitness*, 118, 119). Touting his workout as "easy-to-do coordination, strengthening and isometric Yoga exercises especially designed for office workers and housewives," Hittleman sets aside an entire chapter, "Muscle Tone and Firmness," for presenting four yoga strengthening exercises that target hip and lower spine muscles: Side Raise, Back Push-up, Locust, and Lie Down–Sit Up. Addressing those readers who aren't inclined to perform "heavy muscular work requiring a great deal of effort" and therefore "end up doing no real muscular exercise at all," Hittleman assures his readers that these yoga strengthening exercises "require a minimum of effort and time for a maximum return in firming" (ibid., 118). A more forthright claim would've been that these four yoga postures—calisthenics exercises, really—are easy, mildly effective strengthening—and therefore toning—exercises that can be realistically adopted by the slothful and prudently adopted by the unconditioned elderly.

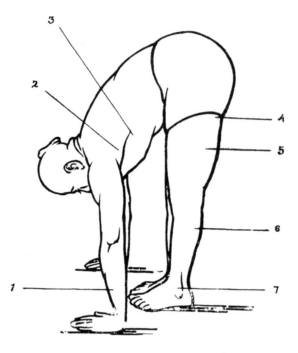

1 Brachio radialis. 2 Trapezeus & subscapularis.
3 Latissimus Dorsi. 4 Gluteii muscles. 5 Biceps Fimoris.
6 Hamstring (Lateral.). 7 Tendo Achillis.

Figure 15.1. Illustration of muscles that receive "strain" in the second position of *surya namaskar*

(From *Surya Namaskars [Sun-Adoration] for Health, Efficiency & Longevity*)

culturist Eugene Sandow," if, by *theory,* Alter means "the basic principles of muscular development upon which a bodybuilding program is built."[18] Bhavanarao's conception of *surya namaskar* was inspired not by a theory but by a *goal,* and not the goal primarily of bodybuilding but of strength training. Even though *surya namaskar,* like yogasana, clearly primarily develops flexibility, Bhavanarao declared that it develops strength. Whether deliberately or out of ignorance, he simply glommed the desired results of Western strength training onto *surya namaskar.*

Cardiorespiratory Endurance

Bhavanarao's touting of *surya namaskar* as strength training is even more puzzling because of his familiarity with the strength-training exercises of *vyayam.* "When young we studied wrestling under Imam Uddin, a well-known professional wrestler from the Punjab. We also practiced 'Jor,' 'Baithaks' and Indian clubs." (A common part of the contemporary Indian wrestler's exercise regimen, *surya namaskar* is conspicuously absent in the *vyayam* regimen that Bhavanarao was taught in the late 19th century, evidence that it became a part of the modern wrestling routine only after Bhavanarao promulgated it.) Bhavanarao gave up wrestling and the preparatory exercises because "in accordance with the accepted doctrines of the old school of wrestlers, we used to partake of unnecessary fatty foods and thus put on an excessive amount of fat."[19]

After rejecting Sandow's system for body-building, why didn't Bhavanarao take up the strength-developing exercises of *vyayam* again, this time without the fatty foods in a wrestler's diet? For one thing, the exercises aren't convenient. "To make . . . a physical exercise universally popular and acceptable," Bhavanarao explained, "there should be no necessity of apparatus or appliances; it should be easy to do; it should take a short time to perform; it should be of such a nature as to enable it to be taken anywhere and by anybody; and it should not necessitate a partner or companion."[20] *Surya namaskar* was handy. And if it didn't basically develop strength, well, Bhavanarao could get away with saying it did.

For another thing, the strength-training exercises of *vyayam,* like *asanas,* don't benefit the cardiorespiratory system. To effectively improve cardiorespiratory endurance, an exercise must rhythmically utilize large muscle groups for a minimum sustained period (at least twenty to thirty minutes) at a moderate to high intensity (between 40 to 85 percent of one's functional capacity). *Surya namaskar,* as advocated by Bhavanarao (as a strenuous repetitive movement performed over three hundred cycles) does.

For Bhavanarao, this was a critical benefit. It was what enabled him to promote *surya namaskar* not only as an Indian strength-training system but also as an Indian alternative to a vigorous form of calisthenics used as cardiorespiratory endurance conditioning. When performed in quick succession, calisthenics exercises tax the heart and lungs, improving the ability of the cardiovascular and respiratory systems to work together to sustain oxygen levels. The same holds for *surya namaskar.* While each

position is beneficial in itself, the flow of the series of positions, repeated many times, makes for cardiorespiratory endurance conditioning. (Which is why some who are deliberate and unhurried by nature dislike doing *surya namaskar.* They can't keep up. And it may remind them and others of the excruciating calisthenics exercises—jumping jacks, push-ups, alternate toe touchings, and such—they had to endure in school gym class.) With *surya namaskar,* "the heart, the lungs and the respiratory organs [are] fully developed and strengthened," Bhavanarao declared.[21]

Dynamic Flexibility

The most significant fitness aspect of *surya namaskar,* however—and the one that Bhavanarao didn't grasp—was another element totally absent in its rival Indian popular exercise, hatha yoga: dynamic stretching. Formed by bringing its previously preparatory conditioning poses to the fore, hatha yoga is based on static stretching, which involves holding a pose. *Surya namaskar,* in contrast, is based on the kind of dynamic stretching that involves rhythmic motion. The series of movements of *surya namaskar* are vigorously repeated in order to increasingly deepen the sequence of stretches. In time, some yogins would come to incorporate this form of dynamic flexibility into their yoga regimes—tagging it onto or even infusing it into their regimes—as a necessary means of obtaining overall flexibility.

Religion

In raising the body's temperature, making breathing arduous, and producing sweat over a sustained period, *surya namaskar* alters one's mood. Bhavanarao described this result as "a most remarkable lightness of body, buoyancy of mind, and a general feeling of youthfulness which must be experienced to be understood."[22] This sounds remarkably like the "runner's high," the euphoric state that sometimes occurs when a threshold is crossed during long, continuous, rigorous exercise. (Bhavanarao bolstered his argument with testimony from Macfadden on the effects of exercise in general: "Your emotional reaction to everything with which you come in contact in life [when you take up sufficient exercise] is tremendously multiplied and intensified. Life becomes a vivid, keen experience to you every day. You feel everything more keenly."[23]) But for Bhavanarao, this change in mood was perhaps the least of his goals. What he set out to do each morning was to change his state of consciousness.

Wanting everyone to reap the health and fitness benefits of *surya namaskar,* Bhavanarao reassured "some atheists and non-Hindus [who] shun the exercise of Namaskars on the ground that it is a religious rite [that] the Namaskar exercise has an appearance but an appearance only of a religious rite. But it is not essentially a religious rite."[24] He knew that the recitation of mantras was especially off-putting. "A great majority of the present generation say that Mantras and Tantras are all humbug," he conceded. "'I have,' said a gentleman to the writer recently, 'absolutely no faith in the mantras. I won't say any mantras in doing Namaskars.'"[25] To those who objected to chanting *bija* and Vedic mantras during their *surya namaskar* practice, Bhavanarao replied that they "might drop them without detracting much from the exercise. Exclusion of these mantras from the Namaskars will, we hope, smooth the [rational Hindus and] non-Hindus' path to health, efficiency and longevity."[26]

Yet in his own practice Bhavanarao "regarded [*surya namaskar*] more as religious duty . . . than as mere physical exercise or training."[27] And the vehicle for *surya namaskar* as religious experience was the recitation of *bija* and Vedic mantras. Although he also described them as a tool for obtaining good health, he chiefly perceived the *bija* mantras as a means of transcendence. In a cosmos that's vibratory in nature, Bhavanarao believed that it's through making vibrations that one identifies with the cosmos: through chanting mantras, the core of one's being, one's very self, becomes the same as Being or Self. Bhavanarao singled out one *bija* mantra, "Om," as the "sacred syllable," "the essence of all Vedic learning." After telling us that its utterance should precede the other *bija* mantras, he further underscored its importance by quoting Shri Krishna in the *Bhagavad Gita:* "He, who, reciting "Om!", the one syllabled Brahman, (and) meditating upon Me, goeth forth, abandoning the body, reacheth the highest goal."[28]

Since "the sun is regarded in the Vedas as the soul of all that is movable and immovable," Bhavanarao reasoned, the sun adorer who identifies with the sun ultimately comes "to identify himself or herself with the Soul or Jivatman [the human soul, which only appears to be different from *atman,* the ultimate reality, the Soul]."[29] Quoting the *Yajurveda,* he incants, "The Spirit yonder in the Sun, / The Spirit dwelling there am I."[30]

16

BHAVANARAO PANT PRATINIDHI

Making *Surya Namaskar* a Part of Physical Education

Mass Exercise

Surya Namaskar as State Exercise

There were 565 princely states in British India before the independence of India and the establishment of Pakistan in 1947 (after which, over a two-year period, these constituent units were absorbed into their mother countries). Ruled by rajahs, they were exempt from direct British rule. The Princely State of Aundh was founded in 1699 by the warrior Parshuram Trabak Pant, who had received the title *Pratinidhi,* meaning "representative of the king" or "viceroy," in 1689 from his Maratha ruler (all subsequent Hindu rajahs of Aundh took the title *Pant Pratinidhi*). Situated approximately a hundred miles southeast of the city of Pune, the dry, hilly territory was about five hundred square miles in area. Its population in 1921 was 64,504. It was one of only twenty-one princely states with a state government.

Early in his reign, Bhavanarao Pant Pratinidhi, who had become the rajah of Aundh in 1909, initiated a series of steps to found a constitutional democracy in his state. Landmarks included establishing the Rayat Sabha (a people's assembly, with representatives from all seventy-two of Aundh's villages) in 1917; holding statewide elections for the Rayat Sabha in 1923; and forming *gram panchayats* (village councils) in many villages in the 1920s and 1930s. The culmination of his efforts to establish constitutional democracy was the Aundh Experiment, launched in 1938 with the declaration of his intention to relinquish all his powers, followed by the Aundh State Constitution Act of 1939, a law that laid out plans for a legislative assembly, which "shall be the supreme authority in the State and will pass such laws and rules as are necessary for the good Government of the State."[1]

Believing that the decentralization of power and institution of democratic reforms could only be ensured through education, Bhavanarao had introduced compulsory and free education throughout the state in 1923. "Scholarships, free boarding and lodging," writes Apa Pant, the rajah's closest confidant among his fourteen children, "enabled the poorest of the realm to 'aspire for the moon.'"[2]

"The Raja wanted an education that would bring about all-round development of man as a responsible and 'complete' citizen," writes Indira Rothermund, scholar of modern South Asian history, in *The Aundh Experiment: A Gandhian Grass-roots Democracy.* Toward that end, "the curriculum was properly scrutinized and evaluated, and besides regular courses in mathematics, languages, history, etc., there were classes in drawing, carpentry, hosiery, typing and weaving. Considerable importance was given to spinning and weaving in keeping with the Gandhian spirit of austerity and self-sacrifice." *Kirtans,* or religious concerts, were introduced. "Physical education through various gymnastics, *yogasanas,* suryanamaskars, wrestling and other sports, as also lectures on the importance of hygiene and cleanliness, were organized."[3]

Taking issue with Rothermund, cultural anthropologist Joseph S. Alter contends that *surya namaskar*—not a rounded education in general or spinning and weaving in particular—was "the mechanics of inculcation"[4] of the self-control and self-sacrifice necessary to ensure that the people of Aundh were capable of self-government: "[Bhavanarao] operationalized self-rule as an institution of the state by making *surya namaskar* a compulsory feature of public education. In this respect, *surya namaskar* may be compared . . . to Gandhi's operationalization of spinning as a concrete project for political, economic, and moral reform."[5] Alter singles out two aspects of *surya namaskar* that account for its ability to instill democracy: rhythmic breathing and beautiful and harmonized movements.

"A consideration of what the rajah said about rhythmic breathing takes one to the heart of the matter—the embodiment of self-rule and the physiology of democracy," Alter asserts. In support of his argument, he quotes a rhapsodic passage from Bhavanarao's second book, *The Ten-Point Way to Health,* that extols the "wonderful sensation of self-control and self-awareness when you can match the rhythm of your breathing with the rhythm of the exercise [while performing *surya namaskar*]. . . . You will know more about yourself than years of jungle-hunting or dealing with international affairs, big business or worldly success would ever give you."[6] But this is flimsy support for the grand thesis that Bhavanarao considered *surya namaskar* to be "the democracy of exercise and the exercise of democracy."[7] Besides, Bhavanarao didn't write the passage. Like most of the text in *The Ten-Point Way to Health,* published in 1938, that differs from Bhavanarao's first book, *Surya Namaskars,* published in English in 1928, this passage was penned by his ghostwriter, *Daily News* journalist Louise Morgan, for a middle-class British audience that entertained misguided fantasies about finding happiness in the outer-directed lives of the elite (with their safaris, diplomacy, big business transactions, and great wealth).

Alter's second argument to support his thesis that Bhavanarao championed *surya namaskar* as a means of instilling democracy is that "in the beautiful and harmonized movements of surya namaskar, Bhawanrao clearly saw the harmonized body of a united Indian polity that would turn, collectively, away from the gross sensations of modern life—sex, drugs, power, pride, prosperity—and toward the pure experience of self-realization."[8] Alter supports this argument with a quote from *Surya Namaskars: An Ancient Indian Exercise,** Apa Pant's book published in 1970: "[*Surya namaskar* exercises] have a deep spiritual content and they open up a new, more profound, more powerful dimension of awareness. Slowly but surely as you continue regularly to practise them things change in you, around you. Experiences miraculously come to you and you feel the full force of the Beauty and Harmony, the unity, the oneness, with all that is."[9] "It is precisely this kind of experience which Bhawanrao was attempting to transpose onto a national level to the end of ethical and moral reform," Alter writes.[10]

But the views of Pant cannot be conflated with those of Bhavanarao. The son and father aren't the same person. Even if he were express-ing his father's views about what one comprehends while performing *surya namaskar,* Pant was referring to the beauty and harmony of the universe, not of the *surya namaskar* movements. And furthermore, as one might expect in a discussion of those who would be helped by *surya namaskar,* it wasn't Bhavanarao, writing strictly for Indians of the 1920s, "a very large majority [of whom] are weak and ill and rarely enjoy normal health,"[11] but the cosmopolitan Pant, a diplomat writing for both Indians and Westerners in 1970 at the apogee of hippie culture, who, looking around him at "the way we live now in the modern world," condemned (very tactfully, as was his nature) the hedonistic impulses "to smoke, drink, keep late hours, eat all kinds of food, be agitated with sex."[12]

Bhavanarao did single out *surya namaskar* from the other subjects in the school curriculum—not, however, for its unique ability to promote democracy in his state but for its capacity to improve the declining health of his people and, as a consequence, the economic well-being of the body politic. "Time has now come that some strenuous effort be made in all seriousness to overcome this national degeneration and economic inefficiency," he bluntly wrote in a chapter of *Surya Namaskars* titled "Cash Value of Health." "Some scientific and systematic form of bodily exercise, therefore, should be *enforced* upon the young generation in general and upon the school and college going students in

---

*This book isn't to be confused with another book with (according to its copyright page) the same title, author, publisher, and original date of publication—but with an entirely different text! If this twin publication took place, it would perhaps be a singular oddity in publishing history. In all likelihood, though, the other book, published in 1989 as a so-called third edition, replaced the better-known 1970 original. The cover of the earlier book shows an orange sun with animated rays, while the cover of the later book shows a circular yellow sun with a woman performing *surya namaskar* around its perimeter.

particular" (emphasis added).[13] He trenchantly and dispassionately presented the rationale for his public health policy:

> The annual loss to industry and commerce, not to mention the privation entailed on private families, brought about by illness and physical inefficiency on the part of the individual workers alone is beyond computation. . . .
>
> As no other sport or exercise but Surya Namaskars can . . . achieve the innumerable benefits to be derived from the systematic practice of Surya Namaskars, we recommend with all the emphasis at our command that the Namaskar exercise be made compulsory in all schools and colleges throughout India.[14]

In vigorously and persistently advocating the compulsory practice of *surya namaskar* in schoolyards throughout India, Bhavanarao was seeking to implement a strategy of propagating good health through social networks—to, in effect, spread good health like a virus from student to family member, relative to friend and neighbor, friend and neighbor to community, community to nation. "It is our dearest wish," Bhavanarao wrote in a chapter titled "A State at Exercise," "that the students of our schools should carry the benefits of the system not only to their families, but extend them to all with whom they come in contact."[15]

Bhavanarao's final words in *Surya Namaskars* reinforced his view of *surya namaskar* practice as social policy to promote national health: "In conclusion, we have no hesitation in assuring our readers—men and women, old and young, rich and poor, strong and weak—that a faithful practice of the Surya Namaskars in accordance with directions laid down above, and coupled with proper diet and fasting, will reward them not only with individual but with National Health, Efficiency and Longevity."[16]

Prime Minister Indira Gandhi recognized the rarity of Bhavanarao's compassionate governing. "His concern for the health and welfare of his people," she recollects in 1974, "stood out in sharp contrast to the attitude and behavior of the majority of Maharajas and Rajas."[17] It may be argued that his objectives (to increase the health and prosperity of his people) in inserting *surya namaskar* into the school curriculum indirectly promoted democratization. But in actuality there was something about the way this remedy for degeneration and economic wastefulness was implemented that, at the least, uncomfortably flirted with the anti-democratic.

In introducing physical exercise based on an Indian exercise system into the schools of Aundh, Bhavanarao was hardly unique. He was part of a broader revival of indigenous exercises in India during the 1920s, which consisted of compulsory physical education in schools and colleges, physical instruction training, sports tournaments for students, standardization of rules for games, and uniform physical education programs among the provinces and princely states. This revival took place in a political context. Under British rule, Western exercises and games were brought to India. "There seemed to have been efforts to condemn and belittle Indian activities and glorify and propagate these foreign activities," write Swami Kuvayalananda biographers Manohar L. and Manmath M. Gharote.[18] In advocating indigenous physical activities, Bhavanarao and others were implicitly condemning the practice of Western physical activities in India. In this, they were part of the growing wave of nationalist spirit in India.

"Indian games, exercises and various other forms of physical culture . . . from the hoary antiquity to the present day . . . [have a] proper place in the field of nation building," Bhavanarao wrote, probably in 1935. They have played a part "in making the then generations healthy and strong and making them heroes and warriors at a time when . . . individual valour and strength were decisive factors to decide their fate."[19] He exhorted the youth of his day, whose easy lives led them to devalue physical culture and the resultant good health, to surpass the ancient heroes and warriors: "If our boys and girls, men and women will practise daily and regularly the Surya Namaskar Exercise [and other exercises] there will shortly be produced a type of humanity that shall excel in body, mind and soul any that the earth has yet brought forth and shall set a new standard for the race."[20]

Unrealized, it seems, by its evangelists, this nationalist fervor in the 1920s and 1930s for promoting culture rooted in the native tradition to improve the race was an international movement—one that was not only nationalistic and patriotic but sometimes also militaristic and even fascist in character. One of the manifestations of fascism was the performance of synchronized movements by large groups, a phenomenon that entranced the populace of countries both East and West. What may readily come to mind are goose-stepping Nazi troopers in Germany, marching in obeisance to their heroic leader while embodying the unity,

sacrifice, and might of the nation. But there were many manifestations less apparent than orchestrated worshipping of the state. Take, for example, the Busby Berkeley–choreographed film musicals in America, featuring large groups of leggy women performing spectacular dance numbers. Filmed from above, they formed patterns, typically floral patterns, in the movie frame, obliterating our sense of the dancers as individuals—indeed, as human beings. "The rendering of movement in grandiose and rigid patterns," writes Susan Sontag, is an element of fascist art, "for such choreography rehearses the very unity of the polity."[21]

Although mass demonstrations of exercise and sport are associated with Nazi Germany and Stalinist Soviet Union, their roots are the mass displays held at *slets* (from the Czech word for "a flocking of birds"), grand gymnastic festivals (which included elaborate welcoming ceremonies, gymnastic competitions, speeches, and theatrical events) put on by Sokol, the first Czechoslovak physical education organization, founded in 1862. The nationalistic and periodically militaristic Sokol movement was strongly influenced by German *turnverein,* the nationalistic gymnastics societies founded by Friedrich Ludwig Jahn in 1811.

Even Bhavanarao wasn't immune to the appeal of synchronized exercise movements by large groups, so antithetical to democracy. "One of the chief merits of Surya Namaskars," he pointed out, "is that it is best adapted to group exercise or exercise *en masse.* Under proper supervision, hundreds of students—boys and girls—can be made to take this exercise simultaneously, thus affording the double advantage of efficiency and economy of time.

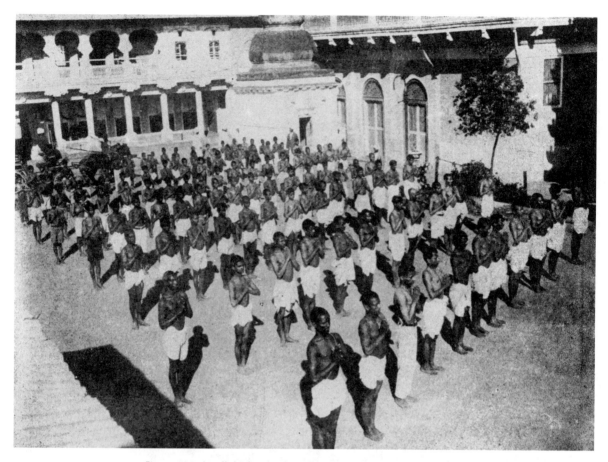

Figure 16.1. Aundh high-school students doing *surya namaskar,* 1924
(From *Surya Namaskars [Sun-Adoration] for Health, Efficiency & Longevity*)

The students may be grouped according to age, height or capacity" (fig. 16.1).[22] To support his position, he quoted Kaiser Wilhelm II from an article in Bernarr Macfadden's February 1927 *Physical Culture:* "It is much more important to see 10,000 men, women, and children to go through a series of carefully planned exercises than to watch some professional athlete beat the world's record in some useless attainment by one-tenth of a second"[23]—a statement that's alarming not only for its needless discrediting of individual athletic accomplishment at the expense of the achievement of good health (the two aren't dichotomous) but for its weirdly displaced emphasis on the importance of viewing (not participating in) synchronized mass exercise. Is pageantry all?

"Mass athletic demonstrations, a choreographed display of bodies," a valued activity, Sontag argues, in all totalitarian countries (but, I would add, not exclusively in totalitarian countries), took place throughout India in the form of vast groups of uniformed exercisers standing as if in battle array in the open air, performing indigenous physical exercises in squad drills.[24] D. C. Mujumdar, editor of the *Encyclopedia of*

Indian Physical Culture, proudly describes this phenomenon: "Mass physical activities led to the introduction of uniforms in Mass Drills and thus the movement of Indian physical activities was revolutionised on military lines followed by the western people."[25] Why give even schoolchildren's exercise the air of military pomp? The goal of imposing mass exercise drills wasn't hidden or unconscious. Mujumdar proclaims:

> Union is strength. Such an adage evinces the paramount importance of strength of mass organization. In the hoary past, the Aryans were aware of this and they used to organize many group games. Group games always presuppose the importance of discipline. They lead to the formation of habits of acting simultaneously in groups which is the backbone of Mass Drill. As a result of regular practice in group games and Mass Drills, the body and mind of players become habituated to obey the general orders meant for enforcing uniformity in Mass Physical Activities. Hence training in giving and practicing orders of Mass Drills is absolutely essential to enforce impressive discipline among masses.[26]

Why call for instilling discipline with military trappings among the masses? Each country that turned bellicose during the 1920s and 1930s had its reason. For India, it was to prepare for the battle of liberation against its British colonizers.

The *Surya Namaskar* Craze

In the 1920s gymnasiums, called *vyayamshalas,* flourished throughout India. Members practiced a variety of physical exercises, such as gymnastics, indigenous strengthening exercises, yogasana, and wrestling.*

It was in these neighborhood *vyayamshalas* that *surya namaskar* was taken up with zeal. Occurring outside the controlled environment of compulsory classes in schools, the *surya namaskar* craze led to competitive misuse by excessive repetition. The cover of the July 1928 issue of the English-language *Vyayam* shows a proud young man, his arms crossed in a regal manner, who developed his toned body by performing 1,200 *surya namaskars* daily. Even Bhavanarao felt compelled to caution against taking *surya namaskar* to such extremes. "To do about a thousand Namaskars a day for a few months and then to come down to about twenty-five or to give them up altogether is positively harmful."[27] Mujumdar puts the dangers more bluntly: "It is always congenial to one's health to practice a few Namaskaras daily and regularly rather than practicing 1000 or more Namaskaras in a slip-shod way i.e. at times many and at times none. This latter mode is decidedly detrimental to one's health, leading to abrupt life end."[28]

In 1924 Bhavanarao published *Surya Namaskars (Sun-Adoration) for Health, Efficiency &*

---

*Just as yoga practiced in *yogashalas,* or yoga schools, was largely separated from its spiritual path, wrestling practiced in *vyayamshalas* was severed from its traditional ethos, ritual, and performance, which had been preserved for centuries in *akharas,* or training halls. Its attack tricks and counters were revealed. This impulse to disclose ancient secrets was also a critical ingredient in the formation of modern hatha yoga.

Longevity, a compilation of articles that he'd written for the Marathi magazine *Purusharth.* Reinforced by a rhetorical strategy of heavily quoting Western physical culturists (beginning on page one with the words of the ex-kaiser from his *Physical Culture* article: "The toxins with which modern civilization poisons our lives are such that man cannot survive without an antidote. The best antidote to the poisons of civilization is a harmonious system of physical culture"[29]), Bhavanarao squarely placed *surya namaskar* within the physical culture movement. But not as an equal system of natural preventive health care among physical culture rivals. His intent was to establish *surya namaskar* "of all exercises, Indian and foreign, intended to impart health, strength and longevity [as] the first and foremost."[30]

Surya Namaskars was met with great enthusiasm. Because of the ensuing large demand in non-Marathi districts, in 1928 the rajah published an English edition of two thousand copies. No doubt the publication of this book and the other steps that he took to revive *surya namaskar* inspired many Indians to improve their health through taking up this indigenous exercise. Yet when all is said and done, the greatest influence of *surya namaskar* would be not on the health of the nation (at least, not directly) but on the course of yoga in the 20th century. Not at first, however, without resistance.

In the July 1926 *Yoga-Mimansa* article "The Rationale of Yogic Poses," an examination of the general principles underlying yogic physical culture, Kuvalayananda, the most acclaimed advocate of the other exercise craze in India in the 1920s, yogasana, made a strong case against *surya namaskar*: "The advocates of Namaskaras . . . have tried to accomplish everything within the narrow compass of one exercise and as they want to ever tack that exercise onto Sun-worship, there is little chance of their system ever being accepted as a system of Physical Culture in the modern sense of the word" (by which he meant that *surya namaskar* was an exercise designed for spiritual rather than solely for bodily development).[31] A footnote, however, softened the critique of the limitations of *surya namaskar*: "This statement has been made from a particular point of view and as such should not lead to misunderstanding. The exercise of Namaskara, as it is being developed by its advocates, has a definite purpose to serve and has certainly a large scope in India. We wish them success from the bottom of our heart."[32] In this rapprochement we have an inkling of the later embrace of *surya namaskar* by yogasana teachers of differing styles.

Beauty

People commonly exercise to look good. What are we to make of this goal? Is the pursuit of physical beauty to be admired and emulated or spurned? This issue bedevils even those yoga practitioners who struggle to loosen all vanity from their ego. They feel they should overcome the superficial desire to look good, yet they find themselves wanting to look good.

Even Bhavanarao was concerned with pursuing a beautiful body. He wrote that in addition to giving superb health throughout one's life, "the Surya Namaskar Exercise also makes a body beautiful."[33] But isn't it possible that the longing for the physical perfection of the gods is a good thing? If by physical beauty we mean not a muscle-bulging Sandowian body but the taut, lithesome body, stately bearing, joyous face, and robustness possessed by a Bhavanarao (a generic term that could be used to refer to votaries of *surya namaskar*), then the answer is yes.

It goes without saying that Bhavanarao looks regal in a photo in which he's presenting him-self in all his splendor as the rajah of Aundh, seated on his gilded throne, bejeweled, dressed in a flowing silk robe and tasseled turban (red, according Pant), and clasping his ceremonial sword in his lap (fig. 16.2). But he's downright stunning in a photo of him wearing just a *dhoti* and sacred thread (fig. 16.3), peering out at us, drawing himself up, his gray handlebar mustache a formal horizontal balance to his erect

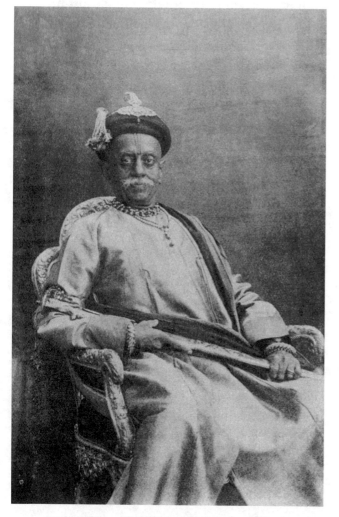

Figure 16.2. Bhavanarao Pant Pratinidhi, dressed in his royal robes, 1928

(From *Surya Namaskars [Sun-Adoration] for Health, Efficiency & Longevity*)

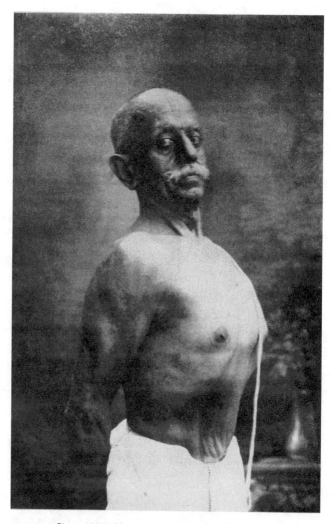

Figure 16.3. Bhavanarao Pant Pratinidhi, wearing a *dhoti*, 1928

(From *Surya Namaskars [Sun-Adoration] for Health, Efficiency & Longevity*)

posture. And, despite his body being largely exposed (nakedness is the great leveler), he's still clearly regal. Indira Gandhi remarks about Bhavanarao: "I met this remarkable human being as a young girl and have a vivid recollection of his enthusiasm for *surya namaskar*. What an upright man he was—in every sense of the word."[34]

Coda

Each morning, after *surya namaskar* practice, Bhavanarao would walk up an approximately eight-hundred-foot hill that rises from the stark and arid Aundh plateau to an ancient temple. Inside this *kuldaiwat* (family shrine) were a carving of Nandi (the divine bull, who represents Jivatma, the human soul), a Shivling (Shiva represented in phallus form), and an over six-foot-high statue of Devi Mahishasur Mardini Yamai—the goddess Jagadamba. There he prayed to Jagadamba, the Goddess on the Hill, with whom his family had been linked for at least four hundred years. Pant describes his father's faith in Jagadamba, Mother of the Universe, as both mystical and practical. "[My father] had total faith in that emanation of the Absolute that was the Deity of the temple on the hill," Pant reminisces. "For him it was SHE who protected him and he was HER child. . . . From my earliest years it was a special experience to hear my father's voice raised in prayer, entirely absorbed and full of deep emotion. At the worst moments of danger and disappointment he would only say, 'It is HER wish. It must be good for us though we do not know it.'"[35]

But Bhavanarao couldn't find consola-tion even in Jagadamba when he lost Aundh upon Indian independence from British rule in 1947. Though he'd spent decades of his life gradually and voluntarily giving up power, after his princely state was absorbed into the new sovereign, democratic nation-state, the Republic of India, this most progressive of rajahs "was no longer what he had been"; without the strong sense of fatalism, born by his faith in Jagadamba, to sustain him, he lost his will to carry on. In 1950, when he and his wife visited Pant and his family in Nairobi, Kenya, for the first time Bhavanarao wasn't happy to have his grandchildren about him. "I could see," observes Pant, "that the life-force that had inspired me and kept me close to him was ebbing away."[36] At the end of the year, Bhavanarao returned to India, where he expired a few months later, in April 1951, in Room 9 of St. George's Hospital in Bombay, while his family looked on.

Pant, who was the child designated to go with his father on his travels, accompanied Bhavanarao's body back to Aundh on his last journey, taken in a black Chrysler driven by the son of Pant's elder deceased brother (and hence the heir to the now empty title of rajah). Over the eight-hour, 220-mile drive, the rajah lay with his head resting on the rani's lap in the back seat. The family arrived in Aundh at night. Pant describes the funeral service: "His body was placed in a beautiful palanquin [in the main temple], in which we usually carried the image of the deity at sacred festivals. There was a constant, lamenting chant of prayers. Eyes were red with tears, and a red and beautiful dawn heralded the departure. The journey was half-way up the hill which he used to climb every morning for sixty-five years to pray at the shrine of the goddess."[37]

Bhavanarao's body was placed on a funeral pyre constructed by the side of his museum, built in 1938 to house his vast art collection.

"As the sun rose, I set fire to the pyre of this great sun-worshipper," Pant recollects.[38] "In a few minutes the departure was complete as his mortal remains were dispersed in the five elements from which they had gathered for his arrival eighty-five years before."[39]

17

T. KRISHNAMACHARYA

Keeping the Flame

Yoga at the Palace

Makings of a Yoga Master

During the mid-1930s, Tirumalai Krishnamacharya (1888–1989) propelled himself so furiously down the sidewalks of Mysore, the capital city of the Princely State of Mysore, that even the elite of society crossed the road to get out of his way.* But then, Krishnamacharya's manner was intimidating even while he was standing still. Just as a tall person's perpetual slouch may denote a kind of courtliness (a slight tipping down toward others in order to listen more attentively), Krishnamacharya's straight back was telling of his rigidity and arrogance: it warned people to keep away. As did his lizard-like countenance, which was so frightful that people were afraid to look him in the eye, never mind engage him in debate. And with good reason. Even in casual discussions, he belittled the views of those who disagreed with him—and those who agreed with him (fig. 17.1).

Krishnamacharya was born on November 18, 1888, in Muchukundapuram (about 150 miles north of Mysore) into a distinguished Vaishnava Brahmin

---

*This is one of three versions of B. K. S. Iyengar's recollections of Krishnamacharya's perambulations in Mysore. In a second, more benevolent version, he says that Krishnamacharya "has his own peculiarity. For instance, while walking he does not see hither and thither. So people who see him on the road often have mistaken notions about his pride" (Iyengar, *Body the Shrine,* 4). In a third, perhaps more damning version, he says, "Due to my Guru's [unpredictable] nature, his acquaintances and friends were avoiding him. I remember very well that people would walk on the left footpath, if he was on the right side" (Iyengar, "My Yogic Journey," 6).

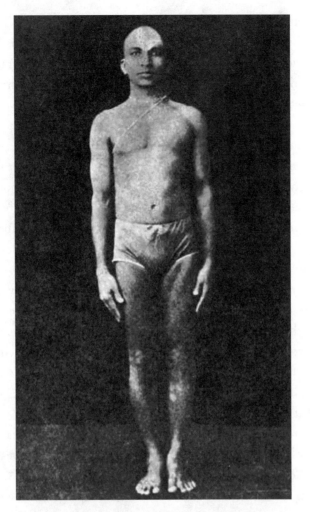

Figure 17.1. T. Krishnamacharya demonstrating
Yogasana Samasthiti Kramam, Equal Standing Pose, 1934

(From *Yoga Makaranda,* by T. Krishnamacharya)

family. Under the strict instruction of his scholarly father, he began to speak and write Sanskrit, chant Vedas, learn Patanjali's *Yoga Sutra,* and practice *asana* and *pranayama* at an early age. When his father died in 1898, his mother took her ten-year-old son and five younger children to Mysore, where her grandfather was the head of the Parakala Math (the first Vaishnavite math, a monastic Hindu institution, established in the 13th century).

In Mysore Krishnamacharya received more formal schooling.

In 1906 Krishnamacharya embarked on a nearly ten-year-long academic pursuit of knowledge of diverse Hindu disciplines, including logic and Sanskrit at the university at Benares (Varanasi), Vedanta at the Parakala Math in Mysore, and the *darshanas* (six orthodox Indian philosophies) at Patna University in Bihar (he would eventually attain degrees from six universities). In 1915, when he was twenty-seven years old, in order to further his yoga studies he decided to seek out the yoga master Rammohan Brahmacari, who lived in the mountains of Tibet. To get the documents required to travel to Tibet, Krishnamacharya sought out the viceroy stationed in Simla, located in the northwest Himalayas. In exchange for six months of yoga lessons (or perhaps of yoga treatment for diabetes), the viceroy granted approval, paid all expenses, and supplied two servants for Krishnamacharya's pilgrimage.

As reported by his son, T. K. V. Desikachar, after trekking for twenty-two days over two hundred miles of "some of the most barren, rocky terrain on the earth," Krishnamacharya "reached Lake Manasarovar at the foot of Mount Kailash, the eternal abode of Lord Shiva," where he found a nearby cave.[1] "A tall, long-bearded saint stood at the entrance," Krishnamacharya recalled. "With deep reverence and respect I prostrated and told my name in Hindi and requested him to take me as his disciple." Brahmachari invited him inside, where "I saw the saint's wife and three children. The saint gave me fruits to eat and I, meditating on Lord Narayana, ate them and drank a cup of tea." The guru took the aspirant down to the lake, showed him the environs for about an hour and a quarter, and, "lifting up his little finger which had turned blue on account of touching the water," warned him not to touch the water. "He told me that many who did not know this had become deformed."[2] This admonitory sermon, with its subtly dramatic gesture, was apparently Brahmachari's way of informing Krishnamacharya that he had met expectations and been accepted for study.

After seven and a half years under Brahmachari's tutelage, Krishnamacharya, according to Desikachar, "embraced . . . [yoga's] use in diagnosing and treating the ill, . . . not only learned Patanjali's *Yoga Sutras* by heart, but also learned to chant them with an exactness of pronunciation, tone and inflection that echoed as nearly as possible their first utterance thousands of years earlier, . . . gained uncanny powers, of which stopping heartbeat and breath were only a part, . . . [and] of about seven thousand *asanas* [that his guru knew] mastered about three thousand."[3]

However, it's likely that most, if not all, of Krishnamacharya's account of his discipleship is fabricated. Its appeal is explained by author Elizabeth Kadetsky, who researched this period in Krishnamacharya's life after writing about B. K. S. Iyengar's yoga journey:

Krishnamacharya's story about discovering a hermit in the caves of Tibet in the deep Himalaya, circa 1915, and imbibing the wisdom of yoga as preserved in the caves since the tenth century, does not really stand up to investigation. Details of the pre-trip and trip don't add up, and there are many obvious embellishments to the experience of the discipleship itself: the whole story is laced with mystical details. So maybe Krishnamacharya never went to Tibet. But the story resonates in a visceral way, and perhaps this is its truer value.[4]

This appealing image of the yogin as a reclusive ascetic who withdraws from society (even from the society of brothers at an ashram or from groups of wandering mendicants) to pursue the path of self-realization (i.e., realization of the supreme Self, Brahman, or god-self within) was, as scholar of South Asian religions David Gordon White shows, a construct of 19th-century British romanticism.

Like postmodern man, who has in recent decades been smitten by a sort of remorse and nostalgia for the various plant and animal species he is responsible for having annihilated, in the latter half of the nineteenth century the British in India began to romanticize the yogis whose lifestyles and livelihoods their policies had largely contributed to wiping out. In urban middle-class society in particular, the bogey of the wild, naked, drug-crazed warrior ascetic was gradually airbrushed into the far more congenial image of a forest-dwelling meditative, spiritual renouncer, something far closer to the ideal of the sages of vedic lore. This romanticization—indeed, this reinvention—of the yogi and his yoga occurred not only among the British but also within an increasingly Anglicized Indian urban society.[5]

In a time when it was still thought that authentic yoga had disappeared from India and could only be found in the forests of Tibet, perhaps Krishnamacharya believed that a résumé that fit this idealized and fashionable model of hermit in Tibet was of value to him.

In 1924 Krishnamacharya returned to live in Mysore. In 1925 he traveled to nearby Bangalore to give religious discourses. "One day he came to our house with some of his relatives," B. K. S. Iyengar recounts matter-of-factly. "My maternal uncle was also with him." The uncle suggested marriage between the nearly thirty-seven-year-old bachelor and Iyengar's twelve-year-old sister, Namagiriamma. "My uncle was keen on this alliance and so my father consented and the marriage was celebrated."[6] (There's a long, dreary history in India of child brides.) The next few years were the hardest of Krishnamacharya's life. "The couple lived in such deep poverty that Krishnamacharya wore a loincloth sewn of fabric torn from his spouse's sari," writes yoga historian Fernando Pagés Ruiz.[7] Krishnamacharya took a job as a foreman at a coffee plantation in the Hassan District in Karnataka—work that Iyengar implies Krishnamacharya must've found demeaning: "He used to dress differently [from his customary orthodox Brahmin dress], wearing half-pants and half-sleeved shirt, socks and shoes, a hat on his head and a stick in his hand. It was unimaginable to see a man dressed in such a manner who had studied *Sad-darsanas*. . . . But destiny had played its trick even on him."[8]

On his days off Krishnamacharya earned extra money as a yoga superman busker. His performance consisted of suspending his pulse, stopping cars with his hands, twisting his body into complex *asanas,* and lifting heavy objects with his teeth. (Ruiz believes that these demonstrations were "designed to stimulate interest in a dying tradition. . . . To teach people about yoga, Krishnamacharya felt, he first had to get their attention."[9])

In 1931 Krishnamacharya left the plantation job to begin giving lectures on Hindu philosophy. A lecture on the Upanishads at the Mysore town hall gained him the recognition and acclaim that he'd long sought. In Iyengar's account: "A hidden scholarly personality, in that garb of half-pant, half-sleeve shirt, hat, socks and shoes, was unearthed. His discourses on the *Vedas, Upanishads* and yoga attracted the elite of Mysore."[10] News of this dazzling scholar reached the maharajah of Mysore, Shri Nalvadi Krishnaraja Wadiyar (also called Krishnaraja Wodeyar IV). He hired Krishnamacharya to teach him scriptures and yoga. Soon afterward, the maharajah appointed Krishnamacharya to teach Mimamsa (the *darshana* that primarily interprets the Vedas) and yoga at his Sanskrit Pathasala (Sanskrit College).

The teaching position lasted only two years. Krishnamacharya antagonized his students with his strict discipline and arrogance (he was more interested in flaunting his learning than in transmitting it). According to Iyengar, the breaking point was Krishnamacharya making the Mimamsa test so difficult that the students (and the other teachers!) couldn't answer it. They protested to the maharajah, who removed Krishnamacharya from his post. This reversal of fortunes led to the greatest opportunity of Krishnamacharya's life.

Yoga Craze

In 1933 a yoga craze had been in full swing in India for about a decade, the latest phase in response to the physical culture movement (that salmagundi of natural practices concocted in Europe and America in the late 19th century as an alternative to conventional medicine). According to the July 1926 issue of *Yoga-Mimansa,* Swami Kuvalayananda's yoga jour-nal: "Of late, in Maharashtra [a large region that was formerly the Maratha empire], there is not a single gymnastic institute worth the name that does not undertake to teach Yoga Asa-nas."[11] First published in 1924, *Yoga-Mimansa* helped start the hatha yoga fad, and the very fact that it and other yoga journals were being published was evidence of a fad already under way.

To Swami Kuvalayananda and others, yogasana was more than an exercise rage. It was a nationalistic cause. In the first modern hatha yoga manual, *Yogic Physical Culture or the Secret of Happiness,* published in 1929, S. Sundaram acknowledges that "thanks to Mr. Bernarr Macffadden* [*sic*] and a host of other pioneers in the field of the newly risen Physical Culture creed," exercise was finally being utilized by Europeans and Americans to build resistance to disease.[12] "Yet they are far behind a system perfected thousands of years ago. A few of their best exercises could but be poor imitations of those contained in the ancient one." "Who owns this system?" Sundaram asks, as if inciting a large audience with a fiery speech. "Is the owner reaping its full benefit? And what is it? To the first the answer is India; the second alas, No! And to the last, the reply echoes through centuries of neglect—YOGA-ASANA."[13]

Sundaram was tacitly admitting that until recently Indians as a people hadn't owned yogasana at all; it had belonged solely to hatha yogins, members of an insular sect. However, according to him blame shouldn't be cast on the hatha yogins. "If India has not reaped the full benefits and does not occupy its merited

---

*Bernarr Macfadden was the self-proclaimed "father of physical culture." See chapter 7.

place as the foremost country in the world, it is due to the fault of its citizens." But thanks to Kuvalayananda and those who worked on his journal, word had begun to spread to the populace about the benefits of yogasana: "Perhaps [Indians] would have continued to sleep and—the modern world might neither have known the system nor appropriated its remarkable benefits. But savants have risen, and chief among them are the authors of the 'Yoga-Mimamsa' [sic] Journal, Lonavla (Poona). They proclaim from mountain tops the existence of this lore, far richer than Solomon's mines, and convince the modern skeptics and struggling humanity of its benefits, powers and utility."[14]

One of those convinced was the maharajah of Mysore, Nalvadi Krishnaraja Wadiyar.

Yogashala

Modern yoga scholar Mark Singleton states that Nalvadi Krishnaraja Wadiyar revived Indian exercises, including yogasana, beginning in the late 1910s in the Mysore state. Quoting P. K. Kamath, who published an article in 1933 about indigenous Indian exercise, Singleton posits: "The Mysore government was 'the first to take up the cause of indigenous physical culture as early as 1919,' with a full-time organizer, Professor M. V. Krishna Rao, appointed to oversee its development. Rao's mission was to popularize Indian exercise and games through the state and 'was of great value in resuscitating the indigenous system.'"[15] "Physical culture in Mysore during the 1920s and 1930s was based

on a spirit of radical fusion and innovation promulgated by the Maharaja (via Krishna Rao)," Singleton concludes, "and in which yogasana played a major role."[16]

But *asana* practice wasn't part of this revitalization of indigenous physical education in the Mysore state during this period. Noting its absence, in an April 2, 1934, letter, Kuvalayananda, whom the maharajah recognized as the leader in researching and promulgating yogic physical culture, implores the maharajah: "The Yogic exercises are capable of building supreme vitality. They deserve to be introduced in all educational institutions. There should also be special institutions [training facilities for teachers in yoga physical education] for the study of Yoga exclusively. I would be greatly pleased to see that the Mysore Government think of doing these things in their State."[17]

Yogasana wasn't even part of the exercise regime taught to the royal family in the 1920s and early 1930s. During this period, its members were taught a combination of indigenous Indian exercise and Western gymnastics. As yoga scholar and philosopher Norman Sjoman points out in his description of the exercises in S. Bharadwaj's *Vyayamadipika,* published in 1896, the manual that probably reflected (and may even have been used to prescribe) the regimen practiced by the royal family in the 1920s: "English exercise consists of gymnastics, trapeze, parallel bars and so on whereas the Indian system consists of bodybuilding, wrestling and the use of weapons."[18]* Conspicuously missing in the Indian division of exercises are *asanas.*

---

*In his book, Bharadwaj acknowledges the help of Veeranna, who was probably his teacher. Veeranna supervised the exercise routine of the maharajah when he was crown prince (his reign began in 1902), so in all likelihood the routine in Bharadwaj's book would've been based on Veeranna's routine.

In 1933 the maharajah sought to remedy this omission by introducing yogasana into the physical culture routine for the boys of the extended maternal royal family, the Arasus. (Kuvalayananda expressed his approval: "It is a matter for congratulations that the members of the Royal Family at Mysore feel keenly interested in Yogic culture."[19]) Knowing that he couldn't very well send them to a neighborhood gymnasium, he decided to open his own yoga facility. He reassigned Krishnamacharya from the Pathasala to a *yogashala* (yoga school or yoga hall), converted from the gymnastics hall, in the Jagan Mohan Palace,* near the Mysore Palace, where the royal family lived (fig. 17.2). "During the latter part of the year," the 1932–1933 administrative report of the Jagan Mohan Palace reads, "the Physical Instruction Class was under Mr. V. D. S. Naidu, and during the latter part of the year Mr. Krishnamachar was appointed to teach the Yogic System of exercises."[20] Iyengar remarks about Krishnamacharya's good fortune: "From a plantation worker Guruji had become an *Asthana Vidwan* [a scholar with a royal position] and a *Yogacharya* [yoga teacher]."[21]

On August 11, 1933, the forty-five-year-old Krishnamacharya began teaching yoga to the young boys of the royal family. By the second school year, 1934–1935, he was teaching thirty-two boys, including a selected few outsiders permitted on special request to attend classes. He would go on to run the *yogashala* at the palace until 1950. For someone with

Krishnamacharya's makeup, this was the perfect job: bullying children in the name of a good cause. But, as is often the case with those who enjoy mistreating others, he turned out to be a servile—and exceptional—employee.

Yogasana as Physical Culture

Sundaram defines yogasana in *Yogic Physical Culture* as "that system of poses which enables the merging of the individual in God-consciousness. This has to act through the God-given instrument, the human body. It perfects the human body, purifies it of all dross, disease and defect, and prepares it for the rousing reception of spiritual powers—the final stage in becoming the Christ-Man, the Jivan-Muktha." But could yogasana's ability to provide "vibrant Health, dynamic Health—Health, the equal of which *no other system in the world has given or could give*"—be separated from its role in spiritual liberation?[22] Sundaram answers affirmatively:

Whatever the object of the sages—the perfection of the human body [through performing conditioning *asanas*] as a means to the end of God-realisation—*it is not against reason to use it as almost an end in itself* [italics added]. For those who are not born for anything higher, limited by fate or fortune, could they not utilize it as a system of physical culture? May not the curse of drugs and diseases be removed through this? Should not the suf-

---

*Constructed in 1861 as a alternative retreat for the royal family, who lived in the nearby Mysore Palace, about a ten-minute walk away, the Jagan Mohan Palace became the temporary home of the Wadiyars from 1897, after the Mysore Palace burned down in a fire that broke out during a royal wedding, until 1912, when the new palace was completed. The Jagan Mohan Palace was primarily converted into an art gallery in 1915.

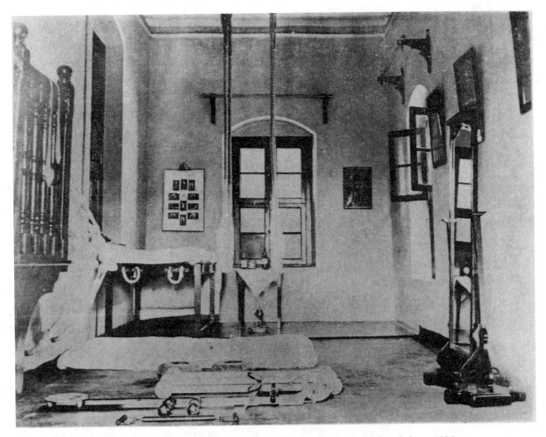

Figure 17.2. T. Krishnamacharya's *yogashala* at the Jagan Mohan Palace, 1934
(From *Yoga Makaranda*)

fering humanity be made properly the trustees of this ancient secret unventilated to the world at large through centuries of hoarding and neglect?[23]

Sundaram and the other pioneer modern yogins proclaimed that hatha yoga, in its capacity (as described by the 15th- to 16th-century *Hatha Yoga Pradipika*) as a "destroyer of disease," should be made available to the Indian masses and, indeed, shared with all humanity (albeit as a reflection of India's glory).

When hired to teach yoga to the royal family, Krishnamacharya, who'd spent nearly his entire life in pursuit of scholarly knowledge and spiritual enlightenment, was probably ignorant of trends in physical culture. If so, the maharajah (or an emissary, who most likely would've been V. D. S. Naidu, the person in charge of the physical instruction class) would've had to inculcate in Krishnamacharya the value of *asanas* as exercise, not as an aid to spiritual realization. Astoundingly, Krishnamacharya, who, one would think—considering his age (mid-forties), rigid personality, and background in erudite study and orthodox yoga practice—would've resisted abandoning his concept of hatha yoga as soteriology, created inspired approaches to teaching *asanas* as exercise that were and would remain unparalleled in yoga history.

First Stages of Discipleship

Kaivalyadhama, Kuvalayananda's yoga ashram at Lonavla, had opened in 1924, and the Bombay branch, Pranavakunja, in 1932. While the Lonavla ashram was the center for scientific research on yoga, both ashrams were training camps for medical doctors and physiotherapists in yogic therapy. In Kuvalayananda's "health resort," Rugna Seva Mandir, in Lonavla, and his Health Centre in Bombay, certified yoga doctors examined patients and prescribed protocols consisting of techniques such as *asanas, kriyas, pranayamas,* and meditation. Certified yoga physiotherapists then taught the prescribed protocols individually to patients.

The ashrams were also facilities for training teachers in yogic physical culture. The *Report of the Physical Training Committee of the Government of Bombay, 1927–1929,* states:

> An experiment unique of its kind is being conducted by Mr. J. G. Gune [Kuvalayananda's real name] . . . at Lonavla. . . . The principles adopted in that school are . . . principally based on Hatha Yoga. It is well known that the Yogis of India have by long experimentation evolved a system of physical training which, if pursued under proper guidance, is sound and beneficial. . . . We are not here concerned with the spiritual side of the Yogic practices but the breathing and abdominal exercises and some of the poses are worth a study in order that they may be exploited for the purposes of corrective and hygienic physical training.[24]

Students at the ashrams took classes with teachers certified in yogic physical culture. Instructions in yoga for maintaining good health and achieving fitness were given free of charge. The assistant director of public health for the government of the United Provinces (a British province corresponding approximately to the combined regions of the present-day states of Uttar Pradesh and Uttarakhand, bordering Nepal) reported on his visit to Kaivalyadhama in 1929: "There are two hostels connected with the Ashrama and they were both full during my stay here with students and patients and some had to be refused admission."[25]

Dissatisfied with the frivolous life she was leading as a diplomat's wife, Indra Devi, who would later become a renowned yoga teacher in America, attended Kaivalyadhama in 1937 (or possibly 1936) to learn yoga. After an interview with Kuvalayananda and an examination by a doctor, she attended a women-only class where she learned yoga as physical culture taught by a female instructor and spent the rest of the day doing as she pleased.

In mid-1938, upon going to the Mysore Palace for a royal wedding, Devi dramatically rejected the social whirl of the wedding celebrations to pursue training at the *yogashala,* where, in contrast to her experience at the Lonavla ashram, she had to devote herself to an austere existence with a very strict daily discipline and diet imposed on her by Krishnamacharya. "Here," she would proudly recall fifteen years later, "[I] underwent the first stages of the training for discipleship."[26]

Devi got up before sunrise, took a bath, practiced *asanas,* and meditated; meditated again at noon; performed *asanas* at the school in the late afternoon/early evening; took her last meal before sunset; and went to sleep at

9:30. She was required to eliminate excitement and bodily exertion (no going to those cocktail parties and dances at the palace), remain celibate, bathe in tepid water, and wear clean and comfortable clothing. She had to vow to obey *niyama* (interior discipline) for the period of her discipleship. "Nyama," she explains, "means internal and external purification, contentment, strength of character, patience, calmness of mind and charity."[27]

Krishnamacharya had left Devi's yoga training to one of his assistants. But when the master saw her dedication, he began giving her personal instruction. He modified the traditional hatha yoga teachings for her, making them suitable for a neophyte European. Her *asana* routine, in particular, was decidedly customized: a version of the anodyne canon formulated by Kuvalayananda, it consisted of a relatively small number of mostly simple *asanas*. The *asana* regime that Krishnamacharya taught the boys of the royal family was far more expansive and difficult.

Keeper of the Flame

A February 24, 1941, photo essay titled ". . . This Is Real Yoga" in *Life,* the American news magazine that dominated the photojournalism market in the 1940s, showed twenty yoga poses demonstrated by four of Krishnamacharya's pupils in the courtyard of the Jagan Mohan Palace.* It's not surprising that the *Life* photojournalist, Wallace Kirkland, turned up at the yoga school at Mysore. According to Devi, the school was already famous in the mid-1930s, and demonstrations by Krishnamacharya's pupils for Westerners were common. (She herself had attended such a presentation, at the end of which Krishnamacharya, making a star turn, lay down and "stopped" his heartbeat for several minutes to the astonishment of Western guests, including physicians armed with watches and stethoscopes. After making his examination, a German doctor said: "I would have pronounced him dead.")[28][†]

Located in the running feature "Speaking of

---

*The *asanas,* in Iyengar's nomenclature, are as follows:

- Arm Balances: *Mayurasana,* Peacock Pose; *Bakasana,* Crane Pose; *Kukkutasana,* Cock Pose, Lotus Pose below torso; *Kukkutasana,* Cock Pose, with variation 1 (one leg in Half Lotus and one leg bent behind the head); *Kukkutasana* with variation 2 (Lotus Pose behind the torso)
- Leg Balances: *Durvasasana,* Durvasa (name of a sage) Pose
- Inversions: *Salamba Sirsasana* II with *Padmasana,* Headstand with Lotus Pose; *Adho Mukha Vrksasana* with *Padmasana,* Handstand with Lotus Pose
- Backbends: Variation of *Vrischikasana,* Scorpion Pose, and *Ganda Bherundasana,* Formidable Side of the Face Pose; *Tiriang Mukhottanasana,* Head Upside Down with Intense Stretch Pose; *Eka Pada Viparita Dandasana* II, Intensified One-Legged Inverted Rod Pose; *Eka Pada Rajakapotasana,* One-Legged Pigeon Pose; *Dhanurasana,* Bow Pose; *Padangustha Dhanurasana,* Intensified Bow Pose
- Seated Poses: *Kandasana,* Knot Pose; *Eka Pada Sirsasana,* One Leg behind Head Pose; *Garbha Pindsana,* Embryo Pose; *Samakonasana,* Split
- Twists: *Marichyasana* III, Sitting Lateral Twist; *Paripurna Matsyendrasana,* Complete Matsyendra (name of hatha yoga founder) Pose

†In another (earlier, and therefore probably more reliable) account, Devi writes that she was told about the demonstration by a doctor friend.

Pictures," the *Life* photos were accompanied by text (without a byline) that describes the *asanas* as "contortion postures." With one or two exceptions, they're simply advanced postures that must've seemed to be contortion stunts to Americans. Even while described as contortions, however, the *asanas* aren't characterized as bizarre, injurious, amusing, heathen, or penitential. In fact, in a surprisingly sympathetic and sophisticated portrayal (especially considering that *Life*'s target readership was primarily middle-class Christian Americans), "real yoga" is presented as soteriological discipline: "Yoga seeks literally to yoke the soul of the individual to the all-pervading soul of the universe. Unlike other Hindu cults, yoga postulates no mere ascetic subjugation of the body to the yearning of the soul. Its catalog of contortions is best understood as exercises which seek to make the body healthy, serene and free from disease and disorder that distract the soul with carnal concerns."[29]

The caption for the variation of *Ganda Bherundasana,* Formidable Side of the Face Pose, reinforces the benefit of a conditioning *asana* practice to aid meditation (not identified as such) and, taking the discourse to another level, even implies that a conditioning posture itself, when properly assumed, is the vehicle for spiritual realization: "Relaxation is attained in this position by [a] practiced yogi. The hands and feet both are in [an] attitude of devotion, the face shows no strain. Yogi[s] work out balanced series of postures for [their] daily routine, perform[ing] them faithfully morning and evening."[30] As is shown in the illustrations in the *asana* section of his 1934 book *Yoga Makaranda* (variously translated as *The Nec-*

tar of Yoga, The Secrets of Yoga, or *The Essence of Yoga*), from the beginning of his tenure as teacher at the *yogashala* Krishnamacharya had been teaching his students to assume even the most difficult postures in tranquillity, a state that was sometimes reinforced by incorporating the palms-pressed-together devotional gesture into a posture such as *Durvasana,* Durvasana (the name of a sage) Pose (fig. 17.3).

Yet, while not showing emaciated ascetic yogins who treat their body as an impediment to enlightenment, the photos in *Life,* as well as the very similar photos in *Yoga Makaranda,* don't truly capture yogins using their body as a tool for spiritual development either. In fact, the photos demystify whatever spirituality may obtain to the exercises. Rather than presenting grown men, dressed in robes or *dhotis,* candidly captured preparing for or already deep in meditation at an ashram, the photos simply present boys in shorts demonstrating physical exercises for a photo shoot set in a picturesque courtyard (with snippets of the palace in the background meant to impress)—attributes that don't bring the viewer into the realm of the spiritual. The text accurately reads: "Demonstrated are advanced postures, such as few yogi[s] today take the time to master. They are assumed in calm, deliberate fashion, held for long intervals. Each pose is thought to bestow its own special benefit, but the general result is a physique as well-toned as any U. S. Athlete's."[31]

No matter how matter-of-fact the presentation of these exercises is, though, there's no getting around that the poses remain unnatural and exotic, at least in the eyes of most *Life* readers. It's easy to understand why the pioneer yogins largely omitted them from their routines

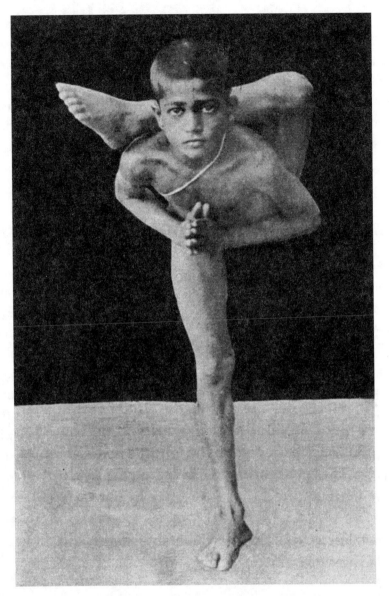

Figure 17.3. Keshavamurthy, T. Krishnamacharya's favorite student, demonstrating *Durvasana*, Durvasana Pose, 1934

(From *Yoga Makaranda*)

for Indians. In general, they require great coordination, control, and concentration; demand limberness far beyond the ready capacity of most adults, especially males; are strenuous; risk injury; and take courage. When she became a yoga teacher, Devi included only the three easiest of these postures (simplified versions of Bow Pose, Peacock Pose, and Headstand) in her routine. Knowing that they were unsuitable for her, Krishnamacharya probably never even tried to teach Devi the other postures. But they were perfect for his young charges.

In *Mystics, Ascetics, and Saints of India,* published in 1905, sociologist of Indian religions John Campbell Oman quotes an 1894 description of a yoga street performer, probably one of the disenfranchised Naga people (tribes inhabiting the northeastern part of India) forced into mendicancy through British actions in the 19th century:

> Many religious mendicants earn a meal or a penny by disclosing, as fortune-tellers, palmists, and interpreters of dreams, the hidden things of the future. Others astonish the world by acrobatic feats—as the following extract from the Allahabad *Pioneer* will show:—
>
> "A wonderful *faquir* was in view in the main street, who all the time he says his prayers goes through acrobatic performances that would earn him a fortune in England. As we approached he was standing on one leg with the other curled round his waist; in another second he was on his hands, head downwards, and his legs round his neck; when we left him he was tied up in something resembling a reef knot and clove hitch combined." ("A March through the Cow-rioting Districts," *Pioneer* [Allahabad], 7th February 1894.)[32]

Asanas that forcefully twist the body out of its natural shape could still be found performed by fakirs in the streets and practiced by devout yogins at ashrams, temporary encampments on beaches, and other locations in India in the 1930s. But Krishnamacharya was using these punishing *asanas,* which he probably carefully observed in South India,

as exercises in the physical culture routine that he developed for his students. In this act of preservation, Krishnamacharya was the keeper of the flame: within the development of modern hatha yoga, he kept alive the entire weird *asana* tradition (which had been greatly diminished by Kuvalayananda in order to form an easy, one-hour yogic physical exercise routine, resembling calisthenics regimens, for middle- and upper-class Indians).

Not that Krishnamacharya was preserving a tradition that was by any means ancient and pure. There was a rapid expansion of the *asana* repertoire, especially of advanced postures, in the 17th and 18th centuries—that is, in the pre- or early modern period in India. (Current scholarly investigations, including one undertaken by the Hatha Yoga Project at the School of Oriental and African Studies in London, are hoping to answer a number of questions about this phenomenon: Exactly which *asanas* were introduced into yoga during this period? What were their origins? What were their aims? Were they preparation for—and therefore totally subservient to—sitting in meditation? Or did they veer off into having their own purposes, such as harnessing subtle energies in the body?)

And not that it was Krishnamacharya's intent to preserve tradition. He was not acting out of a higher purpose, such as devotion to his country. In this, he is perhaps best contrasted to D. C. Mujumdar. In the foreword to the English-language one-volume abridgement of Mujumdar's ten-volume *Encyclopedia of Indian Physical Culture: A Comprehensive Survey of the Physical Education in India Profusely Illustrating Various Activities of Physical Culture, Games, Exercises Etc., as Handed Over to Us from Our*

Fore-Fathers and Practised in India, the first volume of which was published in 1935, Bhavanarao Pant Pratinidhi, the rajah of Aundh, who himself revived, codified, and promoted *surya namaskar,* writes about the encyclopedia, "The work has been carried out on a very ambitious scale and on the lines of a similar work done by Bernarr Macfadden in America." The accomplishment of editor Mujumdar, Bhavanarao continues, rebounds to the glory of India. "[He] has shown to the whole English knowing world what sports, pastimes and various forms of bodily exercises in India have been in vogue for a long time, i.e. since 1000 A. D. at least. Some of them are Mallakhamba or a wrestler's pole, wrestling, Danda and Baithaks, Khokho, Langdi, Viti-Dandu, Chendu-Larori, Atya-Patya, Kite-Flying [and] Lathi."[33]

Bhavanarao (in a nationalistic and racist argument common in the pre–World War II era) advises that if the males and females of India practiced daily *surya namaskar* and the exercises in the encyclopedia, "there will shortly be produced a type of humanity that shall excel in body, mind and soul any that the earth has yet brought forth and shall set a new standard for the race."[34]

Unlike Mujumdar and Bhavanarao, whose passion was to preserve India's exercise past (in order to shape India's future as an independent nation), Krishnamacharya had no interest in preserving the past (or shaping the future). For this reason, it can be said that in teaching the full panoply of *asanas* (instead of the popular limited canon developed by Kuvalayananda and other modernists) to the boys of the royal family (and gradually to other boys, as well) Krishnamacharya was the accidental preservationist of *asanas.*

❦

When the expansive *asana* tradition that Krishnamacharya transmitted to his young students was introduced to the West in the 1960s by Iyengar in his manual *Light on Yoga* and his demonstrations, it astonished, challenged, and exhilarated yoga practitioners. It seemed new. And in some ways, it actually was new. In addition to preserving the complete postural yoga tradition, Krishnamacharya expanded *asana* practice by turning to sources outside the yoga tradition for inspiration. He developed his grueling *asana* routine not solely by incorporating the existing *asanas* performed by fakirs and yogins but also, as Sjoman shows, by creating new *asanas* using the modern Western gymnastics floor exercises found in the *Vyayamadipika,* "the western gymnastics manual [compiled by S. Bharadwaj and] written by the Mysore Palace gymnasts," as "source material."[35]

Krishnamacharya also developed a collaborative form of yoga probably influenced by the long tradition of street acrobatics in India. "Acrobats can traced in Indian literature as far back as Kautilya's *Arthasastra* (ca. 396–312 B.C.E.), where *plavaka* (tightrope walkers) are mentioned among the names of artisans," writes folklorist S. A. Krishnaiah. "A fee (audience tax) was charged for their show."[36]

The group yoga that Krishnamacharya created is displayed in the showy centerpieces of two photos from *Yoga Makaranda* of his students performing *asanas* in the Jagan Mohan Palace courtyard. These eye-catching tricks are performed by three boys, each of whom is doing a familiar *asana,* in a pyramid structure. Two older boys form the base by doing near back-to-back shoulder stands, while at the top a younger

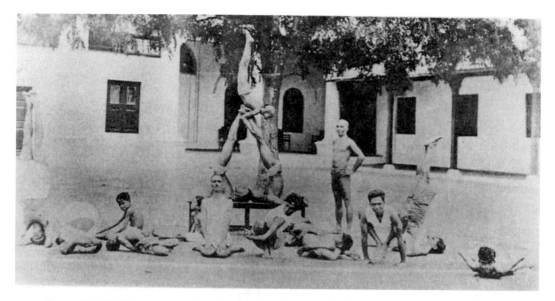

Figure 17.4. T. Krishnamacharya's students performing *asanas* in the Jagan Mohan Palace courtyard, with Krishnamacharya standing at center-right, 1934

(From *Yoga Makaranda*)

boy, supported by the feet of the others, performs an advanced yoga posture. In one case, it's *Pincha Mayurasana,* Feathered Peacock Pose or Forearm Stand, in which balance is maintained on the forearms while the legs are swung up and kept straight (fig. 17.4). In the other case, it's *Vrschikasana* I, Scorpion Pose, in which balance is maintained on the forearms while the legs are swung up and dropped over the head, with the feet coming to rest on the crown of the head. (The poses are somewhat modified due to the assistance of the boys below.)

Krishnamacharya may have seen an acrobatic pyramid feat performed in a marketplace to a mesmerized crowd and created his own versions using yoga poses. The identity of the source of his eye-catching yogic versions of acrobatic performances, though, isn't nearly as important as the fact that he put together disparate elements—from inside and outside the yoga tradition—in an unexpected way to come up with a flashy collaborative yoga.

Krishnamacharya also borrowed from another popular entertainment—one that would provide him with his most difficult and breathtaking advanced postures.

18

T. KRISHNAMACHARYA

Incorporating Contortion into Yoga

Contortion as Entertainment

T. Krishnamacharya wasn't just the keeper of the flame for the old, weird *asana* tradition; as part of his teaching to the boys at the Jagan Mohan Palace in the early 1930s, he made the *asana* repertoire weirder by including several poses—in particular, *Natarajasana, Ganda Bherundasana, Sirsa Padasana,* and *Tiriang Mukhottanasana*—that weren't part of the hatha yoga reclusive or mendicant performance tradition. These *asanas* aren't in the early hatha yoga texts (*Hatha Yoga Pradipika, Gheranda Samhita,* and *Shiva Samhita*). They aren't described in pre-20th-century Western travelers' eyewitness accounts of yogins. And there's no depiction of them in yoga art (e.g., the murals depicting 84 *asanas* that decorate the walls of the sanctum of the temple in Mahamandir, just outside Jodhpur, possibly painted in 1810 and the 121 illustrations of *asanas* in the yoga section of the *Sritattvanidhi,* a manuscript compiled at the Mysore Palace sometime between 1811 and 1868). These new poses, which twist the body into jaw-droppingly difficult and unnatural shapes, were adapted by Krishnamacharya from contortion acts.

Natarajasana, Lord of the Dance Pose, is a standing posture that includes balance and backbending. Beginning in *Tadasana,* Mountain Pose, one brings a leg up behind the back and rests the foot on the head. In his treatise on contortion, *Stage Tricks and Hollywood Exercises: How to Develop Skill in Suppleness and Acrobatics,* Nelson Hall suggests accomplishing this pose by "back kicking" and "catching the foot and pulling it high as possible." "It is another stunt that must be held," he observes, "if the audience is to get it."[1]

Ganda Bherundasana, Formidable Face Pose, is a prone backbending posture. Beginning with the chin and chest, on the floor, the elbows bent, the buttocks tipped up, and the knees and tops of the feet on the floor, one brings the legs up and overhead until the feet rest on the floor beside the head. Hall recommends accomplishing this pose by "lying face down on the floor and doing a rocker roll of the feet over the head to the floor."[2]

Sirsa Padasana, Feet-to-Head Pose, an inverted backbending posture, was considered by Iyengar to be "the hardest of all the back-bending poses."[3] Beginning in *Sirsasana,* Headstand, with the forearms on the floor, one brings the legs over the back until the feet rest on the back of the head. Hall notes that "patting the head with the feet and reaching around the throat with the toes always gets good response."[4]

Tiriang Mukhottanasana, Intense Upside-Down Face Pose, is a standing backbending posture. Beginning in *Tadasana,* Mountain Pose, one bends back and grasps the ankles. After recommending that "you can usually negotiate the position . . . by bending the crab position," Hall suggests "walking the hands to grasp the ankles before waddling about the room."[5]

Contortionism

Contortion, as defined by Hall, is "writhing, twisting and bending movements under control and executed in a pleasing and surprising manner."[6] ("We all start off being contortionists," he maintains, "doing a lot of wiggling, twisting and squirming in the cradle and getting acquainted with our new bodies."[7]) As the art of the Egyptian, Greek, Roman, medieval, and Renaissance eras shows, "contortion work," or the "art of the bender," began in ancient times and continued for centuries. The heyday of contortion, though, surpassing even the period of the Roman and Renaissance circuses, can be found in the circuses, fair sideshows, vaudeville theaters (called music halls in Great Britain), and nightclubs in Europe and America in the late 19th and early 20th centuries.

On the one hand, contortion during the Victorian and early modern era was the same as it was through the ages. After all, the body doesn't bend itself into infinite variations. On the other hand, no other period could match the diversity of presentation (contortion mixed with pantomime, clowning, acrobatics, and comedy); lavish venues (such as the Empire in Paris, the Alhambra in London, and the Wintergarten in Berlin); wide range of roles (contortionists appearing as animals, such as fish, snakes, toads, lizards, and crocodiles, but also characters, such as Mephistopheles, and types, such as a Chinaman); inspired props (such as a pivot, made to cradle a chin, for spinning); unique stage business (such as a contortionist stuffing himself into a small suitcase); narration (shifting effortlessly from one shape into another, contortionists sequencing their complete inventory of tricks like a story); and probably professionalism (consistently high levels of performance, no matter how tired the contortionist was), skill (effortless performance of extreme backward-bending and forward-folding stunts), and star power (the charm and charisma of the contortionists).

In the vaudeville circuit, contortionists—along with pantomimes, dancers, jugglers, and acrobats—were classified as "dumb acts": performers who don't speak. What their contortion work says to us is hard to discern because it's difficult to explain our response to it. We find the display of the adult male and female body in a variety of extreme configurations riveting but also ridiculous and even repugnant. We're delighted by the gracefulness of the movements and poses, yet we're also repulsed (or at least made uncomfortable) by the seemingly haphazard, violent, and gruesome arrangement of body parts, the consequence, perhaps, of some horrific bone disease, birth defect, or accident.

And we're turned on. By violating some natural law of how bodies twist and bend, contortion seems to especially transgress normative sexual practices. We're sexually stimulated by performers seeming to strut their stuff as an invitation to kinky, delirious sex. Or, even though we're openly observing public entertainment, we're sexually excited by what feels like secretly looking at the performers' intimate sexual acts: self-pleasuring that goes beyond ordinary (prehensile) self-sufficiency. In either case, seduced or voyeuristic, we're sinful. We're erotically aroused when we shouldn't be. Perhaps this accounts for both the thrill and discomfort we experience upon watching contortionists.

Both the performers and the audience members, of course, are forbidden from acknowledging the nature of our relationship. We agree to pretend that the performance is innocent light entertainment, some kind of aestheticized athletic exhibit. But "the spectacle of a body twisting into 'unnatural' configurations invariably haunts the spectator, for it appears as if the contorted body transcends either a normal threshold of pain or an acceptable juxtaposition of body parts," observes scholar of body culture Karl Toepfer. "Contortionism therefore constructs a complex, contradictory image of the body as a site of extreme pliancy, extreme strength (or boldness), and extreme vulnerability, and it is this tension between extremes of physical expression that accounts for the visceral excitement of the spectator."[8] In a view of contortion more as public perversion than resonant theater, historian G. Strehly, perhaps the most keen advocate of contortion, remarks in his famous 1903 book *L'Acrobatie et les acrobats* that contortion is "a kind of monstrosity. . . . At performances of these phenomena [the spectator] experiences only the feeling of unhealthy curiosity comparable to what one has for everything which is a deviation from the laws of nature."[9]

Contortion as Physical Culture

In the early 20th century, some physical culturists recognized that contortion work—bending the body into extreme postures—was more than the cultivation of a God-given talent based in double-jointedness (a misnomer). They appreciated the endless practice that went into attaining the high degree of muscular control and flexibility necessary to perform contortion tricks effortlessly and gracefully. They certainly weren't the only customers to be impressed, or even awed, by the sheer athleticism and professionalism of what most considered freak-show entertainment. But they were the first to perceive the ability to perform contortion tricks as a new norm for flexibility.

Instead of viewing many contortion postures as exceptions to the norm—as a going beyond the limit of how the body could (or should) ordinarily stretch—physical culturists viewed many contortion poses as the standard (i.e., ideal) bodily extension that could be attained by anybody with enough training and discipline. (Once the standard joint range of motion was expanded to include contortion movements, deviations from this standard—that is, any capacities less than the full range of contortion movements—were considered impairments of movement. A truly supple person should, for example, be able to bend backward and grab his or her ankles.) This shift in perception led the physical culturists to incorporate contortion stunts into their physical exercise regimes.

By the late 1920s and early 1930s, physical culturists were championing the benefits—especially to the spine and nervous system—of contortion work for the average adult and child. In a 1931 article titled "Should We Do Acrobatics?" (with the teaser "A Discussion of the Good and Bad Results to Be Found by the Average Person in the Use of Ordinary Acrobatics in His or Her Exercise Program—An Article for Both Sexes") in *Strength,* a prominent American physical culture magazine, Bobbie Trebor contended that "such stunts as cartwheels and handstands are perfectly all right" not only for "chorus girls and stage and circus women" but for "most of the gentler sex and the majority of the strong and sturdy oak species, too"—the average woman and man who would probably respond with "holy horror at the idea of doing any of 'that crazy foolishness.'"[10] Aside from the cartwheel and flip-flap (back handspring), the article is actually about contortion stunts, not acrobatic feats.* The contortion stunts featured are the split, headstand, crab (backbend from standing), handstand, limber (from the handstand, the feet fall over forward), front walkover (the limber with the feet brought over separately), and elbow balance.†

Trebor made clear that he was promoting contortion not as a job skill but as health exercise: "Now do not misunderstand me—this magazine is not advocating a nation of professional acrobats, and in presenting this article in favor of acrobatics as a national health builder we are not endeavoring to develop even a single stage performer. But we do hope to bring about a healthier condition in many, many men and women in the everyday walks of life by interesting them in including this . . . health building exercise in their daily program."[11]

What makes contortion exercises beneficial for health, Trebor maintained, is that they bend, twist, and stretch the waist, "the most vital region in the body,"[12] which contains the stomach, liver, and intestines, the three "most

---

*Acrobatics involves short, highly controlled bursts of activity (jumps, twists, flips, and such), sometimes on the run, such as somersaults and handsprings. While acrobatics, like contortion, may also involve static poses that require balance, agility, and coordination, contortion primarily involves the display of dramatic bending and flexing of the body.

†All but one of these contortion stunts are included in B. K. S. Iyengar's *Light on Yoga* as yoga postures: the split is *Samakonasana;* the headstand is *Salamba Sirsasana* II; the crab is *Urdhva Dhanurasana* II; the handstand is *Adho Mukha Vrksasana;* the limber is *Vrschikasana* II; the front walkover, a variant of the limber, is absent; and the elbow balance is *Pincha Mayurasana.* Most astonishingly, even the flip-flap is included as *Viparita Chakrasana* in *Urdhva Dhanurasana. Light on Yoga* documents the full repertoire of yogic poses taught by Krishnamacharya to Iyengar and the other students at the *yogashala.*

utterly neglected and abused organs we possess."[13] In a 1929 *Strength* article titled "Can Your Child Do These Stunts?" (with the teaser "If Your Child Is Not Up to the Average in Strength and Pep You Will Find Teaching Him or Her These Stunts an Easy Way of Administering 'Exercise'"), Robert L. Jones made a similar claim for contortion work: "As for the [specific] benefits of the work, suppleness and the well being of the internal organs are of prime importance"[14] (see fig. 18.1 on page 228).

These articles in *Strength* are evidence that the reframing of contortionism from entertainment to physical culture, while probably not enjoying widespread popularity, was part of the times in the late 1920s and early 1930s. So Krishnamacharya's incorporation of contortion stunts into an exercise routine wasn't unusual. Still, it seems unusual for a yogin. Where, we wonder, did he learn about the contortion stunts that he adapted for his yoga regimen? Unlike Shri Yogendra, Swami Kuvalayananda, K. V. Iyer, S. Sundaram, and Bhavanarao Pant Pratinidhi, who were keen followers of the latest trends in Western physical culture, he probably didn't read books and magazines on physical culture. And it's even more unlikely that he attended nightclubs, musical theaters, palladiums, sideshows, or carnivals.

The Indian Circus

The modern circus began with the official opening of Philip Astley's New British Riding School in London, England, in 1770. After classes were over, Astley held equestrian shows in the afternoons for awed spectators and soon hired acrobats, ropewalkers, and musicians to add to the entertainment. Equestrians with trick-riding skills and trained horses dominated the early circuses. (*Circus* is Latin for "circle" or "ring"—the place where horses ride in a circle.)

Over the next century and a half, circuses—housed in permanent buildings or traveling—evolved into wildly popular extravaganzas with trained animals, acrobats, jugglers, tightrope walkers, trapeze artists, strong men, and clowns. In its heyday the circus included exhibitions of "freaks," educational pageants, menageries, large tents, three-ring arenas, colorful posters, gala parades, and trains designated to carry its personnel, animals, and equipment. In the late 1800s European and American traveling circuses visited countries around the world. Eventually, countries around the world formed their own circuses.

The inspiration for the first circus in India was Giuseppe Chiarini's Royal Italian Circus, the first circus, in December 1879, to tour India. In one version of events, Vishnupanth Moreshwar Chatre, the famed horse trainer, equestrian, and superintendent of the stable at the Kurundwad Palace, and Balasahib Patwardhan, rajah of Kurundwad Senior, sat in front side boxes of the ring to watch the show on Christmas night in Chiarini's arena, camped near a railway station in Bombay. Chiarini, accompanied by two stallions, welcomed the audience with an invitation. He challenged the members of the Indian audience to imitate with their own horses the equestrian feats they would see later on, matching the elegance, precision, and discipline of his horses' movements. He set the wager at one thousand rupees, offered to give the Indian who took up the challenge six months to prepare, and, if he lost, pledged to give up any one of his horses.

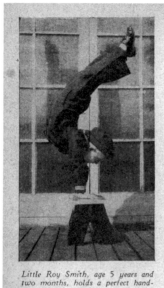

Little Roy Smith, age 5 years and two months, holds a perfect handstand as long as ten seconds.

Can Your Child Do These Stunts?

If Your Child is Not Up to the Average in Strength and Pep You Will Find Teaching Him or Her These Stunts an Easy Way of Administering "Exercise"

By ROBERT L. JONES

TWENTY, or thirty, or forty, or whatever the number may be, years ago when you and I were young, our parents thought us just the grandest thing out if we could beat any youngster in the neighborhood reciting "The Boy Stood On the Burning Deck" or "I'm a Little Curly-Head," or something else of like tenor. For a tot of three to five or more to recite some such nonsense with gestures of sufficient number and violence was considered the acme of infantile and juvenile accomplishment, and more than one great orator or wig-wag expert doubtless owes his success to such early training.

But time changes things, and today even the dullest youngster can, after listening to parents, the radio and the neighbors, discourse on any subject from stocks and bonds to torch murders and bridge with more fluency and much greater intelligence than his grandparents "could say a piece" when they were twice his age. So it has come to pass that the infant prodigy who used to startle the neighborhood by re-

citing perfectly a "speech" longer than any other kid could handle no longer has much of a place in the sun. Today we are interested in what the youngsters can do with their bodies—they do not need any particular vocal encouragement—and fond mothers and proud fathers trot out Sister and Junior to "do your butterfly dance for Mrs. Smythe-Browne" and to "show Mr. Smithkins what Dempsey did to Firpo." And because parents are now taking not a little interest in the physical activities and accomplishments of their offspring the said offspring is a healthier and happier set of youngsters than were the children of other years, and they will make a fitter, more active and more capable generation of adults than were their grandparents and parents.

The last few years have seen countless steps taken for the betterment physically of the youth of the nation. No longer is the underweight child condemned to a sickly life because "he is just that way"; we know in almost every case exactly why a certain child is underweight, or seemingly dull and stupid, or lacking in interest in the things which should be of most concern to him. And knowing these things, we know how to approach rectifying the condition in order to give that child a fair start in the game of life. Per-

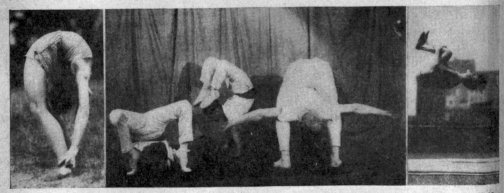

Betty Protz, thirteen, does a great somersault. She is all-round tumbling champion of the Middle Atlantic Division, A. A. U. competition. In the center are the three Duncan Brothers, Harold, Joseph and Marion, of Columbia, Mo., doing their stuff, while at the right Betty Saunders is demonstrating what a limber back looks like.

Figure 18.1. "Can Your Child Do These Stunts?"

(From *Strength*, October 1929)

After that, he cracked his whip, which spurred the horses to furiously run around the circular area. Then he and the horses ran out of the ring.

Chatre and the rajah greatly enjoyed all the acts that followed. When they were over, Chiarini reentered the ring with the two stallions. He repeated his challenge. With Chatre and the rajah watching closely, Chiarini led his horses through their feats: fancy dressage trotting (the horses paraded back and forth), rearing (the horses circled the ring on their hind legs), dancing to the beat of a drum, and probably bowing at the event's conclusion. When Chiarini turned to audience, Chatre, with the rajah's permission, stood up and declared that he accepted the challenge. "My horses can do the items which your horses did and even better than that. I don't need six months, but only three months. If I do not, I promise you ten thousand British Indian rupees and ten horses of the best breed." Then he vowed to form his own circus within a year. The audience cheered, while, according to Sreedharan Champad, author of a book about the history of the Indian circus, Chiarini glowered at Chatre and muttered, "The Black's arrogance. . . ."[15]

Chatre staged his horse show on March 20, 1880, in an arena built on the grounds of the Kurundwad Palace. All of the invited distinguished guests were present—except Chiarini.

Chatre's Great Indian Circus debuted on these grounds on Christmas night 1880.[*]

Chatre's circus was dominated by animal acts. When it came to Tellicherry (also called Thalassery), a city on the Malabar Coast of Kerala, in South India, in 1888, Keeleri Kunhikkannan, an avid enthusiast of athletic endeavors (indigenous wrestling and the South Indian martial art kalaripayattu, as well as gymnastics and sports practiced by the British officers stationed in town), proposed teaching acrobatics (jumping, tumbling, and balancing), juggling, and contortion skills to students if Chatre would employ them. Chatre agreed. Kunhikkannan was soon providing trained child performers to the circus. In molding his young performers, Kunhikkannan was taking advantage of the fact that children tend to be more limber—and more daring—than adults. Children's joints are hypermobile compared to adult joints; as a result, their spines give more. Their tendons, muscles, and ligaments gradually tighten as they age (increasingly so from ages eight to sixteen), steadily decreasing their joint range of motion (unless they practice stretching exercises to make their stiffened bodies flexible). And Kunhikkannan was taking advantage of a ready pool of recruits: to create his circus stars, he used village urchins, establishing a practice that continues into the present.[†]

---

[*]In another even more dramatic telling of these events, after having his best horse perform tricks, Chiarini challenged members of the audience to get his horse to duplicate them. Accepting the challenge, the rajah of Kurundwad sent Chatre into the ring. Under Chatre's commands, the horse surpassed its previous performance. Inspired by his success, Chatre got the idea to form his own circus.

[†]A window into this practice in recent times is Martin Bell's 1993 documentary *The Amazing Plastic Lady.* Its major focus is the relationship between Pratap Singh, a dedicated trainer of a troupe of child acrobats and contortionists, and ten-year-old Pinky, his most talented female contortionist, known in India as a "plastic lady." While capturing the great charm of the circus, the film is primarily a moving document about the powerful *guru-shishya* (or *chela*) *paranpara,* master-student relationship—a four-thousand-year-old tradition in Indian culture. Whether Pinky and the other young performers are considered to be indentured servants or village urchins rescued from a life of poverty, there's no doubt that they take great pride in what they do.

Thus, at the turn of the century, when contortion, acrobatics, and juggling, which had long been performed in India at feasts and celebrations and in the marketplace, became circus acts—that is, became show business—child entertainers were showcased as never before. The circus contortion acts, especially those performed by children, were the likely source of inspiration for Krishnamacharya's incorporation of contortion stunts into yoga. During the 1920s and 1930s more than fifty Indian circuses were performing throughout the country, so there was ample opportunity for Krishnamacharya to have attended shows. But we have no ticket stubs, diary entries, eyewitnesses, or even secondhand reports to prove it. That doesn't mean, however, that it can't be proven that Krishnamacharya's new extreme postures were borrowed from contortion acts, whatever their source.

Borrowings from Contortion Acts

While admitting that the similarities between Krishnamacharya's contortion *asanas* and Western contortion stunts are "suggestive," yoga scholar Mark Singleton abjures any cause and effect: "I point out these similarities not to suggest any *causal* link between the postural forms of the Western sideshow contortionist and the *asanas* of modern postural yoga." How does he explain that the sameness or near sameness of show-business contortion poses and Krishnamacharya's yogic contortion poses? That "many of the most common positions are a perfect match with the advanced postures of popular postural yoga today," Singleton reasons, is a result of "coincidences that may be at least partially due to the structure and limitations of the human body itself."[16] He's arguing that Krishnamacharya's creation of contortion yoga exercises for the boys in his classroom laboratory is, in effect, an example of simultaneous innovation, not cross-fertilization. As the well-known phenomenon of multiple discovery in science and technology shows, discoveries, inventions, and innovations in the same area can occur to different people from different places at the same time—for example, in calculus (Newton and Leibniz), in the theory of natural selection (Darwin and Wallace), and in motion pictures (the Lumière brothers, Dickson, and others).

But each of these scientific and technological innovations evolved from an accumulated knowledge base. There are no postures in the yoga tradition (whether in manuals, on temple murals, or in descriptions of mendicant street practice) from which Krishnamacharya could've developed the shape and range of motion of *Natarajasana, Tiriang Mukhottanasana,* and the other new advanced poses. The closest resemblance to *Natarajasana* of any of the 121 illustrations of *asanas* in the yoga section of the *Sritattvanidhi,* the 1880s manuscript from the private library of the Mysore Palace to which Krishnamacharya had access, is *Trivikramasana* (the name of a different posture in Iyengar yoga), a pose in which the yogin stands on one leg while the other leg is in front of the shoulder and the foot behind the head. (And the only resemblance of *Natarajasana* to the bronze temple statues of Nataraja widely disseminated during the South Indian Chola dynasty is that Nataraja is shown standing on one foot while sprightly lifting the other leg mid–dance step.) The closest resemblance to *Tiriang Mukhotta-*

nasana is *Urdhva Dhanurasana* II, Upward Bow Pose from *Tadasana,* Mountain Pose, in which the hands are placed on the floor far behind the legs.

In addition to having virtually the same configurations and intense extension as the contortion stunts, the contortion yoga postures have two telltale features of contortion performance totally absent (and irrelevant) in the hatha yoga tradition but critical to the performance (i.e., showmanship) aspect of contortion. The first feature is elegance. There are no previous yoga poses with anything like the stylistic flourishes of the curved trunk and arms flung over the head in *Tiriang Mukhottanasana* and the outstretched arm in the early stage and the head tipped back in the final stage of *Natarajasana* (no wonder Iyengar would regularly perform these postures in his demonstrations to drum up interest in yoga in the 1960s in the West!).

The second telltale feature is fluidity—actually, subtle tricks of stage technique that facilitate fluidity—a key aesthetic element in the graceful presentation of a contortion performance. *Tiriang Mukhottanasana* involves bending back to grasp the calves, which is what enables the contortionist performing the stunt version to seamlessly move into the next pose by bending the knees and elbows and then rolling forward or backward, waddling about the stage, or simply poking the head out from between the legs. In the yoga pose, gripping the calves is merely a means of extending the pose by using a prop (in this case a part of the body, not a wall, chair, strap, or the like). (In the stunt version of *Natarajasana,* the contortionist clutches the shin of the raised leg, bends backward, plants the legs wide, and slips down into a split.) Furthermore, in a contortion act, unlike in the yoga session, this elegance and fluidity often serve a unique and affecting aesthetic.

The contortionist Barbara La May, an American expatriate who settled in Paris in the early 1930s, was successful in her prime, writes scholar of body culture Karl Toepfer, because of the tragic nature of her aesthetic: "She combined heroic, dangerous stunts with a voluptuously melancholic display of vulnerability."[17] There's very little in Krishnamacharya's practice, it seems, that turned his performance (or that of his students at demonstrations) into such intense drama (see figs. 18.2 and 18.3 on page 232).

Krishnamacharya and Western physical culturists may have synchronistically turned to contortion as exercise, but Krishnamacharya no more created contortion stunts than the physical culturists did. Like them, he picked up the stunts elsewhere (in his case, probably the Indian circus). The evidence for this—a kind of strong argument from silence—is found in the absence in the hatha yoga tradition of both precursory contortion-like *asanas* and of the particulars of the elegant and fluid contortion performance style.

This leaves the final question: What motivated Krishnamacharya to incorporate contortion stunts into yoga in the first place?

Krishnamacharya's Motivation

While both Trebor and Jones reframed the stunts as physical culture exercise to maintain and improve health, Trebor advocated contortion as "a sport which has a sufficiently

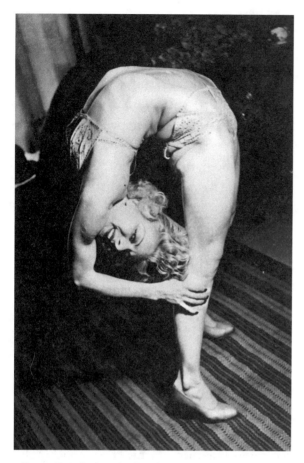

Figure 18.2. Barbara La May demonstrating grasping the ankles from the crab position, circa 1950

(From *Contortionists,* by Michel Louis)

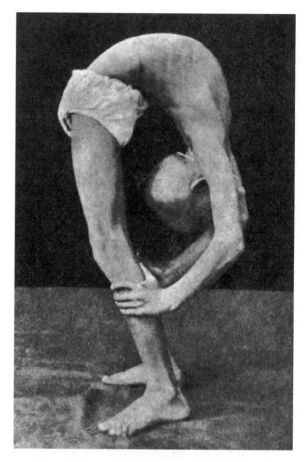

Figure 18.3. One of T. Krishnamacharya's students demonstrating *Tiryangamukha Uttanasana,* Standing Backward Bend, 1934

(From *Yoga Makaranda*)

attractive and pleasant 'sugar coating' to be taken by Mr. Mrs. and Miss Average Citizen," and Jones advocated contortion as an activity that would entice children to exercise (something ordinarily anathema to them).[18] Jones reasoned that children would take to contortion work first because it involves extreme bending and twisting and children are inherently elastic ("Bending and twisting, or, if you prefer to classify the work correctly, contortion work, comes very naturally to young children, for at their age their joints are very

supple") and second because it involves the spirit of play and children are inherently full of high spirits.[19]

It is only the dull, monotonous routine exercise movement that meets opposition from the youthful camp, and . . . it is almost always possible to introduce "exercises" having sufficient of the "play" element present to render them attractive to childish minds. Tumbling and acrobatics were two such agencies mentioned, and in this article are presented a number of [contortion, balancing, and tumbling] stunts of varying degrees of difficulty suitable for teaching to kiddies from the earliest years upward. Contortion work—bending and twisting—balancing, both easy and difficult, and tumbling tricks are illustrated and described so that without the assistance of an instructor you can teach your youngster something interesting which will be at the same time beneficial to his mental and physical well being.[20]

But Krishnamacharya probably didn't add contortion stunts to his yoga regimen for the sake of his students. Blind to the needs of others, he wasn't interested in providing his wards with "the well being of the internal organs" or inserting "the 'play' element" into the work of exercise to "render [it] attractive to childish minds." Nor was he interested in adding contortion stunts to challenge himself or to cultivate disciples who would only want to carry on a legacy that was daring and innovative (although later on one student, B. K. S. Iyengar, would create Iyengar yoga, and another student, K. Pattabhi Jois, would create Ashtanga yoga—both styles derived from Krishnamacharya's teachings). Although he wasn't the first person to incorporate contortion stunts into physical culture, Krishnamacharya was the first to adapt contortion stunts (tricks that twist the body into unnatural shapes, perfected by highly skilled performers to entertain crowds at the circus) to an Indian physical culture regimen (modern hatha yoga, perfected by modern yogins to provide optimal fitness and health to the populace) for a novel purpose: to entertain audiences at yoga demonstrations.

19

T. KRISHNAMACHARYA

Infusing Yoga
with *Surya Namaskar*

Yoga as Performance

Creation of Vinyasa Yoga

In the early summer (the season that spans March to May in India) of 1934, the maharajah of Mysore, Shri Nalvadi Krishnaraja Wadiyar, sent the yoga teacher of the royal family (and other) male youths, T. Krishnamacharya, with his students in tow, on a two-month pilgrimage, whose purpose, according to his student and brother-in-law B. K. S. Iyengar, was "to meet Swami Sri Kuvalay-ananda and to see for himself the Yogashrams conducted by Swamiji at Lonavla and Bombay."[1] Probably the maharajah thought that visiting Kuvalayananda's facilities, especially Kaivalyadhama, the ashram—actually a yoga fitness and health resort—in Lonavla, would afford Krishnamacharya, who was suppos-edly schooled in the traditional esoteric *guru-chela* system of transmission of yogic spiritual knowledge in a cave in Tibet, the opportunity to observe and imitate Kuvalayananda's new model of yoga, in which yoga was made available as convenient exercise and natural health cure at facilities open to the public (or, at least, to those members of the middle class who could afford to temporarily abandon their normal lives to go take advantage of the services). But the central event of the trip turned out to be the demonstrations at Kaivalyadhama given by Krishnamacharya's students of a flowing *asana* format that he'd recently created: Vinyasa yoga. (Although he referred to the repetitive linking sequences in his system as *vinyasas,* Krishnamacharya himself didn't use the term "Vinyasa yoga"; it was coined decades later.)

In a letter written on April 2, 1934, soon after Krishnamacharya's visit, Kuvalayananda reported to the maharajah: "T. Krishnamacharya came to Lonavla and stayed here for three days with a view to study the working of the Ashrama Kaivalyadhama." Instead of then enumerating what Krishnamacharya learned, Kuvalayananda gave an account of what evidently most struck him about Krishnamacharya's visit: "During these three days, he gave two demonstrations of Yogic Asanas to the members of the Kaivalyadhama." After politely giving an obligatory compliment ("Obviously, the Shastriji [learned teacher] has bestowed much attention and labour on his pupils"), he bluntly expressed his disapproval of Krishnamacharya's newfangled yoga, in which very difficult *asanas* were linked by transitional movements. "I have advised the Shastriji to simplify his exercises when they are to be given to the generality of students and grown up individuals. I have also recommended him to keep the Yogic exercises unadulterated by the admixture of non Yogic systems of physical culture." Kuvalayananda courteously concluded, "I wish the Shastriji every success in his mission."[2]

The shrewd Krishnamacharya largely ignored the teaching practices he observed at Kuvalayananda's facilities and the advice about his own teaching practice.

Krishnamacharya created Vinyasa yoga during the time when Swami Kuvalayananda's staid, simple course of hatha yoga and its variants, developed as suitable indigenous exercise for the primly self-restrained emerging Indian middle class, were dominant. Kuvalayananda's regimes consisted of a full course, based on the "Full Course of Yogic Physical Culture for an Average Man of Health" described in his 1931 book *Asanas,* which, in turn, is based on the nearly identical original version of the regime in the October 1925 *Yoga-Mimansa* (eleven *asanas,* one *bandha,* one *mudra,* two *kriyas,* and two *pranayamas*); a short course, developed in 1930 (eight *asanas* and one *pranayama*); and an easy course, developed in 1931 (seven *asanas* and one *pranayama*). The first graded courses of yogic exercises based on the principle of progression (in number, repetition, and duration), they were categorized as physical culture because they had a preventive, not a curative, value (not that Kuvalayananda didn't also use *asanas* and the other yoga exercises for therapeutics).

Contrasting Krishnamacharya's flowing yoga (performed solely by the boys of the royal family at the Jagan Mohan Palace *yogashala*) to Kuvalayananda's stop-and-start yoga canon (increasingly performed by middle-class adults in their homes in "any well ventilated place" on "a carpet large enough to accommodate the length and breadth of the individual practising Yogic exercises"[3]) emphasizes the uniqueness of Vinyasa yoga. Placing the creation of Vinyasa yoga in the context of physical education routines for children in schools across India, yoga scholar Mark Singleton emphasizes instead the ordinariness of Vinyasa yoga: "Krishnamacharya's 'Mysore style' was far from out of step with the dominant forms of physical education in late colonial India and was in fact a variant of standard exercise routines of the time."[4] To make his case, Singleton audaciously claims that a proto–Vinyasa yoga style—characterized by *asanas* combined with mass exercises based in drill techniques—was widespread in educational institutions in India and that the homegrown version was created by none other than Swami Kuvalayananda.

Trends in Indian Physical Education

After the measures taken by government of the United Provinces the previous year to implement Kuvalayananda's curricula of yogic physical culture in its educational institutions "result[ed] in nothing," in November 1933, at the request of the minister of education, Kuvalayananda submitted a proposal to the U.P. government with a new strategy: establishing a school of yogic physical education in Lucknow (now the capital city of Uttar Pradesh).[5]

To serve the needs of the teacher training program at the school, in 1936 Kuvalayananda wrote a booklet in Hindi, *Yaugic Sangha Vyayam* (Yogic group exercise), that included detailed instructions for two group exercises: a simple yogic routine consisting of eight *asanas* (with one variation) and one *kriya,* followed by a calisthenics routine embedded within a drill. At odds with our contemporary purist yoga sensibilities and proposed by, of all people, the most prominent and influential founder of modern hatha yoga, this physical education program startles. It jarringly juxtaposes (emphasizing both a contrast and a link between) the exercises of hatha yoga, a spiritual practice associated with solitary withdrawal from everyday life, and drill, based in military training used to foster a fighting force's ability to think and act at maximum efficiency as a team.

But before he turned his attention to yoga, a young Kuvalayananda, caught up in the nationalistic fervor of the times, performed these drills from 1907 to 1910 as part of his *shastar vidya* (the art of using weapons) training under the guidance of his beloved teacher Rajratna Rajpriya Professor Manikrao. Group drills (*sangha vyayam*) with commands in Hindi (Hindi *aganya shabda*), considered to be Manikrao's most significant contribution to Indian physical education, appealed to the youths performing them and the observers watching them on an aesthetic and a political (i.e., nationalistic) level. This revolutionary approach to teaching martial arts, calisthenics, and indigenous physical exercises so changed attitudes toward physical education that even wealthy families began sending their children to Manikrao's institution, the Jummadada Vyayam Mandir, in Baroda.

The opening phase of the calisthenics/drill in *Yaugic Sangha Vyayam* consists of eleven traditional drill commands (beginning with "Fall in," "Right dress," "Eyes front"). The middle phase—the exercises proper—is nine exercise commands, broken into steps: "Lie on the chest," "Get up," "Sit down," "Lie on the back," "Right roll," "Left roll," "Sit up," "Sit on the heels and toes," and "Stand up." The closing phase is eight traditional drill commands (ending with "Attention," "Salute to the front," "Dismiss").[6]

Singleton notes the similarity between the first two steps of the "Lie on the chest" series and the two steps of the "Sit down" series with, respectively, the "jumping back" and "jumping through" movements of Vinyasa yoga. But the performance of yoga postures followed by calisthenics exercises, even those with snippets that resemble Vinyasa yoga, don't constitute a synthesis of calisthenics and *asanas* into one flowing exercise. Besides, the instructions in the booklet weren't put into practice throughout India or, for that matter, even in the United Provinces. "It was unfortunate that the scheme of starting a school of Yogic Physical Education in U.P. could not be implemented," Kuvalayananda biographers Manohar L. and Manmath M. Gharote report.[7]

In further support of his claim that *vinyasa*-like yoga was prevalent in India in the early 1930s, Singleton makes a similarly inflated use of his other piece of evidence: *Our Physical Activities,* the syllabus created for the Training Institute for Physical Education, established by Kuvalayananda. Singleton writes, "The Bombay Physical Education Committee syllabus—based on Kuvalayananda's work, and compulsory in the province's schools from 1937—shows striking similarities with the system enshrined in postural modern yoga as Ashtanga Vinyasa."[8] (Created by Krishnamacharya's student Krishna Pattabhi Jois, Ashtanga Vinyasa yoga, often simply referred to as Ashtanga yoga, is derived from Krishnamacharya's Vinyasa yoga and closely resembles it.) "The drills often closely match the 'vinyasas' of Krishnamacharya's method," Singleton argues, "such as in the 'Calisthenics' section, which contains a drill called 'Kukh Kas Ek,' close in form and execution to Ashtanga Yoga's *utthita trikonasana.*"[9]

Singleton goes on to describe the similarity between Ashtanga yoga sequences and exercises in another chapter of the syllabus, devoted to "Individualistic Exercises, Dands, Baithaks, Namaskars and Asanas." "It is clear," Singleton states, "that these sections of the syllabus represent a fusion of popular 'indigenous' aerobic exercises with *asana* to create a system of athletic yoga mostly unknown in India before the 1920s."[10] Yet Singleton himself admits elsewhere that the *asanas* and aerobic activities described in the syllabus aren't primarily fused: the "*asanas* are [largely] presented separately from the other exercises."[11]

But once again, it doesn't matter. Singleton's own evidence, when fully examined, undermines his own premise that Kuvalayananda's pedagogy was widespread. The recommendations in the syllabus barely saw the light of day. Swami Kuvalayananda's Physical Education Committee of 1945–46, the Gharotes remark, "observed that the measures recommended by his 1937 Committee for making physical education as [sic] compulsory subject in the school curriculum were neither generally carried out nor the Committee's expectations fulfilled. . . . A few schools . . . had taken up physical education seriously and with enthusiasm. . . . In most schools, however, . . . physical education was either indifferently organised or sadly neglected."[12]

The problem was not only inadequate facilities and equipment but also unqualified physical education teachers, who were largely ex-service men, gym aficionados, and scoutmasters. Another problem was the lamentable state of the very facility for which the syllabus was written: the Training Institute for Physical Education, established in Kandivli, a suburb north of Bombay, for training the physical education teachers. "The short-comings of the institute were many," the Gharotes report. "Firstly, the site was malarious and the incidence of sickness due to malaria became scandalous. . . . The most disappointing feature of the Institute was the extremely poor recruitment of students."[13] This is the educational milieu to which Singleton points in making his strongest claim for the widespread existence of proto-*vinyasas* created by an Indian in schools throughout India. (Physical education in India remained in a lamentable state until after World War II.)

Without realizing that he has failed to make a convincing case that Kuvalayananda's pedagogical recommendations are "a fusion of popular 'indigenous' aerobic exercises with *asana* to create a system of athletic yoga" and that he has overlooked the Gharotes' findings that show that Kuvalayananda's recommendations were never successfully implemented anyway, Singleton posits the existence of a proto-*vinyasa* movement in physical education throughout India initiated by Kuvalayananda as the basis for concluding that "Krishnamacharya's dynamic teaching style in Mysore is of a piece with this trend, and his elaborate innovations in *asana* represent virtuoso additions to what was, by the time he began teaching in Mysore, becoming a standard exercise format across the nation. Although the evident proficiency of his young troupe was probably unsurpassed at the time, the *mode* of practice was in itself by no means exceptional."[14]

Krishnamacharya's *vinyasa* system—described in his yoga manual, *Yoga Makaranda,* composed in 1933 and published in 1934—with its light, nimble movements connecting difficult *asanas,* was spectacularly different from any yoga practiced in India by adults or children in the 1930s, especially the prevailing form of hatha yoga, Kuvalayananda's canon, with its easy, discrete postures. Krishnamacharya was a brilliant innovator. His Vinyasa yoga was a singular achievement within the history of yoga.*

Not that Vinyasa yoga should be seen as an anomalous, souped-up exercise. Singleton convincingly argues that this flowing style of yoga was of a piece with some Western gymnastics. He highlights Primitive Gymnastics, a physical education regime developed by the Dane Niels Bukh that emphasizes intense stretching exercises connected by rhythmic movements, which was imported from Europe and enjoyed widespread popularity in British army training in India in the 1920s and 1930s. "At least *twenty-eight* of the exercises in the first edition of

---

*There's one exception—and it's significant—to the singularity of Krishnamacharya's *vinyasa* system: Shri Yogendra's yoga system. Yogendra's routine, with its simple *asanas* and their dynamic variations, and Krishnamacharya's routine, with its *asanas* and their *vinyasa* variations, both involve yogic postural variations and near continuous movement.

In creating his flowing yoga, Krishnamacharya may even have been influenced by Yogendra's dynamic yoga, which was derived from J. P. Müller's calisthenic routine (see chapter 3). Krishnamacharya could have learned about Yogendra's system by attending one of Yogendra's lectures in Mysore in 1927 about the value and validity of yoga in the lives of householders; by reading Yogendra's *Yoga Asanas Simplified*, published in May 1928, probably as a pamphlet; or by speaking with Mirza Ismail, the diwan (prime minister) of the Kingdom of Mysore (appointed to the position in 1926), who was an admirer of Yogendra's. But it isn't known if Yogendra demonstrated or even described his "perfect course" of yoga exercises at his lectures (let alone that Krishnamacharya attended one of them). There isn't any evidence that knowledge of Yogendra's style of yoga was widespread (let alone that it reached Krishnamacharya through Yogendra's writings). And no record exists of Krishnamacharya speaking with Ismail (let alone about Yogendra's teachings).

Bukh's manual [published in English in 1925] are strikingly similar (often identical) to yoga postures occurring in Pattabhi Jois's Ashtanga sequence," Singleton writes (referring again to Jois's system, which is derived from and closely resembles the flowing yoga of Krishnamacharya's system). "There are several more in the second edition of 1939. Not only do Bukh's positions suggest modern yoga postures but the linking movements between them are reminiscent of the jumping sequences of Ashtanga Vinyasa."[15] "I point out these similarities not to suggest that Krishnamacharya borrowed directly from Bukh," Singleton makes clear, "but to indicate how closely his system matches one of the most prominent modalities of gymnastic culture in India, as well as Europe."[16]

Direct Influence on the Creation of Vinyasa Yoga

Singleton strains to argue not only that Kuvalayananda's pedagogical recommendations, which resembled Vinyasa yoga, were widely implemented in India, thereby making Krishnamacharya's style merely a variance of a commonplace practice, but also that these recommendations were a direct source that influenced Krishnamacharya's creation of Vinyasa yoga. "By the time of Krishnamacharya's visit [to Kuvalayananda's facilities in 1934]," Singleton writes, "Kuvalayananda's *asana* regimes were *the* paradigm of pedagogic yoga instruction in India, and it is reasonable to suppose that Krishnamacharya absorbed some of their core elements and applied them to his work with the children in Mysore."[17] "While Kuvalayananda limits himself in *Yaugic Sangha Vyayam* to simple, dynam-ically performed calisthenic postures and some easy *asanas* (referring the interested reader to his *asanas* of 1933)," Singleton continues, "it would seem clear that Krishnamacharya adopted this format and wove in other, sometimes advanced, yoga postures, much as Kuvalayananda himself would do."[18] As shown above, Kuvalayananda's regimen in *Yaugic Sangha Vyayam* didn't weave calisthenics and *asana* together (if it did, Krishnamacharya's Vinyasa yoga demonstration wouldn't have raised Kuvalayananda's hackles) and wasn't the paradigm of pedagogic yoga instruction in India, so it's not reasonable to suppose that Kuvalayananda's pedagogic proposals influenced Krishnamacharya's teachings.

Singleton also argues "Ashtanga Vinyasa is a powerful synthesis of *asanas* and *dands,* after the manner of Kuvalayananda's national physical culture programs [found in *Our Physical Activities*]."[19] In 1933, when Krishnamacharya created (or at least wrote about) Vinyasa yoga, *dands* were, however, commonly practiced in *akharas* (wrestling gymnasiums), where, combined with *bethaks* (deep knee squats), they comprise the core wrestling *vyayam* regimen (the Indian system of physical training designed to build flexibility, strength, and bulk). So Krishnamacharya could've seen them in neighborhood *akharas*.

But the simple movements of *dands* aren't complex enough to be a model for the linking movements of Vinyasa yoga. The *dand* consists of three positions. In the preparatory position, one lies prone on the ground with the feet placed close together and the palms flat on the ground directly below the shoulders. In the first position, one raises the hips (the buttocks are thrust up) while straightening the arms and legs in a posture that resembles *Adho Mukha Svanasana,* Downward-Facing Dog. In the second position, one bends the arms and legs, pushes the body forward and down, brings the chest (gliding close to the ground) between the hands, straightens the legs, and tilts the head up, with only the palms and the toes on the ground. In the third position, one arches the torso, with the head up and chest out, into what in yoga would be a modification of *Urdhva Mukha Svanasana,* Upward-Facing Dog, and *Bhujangasana,* Cobra Pose. One repeats these movements.

There was, however, a perfect model, whose complexity includes movements that closely resemble *dands.*

The inspiration for Krishnamacharya's creation of Vinyasa yoga wasn't the synthesis of *asanas* and drill exercises in *Yaugic Sangha Vyayam* or of *asanas* and *dands* in *Our Physical Activities* but *surya namaskar* (sun salutation exercises). Singleton himself, in addition to his other theories, recognizes *surya namaskar* as the model for Vinyasa yoga. He flatly states: "Krishnamacharya was to make the flowing movements of Suryanamaskar the basis of his Mysore yoga style."[20] *Surya namaskar,* with its continual movement linking a small set of *asanas,* is a simple form of Vinyasa yoga.

Singleton argues that by 1933, when Krishnamacharya first began teaching Vinyasa yoga,

surya namaskar and *asanas* were already commonly fused together: "Krishnamacharya's addition of *suryanamaskar* to his *yogasana* sequences was simply in keeping with a growing trend within postural modern yoga as a whole." This trend is "evidenced," Singleton maintains, "by Yogendra's admonition"[21] in his *Yoga Asanas Simplified:* "Suryanamaskaras or prostrations to the sun—a form of gymnastics attached to the sun worship in India—indiscriminately mixed up with the yoga physical training by the ill-informed are definitely prohibited by the authorities."[22] But Shri Yogendra's dictum, found in the 1956 edition of his book, was probably made in reference to the use of *surya namaskar* as a warm-up exercise in Swami Sivananda's regime of the 1950s.*

Surya namaskar was ubiquitous in India in 1933, especially in the flourishing *vyayamshalas* (gymnasiums), where *surya namaskar* was taken up with zeal. However, it wasn't a part of yoga; it was an equally trendy rival method of physical training. Which made it easily accessible to Krishnamacharya. He could've picked it up visiting local *vyayamshalas* or *akharas,* where it was part of the wrestling routine, or simply by reading the groundbreaking *Surya Namaskars,* by Bhavanarao Pant Pratinidhi, the rajah of Aundh, published in English in 1928. Krishnamacharya even could've observed *surya namaskar* at the Jagan Mohan Palace. The palace's administrative report for the 1934–1935 school year shows

---

*The Yoga Institute claims that *Yoga Asanas Simplified* was first published in 1928; however, no copies of such an edition exist. The institute archivists say it's lost. If it was published in 1928, in all likelihood it was as a pamphlet. The 1932 (second) and 1947 (fourth) editions also no longer exist. The 1936 (third) edition is currently unavailable; it's been preserved, though, in the Crypt of Civilization in Brookhaven, Georgia, to be read in 8113, when the chamber, sealed in 1940, is opened. The 1956 (fifth) edition is the basis for all subsequent editions. It appears that this edition is the product of several revisions, making the text a palimpsest.

that, amid the gymnastics, military exercises, Western sports and games, and yoga that made up physical culture instruction for the Arasu boys, "thirty-two boys attended the Yogasana Classes and a large number of boys attended the Suryanamaskar Classes."[23] (There's no entry, however, for *surya namaskar* classes in the report for the 1933–1934 school year, when Krishnamacharya began teaching at the *yogashala* and wrote *Yoga Makaranda*.)

Wherever the provenance of his having first learned about *surya namaskar,* there's no doubt that Krishnamacharya incorporated the linking movements of *surya namaskar* into yogasana (or, from another view, expanded and made more challenging the type of linking movements and positions of *surya namaskar*) to create Vinyasa yoga. Yet he took no credit for creating this new style; instead, he claimed to have learned Vinyasa yoga from a *shastra* (sacred text), the *Yoga Korunta,* written on palm leaves, which subsequently disintegrated. (Traditionally, texts were written on dried palm leaves, and after a time, when the manuscripts inevitably became worn and brittle, they were copied onto new sets of palm leaves, thus perpetuating a cycle of copying.) "The *vinyasas* handed down from ancient times should be followed," Krishnamacharya wrote in *Yoga Makaranda*. "But nowadays, in many places, these great practitioners of *yogabhyasa* [yoga practice] ignore *vinyasa krama* [the yoga of sequencing sustained postures linked by transitional movements] and just move and bend and shake their arms and legs and claim that they are practising *asana abhyasa* [asana practice]."[24]

It might be argued that someone might've appropriated *surya namaskar* to create Vinyasa yoga in ancient times. But not only is *surya namaskar* not ancient (nor, for that matter, are conditioning *asanas*), but the form of *surya namaskar* used in Vinyasa yoga was developed only in the early 20th century. While *surya namaskar* (the exercise, not the ancient sun ceremony from which the exercise is derived) is probably a few hundred years old, *surya namaskar* in the standard form that we know it is the result of four modifications made by Bhavanarao in 1909: standing fully erect in the first position (anachronistically called *Tadasana,* Mountain Pose); keeping the knees straight while bending forward in the second position (anachronistically called *Uttanasana,* Standing Forward Bend); bringing the foot in line with the palms in the lunge position; and regulating the breath in accordance with stomach contractions. To create Vinyasa yoga, Krishnamacharya incorporated this new style of *surya namaskar*—with its more alert, angular positions, crisper movements, and multiple inhalations and exhalations—created by Bhavanarao (see fig. 19.1 on page 242).

Why did Krishnamacharya feel obligated to make his spurious claim for the ancient origin of Vinyasa yoga? Singleton suggests that Krishnamacharya was acting out of humility: "I think Krishnamacharya merged and experimented and tinkered with whatever forms he could find during his time in Mysore. What's important to realize, however, is that he was perfectly at liberty as a pandit to innovate within the tradition. There is nothing shocking about it. His 'version' of where he derived his yoga from (guru and *shastras*) is in keeping with the convention of effacing one's own personality when creating new methods or interpretations."[25]

It seems equally likely, though, that Krishnamacharya acted out of self-aggrandizement

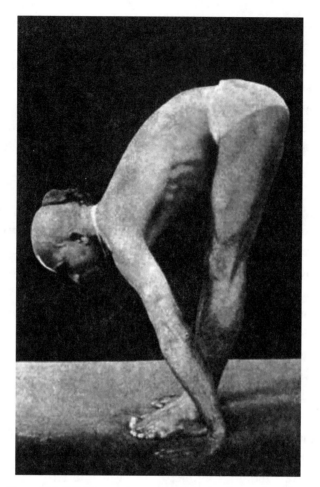

Figure 19.1. T. Krishnamacharya demonstrating *Uttanasana Sthiti,*
Flat-Back Standing Forward Bend, 1934

(From *Yoga Makaranda*)

and self-protection: he wanted to put the imprimatur of the yoga tradition on Vinyasa yoga to lend it prestige and to forestall criticism that it broke with tradition.

One thing isn't in doubt: hatha yoga is centuries old, but it's a growing, changing tradition. Although assumed to be part of yoga for five thousand years, *surya namaskar* was first incorporated into yoga to create Vinyasa yoga only about eighty-five years ago, making the mixture of *surya namaskar* and yoga not as "ancient" as

electric street lights, jazz, Nazism, the general theory of relativity, talking pictures, and commercial passenger air travel.

Motivations for Creating Vinyasa Yoga

Singleton rightfully credits the maharajah with providing the necessary conditions for Krishnamacharya to develop his own system of hatha yoga: "The Maharaja actively fostered a climate of eclectic, creative physical culture in Mysore State, establishing the material and ideological conditions that would directly facilitate . . . synthetic *hatha* experiments."[26] But Singleton also argues that the maharajah's influence on Krishnamacharya was direct. The maharajah encouraged, pushed, or pressured Krishnamacharya to create a kind of yoga that would be popular with the masses: "Thanks largely to the efforts of the Maharaja Krishnaraja Wodeyar IV [more commonly called Nalvadi Krishnaraja Wadiyar], Mysore had, by the time Krishnamacharya arrived, become a pan-Indian hub of physical culture revivalism. Krishnamacharya, working under the personal direction of the Maharaja, was entrusted with the task of popularizing the practice of yoga, and the system he developed [Vinyasa yoga] was the product of this mandate."[27] Singleton seems to be implying that the maharajah charged Krishnamacharya with inventing a kind of "crossover" yoga, a revved-up version that would appeal to the masses.

But Krishnamacharya probably developed his new form of yoga more for a reason other than popularizing yoga. Teaching the centuries-old ascetic discipline of hatha yoga (which involves withdrawal from the everyday world and the application of bodily techniques to harness mental activity as a means of enlightenment) as physical culture to children presented special challenges to him. Writing in 2007 about Krishnamacharya's legacy, journalist Fernando Pagés Ruiz speculates: "As [his] pupils were primarily active young boys, he drew on many disciplines . . . to develop dynamically-performed asana sequences aimed at building physical fitness."[28] Krishnamacharya, as Ruiz implies, may

have injected an element of play (flowing movements) into the yoga exercise regimen at the *yogashala* in order to keep up the interest of his young students—perhaps not even for their sake but to please their parents. It's even more likely, though, that he created Vinyasa yoga, with its twisting of the body into highly unnatural shapes (including newfangled contortion-influenced poses) combined with elegant, continuous moving of the body (like folk dance and circus contortionist and acrobatic acts), because it's particularly suited for making an impressive public performance.

Although Nalvadi Krishnaraja Wadiyar sent Krishnamacharya and his students on tours to demonstrate yoga in order to stimulate interest among the populace in yoga as fitness and health exercise, the groundbreaking demonstrations were those held at the Mysore Palace. These were probably the first yoga demonstrations whose primary goal was to entertain. The maharajah wanted yoga performances to delight and gain the admiration of his distinguished guests, and Krishnamacharya wanted, above all, to please his employer.

In his account of these palace demonstrations, Iyengar describes Krishnamacharya's role as court entertainer: "One of the duties I was often called upon to perform during this period of my life was to give demonstrations of yoga for the Maharaja's court and for visiting dignitaries and guests. It was my guru's duty to provide for the edification and amusement of the Maharaja's entourage by putting his students—of whom I was one of the youngest—through their paces and showing off their ability to stretch and bend their bodies into the most impressive and astonishing postures."[29]

Singleton describes these demonstrations as "a coordinated, high-speed showcase." Students were assigned primary, intermediate, and advanced categories of *asanas* to perform. "These sequences were, according to Jois [who participated in a large number of the demonstrations], virtually identical to the aerobic schema he still teaches today: that is, several distinct 'series' within which each main *asana* is conjoined by a short, repeated, linking series of postures and jumps based on the *suryanamaskar* model. "Although he would never endorse such an interpretation himself," Singleton continues, "his description suggests that the three sequences of Ashtanga system may well have been devised as a 'set list' for public demonstrations: a shared repertoire for student displays."[30] Krishnamacharya had created a dynamic yoga showbiz act to rival the contortionist and acrobatic circus acts. His audiences, like the crowds at the circus, must've responded with a shudder of excitement mixed with anxiety and wonder.

The boys carried out Krishnamacharya's act with daring and discipline—but not out of a need to entertain. They weren't driven to perform. "I pushed myself to the limits in my practice in order to do my duty to my teacher and guardian," says Iyengar, "and to satisfy his demanding expectations," even to the point of injury.[31] Krishnamacharya drove Iyengar and the other boys to perfect their performances solely for his own self-enhancement. He saw the children as extensions of himself. He taught them flashy yogic postures, which seemed to defy the laws of anatomy, joined with elegant linking movements, and extracted incandescent performances from them to bedazzle audiences in various parts of South India, visitors to

the *yogashala,* and especially spectators at the Mysore Palace in order to glorify himself.

There may also have been a deeper, hidden motivation that drew Krishnamacharya to create this system of nimble and dignified bodily extrications (*vinyasas*) from twisted bodily entanglements (*asanas*). Like stunt performer Harry Houdini wriggling free from a straitjacket while suspended upside-down from a building; or the ghastly, gnarled (phony) cripple portrayed by film actor Lon Chaney in *The Miracle Man,* seemingly affected by a miracle cure, straightening up; or, dusted with white powder and lit to emphasize the chiaroscuro of his sculpted body, showman bodybuilder Eugen Sandow, an apparent statue atop a pedestal on a stage, seemingly bursting to life with rippling muscles; or the eponymous hero of Edgar Rice Burroughs's *Tarzan of the Apes,* unfettered by an effete aristocratic English upbringing because reared by an arboreal ape, leaping and swinging from limb to limb in a forest top in Africa, Krishnamacharya presented a narrative of constraint and astonishing escape—a literal embodiment of the common early 20th-century motif of the male's anxiety over stifling threats to his traditional identity (experienced by Krishnamacharya, the brainy, arrogant, scholarly, orthodox Brahmin, when he was forced to work as a foreman at a coffee plantation) and his fantasies of dramatic escape and empowerment.

Which of these motivations (if any—after all, absent a person's heartfelt confession, candid comment, shared deep awakening, or the like, the attribution of motivation, especially to historical figures, is speculative) compelled Krishnamacharya to develop Vinyasa yoga? Perhaps a mixture of them all. After all, most of us—even yoga teachers!—have complex identities derived from a variety of backgrounds and experiences, so the motivation for our actions, like the determination of the cause of our death, is often multilayered and hence multidetermined.

Krishnamacharya's Legacy

Krishnamacharya is commonly credited with being the founder of modern hatha yoga. "Sometime in the early 1930s . . . Krishnamacharya took it upon himself to champion the beauty and the benefits of yoga asana," claims author and *Yoga Journal* editor Linda Sparrowe, "lifting it up from relative obscurity and placing it alongside its [raja], bhakti, karma, and jnana yoga siblings."[32] Krishnamacharya "transformed hatha—once an obscure backwater of yoga—into its central current," concurs Ruiz. "Yoga's resurgence in India owes a great deal to his countless lecture tours and demonstrations during the 1930s, and his four most famous disciples—[K. Pattabhi] Jois, [B. K. S.] Iyengar, [Indra] Devi, and Krishnamacharya's son, T. K. V. Desikachar—played a huge role in popularizing yoga in the West. . . . He never crossed an ocean, but Krishnamacharya's yoga has spread through Europe, Asia, and the Americas. Today it's difficult to find an asana tradition he hasn't influenced."[33] While it's true, as Singleton observes, "In recent years, Krishnamacharya has attracted the reverence of thousands of yoga practitioners worldwide, and is considered by many to be the grandfather of yoga in the modern era,"[34] Krishnamacharya didn't save yoga *asana;* he merely followed in the path of the hatha yoga modernists who were responding to the physical culture movement sweeping the world. Ruiz writes that at the turn of the century "under the pressure of British colonial rule, hatha yoga had fallen by the wayside. Just a small circle of Indian practitioners remained."[35] Even if hatha yoga had fallen into desuetude, though, *asana* practice as a discipline for attaining fitness and good health for the populace wouldn't have been affected because it didn't exist until the first-generation pioneers, such as Shri Yogendra, Swami Kuvalayananda, and S. Sundaram, created and popularized it in the late 1910s and early 1920s. Thanks to them, *asana* practice was hardly obscure by the time Krishnamacharya started teaching it at the palace in 1933; in fact, a yoga fad had been in progress since the mid-1920s.

Although it shouldn't be forgotten that the creation of Vinyasa yoga was the act of a single person, Krishnamacharya, it also shouldn't be overlooked that the origins of a flowing form of yoga can be placed in a larger context— a far larger context than a gymnastics trend in physical education in India. Vinyasa yoga was part of the modernist fascination with dynamic movement, as manifested by French composer Darius Milhaud's incorporation of jazz (and polytonality) into classical music, first in his 1922–1923 ballet music *The Creation of the World (La création du monde)*; the Italian futurist painter Giacomo Balla's presentation of everyday life as a blur of constant movement in abstract works such as *Abstract Speed + Sound (Velocità astratta + rumore)* in 1913–1914; and the French novelist Marcel Proust's juxtaposition of his narrator's organized presentation of rational thoughts with stream of consciousness in *In Search of Lost Time (À la recherche du temps perdu)*, published from 1913–1927, which reflect, respectively, the swinging, stomping rhythms, accelerated pace and streamlined technology, and wildness and overflowing profusion of thought in the early 20th century.

While sharing the basic characteristic of dynamic movement with these modernist arts, Vinyasa yoga—like *surya namaskar* itself, Bukh's gymnastics, circus contortion (with stunts, such as back-kicking and then catching the foot as high as possible, connected by fluid movements), soccer (with moves, such as the bicycle kick and the bending free kick, erupting amid continuous dribbling and passing), and other physical activities in India in the 1930s—is more closely an expression of modernist exercise, sports, and performance style that is characterized by graceful, energetic, and continuous movement. In this, Vinyasa yoga is related to popular exuberant ways of movement—found in gymnasiums, parks, circus tents, stadiums, theaters, nightclubs, and films around the world—such as the Lindy Hop, the contemporaneous jazz dance that, with its smoothly horizontal, elegantly flailing movements, accompanied swing, the new style of jazz-inspired music that transformed American popular music beginning in 1935 with its fluid, rhythmic momentum.*

Although his shape-shifting fluidity of movement is of a piece with the casual abandon of the body (achieved by a hidden work ethic of obsessive practice) introduced in the Jazz Age, one of the most innovative and daring periods in the history of bodily expressiveness, Krishnamacharya didn't expand the repertoire of idiosyncratic yet timeless bodily gesture and movement. Unlike the fidgety gracefulness of Charlie Chaplin as the Tramp (in his splay-footed walk), the snappily rhythmic insouciance of Fred Astaire (in his ebullient and elegiac dancing), the dainty athleticism of Babe Ruth (in his trot around the bases), the raw emotionality of Martha Graham (in the spare pelvic contractions of her dancing), the vibrancy of Al Jolson (in his slight, galvanic tremblings while belting out a song), and the loopy uninhibitedness of Josephine Baker (in her rubbery-legged dancing), Krishnamacharya's fluid plasticity (in his performance of Vinyasa yoga) wasn't a characteristic so singular that it generated unique movements expressive of universal truths. However, the type of physical activity that he created—moving yogic exercise—allows for an embodied spiritual practice unique in yoga history.

Incorporating *vinyasas* into an *asana* routine was the key achievement of Krishnamacharya's syncretistic fervor. As seen in a 1938 silent home movie, the smoothly rhythmic movements that

---

*Singleton does mention that Bukh's gymnastics, and hence Krishnamacharya's Vinyasa yoga, "reflect[ed] a modernist fascination with dynamic movement." He uses an observation by yoga scholar Norman Sjoman as corroboration of this view: "Sjoman inquires with regard to Krishnamacharya's system, 'are the asanas really part of the yoga system or are they created or enlarged upon in the very recent past in response to modern emphasis on movement?' Given the similarities between Bukh's Primitive Gymnastics and these dynamic yoga sequences, it is the latter scenario that seems more compelling" (Singleton, *Yoga Body,* 201, 203). The subject of Sjoman's question, however, isn't Krishnamacharya's Vinyasa yoga but the great number of conditioning *asanas* found in K. V. Iyengar's *Light on Yoga,* which reflect an emphasis on conditioning *asanas* (in contrast to stabilizing meditative *asanas*) in modern hatha yoga practice.

lead into and out of *asanas,* demonstrated by a shy and compliant teenage Iyengar, transform yoga practice into elegant performance.* Iyengar isn't so much going about his private fitness regimen as engaging an audience—us, the film viewers. Using his malleable body, he's showing off the capacity of Vinyasa yoga for garlanding together a seemingly infinite variety of configurations, and we're filled with surprise and delight.

As Sjoman points out, though, Iyengar created his own system by "discard[ing] the *vinyasa* system" taught to him by Krishnamacharya because he felt that the continuous movement and elaborate breathing "distracted from the asana itself. He held the asanas for extended periods of time. . . . He introduced ideas of precision, penetration and introspection into the asana system."[36] Hatha yoga votaries who seek to incorporate an expansive meditativeness into their practice prefer doing static poses. Moving slowly and deliberately to enter a pose and then yielding to the pose—inhabiting one's body—lends itself to penetrating into the essence of things.

The heated-up style of yoga created by Krishnamacharya, which has its origin in charged performance intended to please an audience and rivet its attention, precludes contemplation. But this doesn't mean it must be concerned at all with appearance. Rapt attentiveness to every motion of the body demanded by the flowing movements of the contemporary forms of Vinyasa yoga—Ashtanga Vinyasa yoga and its various spin-offs—can keep the mind from wandering, and it's this absorption that can become paramount, not demonstrating skills or displaying beautiful movement.

By transforming hatha yoga into a fluid performance of poses, Krishnamacharya bequeathed to later generations an *asana* practice that—like other rigorous physical efforts that demand full absorption in movement, such as ballet, competitive gymnastics, or basketball (but without their ultra speedy movement and gravity-defying leaps)—can prohibit all conscious mental activity. This emptying of *citta* (mind-stuff) from the mind, like filling the mind with comprehensions, is also a true form of yogic spirituality.

Krishnamacharya's *vinyasa*-style yoga was unknown in the West for almost forty years. Jois had been teaching Ashtanga Vinyasa yoga, his version of it, at his institute in Mysore, the Ashtanga Yoga Nilayam, since 1948. Jois was incidentally "discovered" by the Belgian yogin André Van Lysebeth, a devout disciple of Sivananda. In 1971 Van Lysebeth published *Pranayama—la dynamique du souffle* (published in English as *Pranayama—The Yoga of Breathing* in 1979). Of the eighteen photos in the book, three show Jois teaching *pranayama* to an advanced student and one shows the student practicing *pranayama* by himself. The caption on page 118 identifies Jois as "a yoga master in South India."[37] The caption on page 135 identifies the student as "an adept of Ashtanga Yoga Nilayam of Mysore."[38] Thus any readers seeking to learn advanced *pranayama* techniques could

---

*A DVD of the film, *1938 Practice,* may be purchased from the Iyengar Yoga Institute in Maida Vale, London. The film can also be found online using the search words "B. K. S. Iyengar 1938 film."

find the "yoga master in South India" at the "Ashtanga Yoga Nilayam of Mysore."

"It was through Van Lysebeth's book," writes Jois apostle Eddie Stern, "that [Jois's] whereabouts became known in Europe, and thus the Europeans were the first to come from the West specifically to study with Guruji."[39] The adventurous aspirants—in all likelihood followers of Sivananda's calming yoga—who sought out Jois for *pranayama* lessons were probably taken aback at seeing the vigorous yoga he was teaching. But then again, because they were accustomed to having *surya namaskar* as part of their routine (Sivananda was the first to introduce *surya namaskar* as a warm-up exercise to *asana* practice proper), perhaps those brave enough to take up Ashtanga Vinyasa yoga, in which a series of *asanas* are linked by the positions of *surya namaskar,* quickly adapted.

The last twenty-five years, during which Jois's fame came to nearly rival Iyengar's, has seen the rise in popularity of Ashtanga Vinyasa yoga to the extent that in America, all other forms of postural yoga are often branded (and dismissed) as "hatha yoga," as if Ashtanga Vinyasa yoga weren't itself a form of hatha yoga. Most take it up as sweat-inducing weight loss exercise. Some, however, practice it as soteriology. They recognize that Ashtanga Vinyasa yoga, as Ruiz aptly writes, while "originally designed [by Krishnamacharya] for youngsters, provides our high-energy, outwardly-focused culture with an approachable gateway to a path of deeper spirituality."[40]

20

K. V. IYER

Mixing Bodybuilding and Yoga at the Palace

Maharajah of Mysore

In the 1930s Shri Nalvadi Krishnaraja Wadiyar (1884–1940), ruler of the Princely State of Mysore, a region as large as England, was revered, writes historian M. Fazlul Hasan, as a "saintly king" whose "years of glorious rule . . . touched chords in the hearts of the citizens"[1] (see fig. 20.1 on page 250). In his chronicle of the fall of the princely states (they were step-by-step stripped of all autonomy following the transference of power from the British Raj to the Dominion of India and the Dominion of Pakistan in 1947), John Lord describes the maharajah of Mysore as "a man of medium size with an expression invariably calm and a deportment of quiet and dignified grace."[2] "Though Sir Krishnaraja's roots were buried deep and true in the distant past, he was able to assimilate much of the West. In his neat semi-European suits he looked and acted the part of the contemporary maharajah, but always in moderation."[3] He enjoyed royal pomp and privilege too much to totally abandon his role as old-fashioned ruler.

During most of the year, the maharajah lived in the Mysore Palace. Started in 1897 and completed in 1912, the huge, three-story stone building in the middle of the capital city of Mysore has a majestic exterior with domes, arches, and an expansive balcony with a view of the Chamundi Hills, and an even more spectacular interior with opulent halls (with ornately gilded columns, stained glass ceilings, and mosaic floors) and grand pavilions (with sculptures, paintings, and frescoes). At night when lit up with tens of thousands of lights on

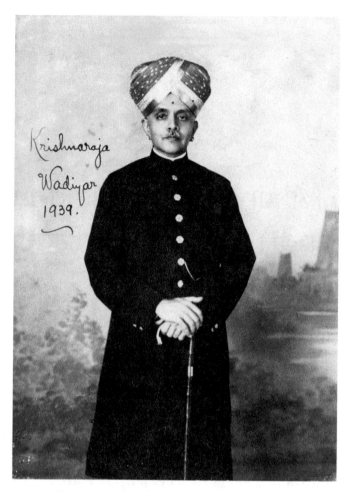

Figure 20.1. Shri Nalvadi Krishnaraja Wadiyar, 1939
(From the author's collection)

its roof edges and abutments, balconies, domes, and towers, the palace appears to glow from within and rise into the air. There, the maharajah governed, held gala events, and carried out his religious duties, most prominently celebrating the ten-night festival of Dasara, which revolved around him almost as a godhead. On the last day, seated atop an elephant, he led a procession out of the palace gates to the nearby hills, where thousands amassed to watch him in a ritual commemorating a mythic epic struggle of the triumph of good over evil. (Ordinarily he traveled in one of his twenty-four Rolls-Royces and Bentleys.)

In the summer, the maharajah led the life of a country gentleman in Fern Hill, Ooty, a hill station (a high-altitude town used to escape the summer heat) in the Nilgiri Hills in southern Mysore, where he stayed in a gabled manor house with sprawling lawns, elegant gardens, and nearby dense forests, overlooking lush valleys. He threw garden parties, took guests on fox hunts and big-game shoots, played tennis and squash, and arranged musical events in the evenings.

Music was his principal delight. He maintained a string quartet to play chamber music. (When he traveled to Europe in 1939 he brought along, in addition to 650 pieces of luggage, a retinue of more than fifty, including ten musicians, a troupe of dancers, and four eminent singers.)

The maharajah also maintained a palace in Bangalore, a city famous for its temperate climate and beautiful gardens. Even with its thirty-five rooms and grand ballroom, where the royal parties and dances were held, the 45,000-square-foot Bangalore Palace, located on 428 acres of land, was small and compact compared to the Mysore Palace.

Despite maintaining this conspicuously lavish style, the maharajah was rightfully beloved for his piety, tolerance (his prime minister was a Muslim, a friend since childhood), and progressivism. He made Mysore into a model state among the princely states of India. He governed through two constitutional assemblies, made primary education compulsory, made medical treatment widely available, founded a university, promoted industry (he erected the first hydroelectric power plant in India), delivered stirring civic speeches at local events, patronized the arts, and financed all state programs with fair taxation.

Kolar Venkatesh Iyer was born in the small village of Devarayasamudram in the Kolar District of Karnataka in 1898. After the death of his mother when he was eight years old, he moved with his father to Bangalore, where his father opened a canteen in Chickpet, one of the city's oldest shopping areas. The eatery served local food (vegetarian fare, such as *idli, dosa, poori, vada,* and varieties of rice) and drink (tea, coffee, and milk) at small tables. While helping out at the canteen after school, young K. V. Iyer learned how to run a business and cook for groups of people.

Emulating the renowned showman bodybuilder Eugen Sandow, "whose non-pereil [*sic*] physique [which Iyer saw only in pictures] is an eternal source of inspiration," Iyer began developing his musculature as a form of body modification (not as a means of improving sports performance) in mid-December 1920.[4] In 1922, at the age of twenty-four, he founded the Hercules Gymnasium. Dedicated to muscle cult and having a flair for self-promotion, he became a world-famous bodybuilder by the early 1930s. In 1933 the maharajah of Mysore asked Professor Iyer (the title "Professor" had been conferred on him to convey the esteem in which he was held) to give him lessons in physical culture. The maharajah was a great admirer of Iyer's physique, which he knew was achieved with a perseverance that he himself would never have. "To build a well-balanced and unique body like yours," he said to Iyer, "is an art, a sacred accomplishment."[5]

Branch Institute in the Jagan Mohan Palace

In 1935 the maharajah, already a grateful student of Iyer's, also became Iyer's patron by inviting him to open the Branch Institute, an offshoot of the Hercules Gymnasium, at Mysore in the Jagan Mohan Palace. Directed by of one of Iyer's pupils, the congenial H. Anantha Rao, the Branch Institute consisted of a large hall, well stocked with equipment, and surrounding rooms. On the walls of the hall, between huge mirrors, were photographs of Greek statues and world-famous bodybuilders, thus, at a glance, connecting modern physical culture to ancient physical culture. (As art historian Tamar Garb observes, photographs were a highly suitable means of establishing the link between modern and ancient because "reproductions of ancient sculptures and modern men could be happily juxtaposed in the two-dimensional world of the photographic print, thereby setting up analogies and invoking comparisons between ancient and modern that were perfectly sustainable in the photographic medium."[6])

The gymnasium was down the palace corridor from the *yogashala* where Tirumalai Krishnamacharya taught. Iyer and Krishnamacharya would "meet every so often socially."[7] As was the custom, they probably had lunch or coffee (the preferred beverage of Brahmins in South India) and snacks at each other's homes or the home of a mutual friend in the company of other men. There's no evidence of their having influenced each other's exercise practices.

Yoga scholar Mark Singleton writes that T. R. S. Sharma, one of Krishnamacharya's students, "relates that while it was fashionable among Mysore youth to attend K. V. Iyer's gymnasium . . . Krishnamacharya's yogashala was considered distinctly démodé."[8] Singleton posits three reasons for Iyer's gymnasium being in vogue and Krishnamacharya's *yogashala* being out of fashion: (1) the absence of celebrities to make yoga trendy, (2) the low opinion in which yoga was held, and (3) the association of yoga with renunciation.

Singleton first posits that "yoga lacked the celebrity luster [necessary for generating popularity] that it enjoys in the West today."[9] But in India in 1935 yoga had been a fad for at least the previous ten years. Yoga didn't need movie stars and supermodels to spark a yoga craze. Although, as it happens, the Princely State of Mysore (perhaps alone among all the territories of India) did have a charismatic celebrity who helped popularize yoga: K. V. Iyer. Iyer's system, at its very inception in 1922, consisted of both yoga and bodybuilding (*surya namaskar* was added later on). His mission in life was to make both disciplines part of everyone's daily exercise routine. Toward that end, he promoted yoga by, among other means, "Physical Culture tours through the Mysore Province" during the 1920s, which included lectures on and demonstrations of *asanas* by S. Sundaram, author of the first modern hatha yoga manual.[10]

In support of his argument that yoga "was subject to ridicule and scorn," Singleton then presents as representative the view, expressed by a friend of Sharma's who was a student at Iyer's Mysore gymnasium, that the gymnasium was more popular than the yoga school because yoga was distained for being (in Singleton's words) "for weaklings, a feminizing force in contrast to Iyer's manly muscle building."[11] This dichotomous view of yoga and bodybuilding certainly wasn't held by Iyer. The combination of yoga cult and muscle cult is exactly what he believed made his system unique and valuable.

At the Mysore gymnasium, yogasana (the practice of yogic postures solely as exercise) was practiced with *surya namaskar* as part of a flexible class curriculum or an independent workout to complement the weight resistance exercises. The two yogic disciplines were informally combined (not synthesized, as in *vinyasa,* into a system of static postures linked by flowing movement). According to Rao: "One may perform the asanas, such as Janu Sirsasana [Head-to-Knee Pose] and Bhujangasana [Cobra Pose], between cycles of Surya Namaskar. Asanas such as Halasana [Plow Pose], Salabhasana [Locust Pose] and Paschimottanasana [Seated Forward Bend] can also be used as part of the physical exercise routine. These are beneficial as they condition the torso. Sarvangasana [Shoulder Stand] is also beneficial. Performance of these asanas increases body suppleness. But development of muscles or body strength does not increase."[12]

Perhaps the youths of Mysore preferred the mixture of yogasana, *surya namaskar,* and bodybuilding at Iyer's gymnasium to the *asana* at Krishnamacharya's *yogashala* because they felt Iyer's all-round exercise program provided superior fitness and/or produced not so much a manly (strong and pumped up) physique but a more pleasingly eye-catching (lithe and toned) physique. Or perhaps they were put off by the particular *asanas* that Krishnamacharya taught. Rao certainly was. In a 1994 essay in tribute to Iyer, he writes that Krishnamacharya was "teaching circus tricks and calling it yoga."[13] In an apparent swipe at Krishnamacharya's teachings, Rao dismisses yogasana that includes poses that violently twist the body out of its natural shape: "Asanas like Garbha Pindasana [Embryo in the Womb Pose, in which one, while seated in *Padmasana,* pulls the legs up and holds the ears], Kukkutasana [Cock Pose, in which one, while seated in *Padmasana,* balances on the hands), or Kurmasana [Tortoise Pose, in which one, while seated with legs crossed at the ankles, bends the head to the floor and brings the arms behind the back] can be performed by a special

few but not by ordinary people. They resemble contortion stunts performed in the circus."[14]

Perhaps the youths found that the *asanas* in Iyer's routine, in contrast to the contortion-like *asanas* taught down the corridor, were challenging but achievable, and therefore aided their flexibility. Or perhaps they simply didn't want to put up with Krishnamacharya's nastiness and volatility.

In further accounting for Iyer's gymnasium being in vogue and Krishnamacharya's *yogashala* being out of fashion, Singleton endorses the belief of sociocultural anthropologist Joseph S. Alter that "yoga's association with asceticism and world renunciation as well as its primary concern with restraint can easily be interpreted as effete and the very antithesis of muscular masculinity."[15] Singleton concedes that yoga's traditional asceticism could also be considered an attraction when he reports that "Sharma qualifies his statements [about yoga's unpopularity in 1930s Mysore] by noting that the brahmical and vedic associations of yoga were in fact a draw to the more tradition-minded youth."[16] But Krishnamacharya's *yogashala* wasn't a retreat for yoga ascetics. His teachings there didn't place his young students' *asana* practice within the context of "brahmical and vedic associations" (although he did hold study sessions for the students on yoga philosophy). Iyer's teachings at his gymnasium in Bangalore, in contrast, contained a ritualized devotional element; once a week he conducted *puja* (formal worship) for members, during which they gave thanks to and invited the blessings of the deity Hanuman for their strength training at the gymnasium.

Another element that reinforced the sense

of Iyer's gymnasium as a sacred place was his relationship with his students. "There existed an intimate rapport between the master and the disciples as one may see in great institutions like Tagore's Shantiniketan," says former student Madhava Rao. This relationship "of mutual love and respect" made the gymnasium a place of "sanctity."[17]

There was yet another way in which Iyer made his Bangalore gymnasium a holy space: his very approach to exercising.

Inspired by his loutish, erudite, bighearted mentor, T. P. Kailasam, the great Kannada dramatist, Iyer was the ringleader for getting his gang of friends involved in various cultural activities. "Prof. Iyer used to go to a great variety of movies and plays in Bangalore," his old friend Shivarama Karanth remembers. "Many times he would drag us with him. And pay for all of us too!"[18] He enticed his pals to come to his home to listen to music after midnight. "Iyer had an excellent short-wave radio set," his lifelong friend V. Sitaramiah recalls. "So we would go his place to listen to BBC programs (lectures and concert programs by such luminaries as Thomas Beecham, Arturo Toscanini, Felix von Weingartner, Fritz Busch and Bruno Walter), which would start at 12:30 a.m."[19] Founder of a theater troupe, Ravi Artists, Iyer mounted plays on weekend evenings on a stage (fronted by a curtain of bright red fabric emblazoned with a golden abstracted image of the rising sun) in the large open hall of the gymnasium. Over 150 different plays, many written by the most prominent Kannada playwrights of the era, were performed. Under government sponsorship, the troupe also traveled to present plays

in cities and villages, primarily in the State of Mysore but also around the rest of the country. The biggest crowd pleaser, H. K. Ranganath's patriotic *Jaagruth Bharathi* (Awakened Mother India), was enacted about 120 times.

Iyer also enjoyed solitary cultural activities at home. He set himself a quota for reading each day in his small private room, where he lounged on a bed. He listened to his collection of records (numbering somewhere from two hundred to three hundred), about half Western music and the other half Carnatic (South Indian style) and Hindustani (North Indian style) classical music. He translated plays, including Ibsen's *A Doll's House, The Master Builder,* and *An Enemy of the People,* into Kannada. And he wrote short stories, a memoir of his adventures with Kailasam (which reads more like a bildungsroman), and three novels (two of them, *Shantala* and *Roopadarshi,* are acclaimed as masterworks)— all in his native Kannada. He read from his short stories and novels to his family (changing his voice to suit his fictional characters).

Yet Iyer was considered a renunciate. His beloved daughter-in-law, Vasantha Karna, says: "Though he did not wear the dress [a saffron robe] suitable to a sanyasi, he lived the life of one."[20] After his only son was born, he asked and received his wife's consent to be celibate. A Vedantist, he performed daily worship. But what made people see him as a renunciate wasn't his celibacy or piousness but his self-regulation. His old friend Ranganath, drama director at All India Radio, comments, "Moving from one task to another was itself a type of relaxation for him."[21] H. Anantha Rao remarks on Iyer's capacity for concentration (he never "worked haphazardly"), self-restraint (he placed "limits on his utterances"), and self-discipline (he exerted "control of the senses").[22] His fellow bodybuilding enthusiast, director of his own gymnasium, and longtime friend K. G. Nadagir recalls that Iyer led "a simple and pure, disciplined and structured life, without any ostentation. This is the spiritual achievement of a dedicated soul."[23]

Iyer's daily activities commenced at 5:00 a.m. He did his ablutions, prayer, and exercise. Then he taught classes at 6:00 and 7:00 a.m. During these sessions he demonstrated and explained exercises at the head of the gymnasium while students followed along. While marking the repetition count for the entire class, he'd go to students to correct their form and then return to his place for the next exercise. He encouraged regulars to complete the full count and told new students to stop early on.

At 8:00 a.m. Iyer ate breakfast and drank half a cup of coffee. Thereafter, he helped members who were exercising on their own, or he treated patients at his clinic. He prepared lunch for whoever was present and sat down to eat with them at 1:00 p.m. He was a strict vegetarian. Lunch usually consisted of *chapathi* (flat bread) or *ragi mudde* (millet balls), red rice (called red after the color of the bran that's preserved in the processing), *sambar* (vegetable stew made with a pigeon pea broth), *rasam* (a kind of spicy thin soup), and spiced, cooked vegetables. "Look at the elephant or the rhinoceros," he said. "They are such strong animals. They are also vegetarians."[24]

In the afternoons Iyer wrote to his correspondence students and set aside time for his reading, writing, and music listening. In later years he taught the evening class while senior students taught the morning classes. He ate a light dinner.

Iyer didn't spend lavishly. He owned three sets of underwear, three pajamas (silk or cotton loose trousers tied at the waist), three *jubbas* (silk or cotton loose shirts that are knee or midthigh length), and two *dhotis* (white cotton garments that are wrapped around the waist and legs and tied at the waist), which were commonly purchased on festival days, cleaned regularly, and replaced yearly or when worn.

Iyer's self-regulation was embodied most of all in his exercise. Take, for example, his manner of executing a biceps curl, as shown in his instructions in *Physique and Figure,* his strength-training manual: "Notice particularly the calm expression of the face, not a twitch or wrinkle, and no hard-set jaw. The biceps muscle is brought into a highly tensed condition. The abdomen is drawn in and held there and all the muscles of the leg[s] are in a state of semi-rigidity. The body is straight"[25] (see figs. 20.2 and 20.3 on page 256).

This seemingly ordinary instruction is actually quite exceptional: it emphasizes concentrating on the muscle most involved (powerfully flexing the biceps), while keeping a sense of the entire body (contracting core muscles of the trunk and securing distant stabilizing muscles in the lower extremities); making subtle, precise movements; holding the body in alignment; and maintaining a placid expression.

Iyer's instructions for yogic postures have a similar emphasis on concentration on the part of the body most involved in the movement; extension of concentration to the whole body; precision of movement; alignment; and calm. Consider his instructions for *Bhujangasana,*

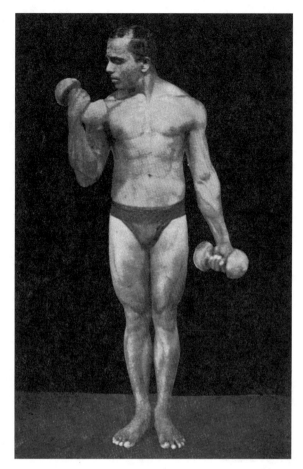

Figure 20.2. K. V. Iyer demonstrating the biceps curl
(front view), 1940

(From *Physique and Figure*, by K. V. Iyer)

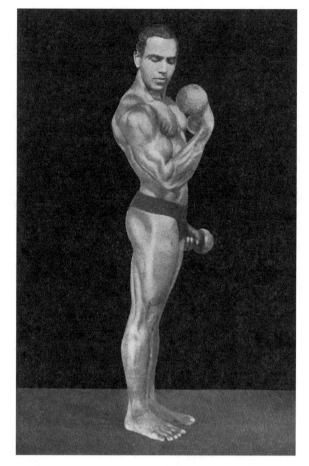

Figure 20.3. K. V. Iyer demonstrating the biceps curl
(side view), 1940

(From *Physique and Figure*)

Cobra Pose, in *Physical Training through Correspondence:*

Lie on the stomach, legs together and toes pointed. Place the palms immediately beneath the shoulder and [lift the trunk as is shown in the illustration] and maintain that position as long as you can, breathing normally all the time.

Take care not to lift the hips off the ground, or to throw the weight of your body on the supporting arms. This posture is maintained by the powerful contractions of the muscles of the back; especially the "Erector-spinae" muscles. The arms only serve to maintain the balance. The head must be thrown as far back as possible.[26]

As Iyer correctly demonstrates, the trunk is pushed up while the pelvis is pushed down (and the arms end up in front of the body). This movement in opposite directions is what creates tension in the lower back and stretches the front of the torso (figs. 20.4 and 20.5).

Iyer also valued "the graceful movement of the limbs while exercising. Not that you should

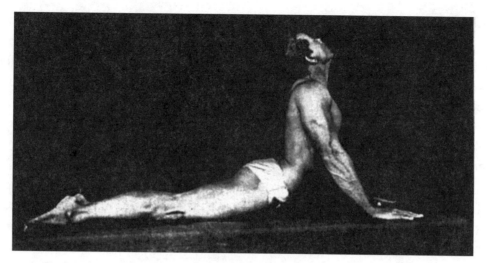

Figure 20.4. K. V. Iyer demonstrating *Bhujangasana,* a photo study for the illustration in *Physical Training through Correspondence,* circa 1940

(With the kind permission of Shashidhar Tokanahalli Nagabhushan Rao)

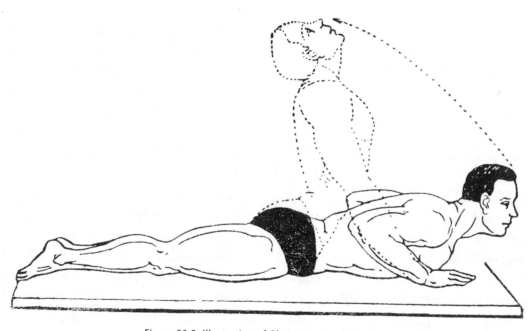

Figure 20.5. Illustration of *Bhujangasana,* Cobra Pose

(From *Physical Training through Correspondence*)

swing and sway to music," he noted, "but while you are using your limbs for exercises let them be used as gracefully as possible. There should be nothing ugly or contortioned either in your movements or in the facial expression."[27] (In banning all grimacing, grunting, lurching, thrusting, and flinging during exercise—and, in all likelihood, preening or swaggering about afterward—Iyer's system is the antithesis of muscular masculinity.)

Perhaps his insistence on intense effort, precise movement, holistic coordination, placidity, and gracefulness in exercise explains why Iyer places self-regulation at the heart of his version of the creation narrative of hatha yoga:

The "Yogic" school of Body-culture is older than 500 B.C. and is based upon the principles of "Hata-Yoga." It was originated and codified by the great Rishis and Yogis of India. . . . This school . . . was meant for the man who was in hot quest of self-realisation—one who wanted to *regulate* his Ahara (Food), Nidra (Sleep), Bhaya (Fear), and Maithuna (Lust); one who was devoted to religious *austerity* and did not like to suffer bodily ills during his Sadhana; one who had *minimized his wants,* and was deeply practicing Yama (*Control*) and Niyama (*Regulation*). . . . This need of the Sadhaka was parent to the Yogic school [italics added].[28]

What Iyer seems to mean by "self-realization" is spiritual liberation—opening oneself up to transcendent Being—through self-regulation, especially in the sense of the second limb of Patanjali's eight-limbed yoga, *niyama* (internal discipline, self-restraint, or observance), which comprises (1) *shauca* (purification), (2) *samtosha* (contentment), (3) *tapas* (austerity), (4) *svadhyaya* (study of self), and (5) *ishvarapranidhana* (surrender to God).

Divine Bodybuilding

"As a system of physical exercise, wrestling is integrated into the philosophy of yoga through the application of two principles: *yam* and *niyam*," writes Alter in his book about wrestling in India. "As Atreya [the guru of a North Indian wrestling gymnasium] explained in an interview, yam and niyam are the root principles of moral, intellectual, and emotional fitness." Not that wrestlers spend much time thinking about the centrality of *yama* and *niyama* to their lives. "For them the intuitive application of these principles to their lives is the primary order of business," Alter continues, using mostly the principles of *niyama* as examples. "To be passive and even-tempered is in accordance with a lifestyle of . . . santosh; to go to a Hanuman temple every Saturday is to be close to god. Exercise is a form of tap, and going to the akhara every morning is an act of internal and external purification. All of this is not to say that wrestlers are yogis in any strict sense of the term. They are not concerned with the metaphysics of their way of life or with spirituality as an esoteric endeavor."[29]

The same can be said for Iyer. Although he wasn't a yogin in the strict sense of the term and didn't consider pumping iron (or even doing yoga exercises) as a yogic spiritual endeavor, his approach to strength training was grounded in—or perhaps more accurately put, conducive to—yoga, and specifically its principles of *niyama*. Using his teachings as a starting point, these principles may be applied to his course of dumbbell and barbell exercises.

Shauca (Purification)

Unique to any bodybuilding/strength-training system, Iyer's regime included *Nauli* and *Uddiyana,* which he considered to be internal purification practices, performed in conjunction with a water enema, that "stir up the 'Lazy

Colon' to activity" by massaging the intestines, and thereby facilitating complete evacuation of the bowels.[30] *Uddiyana* is sharply drawing the diaphragm and abdominal muscles upward and backward. *Nauli* is jutting out the rectus abdominis in the center, where it can easily be rolled from side to side.

But each strengthening exercise in Iyer's system could be considered as a purificatory technique applied to rid the mind of its psychomental muck. In order to be fully absorbed in an exercise, he counseled, one has to expel distractions: "Do not hurry through the exercises because of an urgent call of business or a visit to be paid. The hour of exercise must be kept free from [thoughts about] all other engagements." One must also eliminate all wasteful thoughts of the ego, such as concern about attaining good looks or arrogance over superior bulk. "Beware of developing Narcissism," Iyer bluntly warned his students.[31]

Samtosha (Contentment)

No matter "however difficult the movement may be, or however strongly you may be flexing the muscles, ..." Iyer cautioned, "the face should be normal and calm while exercising. It is better if the face assumes a soft smile instead of being cold or hard."[32] Accepting the discomfort and pain of arduous exercise without complaint—as manifested by a calm expression—is a way of accepting where one's life has taken one, without having regret over the past or fantasies of great change in the future. It's a way of accepting oneself.

Tapas (Austerity)

To act with *tapas* means to be ardent or full of effort (the word is from the root "to heat" or

"to make hot"). Iyer advocated maximal effort: "Physical culture calls for a large amount of concentration, perseverance, physical effort [and] assiduous practice."[33] Instilled with a burning desire to produce maximum performance, one overcomes inertia, lethargy, and despair.

Tapas is also austerity. Like fasting or a taking a vow of silence, going to the gymnasium each day to practice strength training is an act of austerity. Performing exercises with precision and total concentration, a manner that Iyer emphasized, deepens the asceticism: absolute control of the body and mind shuts out the everyday world.

Svadhyaya (Study of Self)

Iyer's son and daughter-in-law, K. V. and Vasantha Karna, note about Iyer: "He told his students that muscular power by itself was useless. To build character and discipline is also important."[34] Iyer understood that character could be built through having the proper attitude about exercise. The way one exercises reflects one's mode of being in the world—one's attitudes toward self and others and even the divine. Through devotion to practice and with the help of a teacher, one can become aware of these dimensions of one's own being and make changes accordingly. In advising "Even the easiest exercise should be performed with all possible care, concentration and correctness," Iyer was guiding students toward changing their mode of being in the world.[35]

Ishvarapranidhana (Closeness to God)

Iyer believed that "each careful repetition takes you nearer to the perfectness of that exercise."[36] He even went so far as to say, "An exercise can be called an exercise, only when done with great care and precision."[37] Performing exercises with care and precision is a prerequisite for perceiving them as a gift from God. As historian of religion and philosopher of yoga Karl Baier writes in "Iyengar and the Yoga Tradition," the second of his groundbreaking examinations of the philosophical dimensions of *asana,* about the application of *niyama* to *asanas,* "Gratitude [for this gift] is realized through complete involvement in the pose, doing it with the utmost attention and precision."[38] Thus, exercise, properly done, becomes worship—an act of surrender to God—through which one becomes close to God. And thus a large space equipped with dumbbells and barbells is transformed into a sacred place.

"The constituent elements of self-restraint (*niyama*) are concerned with the inner life of *yogins,*" explains scholar and popularizer of yoga history and philosophy Georg Feuerstein. "If the five rules of *yama* harmonize their relationship with other beings, the five rules of *niyama* harmonize their relationship to life at large and to the transcendental Reality."[39]

In 1937 the maharajah of Mysore, Nalvadi Krishnaraja Wadiyar, had a mild paralytic stroke while vacationing at the Bangalore Palace. Iyer was called upon to care for His Majesty in the southwest wing of the Tudor-style palace. (By the mid-1930s Iyer's renown in Bangalore as a physiotherapist had come to nearly rival that of his identity as a bodybuilder.) For his "home" visits, Iyer, wearing pants, a long coat, shoes, and a lace turban, was picked up at his gymnasium (then at its Thulaja Bhavan location) in a car belonging to the royal family. Iyer treated the maharajah with a circular abdominal massage that he'd developed. Thereafter, the maharajah would summon Iyer for treatment not only in Bangalore but also in Mysore and Ooty.

Iyer never asked for payment for his services, even in 1940 when he was desperately in need of money. He was building the house/gymnasium of his dreams (an elegant modernist building, called Vyayama Shala, with balanced horizontal and vertical lines, that he designed) on Jayachamarajendra Road in Shankarapuram, a residential area, but lacked the finances to complete it. Construction had stopped halfway. Iyer, who had a great deal of self-respecting pride, rarely spoke to anybody about his lack of funds. Yet somehow knowledge of his financial difficulties reached the maharajah. One day at the end of the massage treatment, the maharajah presented Iyer with an envelope, saying, "This is my *guru dakshina* ["offering to a teacher," given out of gratitude]. Please do not decline it." "The envelope was light," notes Iyer's friend M. H. Krishniah, "but the money inside was quite substantial. The half-finished building was soon completed"[40] (fig. 20.6). (Actually, the gymnasium wasn't completed for another two years.)

In the spring of 1940 Iyer held a large-group demonstration for the maharajah of Mysore. H. Anantha Rao describes the event:

A suggestion was received [from the maharajah] that we should give an exhibition [of the gym activities] in the Courtyard of the Jagan Mohan Palace. We were greatly excited and enthusiastic. Many students came from the Bangalore Gym. We brought all the light-

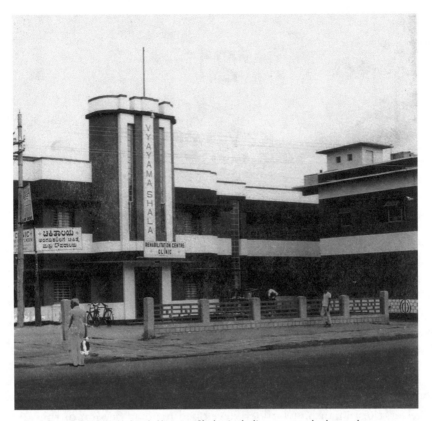

Figure 20.6. K. V. Iyer's Vyayam Shala, including an attached guesthouse, on the right, circa 1950s

(With the kind permission of Ronne Iyer)

ing, curtains etc. needed for the presentation from Bangalore. Prof. Iyer had given many shows by then; so he himself had kept all the required show paraphernalia. He did not have to wait on other suppliers.

On the day of the show, the Maharaja was seated 10 minutes prior to the start. It seems he never used to come so early to any function. . . . Group Surya Namaskaras, with about sixty students participating, and controlled demonstration of muscle flexion were the main items. The Maharaja was quite demonstrative of his appreciation at the end of each item. It looked as though the exhibition made a great impression on him. . . . It was a golden age for us.[41]

This flourishing period in Mysore soon ended with the death of the maharajah on August 3, 1940.

21

K. V. IYER

Presenting *Surya Namaskar* as Stretching Exercise

Surya Namaskar as Flexibility Exercise

After studying Bhavanarao Pant Pratinidhi's manual *Surya Namaskars*, K. V. Iyer, the Indian bodybuilder, developed his own version of the sun salutations, which he presented in *Surya Namaskar,* a booklet published in 1937.* While agreeing with Bhavanarao that *surya namaskar* benefits the digestive, eliminatory, skeletal, nervous, muscular, respiratory, and cardiovascular systems, Iyer had a different understanding of how this occurred. A friend's conversation with Iyer in the 1930s sheds light on the difference.

> I told Iyer that I recently had to go to Athani. I have some friends there who are philosophy professors. An exercise program was going on. A young boy announced, "It is now three hundred." I asked, "What is three hundred?" He said, "Three-hundred surya namaskaras, sir." Imagine a young boy completing 300 surya namaskaras! Me, if I were to do six, I would start hyperventilating, forget about trying 300. I asked Iyer, "Why is this?"

---

*Iyer's *Surya Namaskar* appears to be the first printed work about *surya namaskar* to have been published after Bhavanarao's. The first edition of *Surya Namaskar* in chart form was published in 1934 and a second in 1936. The first edition in booklet form was published in 1937, a second in 1942, a third in 1945, and a fourth in 1949. It's not known how many copies of the chart and booklet were printed and sold or where sales took place, although we can safely assume that the widest distribution and readership was in the Bangalore/Mysore area.

Iyer said, "Endurance for this exercise depends on how one breathes in and breathes out. When one properly bends and stretches the body, the chest is allowed to expand and contract properly. When we are doing all this, we do not know whether the Sun God is pleased, whether we will receive *moksha* [salvation] in our afterlife, but we know for certain that it is beneficial in this life to do the surya namaskara correctly." He told all this to me in a delicate manner so as not to offend me, and then he demonstrated the exercise for me.[1]

Much is revealed about Iyer in this pedestrian story: his attunement to the subtleties of the body, acceptance of his fate, warm sense of humor, eloquence, civility, and dedication to serving others through providing practical, concrete help. What we might not notice is his simple description of how *surya namaskar* works: "one properly bends and stretches the body."

Iyer believed that the stretching involved in *surya namaskar* had a particular role for the skeletal and nervous systems: "The vigorous stretching of the spine, forwards and backwards . . . is of high chiropractic value in maintaining the vigour of the Nervous System."[2] Bhavanarao, in contrast, conceived of *surya namaskar* as a series of strengthening exercises. His description of the benefits of his fifth position, what in yoga would be a modification of *Urdhva Mukha Svanasana*, Upward-Facing Dog (the arms are straight and below the shoulders and the pelvis is off the floor, but as in *Bhujangasana*, Cobra Pose, the thighs and knees are on the floor), shows no understanding of the role that stretching plays. "In this posture the weight of almost the whole body is borne by the arms, hence all their parts, particularly the triceps muscles are fully developed, rendering the arms shapely, strong and supple. The chest also receives the benefit; it becomes wider and deeper. Owing to deep breathing the fat about the abdominal regions is gradually reduced. The girth of the chest increases, whilst that of the abdomen decreases. . . . In this position also most of the muscles of the thighs, back, neck, and throat get strong."[3]

Bhavanarao mistakenly identified the position as a body-shaping/strength-developing exercise, while in fact the pectoral muscles become more expansive from opening up, abdominal fat cannot be targeted by exercise (there's no such thing as spot reduction), and the other bodily segments receive no or only minor strengthening. Once again Bhavanarao was extolling the virtues of a broad-barreled chest and small waist, as well as well-formed arms, which remain his touchstone for the perfect figure.

Iyer exactly understood the primary value of the *surya namaskar* position that resembles *Urdhva Mukha Svanasana*: it stretches the anterior spinal muscles. In this, it complements the position that resembles *Uttanasana*, Standing Forward Bend, which stretches the posterior spinal muscles. In his description of his seventh position, the "Yoga-Asana usually known as *Bhujangasana* (the Cobra pose),"[4] which is actually *Urdhva Mukha Svanasana*, he explained that "the Spine is stretched out just in the opposite direction to that of [what] is usually classed among Yoga-Asanas as *Janu-Sirasan* [what is now commonly named *Uttanasana*]. These two postures stretch out the Spine both

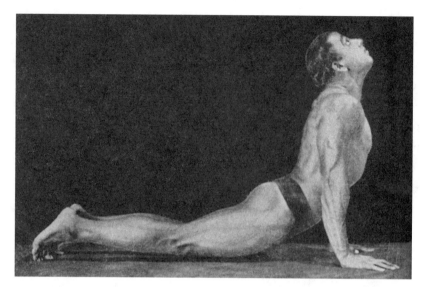

Figure 21.1. K. V. Iyer demonstrating the seventh *surya namaskar* position,
Urdhva Mukha Svanasana, Upward-Facing Dog, 1937

(From *Surya Namaskar,* by K. V. Iyer)

forward and backwards to the limit, drawing apart the Inter-Vertebral spaces and thereby correcting not only the carriage of the body but also the Spinal congestion, if present, *viz.,* the impingement of the Spinal and Sympathetic nerves caused by the close setting of the vertebral bones due either to gradual Ossification or Subluxation"[5] (figs. 21.1 and 21.2).

Perhaps it took a bodybuilder, someone who truly understood how muscles develop, to recognize that performing the positions of *surya namaskar* isn't an efficient means of muscular development. And perhaps it took not just any bodybuilder but one who studied, practiced, taught, and promoted yogasana to recognize that each discrete *asana*-like posture of *surya namaskar* is primarily a means of stretching muscles and other connective tissues: "In my long experience of the Physical Culture life, as student and teacher, I have seen, learnt and taught scores of these spine-stretching exercises.

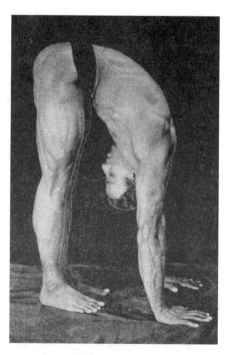

Figure 21.2. K. V. Iyer demonstrating the
tenth (the same as the third)
surya namaskar position, *Uttanasana,*
Standing Forward Bend, 1937

(From *Surya Namaskar*)

After I studied and practiced the 'yogic system of physical culture' I saw that most of these spinal exercises which I knew and taught were at best a poor imitation of the 'yoga-asanas,' intended for the same purpose."[6]

Modification of *Surya Namaskar*

Iyer made modifications to Bhavanarao's *surya namaskar* technique. He incorporated the *Jalandhara Bandha,* the chin lock (the chin pressed against the chest), to his second, third, fourth, fifth, eighth, and ninth positions. He believed that the chin lock powerfully benefits the endocrine system, especially the thyroid glands, "the King of all Glands in the Human system, as they are usually called; they play an important part in the preservation of Youth, Vitality and Vigour in man."* In Iyer's view, the chin lock rejuvenates the thyroid glands through mechanical means: applying the chin lock puts pressure on the thyroids, forcing them to "yield their extract into the blood stream," while releasing the chin lock increases blood flow to the thyroids.[7] This alternate locking and unlocking, he argued, acts to stimulate and revitalize the glands, thereby detoxifying the system.

One great and very important feature of this Thyroid extract is that it has the power of neutralizing certain toxins formed in the sys-tem. Ancient Savants who founded the Yoga methods stated that the Thyroid Glands (*Granthis* situated in the *Visueddhi-Chakra*) can destroy poisonous matter too, which might accidentally get into the system.

The mythological lore says that when Siva (one of the three principal deities of the Hindus) drank the *Kalakoota,* the deadliest of poisons, it was neutralized before it passed down His throat, and that spot where the Thyroids were situated became black. And Siva is therefore known as *Neela-Kantah* [*sic*].[8]

In positing that the mighty thyroid destroys poisons and in recounting the story of Shiva gulping down the great poison that had emerged from the ocean, threatening to destroy the world (the poison is so potent that it turns his throat blue, not black; thus the name Neela-Kantha, blue throat), Iyer has quaintly mixed the (seeming) rationality of pseudoscience with the allure of myth, each validating the other.

The incorporation of the chin lock doesn't seem to have been picked up by many subsequent practitioners of *surya namaskar* (Harvey Day, the mid-20th-century British author of middlebrow and chatty yet erudite and informative yoga books, is a prominent exception). Today its use is discredited. Even if it were of value, it makes performing *surya namaskar* awkward and unsafe because it strains the neck.

---

*The fourth book solely on *surya namaskar*—after Bhavanarao's *Surya Namaskars* (1928), Iyer's *Surya Namaskar* (1937), and Bhavanarao's *Ten-Point Way to Health* (1938)—was *The Secret of Perfect Health: Surya Namaskar* by M. R. Raja Rao, published in 1960. Rao also emphasized the chin lock. This "important detail" is maintained in three of his *surya namaskar* positions. "The followers of Yoga call it *Jalandhara Bandha*. Its effect is to stimulate the thyroid glands situated on the neck" (*Secret of Perfect Health,* 17). Rao had begun studying and practicing *surya namaskar* in 1930. It's not known if his fellow Bangalorean, Iyer, influenced him, or he influenced Iyer.

Healing Power of the Sun

A critical element of the Indian physical culture movement was the assertion by its proponents of not only its superiority to Western physical culture but its antecedence. "In the Vedas and in the various books on Astronomy and Astrology written thousands of years back," Iyer crowed, "great hymns of praise are found in honour of the Sun-God and on the therapeutic effect of His rays upon the human body."[9] "The curative value of Sunlight was known to the early Western world too," he conceded. But the Greeks "learnt of this cult" in India and "carried it back with them to Greece."[10]

It's unlikely that Iyer had any authoritative historical evidence to support his claim that the Greeks learned heliotherapy from the Indians. Almost certainly his assertion that the practice of bathing in sunlight to obtain health originated in India was made out of a feeling of being overshadowed by Western physical culture. (In this he was no different than other Indian physical culturists making similar health claims. Included among their ranks were the modern hatha yoga pioneers, who sought legitimacy for yoga from Western physical culturists, while arguing not only that yoga was the most complete system of physical culture but, having been created by the *rishis,* or ancient sages, was the first exercise system to perfect the human body.)

Late 19th- and early 20th-century Western advocates of the sun cure, in contrast, had no interest in squabbling over the origins of heliotherapy. "They spoke of the ancient heritage [of heliotherapy] for their newly resuscitated practice," says Daniel Freund, a scholar of the 20th-century social history of sunlight. "But these modern supporters never really traced the lines of transmission, as they were far more interested in proving that there was something timeless about sun worship than in proving who taught what to whom. In fact, they usually argued that the fact that sun worship emerged in diverse cultures, was then forgotten, only to be discovered entirely anew was evidence that it's only natural to worship the sun."[11]

Although the therapeutic effect of sunlight may have been known to Indians in ancient times, sunlight—or, rather, the burning concern with the curative value of sunlight—was rediscovered in the late 19th and early 20th centuries in the West. The valorization of sunshine in its varied forms—summer camps and vacations at the beach; sunbathing and nudism; the coveted bronzed look of a glowing tan (previously a sign of lower-class outdoor drudgery); the discovery of the importance of vitamin D, which is manufactured by the skin's exposure to sunlight; sun therapy as an alternative to medicine at tuberculosis sanitariums; ultraviolet carbon arc therapy for the treatment of various common diseases; and the social reform movement to get children out of dark tenements—was a uniquely modern Western creation. The hyping (no matter how sincere) of *surya namaskar* as heliotherapy is yet another instance of the influence of Western physical culture on India. Spurred on by developments in the West, Iyer and other Indian physical culturists rediscovered their sun worship tradition.

Surya namaskar, its proponents claimed, was ancient, yet up to date—the invention of the *rishis,* yet a preventive and cure similar to (but more beneficial than) newly created medical treatments and, by analogy, having the same proven (or so it appeared at the time) scientific efficacy. (These were the same claims that the modern hatha yoga pioneers made for yogasana.) Iyer suggested a protocol for the effective practice of *surya namaskar* as heliotherapy:

> Surya namaskars bestow upon their votaries full benefit if done when the morning Sun is bright and warm, and at an angle between 35 and 50 degrees in the east. In bad weather the namaskars may be performed in one's own room. The evening rays of the Sun are not so effective as those of the morning; for then, the atmosphere will have been soused in dust and smoke, which prevent the ultraviolet rays from reaching our naked skin. While performing the namaskars one should wear only a thin loin-cloth or "langot," as any other cloth on the body—however thin—cuts off these effective actinic rays.[12]

In actuality, instead of using *surya namaskar* for its ability to capture sunlight, Iyer employed it as a warm-up exercise.

Starting no later than the early 1930s, Iyer performed and taught *surya namaskar* as a warm-up to bodybuilding/strength training in his gymnasiums. Although he touted its "rhythmic breathing which is necessary to balance the working of the lungs and heart"[13] when it "alone [is] persisted in,"[14] by using *surya namaskar* as a short warm-up activity to prepare for other exercises, Iyer broke with the common practice of performing *surya namaskar* for a sustained period as a stand-alone dynamic stretching/cardiorespiratory activity. (Despite elevating the heart rate, performing sets of *surya namaskar* as warm-up exercise—moving quickly from position to position for five to ten minutes—doesn't significantly increase cardiorespiratory capacity.) Typically, fifteen to twenty *surya namaskars* were performed at the beginning of his classes.

An article about *surya namaskar* as warm-up activity for weight lifters and bodybuilders appeared in a 1948 issue of *Vigour,* a British physical culture magazine, with "photos posed by K. V. Iyer, Principal, Hercules Gymnasium, Bangalore, India."[15] It's likely that Iyer wouldn't have given permission to use these photos, which are from his booklet, if he hadn't endorsed the views of the author, Mark Lewis. Lewis laid down a challenge to macho muscleheads:

> In a previous article, I mentioned that Surya Namaskars make a splendid warming-up and limbering movement to commence a programme. . . .
>
> All breathing is through the nose. This exercise gives the internals a vigorous massage and the spine a real stretch. The lifter and bodybuilder might well try a dozen or so of these exercises before picking up the weights; I'll be surprised if it doesn't leave even "tough guys" pleasantly "steamed up."[16]

When Iyer wanted to take advantage of the healing power of the sun's rays, he didn't go out in the morning sun in a loincloth; he did so by turning to a Western invention with the ability to replicate sunlight. "What was known and taken full advantage of in Ancient India long before the Christian Era, has been only recently discovered in the Modern Scientific way by

Dr Finsen of Copenhagen (Denmark), the first man of the West to try the curative effect of the Sun's Rays upon the human system," Iyer explained. "He chose the carbon arc for his experiment since he thought that continuity of light of the same intensity as the Sun was necessary, and the carbon arc was very near to the Sunlight in composition."[17]

The valorization of sunshine—or, at least, the touting of the benefits of its transmutation as artificial light from a carbon arc—was one of the critical influences on Iyer's physiotherapy practice, which took on increasing importance for him in the 1930s. Iyer's unconventional medical care—"It could be called 'improvised therapy,'" says his student H. Anantha Rao. "I do not think Prof. Iyer had any fixed treatment for any specific disease"—consisted of an intuitive grab bag of modalities, put together in response to patients' descriptions of their symptoms, that made use of ultraviolet ray, heat, and vibration equipment; massage; *asana, pranayama,* and *surya namaskar;* and dumbbell exercises.[18] Patients were treated with the special equipment and given massages in a therapy room, while the rest of the regimen took place in the main gym.

Salutation to the Sun God

Iyer's system of *surya namaskar* includes a position absent in Bhavanarao's system: the Standing Backbend as the second position (the first position is standing at attention facing the sun). (It's not known whether Iyer created the position or merely adapted it from others; it appears that he was the first to illustrate and write about it.) The Standing Backbend is performed by inhaling deeply as one raises both arms above the head while arching the back "as far back as possible without disturbing balance," keeping the buttocks and legs firmly in place.[19]

Iyer insightfully described the benefits of performing the Standing Backbend: "The backward stretching of the spine . . . overcomes the habitual curvatures, round shoulders and strengthens the neck. In short it tends to improve the bearing of the body. The spine should always be kept supple, lest ossification should occur; and [everyday] spinal movements alone do help to keep it supple. In the daily life there are chances for a person to bend forward and sideways, to the left and right, but there is little chance of bending backwards. Hence this movement is of very great value."[20]

Iyer was so keen on the Standing Backbend that he used it to epitomize *surya namaskar* on the cover of his booklet—not for its benefits to the spine, though. The cover illustration shows a bulked-up man in skimpy posing trunks bending backward, his arms flung overhead, on a mountain ledge that juts out over clouds. He's basking in the spooky geometric rays of the sun or, perhaps, expressing his gratitude to the Sun God for making him into a divine hero or merely into a tanned, massively muscular, virile figure.

The lofty setting, which may very well be the Alps, not the Himalayas, is infused with spirituality. Nature is exalted. We envy the man his immediate experience of intimacy with the immense sun-drenched sky, a manifestation of the divine in nature—while probably preferring our experience of looking at it via a picture rather than standing on a dangerous rock shelf. (As the philosopher Immanuel

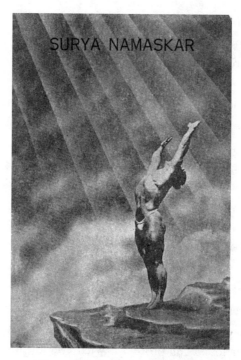

SURYA NAMASKAR

Figure 21.3. Cover, *Surya Namaskar*
(From *Surya Namaskar*)

Kant pointed out, awe and fear of nature are best contemplated at a safe distance.) The man might very well agree with us: the photo of him is superimposed on the scenery. He's in no danger of falling or even of being exposed to severe weather—the bitter cold, severe wind, and thin air or, for that matter, the sun's intense rays (fig. 21.3).

What a ridiculous image! How could Iyer have come up with (or approved) such a florid, sentimental, and superficial Westernized portrayal of Indian sun adoration? Actually, the cover art is his touching homage to someone whom he greatly admired: "The Glorious Physique Portrayed on the cover page is that of my good friend John C. Grimek."[21] Although they never met, Iyer and Grimek, the only bodybuilder to win two Mr. America titles (the

contest organizers changed the rules to prevent him from winning yet again) were longtime pen pals. Grimek described Iyer's letters as "always bright and cheery and they were filled with words of kindness and praise."[22]

And despite its expression of the European and American cult of health and beauty, evocation of the sublime in German romanticism, and displaced emphasis on Grimek, the cover conveys Iyer's genuine belief in the sacred nature of the series of positions that comprise *surya namaskar:* they embody spirituality. "Namaskar is a Sanskrit term for Salutation in respect and devotion, and Surya means the Sun; Surya Namaskar, therefore, simply means Salutation to the Sun-God, Who is the source of all *Light* and *Life* on this Globe."[23] But this short explanation was practically all Iyer wrote about *surya namaskar* as worship, and he never described any of the positions, including the Standing Backbend, as an expression of gratitude or supplication.

The assertion that the series of movements of *surya namaskar* (or, for that matter, of the ancient sun worship ceremony) is an act of respect and devotion to the Sun God isn't a given: in performing *surya namaskar,* we wouldn't know we were worshipping the sun deity unless somebody told us. Worshipping Surya during *surya namaskar* has nothing to do with our actual bodily experience of the movements. It's an ideological accretion. True enough, some of the gestures and positions of *surya namaskar* (e.g., placing the hands together, palm to palm; bowing low; lying prostrate) are traditionally (and inherently) expressive of reverence and submission, possibly even to a Sun God. But an authentic comprehension of the holiness of this series of movements, one that might open us up to Being, would begin with an exploration of our experience of all the positions, not just those associated with prayer: standing upright faced forward, oriented in a particular direction, magisterially surveying our environment; reaching up and back, putting ourselves at risk of losing our balance, falling, and getting injured; bending low, a folding up that averts the eyes; lying close to the ground, nearly prostrate, abject and humble; raising the hips and straightening the legs against the wearying pull of gravity; springing up, in a kind of forceful declaration of our presence; repeating the series of movements in which we end up where we started, thereby obliterating the restless quest for novelty and any sense of progress and history.

A Bhavanarao in a World of Sandows

The December 1937 *Superman,* the British bodybuilding magazine, has an article titled "The World's Oldest P. C. System Part One: 'Surya Namaskar,'" by R. S. Balsekar. (Part 2 is "Yoga-Asanas," "a fully illustrated article divulging further Physical Culture secrets of Ancient India.") Although the byline is Balsekar, most of the text is taken from Iyer's *Surya Namaskar.* (Evidently stealing the writings of others and having complicity in the theft of your own writings weren't unusual practices in those days, at least for Balsekar and Iyer, who were friends. In an April 1939 *Superman* interview with Iyer by Balsekar, most of Iyer's dialogue is actually cribbed expository text from Iyer's 1930 correspondence-course brochure *Muscle Cult—A Pro-em to My System.*) The last paragraph (although not from Iyer's book) concisely expresses Iyer's belief about the strengthening aspect of *surya namaskar:* "Surya Namaskar is perfect in its conception and correct in its application, intended more to ensure health and a moderate development of all the muscles rather than aiming at mere muscular development only. For better development, Surya Namaskars should be combined with other heavier forms of exercise."[24]

Like Bhavanarao, Iyer was a follower of Sandow. But whereas Bhavanarao, disillusioned with the results of Sandow's system, stopped practicing it and began (misguidedly) practicing *surya namaskars* as an indigenous form of bodybuilding/strength training in its stead, Iyer chose to *supplement* Sandow's bodybuilding/strength-training system (and other related systems) with *surya namaskar* (and yogasana). In other words, Iyer, unlike Bhavanarao, perceived *surya namaskar* not as a substitute for strength training but as a complement to strength training. Iyer understood that *surya namaskar* and strength training, as well as yogasana, complete each other.

In 1934 a curious but timid thirteen-year-old high school student named B. S. Narayana Rao, who would later become an actor in Iyer's theater troupe, Ravi Artists, would pass Iyer's gymnasium in Bangalore on his way home from school and stand at a distance from its front window to watch Iyer's exercise classes with great interest. A few years later, after the gymnasium had relocated, Rao finally went inside. What struck him most that day were photos on the walls of "Sandows from different countries" (during this period "Sandow" was the generic term for bodybuilders), as well as of Iyer in various *surya namaskar* positions.[25] What strikes us today is that Iyer chose in his own gymnasium to present himself as a votary of *surya namaskar* (or should it be said "a Bhavanarao") in a world of Sandows.

What distinguished Iyer from most bodybuilders of his time wasn't his well-defined, large musculature; even by 1930s' standards (to say nothing of the standards of today), he wasn't very "cut" or bulked up. Nor was it his self-touted perfect symmetry. What set him apart was his grace and nimbleness, captured in the stop-motion frames of him performing *surya namaskar* (see fig. 21.4 on page 272). Iyer believed that "grace should become your second nature. Feel like being twin born with it. In talk or walk, laugh or smile, let grace and charm show up always."[26] Iyer incorporated

this quality into his most routine activities, such as massaging a patient in his physiotherapy office: "One could see his hands moving very fast and his strong body would move and bend with a supple grace," observes his friend Sumana.[27] Iyer attained his elegance and poise from his daily yogasana practice, and his agility, quickness, and lightness of movement from his daily *surya namaskar* practice.

Upon looking at the photos of Iyer demonstrating dumbbell exercises in his manual, *Physique and Figure,* it's easy to imagine him putting the dumbbells aside and suddenly springing into a gymnast's choreographed routine of balanced tumbles, jumps, cartwheels, and other maneuvers. He seems like somebody who was more at ease—more himself—in moving than at rest. The ancient Greeks, whose notion of corporeal beauty was a body in motion, would've been captivated by Iyer. And so would've been movie audiences.

For a time Iyer strongly aspired to be a movie star. (He was a passionate moviegoer all his life. Even after developing cataracts, he had one of his grandsons lead him to movie theaters. He was crazy about Hollywood films.) If he had succeeded, almost surely he would've been like raffish Douglas Fairbanks in his comedy/adventure movies—an actor whose character extends his personality through his physical prowess. Seeming quite ordinary (and perhaps even less than virtuous) under normal circumstances, he reveals his inner character (brave, clever, self-sacrificing, daring) in amazing acts of strength and acrobatics—what is ultimately nothing less than a transformation of the soul achieved through the body.

❧

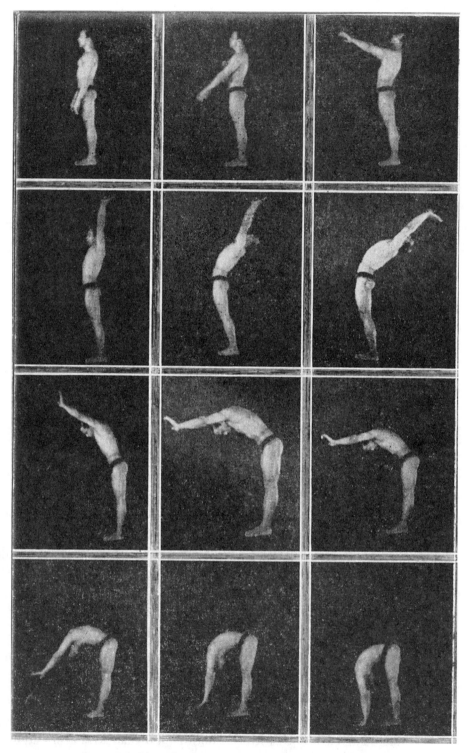

Figure 21.4. Film stills of K. V. Iyer demonstrating *surya namaskar,*
showing continuous movement

(From *Surya Namaskar*)

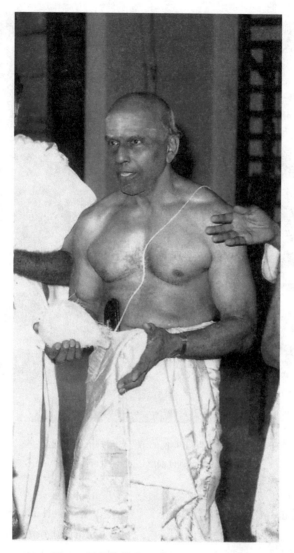

Figure 21.5. K. V. Iyer, age seventy-five,
at a *puja* ceremony held at his gymnasium, 1973
(With the kind permission of Ronne Iyer)

Iyer performed strength training, yogasana, and *surya namaskar* into his old age, although in a limited way (fig. 21.5). "These days, I do not go out of the house, Ayya," he told Sumana. "My eyes have become cloudy. I do not see clearly. I will be run over by some vehicle in the road if I go out by myself. So I don't go out much. I stay in the midst of my students. I keep myself occupied with my classes. My teaching [which included the demonstration of exercises] gives me sufficient exercise. Else, I would not be alive."[28]

Iyer died on January 3, 1980, at about 10:30 p.m. The next morning, his body was placed with his head facing south (the inauspicious direction for the living) in the main hall

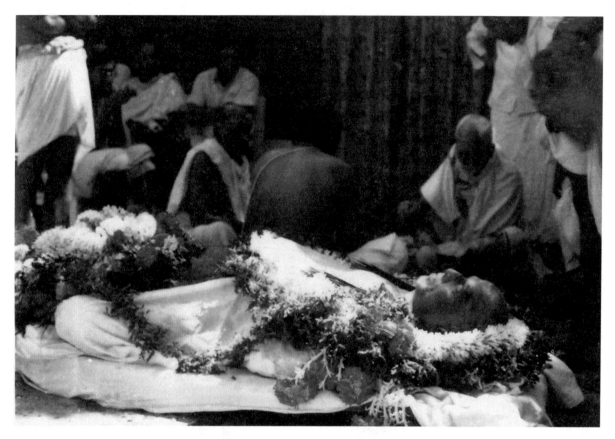

Figure 21.6. K. V. Iyer funeral, 1980
(With the kind permission of Ronne Iyer)

of the Vyayama Shala, where it could be viewed by mourners (fig. 21.6). (Sadly and infuriatingly, the gymnasium was torn down in 1984 and replaced by a car mart; it should have been preserved as a memorial.) On the wall behind the lifeless body was a splendid poster of the young Iyer posing to set off his magnificent muscular physique. Surrounding it were several photos of Iyer from his promotional booklet *Perfect Physique* and from his pamphlet *Surya Namaskar.* Seeing the dead body juxtaposed with the youthful body in the photos prompted Sumana

to ask himself the melancholic question, "Do the beautiful body in the photos and the dead body belong to the same person?" Sumana had observed that even when Iyer was seventy-five, beneath his usual loose clothing one could make out his broad shoulders and chest and his strong arms and legs. Standing over his friend now, Sumana thought, "Even such a strong person can be carried away by death."[29] Upon hearing of Iyer's death, his friend H. K. Ranganath said: "His *kaya* was *kavya*"—his body was poetry.[30]

22

LOUISE MORGAN

Making *Surya Namaskar* into an Elixir for Western Women

Interview with the Rajah of Aundh

In July 1936 Bhavanarao Pant Pratinidhi, the rajah of Aundh, made a trip to England primarily to give lectures and exhibit a film about *surya namaskar* (sun salutation exercises), which he had revivified in India beginning in 1908. (The film, shown at the British Film Institute in London, featured *surya namaskar* demonstrations by the rajah and his family in the palace and by his subjects in state schools.) While in London, Bhavanarao was interviewed at the opulent Savoy Hotel by the well-known journalist Louise Morgan (1886?–1964) for the *News Chronicle,* a London-based national newspaper founded by Charles Dickens. Morgan's reputation was based on her articles focusing on health and social welfare issues and on her celebrity interviews (which, over the course of her career, would include such varied notables as Walt Disney, W. B. Yeats, Paul Robeson, George Bernard Shaw, Field Marshal Sir Bernard Montgomery, and Somerset Maugham). Morgan would recall of her meeting with Bhavanarao: "In my capacity as journalist, I had the privilege of talking with one of the most vital human beings I have ever met—and I have interviewed hundreds of the world's outstanding men and women. He is the Rajah of Aundh."[1] Perhaps part of the reason Morgan was so impressed with Bhavanarao was her low expectations.

> I had discovered beforehand that the rajah was over seventy [actually, he was sixty-seven], and knowing that Indians age early, I was prepared for even more

of the sagging muscles and profound wrinkles which mark the vast majority of "old people" everywhere.

Imagine my astonishment, therefore, when the rajah's secretary presented me to him in the drawing-room of a suite at the Savoy Hotel, to see a man with the agile, supple movements of youth, eyes shining like a boy's, strong, brilliantly white teeth, firm muscles, radiant smile, and a mind that worked like summer lightning.[2]

"You seem surprised not to find me the usual doddering old creature!" the rajah mischievously exclaimed to her.[3]

Morgan's account of her interview with Bhavanarao appeared in the *News Chronicle* on July 6, 1936, the day before the film screening. The splashy headlines and subheads said it all: "'Surya Namaskars'—The Secret of Health"/ "Mothers Look Younger Than Daughters"/ "Rajah's Way to Banish Age and Illness." In the main text Morgan, allowing for no doubt and surely intending to astonish, made a series of astounding claims about the effects of *surya namaskar* practice. It "is banishing old age, pain, disease and worry from [the rajah's] realm." The seventy-year-old rajah is "full of vitality and joy in life. He has not had even a cold for 28 years." The rani (a rajah's wife), aged thirty-six, the mother of eight children, "looks like a girl of 16. Her body is slender, supple, and extremely strong." The wife of the rani's tutor, a sixty-year-old mother of ten children, who had been rheumatic and fat, "is now in perfect health and younger-looking than any of her daughters."[4] This

last claim, especially, must've made a powerful impact on Morgan's readers, especially on mothers with daughters. For many of them, it was an utterance of their most unspoken, shameful wish: to outshine their daughters. (It was thus a sanctioning of a trait that they perhaps despised in themselves: their vanity that spared no one, even their children.) Here, indeed, was a secret revealed!

This newspaper interview was the first instance of *surya namaskar* being pitched solely to Westerners, and in particular, female Westerners. "The effect on women is even more astonishing than on men," the rajah was quoted as saying. "Our women age very rapidly, but now they can keep the vitality and beauty of their youth to an advanced age."[5] Whereas Bhavanarao, in his book, had framed *surya namaskar* as a means of attaining strength and good health, Morgan, in her article, emphasized the powers of *surya namaskar* to extend and restore youth.

Lost Youth and Long Life

In presenting *surya namaskar* as a miraculous Oriental practice that makes people younger and bestows long life upon them and by proclaiming Bhavanarao and his consort as its living exemplars, Morgan was writing for a primed audience. Although people longed for their lost youth and a long life in other times—as evidenced by, among other endeavors, attempts by Christians to locate and return to the Garden of Eden, by alchemists to make or discover the philosopher's stone, and by explorers (although, apparently, not the Spanish explorer Ponce de León) to find the Fountain of Youth—perhaps no period was more defined by these yearnings than the early 20th century in the West. Examples may be found in various aspects of Western culture.

Perpetual Youth

Perhaps the earliest 20th-century expression of the flight from the difficult but pleasurable realities of adulthood (work and mature relationships) was J. M. Barrie's adaptation of his play *Peter Pan, or the Boy Who Wouldn't Grow Up* (1904) into the novel *Peter and Wendy*. "All children, except one, grow up," the book begins.[6] Not only free of cares and responsibilities, Peter Pan is even free from aging, death, and time.

The desire for perpetual youth could also be found in the spike in incidences of anorexia nervosa in the 1920s, when the feminine ideal shifted from plump and voluptuous to thin and flat. But whereas the corsetless flappers, with their cropped hair, mannish clothes, and slimmed bodies, cultivated an androgynous look, the extremely thin anorexics weren't fashionably boyish but simply young girlish. As two of the major theorists of dynamic psychiatry Sigmund Freud and Pierre Janet had already posited between 1895 and 1905, anorexic girls refused food in order to keep their bodies thin and childlike out of a fear of adulthood (in Freud and Janet's simplistic formulation, in order to forestall adult sexuality, in particular). While the trendy flapper ideal may have provided them with a rationale and cover for severely restricting their diet, anorexic girls were actually succumbing to an escapist fantasy of never growing up.

Rejuvenation

In the 1920s and 1930s there was a vogue for medical procedures to satisfy the desire to feel or appear young again. French surgeon Serge Abrahamovitch Voronoff performed his first grafting of "monkey glands" (actually thin slices of testicles from chimpanzees and baboons) onto men's testicles in 1920 in order to reverse aging by restoring vigor and increasing virility.

Another indicator of the desire for rejuvenation was the development of cosmetic plastic surgery. In 1921, when the first North American association of plastic surgeons was organized, plastic surgery wasn't even a recognized medical specialty. Through the 1920s and 1930s, though, it became a cultural phenomenon. The modern techniques of plastic surgery, developed following World War I for use in reconstructive surgery to repair faces mutilated on the battlefield, were adapted to modify the body for cosmetic purposes: in order to appear more youthful, older women had their wrinkles and sagging skin, once considered normal attributes of aging, abolished.

Longevity

The steps taken toward extending the duration of life were sometimes hugely ambitious. In 1930 Dr. Alexis Carrel, in collaboration with Charles Lindbergh, built the Lindbergh life chamber, in which whole organs were kept alive, in Carrel's laboratory at New York's Rockefeller Institute for Medical Research. Carrel thought of the chamber as only the first step in a human storage-vault project that would fulfill the quest to achieve near immortality. Interviewed for an article, "Can Science Make Us Live Forever?" in *Modern Mechanix* in 1936, Carrel said, "Some individuals could be put in storage for long periods of time, brought back to normal existence for other periods, and permitted in this manner to exist for several centuries."[7]

Perhaps the most poignant manifestation of the dreams of eternal youth and extended life during this time was James Hilton's enormously popular novel *Lost Horizon,* published by Macmillan and Company in 1933 in the United Kingdom. *Lost Horizon* wasn't an instant success. The great popularity of Hilton's next novel, *Goodbye Mr. Chips,* in 1934, called attention to *Lost Horizon,* which became a top-ten best seller the following year, 1935.*

Lost Horizon was a mixture of fantasy adventure and utopian novel. A plane carrying minor British consular official and author Robert Conway and a few other passengers is hijacked in India. The plane crashes in the Himalayas, where the passengers are rescued and taken to Shangri-La, a community hidden in a valley protected from the surrounding fierce elements, where residents lead a life of virtue and moderation. Conway eventually learns that he's been brought to Shangri-La to replace the dying High Lama.

It's commonly thought that in creating Shangri-La, Hilton drew on an actual account of a journey to Tibet.† Positing instead that Shangri-La is a mix of Hilton's fantasy and memory, the film critic Andrew Sarris, writing

in the 1990s, quips: "More than ever, Shangri-La evokes a pleasant retirement community in Florida or California, with a restricted clientele limited to Oxbridge and Ivy League types"[8] (Hilton was educated at Cambridge). But in the 1930s, when life for many was bleak—liberal democracies and dictatorships alike were suffering through the hardships of the Great Depression—who can pass judgment on the desire for escapism?

Whatever its source, Shangri-La became a cultural referent for a utopian society, whether an imaginary remote paradise on earth or a real hideaway of great beauty where one could find peace. But the more powerful pull of the novel, the real reason it entered into the dream life of the populace in the 1930s, wasn't in its presentation of an ideal society but in its portrayal of longevity: aging is decelerated in Shangri-La. The High Lama is over two hundred years old.

The heralding in the West of Eastern holy men who possess the secret of longevity preceded the novel. An example in popular culture is "The Tibetan Legend: Recent Confirmations and a Dawn of Hope," an article in the June 3, 1933, issue of *Health & Strength,* a British physical culture magazine, in which "a Physician" reports:

While it is now admitted that the Dalai Lama and the other chiefs or priests of the

---

*Hilton's all-time best seller, *Lost Horizon* went on to become one of the biggest international best sellers of the 1930s and 1940s, thanks in part to it also having been published in America in 1939 as the first Pocket Books title. The publication of *Lost Horizon* as a mass-market, pocket-sized paperback is said to have begun the paperback revolution.

†That account is variously claimed to be "Land of the Yellow Lama: National Geographic Society Explorer Visits the Strange Kingdom of Muli, beyond the Likiang Snow Range of Yunnan, China," published in1924, and/or other articles by explorer Joseph Rock in *National Geographic; Voyage d'une Parisienne à Lhassa* (*My Journey to Lhasa*), published in 1927, or *Mystiques et Magiciens du Tibet* (*Magic and Mystery in Tibet*), published in 1929, by explorer Alexandra David-Néel; or *Shambhala, the Resplendent,* published in 1930, by Russian artist Nicholas Roerich.

Tibetan monasteries are in possession of very considerable knowledge, so far closed to the rest of the world, it has now become more or less generally accepted by Europeans who have studied the subject that these are but comparative novices, and that there are far greater adepts in wisdom and knowledge and power, who are to be found, when they elect to be found, if ever, in the higher plateaux of the Himalayas.

These are stated to be in possession of powers which are, and which have been, most jealously preserved. . . .

Among the remarkable powers possessed by these adepts [Tibetan monks] it is claimed that they are able to control the elements, and also to prolong life throughout many centuries. These stories, which were even regarded as absurd and even wicked, cannot to-day be so contemptuously dismissed, since closer acquaintance with Hindoo *yogis* has satisfied even those observers who were at first most incredulous that there may be solid substance for the claims advanced. It has been recognized that certain *yogis* are unquestionably possessed of powers and abilities of which Europeans are wholly ignorant, while it is also believed that the years of some of these men are patriarchal, in a Methuselahistic sense.[9]

Morgan wasn't just presenting Bhavanarao to the citizens of England as the living incarnation of the High Lama; she was also bringing Shangri-La into their living rooms and yards. People wouldn't have to go live in India to reap the age-retarding benefits of *surya namaskar;* they didn't even have to go for a short stay, as one might to a spa or resort hotel. They could practice the secret of health and longevity right in their home, and for an expenditure of only five to ten minutes a day, just before breakfast. "Surya Namaskars is simplicity itself," Morgan wrote, "and takes only five minutes to do. The hands are put flat on the floor in a bending position and kept fixed throughout the cycle of ten positions."[10] If they would only incorporate this exercise into their daily lives, the British, too, could remain young and beautiful practically forever.

Very soon after the interview appeared in the *News Chronicle,* while Bhavanarao went off to tour pig, chicken, and dairy farms in England, Ireland, and Scotland, where his cameraman took extensive footage of farm processes for educational films to be shown to the people of Aundh, Morgan went on a badly needed holiday to Rodmell Hill, a small village near Lewes, in East Sussex, fifty miles from London (making it an attractive country retreat for Londoners, including Virginia and Leonard Woolf), where she stayed at the cottage of a friend, Evelyn Pember, who was off traveling in France. (Having been under continual stress over the previous few months due to the uproar she had created with her series of articles in the *News Chronicle* in February exposing the accidents and diseases faced by Welsh and English coal miners, the normally energetic Morgan wasn't feeling quite herself.)

Morgan was a sophisticate. She was born in America. In her mid-thirties, while married, she had an affair with Otto Theis, probably while they were working for the same newspaper in New York. In 1923, after Theis became literary

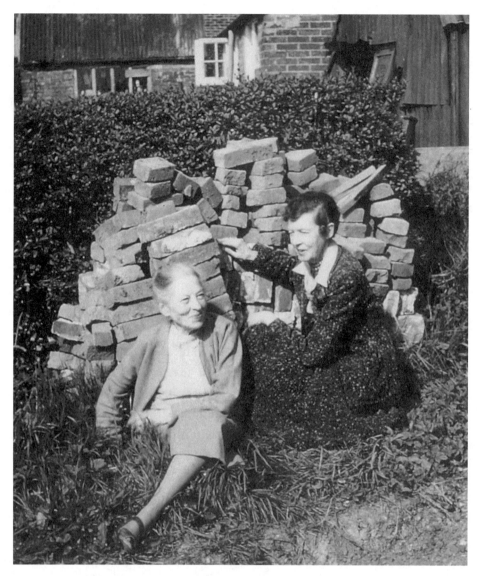

Figure 22.1. Louise Morgan (left) with Nancy Cunard, July 1959

(With the kind permission of Louise Morgan and Otto Theis Papers, General Collection, Beinecke Rare Book and Manuscript Library)

editor of *The Outlook,* an English political-literary magazine, Morgan left her husband to follow Theis to England. They married. After working for *The Outlook* and *Everyman,* Morgan was hired by the *News Chronicle* in 1933. By 1936 Theis had established a career as a literary agent. The couple had a wide circle of literary and high-society friends, including a long, close relationship with the beautiful, rebellious, and flamboyant heiress Nancy Cunard, with whom Morgan shared an ardent commitment to social justice (fig. 22.1). Morgan and her husband would become British citizens just prior to World War II.

For a woman so knowledgeable about the ways of the world, all that gushing over the rajah in Morgan's interview might seem like so much journalistic hype, but Morgan was genuinely gaga over that "bright-eyed lithe old man who looked 25 years younger than his age."[11] As she traveled by train to Rodmell Hill, "the image of that ageless man went with [her]."[12] And her enthusiasm for *surya namaskar* was equally genuine. Arriving at the cottage, she "began the exercises at once."[13] "From the first," she recounted, "I noted a reflow of energy back into my being."[14] Despite straining several muscles and limping around for days, she sedulously persisted in her practice for the full three weeks of her holiday.

Upon returning to work, a refreshed Morgan learned that letters had been pouring into the *News Chronicle* office inquiring about the "fountain of youth" she had written about in her interview with Bhavanarao. As a result of the overflowing reader response, Morgan was asked by her editor to write an entire series on *surya namaskar*.

Series of Articles

The four-part series of articles on *surya namaskar* appeared on successive Thursdays in the *News Chronicle* "Home" page beginning on July 30, 1936. The articles were a step-by-step crash course on how to perform *surya namaskar*. "Five to ten minutes a day, just before breakfast, is ample. . . . All you need is a piece of cloth 22 in. square and gym dress. Trunks are advised for men and brassiere and shorts for women."[15]

The *surya namaskar* articles held prominence of place on the "Home" page otherwise cluttered with advertisements, articles, and notices. The articles were top and center and several columns wide. They had splashy headlines: "Surya Namaskars/A Rajah's 10-point way to health and youth";[16] "Surya Namaskars No. 2/ Have you learnt how to Breathe?/—then you are ready for lesson two in this 10-point way to health and youth";[17] "Surya Namaskars—3/ These exercises may Cure Bad Temper";[18] "Final Lesson in Surya Namaskars."[19] They were illustrated with photos of the debonair Apa Pant (the rajah's twenty-three-year-old son who was studying law at Oxford) elegantly and effortlessly demonstrating the steps. Yet it's the ads, articles, and notices surrounding the *surya namaskar* articles that immediately draw our attention. They all have a certain charm and verve. And there are a lot of them (see fig. 22.2 on page 282).

There are ads for such products as Silf, a tablet that allows you to lose weight without having to alter your diet ("Banish the Shadow of Fatness"); Beechams Brand Powder ("Stop That Pain for 2 D"); Zam-Buk ("Feet won't spoil your pleasure if treated nightly with Zam-Buk"); and Del Monte Canned Pears ("Women are getting wise about canned fruits. . . . They insist on Del Monte"). There are articles on such topics as bedroom furniture ("Modern Bedroom Furnished for Less Than £20"); summer sweets ("cool and acceptable sweets can be made entirely . . . from fruit"); willow woods and twigs ("Those Confusing Willows"); sets of hairbrushes that match the furnishing of a bed or dressing room ("New Accessories for Your Dressing Table"); and fashionable jewelry inspired by speed in the form of elongated greyhounds, dragon flies, seagulls, and aeroplanes ("Speed Jewels"). And there are notices on such subjects as dressmaking advice ("If you have

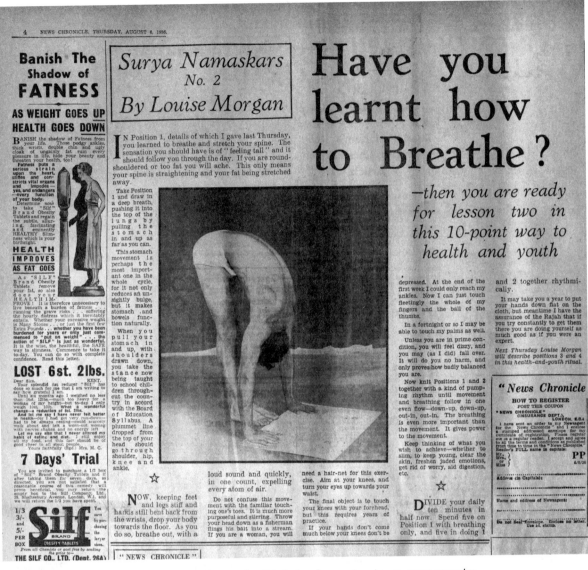
Surya Namaskars No. 2
By Louise Morgan

IN Position 1, details of which I gave last Thursday, you learned to breathe and stretch your spine. The sensation you should have is of "feeling tall" and it should follow you through the day. If you are round-shouldered or too fat you will ache. This only means your spine is straightening and your fat being stretched away.

Take Position 1 and draw in a deep breath, pushing it into the top of the lungs by pulling the stomach in and up as far as you can.

This stomach movement is perhaps the most important one in the whole cycle, for it not only reduces an unsightly bulge, but it makes stomach and bowels function naturally.

When you pull your stomach in and up, with shoulders drawn down, you take the stance now being taught to school children throughout the country in accord with the Board of Education Syllabus. A plummet line dropped from the top of your head should go through shoulder, hip, knee and ankle.

☆

NOW, keeping feet and legs stiff and hands still bent back from the wrists, drop your body towards the floor. As you do so, breathe out, with a loud sound and quickly, in one count, expelling every atom of air.

Do not confuse this movement with the familiar touching one's toes. It is much more purposeful and stirring. Throw your head down as a fisherman flings his bait into a stream. If you are a woman, you will need a hair-net for this exercise. Aim at your knees, and turn your eyes up towards your waist.

The final object is to touch your knees with your forehead, but this requires years of practice.

If your hands don't come much below your knees don't be depressed. At the end of the first week I could only reach my ankles. Now I can just touch fleetingly the whole of my fingers and the ball of the thumbs.

In a fortnight or so I may be able to touch my palms as well.

Unless you are in prime condition, you will feel dizzy, and you may (as I did) fall over. It will do you no harm, and only proves how badly balanced you are.

Now knit Positions 1 and 2 together with a kind of pumping rhythm until movement and breathing follow in one even flow—down-up, down-up, out-in, out-in. The breathing is even more important than the movement. It gives power to the movement.

Keep thinking of what you wish to achieve—whether to slim, to keep young, clear the skin, freshen jaded emotions, get rid of worry, aid digestion, etc.

☆

DIVIDE your daily ten minutes in half now. Spend five on Position 1 with breathing only, and five in doing 1 and 2 together rhythmically.

It may take you a year to put your hands down flat on the cloth, but meantime I have the assurance of the Rajah that if you try constantly to get them there you are doing yourself as much good as if you were an expert.

Next Thursday Louise Morgan will describe positions 3 and 4 in this health-and-youth ritual.

"NEWS CHRONICLE"

Have you learnt how to Breathe?

—then you are ready for lesson two in this 10-point way to health and youth

Figure 22.2. Morgan's second article in her four-part series on *surya namaskar*
(From the *News Chronicle*, August 6, 1936)

any dressmaking renovation query, write to Vanessa, c/o the Home Page Editor, enclosing a stamped addressed envelope for reply. She will help you") and the result of short-wave radio tests ("News Chronicle Wireless Test—Radio Globe-Trotting").[20]

At first the short course on *surya namaskar* seems jarringly out of place amid all these appeals to consumer appetites, these evocations of the comfortable (and anxiety-provoking) middle-class life possessed by some, aspired to by others. Then we realize that's the point. Although yours for the taking, *surya namaskar* is just another accoutrement to the good life.

In postindustrial society, with its greatly expanding consumer market, newspapers had become the primary market intermediary between advertisers and consumers. To appeal to a wider public (boosting circulation spurred ad revenues), 19th- and early 20th-century newspapers covered a wide range of subjects, instead of just politics and business (their traditional focus). Articles on politics, business, sports, crime, entertainment, and health were mixed together, appearing with comics, gossip columns, interviews, and advertisements.

The articles, advertisements, and notices on the *News Chronicle* "Home" page were primarily aimed at a particular segment of the buying market: middle-class women. Although Bhavanarao, too, had argued that women derive benefits from *surya namaskar* practice, he tried to include women in what was basically a male activity; in contrast, Morgan presented *surya namaskar* as an exercise basically for women. And not mere exercise. She presented *surya namaskar* as "a perfect instrument, not only for keeping the body fit, but for warding off old age and disease, invigorating the mind, strengthening the character and will, and increasing to its full limit one's capacity for vital and joyous living. No age up to 80 is too old at which to begin them."[21]

Morgan was the perfect teacher for her audience. She was spunky, reassuring, cajoling, and practical. Her language was vivid, mixing the homely and poetic. Her tone was charmingly chatty. (Bhavanarao's matter-of-fact instructions, compared to hers, seem brusque.) In her instructions to readers for Position 2, *Uttanasana,* Standing Forward Bend, she began with gusto: "Now, keeping feet and legs stiff and hands still bent back from the wrists, drop your [upper] body towards the floor. As you do so, breathe out, with a loud sound and quickly, in one count, expelling every atom of air." Then she admonished her readers ("Do not confuse this movement with the familiar touching one's toes. It is much more purposeful and stirring"), gave a directive with brio ("Throw your head down as a fisherman flings his bait into a stream"), made an eminently practical suggestion ("If you are a woman, you will need a hair-net for this exercise"), and gave a straightforward command with a subtle tip ("Aim at your knees, and turn your eyes up towards your waist").[22] Lastly, out of concern for her readers (she wanted them to know they could carry on despite discouraging setbacks), she selflessly exhibited frankness about her own failures:

> If your hands don't come much below your knees don't be depressed. At the end of the first week I could only reach my ankles. Now [after three weeks] I can touch fleetingly the whole of my fingers and the ball of the thumbs.
>
> In a fortnight or so I may be able to touch my palms as well.
>
> Unless you are in primed condition, you will feel dizzy, and you may (as I did) fall over. It will do you no harm, and only proves how badly balanced you are.[23]

She concluded with motivational advice that, as always, was never less than sunny: "Keep thinking of what you wish to achieve—whether to slim, to keep young, clear the skin, freshen jaded emotions, get rid of worry, aid digestion, etc."[24]

The reader response to the *surya namaskar* articles was overwhelming. Over a year later, Morgan was still receiving letters from England and abroad about the miraculous benefits people were receiving from their *surya namaskar* practice: "They have told me of remarkable cures, of the restoration of faith and hope, and of the intensification of emotional experience which made each waking to a new day a delight." These conversion testimonies were coming from a cross section of readers: "doctors, school teachers, bankers and bank clerks, poets, saxophonists, newspaper vendors, charwomen, typists, retired civil servants, writers, engineers, actors, and dozens of other types."[25] Although Morgan's account of the responses—their content (the salvific overturning of beliefs) and breadth (egalitarian and eclectic)—may be skewed, there's no doubt that the letters showed a surge of interest in *surya namaskar* in England.

23

LOUISE MORGAN

Pointing the Way to Health through *Surya Namaskar*

New Book: *The Ten-Point Way to Health*

In 1938 Bhavanarao Pant Pratinidhi, the rajah of Aundh, published his second book on *surya namaskar, The Ten-Point Way to Health,* in England. Edited and with an introduction by journalist Louise Morgan, who'd interviewed the rajah and written a four-part series on *surya namaskar* for the *News Chronicle,* the book immediately replaced his original book, *Surya Namaskars (Sun-Adoration) for Health, Efficiency & Longevity,* published in 1928, in India, as the manual that defined *surya namaskar.* One reason for this was simply that the earlier book was out of print (published in India in 1928, 1929, and 1931, each English-language edition fell out of print after a few months).

The Ten-Point Way to Health would be continuously in print for about the next thirty-five years. (No wonder it's commonly mistaken in our day as the foundational text of modern *surya namaskar.*) In the correspondence between Bhavanarao's son Apa Pant and Morgan in 1962 that began with Pant writing the book's publisher, J. M. Dent and Sons, to request having a foreword that he'd written be added to *The Ten-Point Way to Health,* Morgan, representing the publisher, told Pant about "the implied tribute to your Father which Dent have been making by keeping his book alive. . . . During the war, sales fell to nothing, but Dent kept the book 'on the stocks' and turned out a cheap edition after the war."* "I feel you

---

*Founded in 1888, Dent achieved its initial success by selling cheap editions of the classics to the working class, beginning with a Shakespeare series.

will be proud of this tribute paid by Dent to your Father," Morgan continued.[1]

Pant related that he himself had kept interest in the book alive by disseminating copies to notables since it was first published: "In the last 24 years this book has seen many editions. I myself have been distributing it to worthy persons from time to time."[2] Morgan replied: "We note with interest and pleasure that you have been distributing copies of *The Ten Point Way to Health* among worthy persons, and we are convinced that your Father would rejoice to know you are following in his footsteps so faithfully."[3] Pant wrote back: "I have had so many good reports about this book from all over the world. One day in 1951 I walked into a book shop in the heart of London. There I saw a pile of 'The Ten-Point Way to Health.' I asked the owner of the book shop whether this particular book sold well. He exclaimed 'Sell well? Sir, this is a classic!!'"[4]

It's understandable that *Surya Namaskars* went quickly out of print and *The Ten-Point Way to Health* was in print for so long. Even when it was first published, *Surya Namaskars* was a fusty (in appearance and attitude) physical culture manual for Indians, while *The Ten-Point Way to Health* was a giddy informal guide to changing everyday behavior—a self-help book—for Westerners. In this, it was strikingly modern, and remains so even today.

The Ten-Point Way to Health was based solely on Bhavanarao's *Surya Namaskars* and lectures given in England. Or so it appeared. Although he's identified as the author and Morgan as the editor, Morgan excised much of his original text and largely replaced it with her own, includ-

ing text taken directly, or nearly so, from her newspaper series, usually to great effect. In the process of including her own material in Bhavanarao's second book, Morgan became more than a ghostwriter. She made the book her own. Even the title, *The Ten-Point Way to Health,* is taken from the catchy tag line for her articles.

Despite being written by two people, the book is no pastiche; it seems nearly seamless. This is especially surprising when you consider that Morgan did nothing to ape the rajah's writing. She maintained her breezy tone, snappy sentences, and vivid figures of speech, with the result that somehow even Bhavanarao's original text sounds uncannily like hers. The new autobiographical passages (probably adapted from Bhavanarao's lectures in England), such as those on making changes to the old system, clearly derive from Bhavanarao's experience. But even they aren't jarring, for they, too, are in Morgan's voice. (Few British readers would've been familiar with Bhavanarao's first book, so they wouldn't have known the difference.)

And it's not just that the new book has Morgan's panache; it expands on the concerns she voiced in the articles. In fact, the entire focus of the book has changed from the previous book: whereas the old book presents *surya namaskar* as an exercise that imparts strength, stamina, and health to Indian men weakened and made ill by their sedentary lives, the new book presents *surya namaskar* as an exercise for Westerners, especially women, whose lives need some spicing up.

Perhaps nothing better represents Morgan's appropriation of Bhavanarao's book than the illustrations. The book reprints not the photographs of Bhavanarao from his 1928 book but the photographs of Bhavanarao's son Apa Pant demonstrating the series of *surya namaskar* positions from Morgan's newspaper articles published in the summer of 1936. Part young, handsome, well-educated, suave prince and part lithe, exotic, scantily clad beefcake, Pant's appeal to the female readership as cultured scion and wild creature is more explicit in the book than in the articles, even though the photos are the same. That's because the book also includes photos of a comely foil, Rita Brynteson, demonstrating the exercises. A blond, pug-nosed, and pert young Englishwoman, Brynteson also serves as a less accomplished adherent (while he performs the exercises with an elegant nonchalance, she "has not done Surya Namaskars for long, and is not perfect"[5]) with whom the female readership can identify—and as a pinup for the male readership to ogle.

Wearing a fetching two-piece costume (halter top and shorts) made of wool and silk (a rather risqué outfit for performing what many people still considered a Hindu ritual), Brynteson practices her exercises in the sunny outdoors on the grass of a spacious lawn with woods in the distance. She's in stark contrast to the darkly beautiful rani (the rajah's wife), pictured in the original book when she was twenty-eight (and the rajah was sixty): bejeweled from earlobe to toe and enveloped in a flowing sari, she's standing on a wooden platform surrounded by a black backdrop. In dress, setting, appearance, and manner, Brynteson represents the modern suburban woman. And, of course, she's in stark contrast to Pant. Morgan's captions reveal the difference in her attitudes toward them. For Pant, Morgan wrote: Position 2: "Feet remain rooted, knees straight, wrists at edge of clothe in line with toes, and stomach is drawn deeply in." Position 4: "Appasahib's heels do not quite touch the ground. They should, but he demonstrates under unfamiliar conditions, and is not up to standard." Position 8: "Position 3 repeated backwards. For balance, put other foot back. Pressure is then exerted against other side of trunk" (see fig. 23.1 on page 288). For Brynteson, Morgan wrote: Position 2: "Hands too far away from feet. Head not touching knees. Compare this position with Appasahib's." Position 4: "Back is not straight. Downward pressure at waist by helper is advisable. Net essential to keep hair in order." Position 8: "By this time, even on a cold day, she was warm, and intends to keep to this costume of wool and silk"[6] (see fig. 23.2 on page 288).

Audience

In the most poignant part of his 1928 book, a section titled "Postponing Old Age," Bhavanarao reached out to his most natural constituency: Indian old men. To those old men who are still energetic, he recommended a moderate course of *surya namaskar* "in order that their life may be prolonged so as to enable them to accomplish the beneficial objects which they have at heart." For those old men who had suffered reverses in life, such as failure in their careers, sickness, and loss of loved ones, he said that *surya namaskar* "ministers not only to the body but to the spirit as well." And for those old men who had behaved recklessly by squandering their health, he offered salvation: "Even to these old sinners there can be held out a promise of redemption, if they be like children and follow

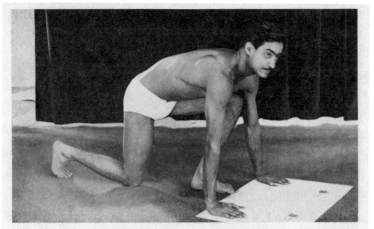

8 Position 3 repeated backwards. For balance, put other foot back. Pressure is then exerted against other side of trunk.

Figure 23.1. "Surya Namaskars Demonstrated by an Expert, Appasahib, Son of the Rajah of Aundh," 1938

(From *The Ten-Point Way to Health,* by Bhavanarao Pant Pratinidhi)

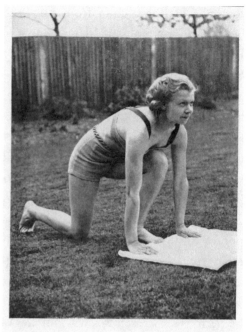

8 By this time, even on a cold day, she was warm, and intends to keep to this costume of wool and silk.

Figure 23.2. "Surya Namaskars Demonstrated by a Learner, Miss Rita Brynteson," 1938

(From *The Ten-Point Way to Health*)

faithfully the course of Surya Namaskars."[7] (Morgan kept much of this.)

In the section titled "Value to Women" in the 1938 book, Morgan addressed her natural constituency: Western middle-aged, middle-class women. "Surya Namaskars have a peculiar importance for women in so far as they more than men depend upon physical attractiveness [to get what they want]," she told them, "and by the harmonious action of these exercises in toning up all their physical processes they acquire a very bloom of personality."[8] The vigorous nature of *surya namaskar,* Morgan seemed to be saying, ensures the good health of the organ systems, which makes even a homely and plain woman vivacious. (In the section "Exercise for Women" in his 1928 book, Bhavanarao, too, advocated *surya namaskar* practice for women. Answering the objections of those who hold that women do not need any exercise, he argued that the primary benefit for women of *surya namaskar* is good health in the service of motherhood.

"It should be emphasized that woman—the mother—is, as the Indian poet says, 'The mine of heroes and great men,' and that you cannot expect a weak and sickly mother to bear healthy, strong and long-lived children."[9] It's hard to decide whether Morgan or Bhavanarao, both of whom possessed a keen sense of social injustice, was the more patronizing—or was it the more realistic?—champion of women.)

The very fabric of the 1938 book reveals its intended audience as Western, middle class, and mostly female. With her innate journalistic sense of detail, Morgan couldn't help but present the minutiae (settings, routines, dress codes, and mores) of middle-class British life when dispensing her commonsense advice. After telling of the need for a square piece of cloth on which the hands should be placed while going through the exercises, she cautioned: "If your floor is polished lino, a square of rubber would be best, to avoid slipping."[10] She counseled: "Take your ten minutes a day without fail, as regularly as you catch the train to town every morning."[11] She recommended practicing *surya namaskar* to "counteract the bad effect of high heels, tight shoes, belts, collars, and other restrictive clothing demanded by custom or fashion."[12] She suggested that when practicing *surya namaskar,* "wear as little clothing as possible, the less the better. Let that little be loose and airy."[13] (In Bhavanarao's 1928 book, intended for Indian readers, the women in the photos wear yards of sari cloth wrapped about their waist and draped over their shoulders.)

Most of Morgan's advice about cosmetic matters was addressed to women. She advocated *surya namaskar* as the panacea for a wrinkly neck, small or droopy breasts, plumpness, and a pallid complexion. "The bending of the head exercises the muscles of neck and throat, filling out the skin and preventing the 'ropy' or 'crêpey' effect so common in older women."[14] "In this posture . . . the bust in women is improved and developed, becoming firm and elastic."[15] "[*Surya namaskars*] reduce redundant fat, especially the fat about the abdomen, hips, thighs, neck, and chin."[16] [*Surya namaskars*] improve the colour and function of the skin."[17]

Warding Off Old Age: Health and Fitness

"Premature old age and premature death are tragedies," proclaimed Morgan in *The Ten-Point*

Way to Health. "The spirit of youth is always and everywhere desirable, nay, absolutely necessary."[18] In most of her explanations for how *surya namaskar* warded off old age, she more or less followed Bhavanarao. She contended that *surya namaskar* maintains or restores youthfulness through providing immunity from disease by aiding the digestive system, developing the lungs, invigorating the heart, toning up the nervous system, and stimulating the glands.

Morgan also maintained that *surya namaskar* exercises "stimulate the uterus and ovaries; remove menstrual disorders and consequent pain and misery; render child-bearing less painful and less dangerous."[19]

Morgan elaborated on the ability of *surya namaskar* to generate weight loss. ("The chief aim of Position Five is to lift the abdomen and hips as high off the floor as possible. This squeezes every fraction of useless fat off, leaving the muscles clean and supple."[20]) Whereas Bhavanarao ascribed *surya namaskar*'s ability to purge the body of toxins to chanting *bija* mantras, she wrote about *surya namaskar*'s ability to "eradicate toxic impurities through profuse perspiration."[21] In her instructions for Position 2, *Uttanasana,* she wrote (elaborating on her instructions in the articles): "Do not confuse this position with the familiar exercise of 'touching the toes.' It is much more purposeful and stirring. Thousands who 'touch their toes' religiously every day have no idea what real exercise is like! How many people, after touching their toes, feel the healthy sweat coming from every pore?"[22]

While giving a nod to *surya namaskar*'s role in developing strength, Morgan emphasized its ability to develop flexibility—a needed corrective to Bhavanarao's relentless emphasis on its ability to build strength. She wrote in the instructions in the book (elaborating on those in her article) for Position 2: "Throw your head down as a fisherman flings his bait into a stream. Aim your head at your knees, and turn your eyes upwards towards your waist. This will in time make your spine beautifully supple and as elastic as a child's."[23]

Morgan's description of the benefit of the *Uttanasana* position—making the spine "beautifully supple and elastic as a child's"—makes clear that she understands the true fitness benefit of *surya namaskar:* flexibility of the joints, and in particular elongation of the spine. "A joint in any mechanism, whether of wood, steel, or flesh, will function stiffly or not at all if neglected," Morgan wrote elsewhere in the book.[24] "It is the spinal cord that represents life. If it is diseased, death will follow; if it is unhealthy, the body will be unhealthy." So a "strong, straight, and flexible spine" is indispensable for "making our bodies young."[25] To emphasize the critical role of flexibility, Morgan concluded her new commentary on the *Uttanasana* position with a homespun (yet plenty sophisticated) take on its value: "The spine in this position is stretched—a fundamentally important action. The animals know the wisdom of this. Watch your cat or dog; it stretches its spine a dozen times a day."[26]

In spelling out these benefits—beauty, youthfulness, alleviation of pain, weight loss, cleansing, and grace—Morgan was making a strong appeal to women to take up *surya namaskar.*

In shaping the content of *The Ten-Point Way to Health,* making it for all intents and purposes her book, did Morgan reflect or effect a profound shift in *surya namaskar* practice from Indian and male to Western and female? That is, was she an exemplum who represented (to an exceptional degree) her times or an exception who influenced her times? It appears that Morgan was an effector of change: she prominently promoted *surya namaskar* in England and stamped it as an exercise for women. But her more important influence may have been on yoga.

It's not that Morgan was influential in women taking up yoga in the West, a trend, begun in the 1890s, that had become, according to Sita Devi, Shri Yogendra's wife, a "growing fashion" in London in the 1930s.[27] ("A London report states that young women have taken to Asanas and other yogic practices in their quest for radiant health," Devi wrote in her 1934 *Easy Postures for Woman* [sic], the first yoga manual written by a woman.[28] These women, it seems, would've been in vanguard of those Londoners receptive to Morgan's entreaties to take up *surya namaskar,* a similar but at that time rival exercise to yoga.) Instead, Morgan was critical in expanding the parameters of postural yoga.

Through significantly shaping a book that generated interest in *surya namaskar* among the populace (as evidenced by the continued sales of *The Ten-Point Way to Health* over decades) Morgan paved the way for the rebranding of the sun salutations as a yogic warm-up exercise, most prominently by Swami Sivananda, who, in the 1950s, incorporated the sun salutations into a yoga routine that he spread around the world. Just as important as her promotion of *surya namaskar* in the West, though, was her full-throttled advocacy of *surya namaskar* as a strenuous and invigorating exercise.

In her yoga manual written for the modern Indian woman (chiefly members of "the middle and well-to-do classes, usually the educated—blessed with fair circumstances—[who] suffer from inactivity and superfluity"[29]), Devi presented a compelling rationale for women to take up yoga: "Yogic exercises since they are non-violent and non-fatiguing are particularly suited to a woman and make her more beautiful."[30] Although progressive in many ways, Devi was advocating a gentle yoga for the fairer sex: "Any exercise, irrespective whether it belongs to modern physical culture of Yoga, which takes away from a woman the grace and charm of womanhood is likely to have very little appeal to a modern woman."[31] Here Devi was referring to such vigorous exercises as the sun salutations.

For men, used to participating in sports and gymnastics, performing *surya namaskar* didn't violate any accepted boundaries. For women, it was transgressive. To them, the sun salutations more nearly resembled the jitterbug or sexual intercourse. Morgan changed all that. She domesticated *surya namaskar,* making it into acceptable home exercise for middle-class women—but without making it less wild. Inspired to take up the sun salutations from reading her articles or *The Ten-Point Way to Health,* women found themselves thrusting about, straining to breathe, sweating, becoming delirious, and ending up drained, yet calmly exuberant. Which means to say, to the extent that she influenced the incorporation of *surya namaskar* into yoga, Morgan helped make yoga (what Devi would consider) "violent and fatiguing." Not that Morgan by any means considered *surya namaskar* to be mere exercise.

Self-Awareness

For Morgan, *surya namaskar* was a means of self-exploration—examining one's values as a means of discovering one's essential nature. When practicing *surya namaskar,* she maintained, almost certainly addressing men in particular, "you will be aware of the wonder of living, and of your power to share in it, as no amount of actual adventurous life in the external world can teach you. You will know more about yourself than years of jungle-hunting or dealing with international affairs, big business or worldly success would ever give you."[32]

Morgan advocated reflection over action (although in her social welfare articles she sought to rile up readers to provoke them into taking action to make the world a better place). She exhorted her readers to forsake the restless quest for adventure (for most of her readers, no doubt, more fantasy than achievement—the travel books of Peter Fleming, Graham Greene, and Evelyn Waugh were extremely popular in Great Britain in the 1930s, providing temporary escape for many) and the single-minded desire for great material success (although, evidently, her notion of crass "worldly success" didn't extend to establishing a career as a journalist, being part of the smart set, publishing four books, and owning a country house in Dallington—her own accomplishments). She implored her readers to take up *surya namaskar* instead as a better means of self-knowledge. In her view, a new type of person emerges from *surya namaskar* practice—one who is positive, empowered, vigorous, and introspective. "You will feel: 'I can do great things. I can and will live to the utmost capacity that God intended me to.' You will, in fact, be meeting yourself for the first time."[33]

What is the power of *surya namaskars* to bring us knowledge of our true selves for the first time? "Some explanation of their power may be found in the fact they are the concentration of hundreds of generations of human experience," explained Morgan, as part of her quirky insight into the movements of *surya namaskar* in her introduction to *The Ten-Point Way to Health*.[34] While not arguing that they were created to evoke the movements of everyday life, Morgan held that the positions of *surya namaskar* "include the full cycle of human activity since the casting-out from the Garden of Eden: the thrusting down of the treader of grapes and the woman in childbirth, the proud stretch of the warrior and the coquette, the swing of reaper and weaver, the tautness of runner and mother protecting her young, the bend of the weeder, the washer, and the human being at prayer."[35]

In this formulation, the positions of *surya namaskar* incongruously embody the instinctive and culturally acquired movements of work, birth, war, sexual desire, sport, motherhood, and prayer. Through inhabiting these various positions, Morgan seems to say, we attain knowledge of our true selves as members of humanity, especially of people who lived in simpler times. She was asking her readers, in effect, to take on various identities, not, as in dance, for display (to entertain an audience) but for recapturing what had been lost in the modern era. "In our mechanized times, these natural physical movements have been lost or distorted, and [*surya namaskar*] restores something of the primitive vigour and oneness of being to revive them."[36]

Actually, the movements described by Morgan that have been lost or drastically changed or become rare are the graceful movements of laborers belonging to agrarian and rural societies whose manual tasks were replaced during the industrial revolution by machinery (iron plows, McCormick reapers, spinning jennies, steam-powered wine presses, and such). In singling out the movements made obsolete by technological advances, she was touting a transformation of self that's achieved by fleetingly capturing the movements of an outmoded holistic agricultural tradition. Like many others in her generation influenced by the prominent 19th-century social critics Thomas Carlyle, John Ruskin, and William Morris, who, in their opposition to large-scale mechanization, sought to make England organic through emphasizing a model of work based on preindustrial society, she championed preindustrial modes of work as being truer to the rhythms of life. (In her yearning for a halcyon past, Morgan omitted even hints of the grimness of preindustrial times, when the lives of most of her European ancestors, whether in villages, towns, or cities, were impoverished, unsanitary, violent, and oppressed.) This nostalgia for the vast period preceding industrialization defines modernity perhaps as much as the aspiration to make everything new.

Not that nostalgia for an unexperienced and idealized rural life (whose eulogized simplicity, serenity, and spirituality contrast positively against the complexity, anxiety, fragmentation, and alienation of contemporary life) is anything new. Although we may associate the origins of pastoralism with Wordsworth, Thoreau, and others, the yearning for previous simpler times in European culture goes back (in literature) at least as far as the bucolic poems of Theocritus, composed in the 3rd century BC.

Nor was admiration for the folk—the common people of society considered to be the representatives of a traditional way of life—uncommon to Morgan's generation. In fact, it was widespread in culture and politics in countries around the world during the 1930s. The concept of *Volk* (which adds to *folk* the idea of the superiority of the entire German culture) had been important in Germany since the early 19th century. In writing about the milieu in which the Grimm brothers collected fairy tales, which culminated with the publication of their two-volume *Nursery and Household Tales* in 1812 and 1815, journalist Joan Acocella writes: "The Grimms grew up in the febrile atmosphere of German Romanticism, which involved intense nationalism and, in support of that, a fascination with the supposedly deep, pre-rational culture of the German peasantry, the *Volk*."[37]

We would be wrong, however, to dismiss Morgan's encouraging us to partake of "the full cycle of human activity" during *surya namaskar* as solely a fantasy about escaping from modern realities by bringing the common people and other human types to life.

It's said that during *samyama*—the three interiorized stages of classical yoga: *dharana* (concentration), *dhyana* (absorption), and *samadhi* (integration)—the advanced yogin acquires *siddhis,* miraculous powers, by assimilating an object or idea through fully identifying with it. The historian of religion Mircea Eliade describes these *siddhis:* "By practicing *samyama* on the distinction between 'object' and 'idea,'

the yogin knows the cries of all creatures. By practicing *samyama* in regard to subconscious residues (*samskaras*), he knows his previous existences. Through *samyama* exercised in respect to 'notions' (*pratyaya*) [ideas], he knows the 'mental states' of other men."[38]

In taking possession of the archetypes present in *surya namaskar,* Morgan unknowingly updated these *siddhis.* Her suprapowers are admittedly a diminished version of the traditional yogic occult powers. But then, the *siddhis* aren't real (they could be the basis for an exciting graphic novel about a yogin superhero), and Morgan's *surya namaskar* practice was limited by reality. What's more, she identified with other human beings through a more radical means than mere thought projection: fleshing out their movements.

One might think that Morgan would've singled out modern dance, which is far more expressive than *surya namaskar,* as a vehicle for inhabiting the being of others. Whereas modern dance can create an infinite variety of detailed, vivid gestures and movements to portray life's diverse fundamental activities, *surya namaskar* is limited to a few crisp, abstract, formulaic movements. In contrast to the swirls and leaps of some modern dance, most of the stages of *surya namaskar*—especially the bending down, kneeling on one knee with the hands on the floor, and lying facedown on the floor positions—are decidedly earthbound. And, unlike most modern dance, the movements of *surya namaskar* form a loop: the same movements are endlessly repeated. But it's exactly their qualities of distillation, groundedness, and repetition that seem to have led Morgan to assert the resemblance of the *surya namaskar* positions to the "full cycle of human activity," making *surya namaskar* a repository of "hundreds of generations of human experience." (Although Morgan herself might be hard-pressed to make an exact correlation between the particular bodily movements she itemizes and the movements of *surya namaskar*.)

When performing the positions of *surya namaskar*, we put aside everyday concerns in order to recollect our fundamental nature as members of the human race. Like attending a play, going to the movies, or reading a novel, performing *surya namaskar*, Morgan wanted people to understand, is a life lesson—not one for making us virtuous (compassionate, courageous, just, and the like) but one for making us spirited and whole.

Blank Slate

Morgan reassured her Christian readers in *The Ten-Point Way to Health* that they wouldn't be committing blasphemy when they practiced *surya namaskar:* "Let us emphasize here, for those who would be inclined to object to Surya Namaskars on the ground that they are religious rite, *that they have the appearance only of a religious rite.*"[39] In order to appeal to those nonbelievers whose health would improve by taking up the exercises, Bhavanarao said much the same thing. But, in truth, as he also proudly acknowledged, his practice was permeated with elements of the Hindu path to salvation, most conspicuously chanting *bija* and Vedic mantras. Despite the inclusion of two abbreviated chapters on chanting in the new book, Morgan reassured her readers in the introduction that "the *mantras* are essentially non-religious, and owe none of their virtues to a religious source."[40]

In stripping *surya namaskar* of all traces of the Hinduism, Morgan wasn't merely making the exercise safe for non-Hindus to perform; she was emptying the mind of the practitioner of *surya namaskar* of any preconceptions about the practice, creating a tabula rasa, upon which impressions could be recorded by the experience of the exercise itself, leading to a transcendence of everyday life. These impressions were based on a new epistemology.

24

LOUISE MORGAN

Becoming Aware of the Body in *Surya Namaskar*

Enthrallment with Human Motion

Between the 1830s and 1860s in the West, there was a rage for optical entertainment simulating motion. Hundreds of toys were manufactured that used phase drawings to produce the illusion of continuity of motion. One of the most popular was William George Horner's zoetrope, which mounted drawings on the inside of a rotating cylinder watched through a series of slots. The faster the cylinder was turned, the more seamlessly flowing the movement appeared.

In his motion studies begun in 1872, Eadweard Muybridge recorded continuous live action in a series of still photographs for the first time—not in order to simulate continuous motion but to dissect motion. Viewers were just as astonished by the successive, separate, minute stages of animal and human motion captured in Muybridge's photographs as they were by the fleeting landscapes seen outside train windows. In his serial photographs of naked people (all seeming to be not models or nudists but victims of an outbreak of contagious sleep walking)—such as a woman walking, sprinkling water from a basin, and turning around, a child ascending steps, and a man (Muybridge himself!) sprinting—Muybridge didn't so much closely observe as analyze bodily movement. He didn't so much slow down or even stop time as reveal moments between time.

An unprecedented fascination with human movement, in particular, was one of the critical elements of modernity. From the mid-19th to the early

20th century, the urge to perform movements or witness the performance of movements was the underlying impulse that led to the proliferation of traveling circuses (featuring acrobats, trapeze artists, and tightrope walkers); the burgeoning of knockabout vaudeville acts; the craze for physical recreation (e.g., bicycling, hiking, and gymnastics) as a means of personal regeneration; the invention of the movies; the revival of the Olympics; the mania for extravagant celebratory parades (the procession as bold social narrative); the popularity of sports spectacles (e.g., boxing matches and football games), in which the cultural conflict between ascendant middle-class values and nostalgia for preindustrial manly values was enacted; and the emergence of uninhibited dances.

This enthrallment with human movement could also be found in an intense scientific exploration of how our body moves. Such groundbreaking research was performed as the German physiologist Adolf Eugen Fick's 1867 differentiation between isotonic contraction (muscle contraction that causes bones to move—roll, slide, and spin—at their joints) and isometric contraction (muscular contraction that is not accompanied by joint movement); the French anatomist Louis-Antoine Ranvier's observation in 1873 that red muscles contract in a slower, more sustained manner than white muscles; and German anatomists Christian Wilhelm Braune and Otto Fischer's experimental studies of human gait (an analysis of subjects freely walking or walking with a heavy and bulky load—the field equipment of a German infantryman), the results of which were published from 1895 to 1904. (In subsequent decades, the application of physiologi-

cal, anatomical, kinesiological, and mechanical principles to bodily movement would be used to improve physical performance in sports, fitness, and physical therapy.)

This captivation with human movement could also be found in a startlingly new direction of scientific inquiry: not into how our body moves but into how we know our body moves.

Proprioception

"The surface field [on which the body's sensory receptor organs are distributed] lies freely open to the numberless vicissitudes of the environment," declaimed the English physiologist Charles Scott Sherrington in a lecture, part of his "Integrative Action of the Nervous System" series given at Yale University in 1905. "It has felt for countless ages the full stream of the varied agencies forever pouring upon it from the outside world. This field, *extero-ceptive* as it may be called, is rich in the number and variety of receptors which adaptation has evolved in it."[1] These receptors are found in the sense organs that detect light, sound, odor, and tactile stimuli: the eyes, ears, nose, and skin. A second receptive field, "though in contact with the environment, lies however less freely open to it": the *intero-ceptive* field.[2] The receptors in this field are located in the taste organs of the mouth.

But there exists a third primary field, Sherrington newly maintained—one fundamentally different from the others and hitherto unexamined because it's totally closed to "the numberless vicissitudes of the environment." "The receptors which lie in the depth of the organism are adapted for excitation consonantly with changes going on in the organism itself, particularly in its muscles and their accessory organs (tendons, joints, blood-vessels, etc). Since in this field the stimuli to the receptors are given by the organism itself, their field may be called the *proprio-ceptive* field [*proprio* is derived from the Latin word *proprius,* meaning "own"]."[3] In coining the term *proprioception,* Sherrington was identifying and initiating an exploration of our ability to sense our body's movement, joint position, and equilibrium—even in the dark.

Along with the sensory system of the skin that detects pressure (light or deep), temperature (warm or cold), and pain (including itch and tickle), proprioception is part of the somatosensory—nonvisceral—system. (Internal sensory information, such as a fluttering heart, an urge to evacuate the bowels, or a stomachache, forms the visceral sensory system.) The somatosensory system, together with the visual and vestibular systems, contributes to the maintenance of upright posture and movement by providing information about the relative location of the body—information that originates with muscles and joints and is aided by the skin, eyes, and vestibules of the ears.

Unlike autonomic reflexes (Sherrington's other major area of study), such as the increase in heart rate when we rapidly rise from a bath, the secretion of saliva when we bite into an apple, and the jerk of our leg when it's tapped with a medical hammer just below the knee, which are automatic, our largely unconscious perceptions of our everyday movements can be brought to consciousness and controlled. This new observation in physiology led to a dynamic conception of bodily movement, orientation, and balance in several applied fields—a concep-

tion that was paralleled in psychology, where an emphasis on the functions of the mind was giving way to a focus on the turmoil of the mind, the powerful unconscious drives and conflicts explored by psychoanalysis. Whereas psychoanalysis aimed to make unconscious motivations, formed in childhood, conscious in order to form rational motivational behavior, various popular proprioceptive disciplines, from types of dance to muscle control (a type of bodybuilding) to physical therapy to postural work, sought to bring habitually underutilized or deformed unconscious movements to awareness in order create a harmonious arrangement between the skeletal and muscular systems. Thusly, the fascination with human movement—in particular, with how the body moves and how we know it moves—developed into a 20th-century preoccupation with treating flawed bodily movements through close observation and resolute remedial action. The seminal figure in this cause was F. M. Alexander.

Attention to Ordinary Movements

After studying the "histrionic arts" (recitation and acting), young Frederick Matthias Alexander (1869–1955) began his career in earnest as a reciter and elocution teacher in 1895 in Melbourne, Australia. (Attaining a cultured voice was part of the Australian fashion for wanting to appear to belong to Great Britain's upper middle class.) His teachings were based on the Delsarte method of public speaking, which emphasized highly stylized gestures.

After a few successful years, Alexander, to his dismay, progressively lost his voice while reciting (but not when conversing). "I was told by my friends that when I was reciting my breathing was audible, and that they could hear me (as they put it) 'gasping' and 'sucking in air' through my mouth," he recalled. "This worried me even more than my actual throat trouble."[4] To relieve his faulty breathing and hoarseness, he turned to doctors and voice trainers. When all medical treatments and advice proved unsuccessful, he began to study his recitation mechanics. Following months of experimentation using full-length and hand mirrors, he discovered that when he kept his head from going back, he was able to perform without being plagued by throat problems. This simple observation by a man who'd lost his voice was part of the historic modernist shift in interest from end result to process (especially flaunted by some painters and novelists, who emphasized representation itself over the thing represented).

By 1910, with the publication of his first book, *Man's Supreme Inheritance* (a reference to the body, consciously controlled through thought and action), Alexander had turned from promoting elocution to ardently studying ordinary activities in order to learn and teach the mechanisms involved in carrying them out. "He occupied himself with breathing, sitting down, getting up, standing, walking and the other humble, inconsidered, and often despised small activities . . . which occupy the time of all human creatures," wrote Louise Morgan in her 1954 book *Inside Yourself: A New Way to Health Based on the Alexander Technique*. "He treated them as if they really were important. . . . He illumined them with the light of his genius, gave them a glow of the freshness which is found in the field flower as well as the exhibition rose."[5]

Alexander used his close observations to help people cure bodily disorders (a stiff neck, restricted breathing, a dragging leg, and the like) by improving their ingrained poor habits of standing, sitting, and moving. The identification of unconscious movement habits as the cause of ailments and, logically enough, of changing muscle patterns as the remedy were part of the modernist impulse to emphasize self-struggle over acceptance of habit, rules, ritual, and tradition (fig. 24.1).

Changing how we stand, sit, and move is an oddly difficult endeavor, even when we receive verbal instructions from someone, watch someone modeling correct movements, and/or look at ourselves in a mirror. "Correcting the movements carried out by our proprioceptive reflexes is something like trying to reset a machine, whose works are intangible, and the net output all we know of the running," Sherrington observed. The great English neurophysiologist recognized Alexander's contribution to finding a solution for bettering our breathing, standing, sitting, and walking, which, although innate, "suffer from defects in our ways of doing them."[6] "Mr. Alexander had done a service to the subject by insistently treating each act as involving the whole integrated individual, the whole psycho-physical man. To take a step is an affair not of this or that limb solely, but of the total neuro-muscular activity of the moment—not least of the head and the neck."[7]

An example of Alexander's attentiveness to the process of an everyday activity that involves the whole body may be found in his meticulous prescription for correctly sitting down in a chair. He instructs us to stand with our head forward and up, neck relaxed, spine lengthened, and

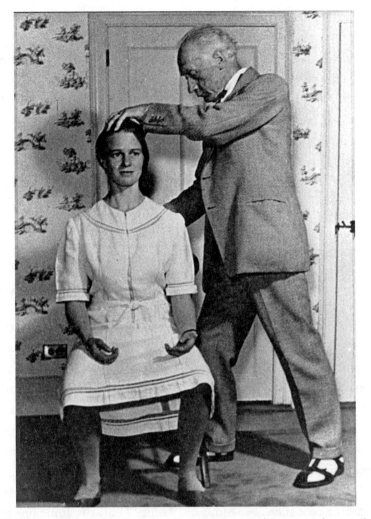

Figure 24.1. F. M. Alexander using light hand contact to guide the posture of a seated woman at the Whitney Homestead in Stow, Massachusetts, which served as his headquarters from the end of January 1941 to September 1942, during his exile from England

(© 2016 The Society of Teachers of the Alexander Technique, London)

back wide. Then place our knees forward and apart, bring our hips back, and, while keeping our spine at its greatest possible length, move our torso forward, at which point, in Morgan's felicitous words, we "glide weightlessly into the chair, feeling very pleased with [our]self."[8]

Recognizing the momentousness of his modest observations, Morgan credited Alexander (whose technique she was first attracted to around 1953 out of her long concern with bodily awareness) with being "the first to experiment on the living human being, noting minutely the behaviour of living tissue over extensive periods of time. It meant a succession of sustained, accurate, and carefully co-ordinated observations requiring the most concentrated attention because the muscles observed were not only alive, but in action."[9]

Morgan also scrutinized our experience of movement, not in any innate activity but in the formalized exercise *surya namaskar,* sun salutations. Like Alexander, she had a utilitarian goal: correcting form. But she also had a wildly more ambitious goal: applying an unprecedented attentiveness to the three elements of *surya namaskar* (standing still, breathing, and moving) as a means of transforming everyday life—at least for a while.

Applying Awareness to *Surya Namaskar*

According to Morgan, *surya namaskar* isn't just exercise but is an experience of "seeming miracles," when we have "a glorious sense of freedom, power, and happiness."[10] Her description of this process of transformation starts with the systematic stiffening of the body during the first position, called *Tadasana,* Mountain Pose, in yoga, but which Morgan visualized as standing like a tree: "Now, stiffen your whole body, beginning with the feet. Push them into the floor as if you were taking root there.... Move gradually up to the top of the head, concentrating on each separate part that is being stiffened, doing it slowly and deliberately. *You will thus become aware of every muscle in your body*" [italics added].[11]

Morgan next recommended the commencement of deep rhythmic breathing (an activity evidently so foreign to her British readers that she was occasioned to wryly remark, "Some never take a deep breath except once a year, while on holiday, and then only a few"[12]). "Without the breathing," Morgan cautioned, "Surya Namaskars . . . would act like a smol-

dering rather than a clearly burning fire."[13] To get them to breathe properly, she challenged her readers to behave in a manner that they surely found uncouth: "Keeping stiff, begin to breathe as you have never breathed before. . . . Breathe in through the nose as deeply and quietly as possible, and then out through the mouth with a loud sharp gust. Grunt a bit at the end to expel the last bit of bad air."[14] But the breathing cannot be mindless. "*You first must become aware of your breath,*" Morgan sternly cautioned (in one of her few uses of italics for emphasis in *The Ten-Point Way to Health*). "*You cannot drink deep of a healing draught that you do not know is there.*"[15]

This deep nasal breathing isn't for the lackadaisical: it's dynamic and forceful. But for those who practice it, the value is great. Right there in the alveolar region of the lungs, not only is pure air exchanged for foul air by diffusion between the gaseous external environment and our blood, but the rhythmic breath, Morgan maintained, permeates through matter into our fundamental or essential nature—our being. "This rhythmic breathing is the secret of the wonderful power of the exercises to revitalize the system. Let it pervade your being."[16]

Then Morgan turned to the movements. We're usually aware of our muscles only when we feel discomfort in them (muscle soreness is a common cause for complaint among those who exercise rigorously). So we'd rather have as little sense of our muscles as possible. But in her instructions for performing the active positions of *surya namaskar,* Morgan cheerily asked her readers to embrace, not avoid, the ensuing discomfort, and thus transform it into pleasure. "By now you will be feeling the existence of muscles you were never before aware of," Morgan enthused.[17]

Morgan brought awareness not only to the sensations of muscular contraction and elongation (tension and relaxation) but also to the movements (permitted by joints) of the trunk, head, and limb in space, as is evidenced by the fervor of her newspaper-series instructions for taking the positions of *surya namaskar:* "throw your head down as a fisherman flings his bait into a stream," "knit [the positions] together with a kind of pumping rhythm until movement and breathing follow in one even flow—down-up, down-up, out-in, out-in,"[18] "raise your body without bending [your] arms, and push [your] left leg back,"[19] "drop flat on the floor, touching forehead, nose, chest, knees, toes, but not the abdomen," and "throw [your] chest out, curve [your] back and look up at [the] ceiling, stretching [your] neck back as far as you can."[20] For her, awareness was gained not through close attention to the subtle movements of the positions of *surya namaskar* (such as, during the *Adho Mukha Svanasana,* Downward Facing Dog, pressing down on the heel and palm of the hands, rotating the arms externally, and keeping the coccyx pointing up) but through performing them with panache.

Surya Namaskar as Vehicle of Meditation

Although the apprehension of ultimate realities may occur at any time, in the Hindu tradition transcendence of the everyday world is systematically aided through meditation. In order to facilitate stopping the mind's fluctuations (the precondition for comprehending realities

underlying appearances), the yogin fixes his body in an immobile, hieratic seated position (thereby putting an end to the functional and expressive mobility of the body) and concentrates on a single thing—a mantra, a mandala, glowing coals, an image of a god, or even parts of the body (e.g., the navel, solar plexus, forehead, tip of the nose, tip of the tongue, or area between the eyebrows). Although based on the sun worship ritual, *surya namaskar* appears to be an unlikely vehicle for meditation because it is, after all, a series of vigorous movements, while meditation is traditionally and typically quiescent. Bhavanarao Pant Pratinidhi primarily compensated for possible distractions caused by the movements by chanting seed mantras. Morgan endorsed their use but assured her readers that "the mantras are essentially non-religious." They're merely used by custom: "The recitation of the *mantras,* which are certain syllables so ancient that they have lost their meaning, invariably accompanies" movement in Eastern exercises.[21]

Bhavanarao also used imagery to secure undivided attention of the mind. When standing with the hands folded in supplication during the first and last *surya namaskar* stages, he said, one should concentrate on "an image of the Sun, a tutelary or guardian deity, a swastika, or a white circular spot, hung up in front."[22] Morgan gave a nod to using secularized imagery to facilitate concentration: "Have a picture of something or someone of significance to you hung up on the wall before you. Or on a piece of cardboard paint a sun or a star or a circle in a vivid colour or colours and put that up in front of you."[23] But her enthusiasm was clearly for attentiveness to something else: the moving body itself coordinated with rhythmic breathing.

Performing the series of flowing *surya namaskar* positions engenders transcendence, Morgan argued, not by concentration—in the sense of focused attention—on a single object, such as a mantra, sacred image, the isolated breath, or a part of the body, but by awareness of an expanded field of attention, in this case, our bodily sensations—in particular, of muscles contracting and elongating and, in general, of movement patterns—as they arise moment by moment in the course of moving into and out of the positions. Whereas previously S. Sundaram, who wrote the first modern hatha yoga manual, drew attention to the still body during *Savasana*, Corpse Pose, making it the object of meditation, Morgan expanded the scope of bodily awareness to the moving body in *surya namaskar* (and, by extension, to the moving body in *asana*), making it the object of meditation.

Embodied Transcendence

Whereas before the late 19th and early 20th centuries knowledge of the human body was primarily gained through authority, rational thought, empirical observation, and experimentation, over the course of the 20th century there was a growing emphasis on the subjective experience of the body—on direct personal awareness of one's still and moving body. From the late 19th century to the present, various disciplines promoting awareness of one's body as the means to becoming truly alive or enlightened have captivated coteries in the West: gymnastics (e.g., Delsarte gymnastics); dance (e.g., Rudolf Laban's teachings); bodywork (e.g., the Alexander technique, Gurdjieff's work, the Feldenkrais method, Hellerwork, the Trager approach, and Rolfing); martial arts (e.g., kalaripayattu and t'ai chi); psychology (e.g., Wilhelm Reich's therapy and Alexander Lowen's bioenergetics); religion (e.g., Zen Buddhism and Taoism); and philosophy (e.g., existentialism and phenomenology). These disciplines all hold (or are interpreted to hold) that the self consists of a mind and body that form a single organic whole and that (sometimes harsh) training (or, perhaps more accurately said, retraining) and (sometimes intense) exploration of the body are needed to transform human beings. As Aldous Huxley writes in his foreword to Morgan's *Inside Yourself:* "Most civilised men and women make use of their organisms in ways which positively guarantee them against the perfect functioning of the mind-body. . . . F. M. Alexander has devoted the greater part of a long and fruitful life to the task of showing his fellows how to maintain, and, where necessary, how to restore the proper use of the self."[24]

In the late 20th century subjective experience grounded in proprioception—drawing attention to the sensations produced by even the slightest of one's movements—became a common feature of modern hatha yoga (which foregrounds *asana*), influenced (directly or indirectly) by bodywork, Taoist meditation, and the like, as well as the profoundly detail-oriented teachings of yoga master B. K. S. Iyengar. This approach is found most prominently in the teachings of the lyrical philosopher-yogin Vanda Scaravelli, an Iyengar disciple, who called on students in her classes to "delight in the body's unfolding."[25] This attentiveness to the body, which keeps the mind from wandering, gave late 20th-century hatha yoga, no matter what the school (whether static or dynamic), an inward dimension—a tendency toward the meditative.

Morgan had already brought this subjective, inward-turning experience of the body to *surya namaskar* in 1938. But whereas the yoga teachers of the late 20th century would have the goal of finding pleasure in one's movements, overcoming unconscious habits of inattention to live more fully in the moment or opening oneself up to one's true self, she used awareness of the moving body, coordinated with the breath, in *surya namaskar* as a meditation technique that connected one to the rhythms of the universe.

In our daily lives, our movements are in service of quotidian needs. We sit down in a chair at the kitchen table to have dinner, step back in the face of implacable danger, run to catch a bus, shrug in bewilderment, point to a landmark, or embrace an old friend. In contrast, the movements of *surya namaskar,* Morgan maintained, when performed in a session set aside during the day, create a time of heightened reality, during which we experience a series of epiphanies. What gives the movements of *surya namaskar* this capacity for amplitude—what distinguishes the movements of *surya namaskar* from the movements of everyday life (and those of most exercises, sports, and dance)—is their strenuous, comprehensive, repetitive, rhythmical, and continuous (some might say boring and exhausting) nature.

The set of yoga-like positions practiced seriatim that make up *surya namaskar* are taxing; they demand from practitioners a great physical effort that is rare in everyday life. Because they're full body movements, they involve all the major muscles of the body. They're repeated in the same order, in the same space (virtually, on the ground we stand on), and at the same tempo. They form a pattern by alternating up and down, back and forth, bending and straightening, and pulling and pushing movements. Springing from each other, they're uninterrupted, so there's no lag time between positions, and therefore no extraneous movement.

Because the pace is always the same, movement and breath in *surya namaskar* can easily be coordinated. Morgan provided a handy list for her newspaper readers that distills the movement/breath pattern for the ten *surya namaskar* positions:

1	Stand (in).
2	Double over (out).
3	Left leg back (in).
4	Inverted V (hold).
5	Flat on floor (out).
6	Trunk raised on arms (in).
7	Inverted V (hold).
8	Right leg back (hold).
9	Double over (out).
10	Stand (in).[26]

Morgan, whose idyllic childhood was spent "in New England, in a small town on the edge of countryside, river, woods and sea,"[27] touted the expansion of consciousness to the natural world that occurs by matching the rhythm of the *surya namaskar* movements with the rhythm of breathing: "You will now feel the first sense of rhythmical well-being, as if your nerves had suddenly 'tuned-in' to the peaceful rhythm of the world of natural things like the stars, the tides, the changing of the seasons."[28] How odd! It's not stargazing, walking along the ocean's edge, or hiking in the woods that brings us closer to the natural world, in Morgan's view, but this weird Indian version of calisthenics that's usually practiced in a living room or studio or other interior space. What's more, Morgan saw *surya namaskar* as connecting us to more than nature. "When you can match the rhythm of your breathing with the rhythm of the exercises," she declared, ". . . you will feel rhythmic all over, and in accord with the great rhythm of life and the universe."[29]

Bhavanarao recommended performing *surya namaskar* while facing east, looking at an image of a Hindu symbol or deity and chanting *bija* mantras to unite with the cosmos. He believed that by uttering sound vibrations, we tune in to the cosmic vibrations. For Morgan, in contrast, attunement to the cosmic vibrations is attained not by repeatedly making a sound that emanates from the larynx and is articulated by the tongue, palate, cheeks, and lips but by repeatedly moving the body through the series of *asana*-like movements that make up *surya namaskar*. The *surya namaskar* movements themselves are a kind of chant. This is what Morgan meant, I think, when she likened the effect of *surya namaskar* to singing. "The great advantage of Surya Namaskars," Morgan exhorted us to recognize, "is that they do not over-develop some muscles and neglect others, but search out every cell and sinew in the body, rousing them and tuning them into harmony. They make the body sing."[30]

Just as song transforms mere words into heightened utterance, *surya namaskar* transforms mere exercise movement into vibrant motion that's in harmony with the vibrations of the universe. To unite with the cosmic vibrations, Morgan believed, we need only set our body aquiver through the vigorous, all-encompassing, repetitive, rhythmical flowing movements of *surya namaskar*. The experience of this vibratory attunement brings an overwhelming feeling of contentment.

25

APA PANT

Making *Surya Namaskar* into a Meditation

Conversion

Apa Pant (1912–1992) learned *surya namaskar* from his father, Bhavanarao Pant Pratinidhi, the rajah of Aundh, when he was four years old. The second eldest son of twelve children, Pant adored his father. "From no one could I have absorbed more 'radiation' [that is, radiance or resplendence] than I did from him," Pant reminisced, "and its source was a personality in which there was always something joyous and optimistic."[1] Even so, Pant, rebellious by nature, felt put upon when made to perform a ritual, or anything resembling a ritual. Throughout his youth, whenever he could get away with it, he avoided practicing *surya namaskars*. When obligated to perform them, he did so "badly, hurriedly, as if I were ashamed of doing them."[2] He preferred riding horses and elephants, hunting, swimming, and collecting mangoes from trees to eat in the summer.

At fifteen, Pant had a conversion to *surya namaskar*. Near death from pneumonia, he was asked by his father to promise that if he survived he would practice *surya namaskar* "as long as you live, everyday."[3] When he recovered, he not only kept his promise to practice *surya namaskar* daily, he found a way to do so without resentment. Having never truly perceived his father's practice of *surya namaskar* as ritual in the strict sense (even though for his father the practice had "a spiritual as well as physiological aspect, and especially so with him, for whom religion was so all-pervasive"[4]), after his illness Pant was able to practice *surya namaskar* wholeheartedly by emphasizing to himself that it was not a part of traditional Hindu observances:

> I gave the promise, and from the time when I got well I have kept it. I have written elsewhere of what these exercises . . . can do to tone up not only the physique but the whole personality. Since I did not see them in the same light as the ritualistic observances, and since I had promised my father, and since experience had taught me to value the *Surya Namaskars,* they were not included [in my mind] with the *pujas* and idol-worship against which I reacted so strongly. . . . What repelled me were the rituals that were carried out, for the most part, with no regard to their meaning . . . and those that were not devotional in a pure sense but carried out . . . to ask favours of some deity.[5]

By the mid-1930s, Bhavanarao seemed to have changed his tune about the necessity of performing large numbers of *surya namaskars* over an extended period of time. In his book *Surya Namaskars,* published in 1928, he advocated an arduous routine: "all persons above sixteen should gradually increase the number up to 300."[6] The exercise "requires from 15 to 30 minutes."[7] He repeated the recommendation of three hundred cycles in his second book, *The Ten-Point Way to Health,* published in 1938. But in her introduction to the book, its editor, journalist Louise Morgan, noted that in her interview with Bhavanarao in London in 1936, he had advocated a less demanding regime for (what she described as) the "series of exercises called 'Surya Namaskar,'

literally translated 'Sun Prayers'": "They were simplicity itself, he explained, taking only five or six minutes to complete a round of twenty-five cycles and requiring no sort of equipment whatever."[8]

This new recommendation of a short stint of *surya namaskar* was more than a reduction in number; it redefined the nature of *surya namaskar.* No longer defined as essentially an experience that enables us to transcend our quotidian existence—a rhythmic movement-plus-mantras that expands one's ordinary state of consciousness or even a long session of cardiorespiratory exercise that profoundly alters one's mood—*surya namaskar* could now be used as an exercise to improve activities of daily living.

Upon interviewing Pant (six weeks after interviewing his father) at a photo shoot for the illustrations for her series of articles about *surya namaskar* (these photos of Pant modeling the steps of *surya namaskar* were subsequently used for Bhavanarao's new book), Morgan learned that Pant, who was studying law in London, had discovered two uses for this shortened version of *surya namaskar:* as a pick-me-up and a calm-me-down. She gave an example of each. "Shrimant Appasahib [Pant] used [*surya namaskars*] as a tonic immediately after a hard day's sport, such as ski-ing [*sic*], to prevent soreness and fatigue," Morgan explained. (Performing a bout of *surya namaskars* is also "a tonic if done immediately after . . . a nerve-straining day in the office," she added.)[9] "They had also kept his nerves in good condition for his law examinations, he told me, removing all trace of uneasiness and clearing his brain."[10] Over time, people came to use a short period of *surya namaskar* not only as a restorative technique and a preventive sedative but as an invigorating wake-me-up morning exercise that boosts alertness throughtout the day.

Ambassador

After finishing his law studies in 1937, Pant returned to India to help his father with state work for the next ten years. On his seventieth birthday in November 1938, the rajah launched his majestic experiment in village democracy, the Aundh Experiment, by declaring his intention to relinquish all his powers in favor of self-rule by the people of his state. His experiment, for which he'd been making preparations for twenty years, was received with great enthusiasm. In the November 12, 1938, issue of his weekly English-language newspaper, *Harijan* (Children of God), Gandhi congratulated Bhavanarao on the "grant of a great charter of sovereignty to the people of Aundh, bestowed upon them without the usual process of struggle and revolution."[11]

Pant, who had encouraged his father to undertake the Aundh Experiment, was named prime minister and put in charge of implementing this extraordinary undertaking in village democracy. The charter stated, "Self-government implies self-control and self-sacrifice." Taking these values to heart, Pant set an example for others by intimately involving himself with the political and practical problems of the enterprise. "The Prime Minister's transparent simplicity and willingness to work hard for the good of all established the sincerity and credibility of the Aundh rulers and motivated the people to work hard too and make

their own contribution to the state of Aundh," Indira Rothermund, scholar of modern South Asian history, notes.[12]

Pant was not unaware of the privileges of his royal birth. He dedicated his memoir "to the proud and poor people of the Aundh villages, who for the first thirty years of my life toiled, sweated, went without food, to tolerate and provide my horses, elephants, cars, gliders, travels, play and study abroad." He considered the ten years he spent working for the people of Aundh—"wandering from village to village, inspired by their faith and dedication to democracy and their determination to do away with poverty"—to be a way of repaying his debts, "even though I may have failed adequately to do so."[13]

Yet the day of Indian independence, August 15, 1947, was met by Pant with mixed feelings. He rejoiced in India's long-sought sovereignty. Still, he wanted everything to continue as he had known it: "the horses, the elephants . . . the rituals, the kind, paternal, relaxed atmosphere of an extended family that allowed the democratic experiment to come into being. I could not think of the absorption of Aundh in an impersonal, bureaucratic system."[14] Aundh was officially incorporated into free India on March 8, 1948.

Perhaps in order to escape becoming an exile in his ancestral homeland, Pant, along with his wife, Nalini, and two children, Aditi and Aniket (he would later have a third child, Avalokita), left Aundh. "I could not believe that I was leaving Aundh for good," he recalled about the actual move, made at the end of 1947. "All the pots and pans, beds and cupboards and chairs were loaded on to an Aundh state red-number-plate truck (official vehicles had a red license plate embossed with the emblem of India in gold)." The family moved to Pune, where Nalini started practicing medicine and surgery. Living in a house that she had built on a family plot, the thirty-five-year-old Pant, who had no job or mission, was lost and depressed. "I tried to settle down to a routine. . . . I did not know what to do." He "retired," as he put it, "into my minuscule ego."[15]

In December 1947, Pant was summoned to meet with Jawaharlal Nehru, the prime minister of the new Indian nation, in Bombay. Nehru offered him the diplomatic post of commissioner of India to East Africa: "Apa, go to East Africa as our first ambassador there."[16] Pant felt unworthy to take the position. Despite his doubts ("The doors that open unexpectedly are not always easy to pass through"), he accepted.[17] "Ambassador? I was to be an Ambassador? I should have shouted for joy, but didn't feel like it. . . . My ego would take a while to assert itself again."[18]

Pant boarded the ship for Kenya in August 1948, with only a private secretary accompanying him. Even before the ship left port, he felt forlorn. He wept. "I missed Aundh, Baba [a term of endearment for a father], Nalini, Aditi and little Aniket, our son who was then just a year and a half old."[19] Sacrificing her position at a hospital and her private practice, his wife, along with the children, would join him in the next year (fig. 25.1).

Pant's career as a diplomat would span Africa, Asia, and Europe. His posts included being India's political officer in the Himalayan states of Sikkim and Bhutan (giving him the opportunity to visit Tibet, where he met the Dalai Lama, whom he would receive in 1959 at Siliguri in India after the Lhasa revolt against the Chinese) and high commissioner to the United Kingdom. These positions provided him with the opportunity to practice *surya namaskar* "almost all over the world—[including] Lhasa [the city in Tibet that's the seat of the Dalai Lama], Svalbard [an archipelago in the Arctic Ocean about midway between Norway and the North Pole], Bhutan, Borneo, almost on top of Mt. Kenya, in deserts, in the open air, on ships, decks, in railway carriages, in palaces and huts."[20]

In India, during the period of the Aundh Experiment, Pant had not only practiced *surya namaskar* but also helped carry on his father's *surya namaskar* legacy by presenting lectures/demonstrations in India. (Upon attending one of the events that Pant gave in colleges in Bangalore in 1938, Swami Sivananda remarked, "The Prince of Aundh, like his father, is a great votary of Suryanamaskar."[21]) Wherever he was assigned as a diplomat, Pant not only practiced but also continued demonstrating and teaching *surya namaskar*. Singapore's ambassador, Lee Khoon Choy, conjures up a picture of Pant and his teaching during his ambassadorship to Egypt from 1966 to 1969:

The Indian Ambassador Apa Pant was from a royal family and was a yogi. He was slim and tall, always wearing a collarless Indian coat. Every Wednesday morning, we would go to his residence for yoga lessons which he described as Surianamaskar [*sic*], and then adjourn to an Indian breakfast. The exercises involved fast breathing which necessitated contracting the stomach and a lot of bending

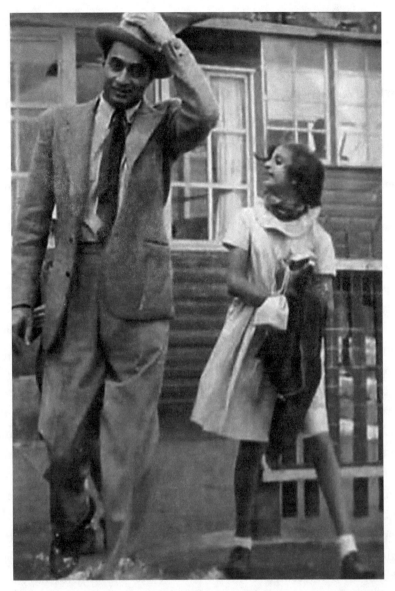

Figure 25.1. Apa Pant with his older daughter and son (behind him) in Kenya, 1954
(With the kind permission of Benegal Pereira)

of the knees. He wrote a book on Suriana-maskar [sic] translated into Arabic. Several Ambassadors from the European countries including the Dutch and Canadian Ambassadors attended the functions. The breakfast consisted of little Indian tit-bits and "Puttumayam" which I enjoyed very much.[22]

From reading this delightful anecdote about Pant imposing the burdensome task of performing this strange exercise, *surya namaskar,* on his fellow ambassadors and then rewarding them with tasty breakfast treats once a week at his living quarters in Cairo, one might dismiss Pant's *surya namaskar* practice—and his privileged life—as a frivolous, blithe pursuit. But one would be mistaken.

World Weariness

Pant said about B. K. S. Iyengar, the renowned yoga teacher (with whom Pant became good friends when, in his retirement, he settled in Pune, where Iyengar taught): "Yoga is to join the limited to the unlimited, the finite to the infinite. The human consciousness when it is circumscribed and limited is full of contradictions, confusion and sorrow. To release human consciousness from this confinement is the task of Yoga. No one can do it better than Mr. Iyengar."[23]

In making this eloquent tribute to Iyengar, Pant projected onto Iyengar's discipline, yoga, his philosophy of his own discipline, *surya namaskar*—and revealed "the contradictions, confusion and sorrow" of his own mental state. He attributed his inner turmoil to the dark side of human nature that he'd relentlessly encountered as a diplomat. "Often among the experiences that have come to me in such variety and abundance I felt myself reduced to despair. I felt exhausted, sad, futile, lost. I asked myself whether it was all worthwhile. I wandered in bewilderment through what seemed endless corridors of corruption and power mania and sorrow and hypocrisy."[24] He also attributed his despondency to modern society: "In the modern world of constant and continuous sensations, noise, hurry, and insecurity, fear and loneliness is the lot of man."[25] Yet one can't help but think that the anguish of this cordial, polished, gregarious diplomat can also be attributed to a more personal etiology from his childhood. He was haunted by the death of his mother (his "real" mother, as he often called his natural mother to distinguish her from his father's young second wife), who died when he wasn't yet three. And he was recurrently overcome by a dread of losing his beloved father "who had protected me ever since my mother had died"[26] ("To imagine that my father would die—an idea that comes sometimes in every childhood—used to put me in a panic"[27]). Having his homeland (as he knew it) taken from him when he was in his early thirties must've evoked in Pant his childhood sense of deep loss and great fear of more loss.

Not that Pant had what psychiatrists diagnose as major depressive disorder. His condition wasn't a biological illness. And there's no indication that his ability to function in the world was impaired. (He didn't stay in bed all morning, have a debilitating sense of worthlessness, have a markedly diminished sense of pleasure in things, make plans to kill himself, or the like.) Quite the contrary. He energetically carried out his duties to family and country throughout his entire middle age and remained spirited into his old age. Although he divulged his loss of hope and confidence in his memoir, the melancholically (or perhaps spiritually) titled *A Moment in Time,* he seems to have tactfully hidden it from others in his private and public life. Pant's despair may be characterized as what from 1869 (when the term was first used to describe a clinical entity) to the early 1940s (when the term fell out of use) was called "neurasthenia," or nervous exhaustion, perhaps caused by his having to deal with endless crises, but it is better characterized, in order to encompass all his life's experiences, as a profound weariness, what we call "a heavy heart."

No wonder Pant was gradually turning to *surya namaskar* as a means of salvation—and turning *surya namaskar* into a means of salvation for all.

"A Short Note on Surya Namaskars"

In the spring of 1962, about twenty-five years after they'd met in London, Pant and Morgan became briefly reacquainted. Pant had written to J. M. Dent & Sons on May 9 to propose a new foreword for his father's second book, *The Ten-Point Way to Health*. The editorial director, E. F. Bozman, handed the matter over to Morgan. In a typewritten memo, Morgan wistfully wrote to "Boz" that Pant, Bhavanarao's favorite son, was "the wonderful creature who posed for the photographs in The Ten-Point Way." Still lost in her reverie, she added in a handwritten postscript that Pant "must be in his 50's. He looked like Eternal Youth."[28]

In her decorous response to Pant's query, Morgan, perhaps assuming that Pant wouldn't remember her, didn't mention having met him. "[The editorial director of the House of Dent] has asked me to reply to you, as one who has met and spoken with your revered Father, the Rajah of Aundh," she wrote, "and I am happy and honoured to do so." She turned down Pant's proposal, though, apologetically explaining that a new edition of the book had just been published.* "This is most unfortunate. If only your offer had come earlier!"[29] She asked if she might read his new foreword anyway.

Clearly excited to hear from Morgan, Pant wrote in his next letter on June 22, "I never imagined that I would be in touch with you again. I well remember the day when you dragged me up to be photographed for the illustrations in the book 'The Ten-Point Way to Health.'"[30] Lamentably, Morgan's June 28, 1962, response to Pant's letter is missing from her papers; I think we can safely assume, though, that it was equally heartfelt and joyous. Their meeting in 1936 was evidently indelible to both of them.

Disappointed to learn that a new edition of the book had just been printed, Pant nevertheless told Morgan, "If you still think that what I have written would be of some interest to you from the point of view of the book, I would send it on to you."[31] Responding to her subsequent reaffirmation of her desire to read the foreword (evidently expressed in the missing letter), on July 13 Pant sent Morgan "A Short Note on Surya Namaskars—A Yogic Exercise." In his cover letter, he justified his reason for having written this introductory note: "The first part of it is a repetition of the description of the exercises which appear in the book, but the last part on realisation and meditation is, I think, somewhat of a new approach."[32]

"Mind is . . . a mere succession of rapidly changing sensations . . . plus a memory . . . of these

---

*"Most unfortunately and tragically for a great many people, the great Liberal newspaper, the News Chronicle, founded by Charles Dickens, that great humanitarian as well as artist, was closed down without warning, overnight, in 1961," she explained. "References to it had naturally to be removed from the text of 'The Ten Point Way to Health,' and as soon as possible. A new edition containing the necessary changes has only just appeared" (Morgan to Pant, May 20, 1962 [misdated], from the Louise Morgan and Otto Theis papers).

sensations," Pant explained in "A Short Note." The "'Ego' or the 'I' which is just a 'habit' or is really fictitious, wants to . . . perpetuate the pleasurable sensations. . . . [and] desires to end, as quickly as possibly, less pleasurable or troublesome or irritable sensations." The desire to continue pleasurable sensations and discontinue unpleasurable sensations "binds the 'Ego' to the sensations. . . . This is attachment."[33] Through concentrating on both the movements of the body and the fluctuations of the mind while performing *surya namaskar,* Pant maintained, "you experience the fact of this matter." You realize that the "I" is "false, empty, impermanent and binding. The moment you realize the Truth of this, there is instantaneous Liberation."[34]

What's utterly remarkable about this run-of-the-mill exposition of yogic philosophy is its application to *surya namaskar,* which Pant redefines as a kind of moving yogic meditation practice—just as critical a turn in the reconciliation between the decades-old rivals *surya namaskar* and hatha yoga as Krishnamacharya's using *surya namaskar* to link yogic conditioning postures to create a flowing yoga (see chapter 19) and Sivananda's using *surya namaskar* as a dynamic warm-up exercise to raise the heart rate and stretch muscles in preparation for performing static yogic conditioning postures (see chapter 26).

What differentiates yoga from other Indian philosophies is its "application of a series of techniques, all of which, broadly speaking, aim at annihilating the psychomental flux,

undertake to 'arrest' it," explains historian of religion Mircea Eliade.[35] Determined and continuous concentration on a single point—the central technique—cannot be obtained without the practice of numerous ancillary techniques. It cannot be obtained, Eliade argues, "if, for example, the body is in a tiring or even uncomfortable posture, or if the respiration is disorganized, unrhythmical."[36] Yoga technique, properly speaking, begins (as described in Patanjali's *Yoga Sutra*) with sitting in a stable and effortless posture and breathing rhythmically.

Pant argued that *surya namaskar*—a sequence of a dozen or so positions performed as one continuous exercise—is a technique that's just as suitable (if not more so) for achieving self-realization as a still, seated position (such as *Padmasana,* Lotus Posture), because performing, say, twelve or even four rounds of *surya namaskar* creates a restricted and concentrated "field of experiment in which you operate for the time being in order to facilitate your . . . realizing of . . . the Real."[37] Thus, "Surya Namaskars can be an instrument, a Path to this Realization."[38]

Pant didn't discount the extrinsic benefits (those occurring after the session—that is, in daily life) of performing *surya namaskar.* The first two, he maintained, are fitness and health. The third is joy in living. Understanding that a long bout of *surya namaskar*—an aerobic exercise—is a natural mood elevator, Pant, sounding like a hippie, described with a giddy fervor the results of regularly performing *surya namaskar* for three months or less.*

---

*Begun in the mid-1960s in America and, within the next few years, spread to many regions around the world, the hippie movement is known for its utopian fantasy of effecting radical changes in societal values, including sexual liberation, the reduction of possessions, self-sufficiency, the exploration of altered states, and communal living. But another critical credo of hippiedom, which further distinguished it from the political activist faction of the counterculture, was the cultivation of a heightened sense of everyday reality.

You will also find that you are not only mentally more alert but that you get a tremendous kick and happiness out of living. You will find that you are capable of feeling the joy of life. You will find that you can feel and experience every moment the joy that a tree, that a cloud, that a breath of wind expresses and experiences. You will feel and experience within yourself the vibrant energy of Creation. Simultaneously, you will start feeling that every thing living and not living (apparently) consists of Karuna or love.[39]

But these changes in the quotidian world, however rewarding, are negligible, Pant argued, compared with the intrinsic benefit of *surya namaskar*: the overwhelming transformation of self that occurs during its performance. When you're totally engaged in the exercise, "the false 'I' and with it all the attachments that this 'I' has built up . . . will just dissolve itself in the Eternal, the Real."[40] The fluctuations of the mind cease, the ego ceases to exist, and you find yourself united to transcendent reality. "Thus, during the exercise you realize that truly in the ordinary way [you go about your daily routine,] you live the life of a 'ghost existence.'"[41]

Pant's *Surya Namaskar* Manual

It's likely that even if a new edition hadn't just appeared, Morgan would've rejected Pant's proposal for a new foreword anyway. It wasn't compatible with the conception of *surya namaskar* presented in *The Ten-Point Way to Health*. (It seems more than likely that she was being polite when she wrote: "Your 'note,' as you so modestly call it, delights and illuminates me."[42])

"A Short Note" didn't fit with the breezy book for women that she had extensively shaped and written.

Even if she didn't feel that the proposed foreword was a good match for *The Ten-Point Way to Health*, that didn't mean Morgan failed to recognize the value of what Pant had written. She encouraged him to write his own book: "It might well be a whole book by itself, signed by yourself as a supplement to your Father's."[43] Pant took her advice. In 1970 he published *Surya Namaskars—An Ancient Indian Exercise* (see fig. 25.2 on page 314). A pamphlet-sized manual, *Surya Namaskars* expands his proposed foreword, "A Short Note on Surya Namaskar," but the message is the same: pursuing the unprecedented number of offerings (most prominently, money, sex, and power) of the modern world to shore up our "I" is a fruitless action that only leads us to sorrow; the key to our salvation is practicing *surya namaskar* as a vehicle for dissolving the ego.

The most surprising aspect of *Surya Namaskars* is the expansion of the seemingly hippie sensibility of "A Short Note on Surya Namaskar." A lyrical passage about the importance of being aware of the moment in daily living begins the section "Art and Science of Waking":

When you wake up, do not get out of bed immediately and start rushing around. As you wake up, be aware of the sounds around you. Be aware of the beauty and harmony, of the birds, of the trees, of the wind or rain or sun. Be just aware. Be aware of your body. Be aware of your toes first and move gently, caressingly, your awareness over your legs, your stomach, chest, arms. Be just, gently,

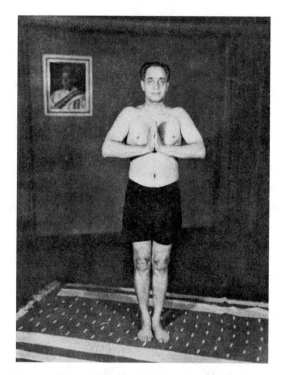

Figure 25.2. Apa Pant demonstrating
the first position of *surya namaskar,* 1970
(From *Surya Namaskars: An Ancient Indian Exercise*)

aware. If there is any pain, cramp, soreness, just be aware—nothing more or less—just be aware.[44]

And Pant's description of how the spiritual nature of the *surya namaskar* exercises affects everyday life concludes:

But they have a deep spiritual content and they open up a new, more profound, more powerful dimension of awareness. Slowly but surely as you continue regularly to practise them things change in you, around you. Experiences miraculously come to you and you feel the full force of the Beauty and Harmony, the unity, the oneness, with all that is.[45]

It's possible that Pant's plea for taking delight in one's body and surroundings (what in the 1960s was called "tuning in"—interacting harmoniously with the natural world in a lively manner) and his advocacy of practicing *surya namaskar* exercises as a vehicle for experiencing ecstasy in everyday life was inspired by his intoxication with the sweet hedonism of the hippie movement in its heyday. It's more likely, though, that his valorization of sensual and spiritual awareness was simply concurrent with hippie beliefs.

In any case, the more critical difference between "A Short Note on Surya Namaskar" and *Surya Namaskars* is that in the book Pant deepens his argument for performing *surya namaskar* as a means to opening ourselves to

Being. This process begins with an awareness of our attempts to continue what is pleasurable and terminate what is unpleasurable.

During these exercises you are just aware of and thus understand and experience how pleasurable sensations are arising, the memory of these suddenly, as it were, takes over as the "I" which has these experiences, and through the false creation of this "Ego" or "I," desires to continue the pleasurable sensations. You must see how the "Ego" hopes to perpetuate itself through this memory. During these exercises you also see how at the moment an unpleasurable sensation arises, your Mind or Ego struggles hard to discontinue it. And you must see how this continuous conflict and struggle wears you out. You become old and dull due to it.[46]

Pant described the process of becoming aware of the psychomental flux—the pleasurable and unpleasurable thoughts and feelings that arise and vie for our attention and construct the ego or I—*during the exercises.* He doesn't make clear, though, whether these desires to continue pleasure and avoid pain pertain to intrusive thoughts and feelings about matters in our daily life or to responses to the rewarding but taxing movements of *surya namaskar* itself. But the point remains the same: during the exercise, we learn to ask, "Who is this 'I' that has longings?" "Who is this 'I' that is complaining?" and even "Who is this 'I' that feels it must persist?" as a means of realizing that the "I" is a fabrication.

The point really is whether one can clearly see and Experience for oneself the process of the building up of the "I," which desires or does not desire; this whole conflict is not only empty, ephemeral and temporary, but also exhausting and utterly ridiculous. Can one realize and experience that 90 per cent of one's conscious existence, or even more, is taken up by this conflict of desiring and not desiring? Have you ever felt that you are hardly aware of the total and immediate reality of the moment? You are never really conscious of the eternal moment.[47]

What is the way out? "Through concentration [on performing the *surya namaskar* exercises]," Pant intones, "that is by being alertly aware, conscious of all that is happening in you at that moment, by, as it were, having a part of you 'as a constant witness,' Sakshi to everything, you realize the fact that 'memory' and . . . 'desire' . . . are false, empty, impermanent."[48]

Becoming aware of the thoughts and feelings that arise is the preliminary stage, a necessary condition for discarding them, which enables one to live in the moment. So it's not stopping the psychomental flux in itself that liberates, but the consequent full living in the moment. In this collapse of the past and future into the present, the now is ever new—and mind expanding: "And the 'new', the ever-New is not restricted by space—it is Everywhere. In the 'now' you live and feel a part of, and not apart from, the Totality of Existence and with the powerful and continuous process of creation. When you are in touch constantly from moment to moment with the New you are really alive. Surya Namaskars will teach you to be really alive."[49]

Living in the moment, Pant argues, expands

consciousness in time (you comprehend being part of the ongoing cosmic emanation—the flow of the manifest universe from nothing) and space (you comprehend being part of the expanse in which all things exist—the manifest universe itself).*

The laid-back hippie belief in living in the present moment was formed by many influences, both Western (such as the Beat poets and Gestalt therapy) and Eastern (such as Zen as interpreted by Alan Watts and the Tao Te Ching). In the early 1970s a movement arose that synthesized these influences and packaged them for Westerners as self-help books or workshops for bettering one's life by methodically banishing ruminations on or changing behavior driven by the past and future, which facilitates living fully in the present moment (and even achieving a state of bliss!). Dick Price, cofounder of Esalen, began teaching Gestalt practice in 1970. Ram Dass published *Be Here Now* in 1971. Werner Erhard, founder of est, Erhard Seminars Training, began giving his workshops in 1971. Ken Wilber completed *Spectrum of Consciousness* in 1973. In publishing *Surya Namaskars* in 1970, Pant unknowingly became part of this movement. No doubt influenced by a mix of his personal experience and Indian heritage, he, however, acknowledged a universal condition of existence that the oth-

ers ignored: suffering. Perceiving everyday life as "futile, confusing, oppressed by sorrow," Pant increasingly found solace in a *surya namaskar* practice rooted in Hindu metaphysics.[50] This *surya namaskar* allowed him to live "without sorrow in the presence of contractions and conflicts,"[51] gave him a "larger perspective and purpose,"[52] and enabled him to abandon the senses (the faculties by which we obtain information about the mundane world) to "merge with the infinite."[53] "The main purpose of life, according to the Hindus," he explained, "is liberation: liberation from the limited, relative, and therefore confusing vision that is available to us when we live on the plane of the senses."[54]

This personal salvation, it seems, is also what allowed Pant to become more involved with others. Through his *surya namaskar* practice he became detached not only from sorrows but also from "anger, hatred, pride, jealousy, desire."[55] The result of an encounter with the Real, he maintained, was the annihilation of the wish to do others harm or use them to our ends: "The Power of Truth, when it is realised and experienced . . . is so immense that impurities such as anger, hate, lust, etc. disintegrate and dissolve in its power."[56] Pant experienced this dissolution of impurities as an overflowing of compassion: "God, Ishwara, Allah and Buddha are attempts in words to express . . . compassion."[57] All base desires destroyed, we

---

*Indian wrestlers evidently make their core *vyayam* regimen (the Indian system of physical training designed to build flexibility, strength, and bulk), consisting of *dands* (jackknifing push-ups) and *bethaks* (deep knee squats), into spiritual exercise without even trying. Sociocultural anthropologist Joseph S. Alter gives this account of their practice: "The most important feature of dands and bethaks is that they be done rhythmically and at a steady pace. The performance of thousands of these exercises produces a mental state not unlike that of a person who has gone into a trance through the rote recitation of a mantra or prayer. Thus, dands and bethaks transport the wrestler into an altered state of consciousness from which he derives psychic and spiritual purification. Vyayam is very much like meditation in this respect" (Alter, *Wrestler's Body,* 104–5).

find ourselves able to consider others: to tend to their needs, to attempt to alleviate their distress, and to wish them well. Through the isolating and lonely liberation gained by his *surya namaskar* practice, Pant was able to spend his life in noble service to others.

Coda

Even as a young man, Pant never lost his aplomb. Morgan remarked upon meeting him in 1936 in London that he "was a magnificent physical specimen, but there was about him a more impressive quality than perfect bodily fitness. He had, in the midst of nerve-ridden London, an Olympian calmness and poise." Not that his godlike physicality was easy to overlook. Upon watching him pose for the photographs used to illustrate *The Ten-Point Way to Health,* Morgan observed: "When he had finished the dozen or so Namaskars necessary he was dripping and radiant as if he had risen out of some eternal spring."[58]

Pant remained impressive his entire life, for both his handsome appearance and his good-humored, gracious manner (see fig. 25.3 on page 318). Scholar of Indian dance Roxanne Gupta, echoing Morgan's encounter with Bhavanarao over forty years before, recounts her first meeting with Pant in the late 1980s:

I met Apa Pant when he was in his mid seventies. He had come to give a talk at Syracuse University [in New York], where I was working as Outreach Coordinator, and I invited him to stay at my home. On the way to the car following his talk, I offered to carry his overnight bag. With all the charm that comes naturally to an international diplomat, he said, "Madame, I can not only carry this bag. I can carry you along with it if you like." From that moment on I was totally infatuated.[59]

Pant's aplomb and charm, while surely accounted for by his breeding and nature, were also hard-won. Each day he had to overcome his tendency to withdraw into a state of darkness. From an early age he had brooded about dying. "As a child and a youngster I had a terror of dead bodies, funerals, ghosts," he recollected.[60] No wonder. During the three-year influenza pandemic that began in 1918, when he was six, he witnessed hundreds of funeral processions, with their chanting, lamenting, and music of death, parade past his ancestral house in Pune on route to the nearby burning *ghat,* where the bodies were cremated and the ashes allowed to be washed away by the river. (The impact of the pandemic on India was particularly appalling: seventeen million deaths from the flu occurred there.) Throughout the rest of his life he saw many deaths, including that of a friend who died (from a heart attack or stroke) in the garden of Pant's home. The death of his mother (with whom he powerfully identified, at least in her dying: "I felt deep, deep down inside me . . . a sense of unity [with] my mother and her release from a body which—though this I could not have understood—was diseased"[61]) was his earliest (and most indelible) memory. And, of course, there was the death of his beloved father.

Pant himself nearly died a few times, once from the bout with pneumonia that led to his conversion to *surya namaskar* but mostly from youthful feats of derring-do. He twice

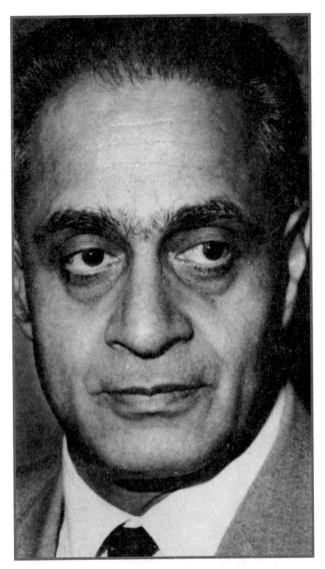

Figure 25.3. Apa Pant, 1974

(From *A Moment in Time,* by Apa Pant)

crashed old Puss Moth planes he was piloting while doing aerobatics; he tumbled eighty-five feet to the ground when his homemade glider fell apart in midair; and he plunged over a two-thousand-foot precipice in Tibet when he was thrown by a horse (his fifty-foot fall was arrested by a ledge).

Pant wasn't afraid of death per se. What he feared was knowing that his spirit was separating from his body. The Indian funeral rituals that frightened him as a child, he realized, "were associated with the agony of soul and spirit of the living person in the period just before death." Death itself was merely a mystery to Pant. But the awareness that the spirit and body will be separated . . . "*this* was a terror."[62]

Pant searched for a way to come to terms with his fear. "I put questions about death to many a mystic in many a land, and I pored over sacred and secret and mythological texts."[63] What he came realize was that "the dead weight of memory and sensation-habits [which constitute the "I"] presses constantly on living." Each day he removed that weight by destroying his "I" through performing *surya namaskar*. During *surya namaskar* practice "the idea of death [had] no power to disturb the joy and harmony of living in the timeless instant."[64]

In mid-1992 Pant suffered a heart attack or stroke, and a few months later, after a recurrence, he died on October 5, 1992.

26

SWAMI SIVANANDA

Using *Surya Namaskar* as a Warm-up Exercise for Yoga

Opening the Sivananda Yoga Vedanta Centre in Boston

In the early summer of 1962 Marcia Moore, a lithe gamine who possessed the crystalline beauty of a movie star, was teaching postural yoga at the YMCA in Boston and at her house in Concord, a small town about nineteen miles northwest of the capital, notable for its mid-19th-century transcendentalist circle. Among its members was Henry David Thoreau, best known for writing *Walden; or Life in the Woods* but revered by Moore as the first American to practice yoga (as he understood it). Of course, his ethereal yoga, she acknowledged, was different from her yoga, grounded in *asana*. (As she cheekily put it: Thoreau's mentor and friend, the center of the circle, Ralph Waldo Emerson, who himself was immersed in Hinduism, never said to him, "'Now Henry, a headstand, please.'"[1]) Nevertheless, it could be said that she was bringing yoga back to Concord, where it originated in America (fig. 26.1).

Considering her experience teaching yoga, it's no wonder that when Moore called up the Dance Circle (an organization that was playing a vital role in fostering interest in modern dance in Boston through artistry and education) to ask about taking dance lessons in August, the transaction turned into her being invited to teach yoga at the Dance Circle. She leapt (a barrel jump, no doubt!) at the opportunity.

The Dance Circle occupied a floor of a building on Boylston Street, near the Fenway Victory Gardens. Most of the space was used by the organization, but

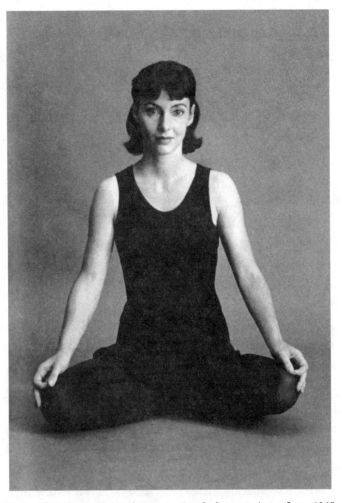

Figure 26.1. Marcia Moore demonstrating *Padmasana*, Lotus Pose, 1965
(From *Yoga, Youth, and Reincarnation,* by Jess Stearn)

Moore was offered a large room for the yoga classes at a small rent. The dance organization retained the option of using it as a smaller studio when it was available. "But it will be ours to fix up and run as we please," Moore exclaimed, referring to herself and her new husband, Louis Acker, in a letter to Katharine and Wilmon Brewer, the couple who were her benefactors and friends.[2] (From prominent families, the Brewers were well-known philanthropists. But they had personal connections to Moore: they were long-time friends of her parents, as well as godparents to her children.) What especially pleased Moore was being able to found Boston's first yoga center where members could pursue spiritual goals primarily through practicing hatha yoga. (A chapter of the Vedanta Society, which promotes union with the divine Self through the karma, jnana, bhakti, and raja paths of yoga, had been established in Boston in 1910.)

Supplemented with publicity provided by the Dance Circle, Moore promoted the September opening of the yoga center by sending out mailings, giving lectures, and speaking at seminars during the summer. She also appeared on a popular women's TV program, the *Louise Morgan Show,* in an episode that aired on August 17, 1962.* Called *Shopping-Vues* when it was first broadcast in 1949, and then *Dear Homemaker,* the afternoon talk show targeted Moore's most likely potential students: wives who stayed at home to rear the children and manage the household.

Moore opened the Sivananda Yoga Vedanta Centre on September 19, 1962. Although she had first studied hatha yoga in Calcutta with Roman Datta, an English-speaking businessman and Theosophist, during her travels in India with her first husband between 1955 and 1957, she received her critical instruction in a teacher training course taught by Swami Vishnudevananda, Swami Sivananda's first emissary to the West, at the first Sivananda Ashram Yoga Camp in Val Morin, Quebec, near Montreal, in 1961.†

Born in Kerala, South India, in 1927, Vishnudevananda went to the Sivananda Yoga Vedanta Forest Academy in Rishikesh, in the Himalayas, in 1947. Working with Sivananda, he mastered the most advanced hatha yoga techniques (*asanas, pranayamas, mudras, bandhas,* and *kriyas*). He was appointed the first professor of hatha yoga at the ashram (fig. 26.2).

In 1957 he was sent by Sivananda to the West, where he founded yoga centers in the United States and Canada, and then settled in Canada.

"We are but one of many branches of this new, dynamic and authentic movement [created by Sivananda] to bring yoga to America," Moore announced about her center, "both to help individuals and to promote closer understanding between East and West." Toward this end, she sponsored lectures on yoga and related matters, arranged demonstrations, and taught raja yoga, which involved meditation and study of Vedanta. But her specialty, she explained, was a part of raja yoga called hatha yoga, which she, following the teachings of Vishnudevananda, defined as "a manifold discipline designed to develop the body through a five point program of exercise, breathing, diet, relaxation, and positive thinking. Since flesh and spirit are so inextricably mingled we try to take account of both in our over-all program of self-unfoldment."[3]

Classes were initially held on Wednesdays at 1:00, 3:00, 5:30, and 7:30 at the Dance Circle studio. A Thursday morning class was held at the Freniere Studio, another borrowed artistic space, in Concord.‡

A demonstration/lecture by Vishnudevananda at the Concert Hall of Boston University on the evening of October 5th was used to further publicize the new center. A brief dedication

---

*The host, Louise Morgan, one of Boston's most well-liked TV personalities, wasn't the English journalist of the same name who played a key role in popularizing *surya namaskar.*

†When he learned that summertime attendance among his Montreal students was dropping off because they were heading fifty miles north to the Laurentian Mountains to get away from the city, beat the heat, and relax, Vishnudevananda founded a retreat there for yoga vacations. The first yoga camp was set up in Saint-Hyppolyte at the summer home of the parents of his right-hand person, Sylvia Heck, in 1960. The first camp in Val Morin was held in the summer of 1961 on 11th Avenue. In February 1962 the camp moved to its present Val Morin site, on 8th Avenue, amid 250 forested acres.

‡The studio was founded in 1954 by E. Richard "Dick" Freniere, who worked as a graphic artist and illustrator and taught art to the community.

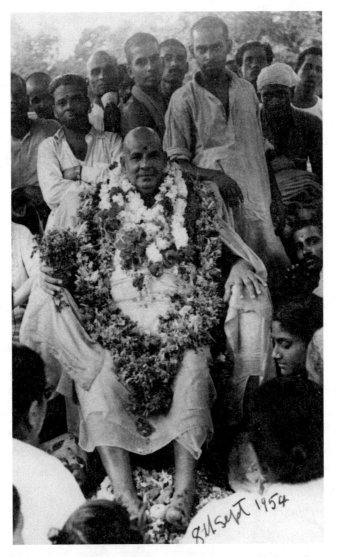

Figure 26.2. Birthday celebration for Swami Sivananda (center),
with Swami Vishnudevananda standing behind him to his left, 1954
(With the kind permission of the Sivananda Yoga Vedanta Center, New York)

ceremony took place beforehand, presided over by Vishnudevananda. The always loyal Brewers braved the severe flooding and damage caused by the combined impact from a nor'easter and Hurricane Daisy to attend the opening, bringing yellow roses from Great Hill, their estate (his family's estate until it was purchased by her family in 1920, when they were young adults who were falling in love!) in Hingham, about sixteen miles south of Boston.

The journalist and author Jess Stearn notes that the classes Moore held at the Sivananda Yoga Vedanta Centre in 1964 were wholly attended by upper-middle-class fortyish housewives. Stearn speculates why the husbands didn't attend Moore's classes at the center: "[They] had turned up out of curiosity, but once they saw the ease with which their wives did the exercises they seemed to lose interest. Most had sedentary office jobs, and felt they would lose standing by not being able to compete with the weaker sex in the physical sphere."* He was at a loss, however, to explain why the women wanted to take better care of their bodies than the men. Moore gave him an answer: "This is the package they've been selling all their lives, and they don't like to see the wrapping wrinkled and spoiled."[4]

Moore's explanation for why the mature upper-middle-class housewives practiced yoga didn't take into account why they preferred to practice yoga in classes rather than at home. Perhaps the appeal of going to yoga classes lay not only in the expertise and motivation provided by a teacher but in the modest autonomy it offered to women whose lives largely revolved around their families. Participating in yoga class provided homemakers with a separate identity. They could undertake this activity with the bemused permission of their husbands and schedule it around sending their children off to school and completing household chores.

Perhaps the attraction also lay in being involved in an exotic exercise practice with a group of other daring women. They became a subculture defined by yoga classes, girlfriends, books, lectures, and even a uniform (commonly black leotards and seamed or fishnet stockings, mixing the hip severity—if not gloominess—of the modern dancer and beatnik chick with the ostentatious allure of the chorus girl and prostitute).

The Sivananda Class

Stearn immersed himself in Sivananda-style yoga classes with Moore for three and half months in the studio in her house in Concord in 1964. (Stearn's work for the *New York Daily News* focused on people marginalized in society. In taking yoga classes with Moore, for the first time "as a reporter [I] experienced the strange and esoteric that I researched and wrote about," he confides in his best-selling *Yoga, Youth, and Reincarnation,* published in 1965. "Otherwise, I might well have been a juvenile delinquent, prostitute, drug addict, homosexual."[5]) He was also a houseguest in her rather unconventional household, consisting of Moore, her young husband Acker, and her three children from a previous marriage.

Moore and Acker seemed an odd pairing, at least to Stearn. She was a Boston Brahmin whose father had founded the Sheraton Hotel chain and whose mother was an artist and book illustrator. Acker's father was alcoholic and his mother was wacky. Moore, at thirty-five, was the mother of three, and Acker was a twenty-three-year-old student at Boston University.

---

*The history of how yoga classes everywhere became predominantly the domain of women (now mostly young women) has yet to be written. Various reasons for why men generally don't take up yoga have been posited. Valuing strength over flexibility, men prefer weight lifting. They favor competitive sports over group classes. They don't want to be shown up by women, whose wider pelvic bone structure makes them naturally more flexible. They're less likely to try something—especially something as weird as yoga poses—that might make them look foolish. They care less about having a trim figure, which yoga is said to promote.

(Moore's two boys, who fancied themselves as Beatles, treated Acker as a member of their band.) "But standing on their heads, a frequent posture in the Moore-Acker household," Stearn observes, "they seemed in complete accord."[6] Moore's infatuation with Acker involved more than a mutual interest in yoga, though. He was handy (he chopped fallen trees for firewood; installed his hi-fi in the cabinet; painted the house; and made paddle wheel boats for the boys). He had a keen interest in astrology (which she shared). And, being over six feet tall and bountifully muscled, he was hunky. Moore and Acker enjoyed elementary activities together, like taking walks in the woods, reading aloud in the evenings, and, Stearn implies, having sex. In marrying Acker, Moore confided to the Brewers, she was rejecting the "artificial veneer of sophistication" of her "cocktail party friends" in order to find a simple, new life.[7]

Yoga classes at Moore's home were held in a large room with a picture-window view of the woods where Thoreau, America's proto-yogin, once strolled. Students included men and women from sixteen to seventy-five. The hatha yoga regime that Sivananda assiduously molded into what he described (in the subtitle of his first book) as an "easy course of physical culture for modern men and women" between the late 1930s and early 1950s was the most popular brand of yoga in the West in the 1950s and 1960s. It consisted of a preliminary period of mantra chanting and breathing exercises; a warm-up period of simple calisthenics exercises (focused on building flexibility) and *surya namaskar* (sun salutation exercises); a main series of about ten yoga postures; and a concluding period of relaxation in *Savasana*, Corpse Pose, and brief mantra chanting.

In *Yoga, Youth, and Reincarnation,* Stearn describes his struggles with learning Sivananda yoga, beginning with the breathing exercises. (Never having breathed in and out through the nose while filling up the diaphragm and relaxing the abdomen with each inhalation and contracting the abdomen with each exhalation, "it was a little difficult getting used to the idea of not sucking in the stomach—or gut—with each deep breath."[8])

"Many of the limbering exercises were familiar," Stearn notes. "I had either done them, or seen them done, in gyms."[9] These exercises were the Rock and Roll ("The first instructions were: 'Lie on your back, pull knees up to chest, clasp hands under the knees, and gently rock back and forth as though your back were the bottom of a rocker, trying to reach an agreeable rhythm'")[10]; the Pump ("In the Pump condition, lying flat, I pulled up a leg, stretching it to the sky, yet keeping my back to the floor, breathing in as the leg came up, out as it went down . . . three times with each leg")[11]; and Head Rolling. Nevertheless, these stretching exercises were challenging to him: they had to be done not only with a wider range of motion than he was used to but also with great concentration, slowly and in a controlled manner.

What really flummoxed Stearn, though, was *surya namaskar*—the series of *asana* and modified *asana* positions performed at a fairly quick pace with fluid transitional movements accompanied by rhythmic breathing. The series is repeated for a length of time. Stearn struggled exasperatingly but gamely to perform (what to him was) this peculiar and arduous exercise.

Our opening major [Indian practice] was the so-called Sun exercise, Suryanamaskar, the Hindu salute to the sun. It began with standing erect, hands folded together, legs close, and facing the sun.

It was a warm-up in itself, for it involved a dozen different movements. I started raising the arms way back over the head and stretching, breathing in deeply; then bending forward and touching the toes, releasing the breath as I did so. Then, forward on one knee, chest, neck, and head tilted upward—toward the sun, of course—again stretching.

As I was hoping the exercise was over, came the signal to lie flat, touching feet, knees, chest, and forehead to the mat, but keeping the hips arched upward. Then I flattened out completely, and brought head and chest up. Then—there seemed no end to this one exercise—Marcia ordered me up halfway, feet and palms flat, body hunched up in a pyramid effect, then scrunching forward on the other knee, bringing the feet together between the hands, and finally erect again, arms back over the head, breathing deeply.

It was all as complicated as it sounds, and I couldn't see myself doing it in a million years. "How can I do an exercise when I can't even remember it?" I asked.[12]

Stearn and the other first-time students weren't used to (what they considered) the odd, ungainly configurations and protracted strenuousness of *surya namaskar.* Their frustration was so palpable that Moore abruptly stopped the activity. "We'll put Suryanamaskar away for a while, then come back to it later," she said,

"when the coordination between mind and body has improved."[13]

Surya namaskar was followed by the famous Rishikesh sequence of *asanas:* (1) Shoulder Stand. ("My legs dangled and my lower back sagged, even as I supported it with my hands."[14]) (2) Plow. (The position was directly assumed "from the shoulder stand, by thrusting first one leg, then the other, stiff-kneed over my head."[15]) (3) Forward Bend. ("I stretched vainly for the toes."[16]) (4) Fish. (Kneeling on the floor and bending back while "squatting on my heels grated painfully on my ankles."[17]) (5) Cobra. (6) Locust. ("I was barely able to get both legs off the mat, three inches at most."[18]) (7) Bow. ("I liked the Bow, though I found it quite impossible at first. Still flat on the stomach, I reached back and grabbed my widespread ankles, trying to lift my knees from the mat by pressure of my outstretched arms. It took me three or four days to get the knack of this exercise."[19]) (8) Twist. (9) Stork.

Exercises were performed two or three times, with long pauses in the form of the resting prone position, Corpse Pose, between them. Moore stressed the importance of these rest periods: "You not only absorb oxygen, but you permit your subconscious to assimilate the exercises you have just performed."[20] During the longer relaxation periods, Stearn found that Moore's guided imagery ("Picture yourself on a beach, with the golden sun seeping through your pores with its warm, healing rays . . . soothing, bathing each tired muscle, each straining nerve, with its warm radiance") and voice ("soft as the Concord breeze") "soothed my restless mind and somewhat strained muscles."[21] After nearly an hour, the session ended with a period of total relaxation in Corpse Pose, followed by brief chanting.

The sequence of the *asanas* was balanced: "For every forward sequence, there was a compensating backward exercise," Stearn observes.[22] Sivananda took this principle from the regime of S. Sundaram, whom Sivananda revered as Yogacharya His Holiness Sri Sundaramji for his great contributions to yoga (specifically, his yoga publications, his training and guidance for yoga aspirants, and "his easy and perfect way of performing the difficult yogasanas and kriyas").[23] Sundaram had learned the principle from Swami Kuvalayananda, the most prominent and influential advocate of modern yoga, who had originated it.

The most startling difference between Sivananda's routine and the earlier routines on which it was based is the addition of *surya namaskar*. *Surya namaskar* was a rival indigenous exercise to yogasana, judged by yogins, most prominently Kuvalayananda, to be inferior to yogasana. Sivananda brokered a reconciliation between the two systems by incorporating *surya namaskar* into the yoga routine as a warm-up exercise for *asana* practice. (Previously *surya namaskar* had been used by Krishnamacharya as a means of linking *asanas* into a flowing routine.)

Sivananda may have first gained knowledge of *surya namaskar* from reading one of the rajah of Aundh's books—either the limited-edition first book, *Surya Namaskars (Sun-Adoration) for Health, Efficiency & Longevity,* published in 1928, or the widely available second book, *The Ten-Point Way to Health* (heavily ghostwritten by the unsung English journalist Louise Morgan), published in 1938.* But he himself implied that he learned *surya namaskar* from attending a demonstration by the maharajah's son, Apa Pant, in 1939. "There is a system of physical exercise called Suryanamaskar and the Raja Saheb of Aundh is a great propounder of it," he wrote in 1939. "The Prince of Aundh, like his father, is a great votary of Suryanamaskar. Recently at the request of the students at Bangalore he demonstrated the Suryanamaskar in many colleges there and explained its benefits."[24]

Surya Namaskar as Exercise Compatible with Hatha Yoga

In the earliest incarnation of his system, found in *Yogic Home Exercises: Easy Course of Physical Culture for Modern Men and Women,* published in 1939, Swami Sivananda (1887–1963) provided instructions for practicing yoga: "Get up at 4 a.m. Answer the calls of nature. Wash your face. Then practise your Asans, Pranayam exercises and meditation."[25] He advised practicing *surya namaskar* later on, when the sun came up: "Do Suryanamaskar in the early morning. The morning sun gives out ultra-violet rays as does also the evening sun."[26]

Despite his description of *surya namaskar*

---

*It was the "voice of the Rajah of Aundh" in *The Ten-Point Way to Health* that the Belgian yogin André Van Lysebeth, a devout disciple of Sivananda, cites (as if the maharajah's pronouncements held the same authority as a collection of peer-reviewed randomized clinical trials) to support his claims for the "bountiful effects" of the *surya namaskar* taught at Sivananda's ashram at Rishikesh (Van Lysebeth, *Yoga Self-Taught,* 230). Van Lysebeth's familiarity with this book indicates (but doesn't provide strong evidence) that Sivananda read it and suggested it to his followers.

as "a system of physical exercise," at that time Sivananda didn't conceive of *surya namaskar* as a fitness regime but as a natural health cure effected through sunbathing—basking in the sun's rays—and not by any means the only form of health cure through sunbathing. In fact, he believed, practically any outdoor activity—even if you "lie down on the ground on a blanket or lie on a cot"[27]—performed in the sun cured disease: "If persons suffering from leprosy and other skin diseases strip themselves off all clothing and remain naked in the sun till their body is properly tanned, then the sun rays will penetrate their body and work wonders there. . . . Besides leprosy, tuberculosis, rheumatism, obesity, anaemia, neurasthenia, eczema, colds, coughs, rickets, diseases of the teeth, etc., can also be treated with sun rays."[28]

Like Bhavanarao, Sivananda cleverly buttressed his argument for the benefits of *surya namaskar* (and the superiority of Indian culture) by pointing to how Westerners had recently adapted the sun cure, long known to Indians. He scolded his wayward Indian readers who sought out heliotherapy at sanatoriums in the mountains for adopting derivative Western modalities for using the rays of the sun as a powerful agent in the treatment of disease: "The Rishis and sages of yore who had knowledge of the curative power of the rays of the sun revealed the mysteries of the sun and its beneficial rays and the uses of this radiant energy. But you don't care to read and learn them. You want to borrow everything from the West. What a sad lamentable state! . . . Perform Suryanamaskar daily. . . . You will then have wonderful health and vigour and vitality."[29] Like other Indian physical cultur-

ists, Sivananda invoked the *rishis* not in an attempt to impartially and critically examine India's past but to solidify India's identity as a nation with a great history—exhibited by its repository of superior knowledge and wisdom—and thus deserving of independence. Rejecting, casting doubt on, or merely being indifferent to this history (manifested by going to a sanatorium rather than taking up *surya namaskar*), he was implying, was not merely lamentable but unpatriotic. (In this subtle intimidation, he was like the nationalists of many countries in the 1930s.)

Sivananda's promotion of exercising in the sun was hardly limited to maintaining and restoring good health. By exercising while abandoning oneself to the penetrating rays of the sun, Sivananda proclaimed, one could experience a sensuous ecstasy:

Wear a thin light garment and walk on the western bank of a river, on the west side of the sea, a lake or a tank early morning at sunrise. Run also. You will doubtless enjoy a sun-bath. Practice Asans and physical exercises [presumably, including *surya namaskar*]. Expose your mouth to the rays of the rising sun. Open it wide. Let the rays penetrate your nostrils also. . . . Let the sun's rays fall on the closed eyes. . . . Practice deep-breathing exercises and Pranayam. The various parts of the body should receive a regulated sun-bath. Turn the body round frequently. . . . Bask in the sun. Expose your body to the rays of the sun.[30]

In this expansive directive, deliriously espoused by Sivananda, *surya namaskar* (and

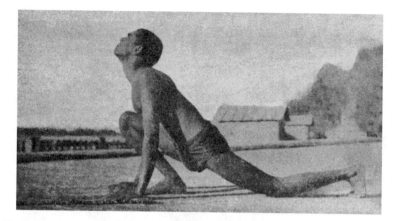

Figure 26.3. Swami Vishnudevananda demonstrating *surya namaskar* outdoors, 1950
(From *Hatha Yoga*, by Swami Sivananda)

other physical exercises) are a means of sybaritically drenching oneself in sunlight in the morning.

Surya Namaskar as Yogic Tonic

The third edition of Sivananda's *Hatha Yoga* (published in 1950), unlike the earlier (1939 and 1944) editions and unlike *Yogic Home Exercises,* includes a short chapter on the technique of *surya namaskar,* with illustrations— photos of one of Sivananda's most renowned followers, Swami Vishnudevananda, performing the positions (fig. 26.3). In this incarnation, *surya namaskar,* while still an activity separate from *asana* practice and practiced outdoors, was no longer capable of generating a euphoric state; it had become mere exercise, albeit now for attaining not only good health but also fitness. "Those who regularly perform Suryanamaskaram early in the morning, facing the sun enjoy radiant health and vitality. It . . . produces lustre in the practitioner's face. . . . It is a Yogic tonic." It cures all disorders of the nervous, digestive, and circulatory systems, Sivana-

nda claimed. "Suryanamaskaram combines the benefits of vigorous physical exercise and Yoga Asanas."[31]

Surya Namaskar as Warm-Up Exercise for *Asanas*

Sivananda incorporated *surya namaskar* directly into his classroom routine sometime in the early to mid-1950s. This diminishment of *surya namaskar,* now subsumed into the yoga session, was antithetical to Sivananda's early advocacy of *surya namaskar* as a means of basking in sunlight to promote health cure, let alone as a means of getting carried away by heated-up bodily sensations to the point of rapture. This new utilitarian conception of *surya namaskar* was first proclaimed in print as part of the Sivananda system with the publication in 1960 of *The Complete Illustrated Book of Yoga,* written by Vishnudevananda. As he did ten years previously for Sivananda's *Hatha Yoga,* the first yoga manual with illustrated instructions for *surya namaskar,* Vishnudevananda modeled

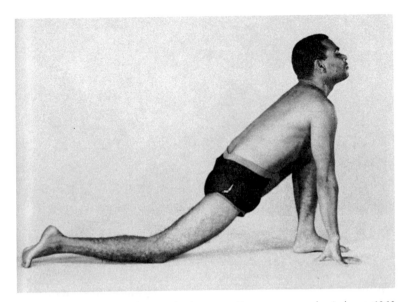

Figure 26.4. Swami Vishnudevananda demonstrating *surya namaskar* indoors, 1960

(From *The Complete Illustrated Book of Yoga,* by Swami Vishnudevananda)

the *surya namaskar* positions for his own book (fig. 26.4).*

Vishnudevananda recognized *surya namaskar* for what it mainly is: not treatment for a host of diseases but fitness exercise. "It reduces abdominal fat, brings flexibility to the spine and limbs, and increases the breathing capacity." And, perhaps more importantly, he identified its function as a warm-up exercise in the Sivananda system: "It is easier to practice *asanas* after doing *soorya namaskar*. Before students practice the more complicated and difficult postures, the spine should acquire some flexibility. For a stiff person, the sun exercise is a boon to bring back lost flexibility."[32] As preparation for *asana* practice proper, *surya namaskar* was presented by Vishnudevananda as the first exercise in the Sivananda routine.

The order of the Sivananda session presented by Vishnudevananda (in his words) is the following:

1. Prayer before beginning exercises, 2. Sun exercises, 3. Relaxation (two to three minutes; longer if required), 4. Headstand, 5. Shoulder stand, 6. Fish Pose (to be followed by a brief period of relaxation), 7. Forward bending exercises, 8. Backward bending exercises, 9. Twisting exercises, 10. Balancing exercises, 11. Leg and foot exercises (sitting), 12. Exercises in standing position, 13. Complete relaxation for ten to fifteen minutes (end of physical exercises), 14. Abdominal exercises, 15. Breathing exercises, 16. Meditation.[33]

---

*Vishnudevananda's book was the third yoga manual with illustrated instructions for *surya namaskar*. The second was Harvey Day's *The Study and Practice of Yoga,* published in 1953. Day's emphasis on the chin lock ("While doing this exercise keep your chin pressed tightly against your chest in a chin lock" [53]) indicates that he picked up the sun salutation exercises from reading K. V. Iyer's *Surya Namaskar.*

In a chapter titled "Suryanamaskar: A Salutation to the Sun" in *Yoga Self-Taught,* first published in France in 1968, Van Lysebeth elaborates on the value of *surya namaskar* in the Sivananda system as a warm-up exercise that loosens up muscles to prepare for *asana* practice.

> You see how I write "A" and not "the" Salutation to the Sun: because there are several variants. I have chosen for this book the one which is taught in Swami Shivananda's ashram at Rishikesh, because it is accessible to everyone and easily learnt. A Salutation to the Sun is made up of twelve successive movements, repeated one after the other, which serve to bring the whole muscular structure into play, warming it up and "conditioning" it for the asanas. It is an ideal exercise to get you moving, with more rapid movements than are customary in yoga. . . .
>
> A Salutation to the Sun however is a complete exercise, which may be practiced outside the daily yoga session. By tradition yogis perform it only at dawn, before their asanas. Roman Catholics need not be alarmed! It is no pagan prayer and I have no intention of forcing anyone to carry out, unbeknownst to themselves, some Hindu ritual or other!
>
> A Salutation to the Sun is a splendid exercise, and a yoga session without it is inconceivable. It prepares for the asanas and completes them, toning up the muscles, quickening and intensifying the respiration and cardiac rhythm, without inducing any fatigue or breathlessness.[34]

By the late 1960s the change to thinking of *surya namaskar* as "an ideal exercise to get you moving," without which the yoga session is "inconceivable," was so complete that Van Lysebeth felt compelled to explain that *surya namaskar* could also be "a complete exercise." This change in the perception of *surya namaskar* can be attributed to Sivananda. Savvy about his audience, he incorporated *surya namaskar* into the yoga class as a heating-up exercise in preparation for performing the somewhat arduous *asanas.* He had discovered (or learned from some source) that a brief aerobic warm-up exercise preceding yogic stretching exercises reduces resistance to stretching. He recognized (probably intuitively) that an increase in the temperature of muscles increases their elastic properties, thereby boosting their ability to stretch.

Some detractors may have objected to the incorporation of *surya namaskar* into the yoga regime. It appears that Shri Yogendra's vehement criticism of this hybrid exercise in the 1956 edition of his *Yoga Asanas Simplified* was directed at Sivananda's increasingly popular new routine: "The most characteristic feature of the yoga physical exercises is their non-violent and non-fatiguing disposition. For pure health, Yoga precludes exercises involving violence, strain or fatigue. Even *suryanamaskaras* or prostrations to the sun—a form of gymnastics attached to the sun worship in India—indiscriminately mixed up with the yoga physical training by the ill-informed are definitely prohibited by the authorities."[35*] But then, Yogendra's attacks on his (perceived) rivals were always less representative

---

*The 1956 edition of *Yoga Asanas Simplified,* the basis for all subsequent editions, may be essentially the same manuscript as the (lost) enlarged 1947 edition. If so, Yogendra's comments about *surya namaskar* were made about a decade earlier, before Sivananda incorporated *surya namaskar* into his yoga routine, and so weren't a criticism of Sivananda's routine.

of the times and more revealing of his cranki-
ness, rigidity, and envy.

Promoting Yoga

In 1936 Sivananda formed the Divine Life Society (DLS). In reframing his community at the
ashram in Rishikesh, on the edge of the sacred
Ganges, as an official spiritual organization,
he did more than solidify his growing following; he created the means for disseminating his
yoga system. The critical evolution of the DLS
took place after World War II, mainly due to
the establishment in 1948 of the Yoga Vedanta
Forest Academy, a formal yoga training center,
located within the ashram grounds. It attracted
not only disciples (residents) but also lay members (visitors). "And, to crown it all," writes Van
Lysebeth in "The Yogic Dynamo," his tribute to
his guru, "[Sivananda] accepted people from the
west, and even females!"[36] A magnanimous and
magnetic spiritual teacher, he encouraged these
students not only to practice yoga but also to
teach yoga by forming small groups when they
returned home (fig. 26.5).

Sivananda published books and pamphlets
through the DLS press, the Sivananda Publication League. (He would eventually author over
two hundred books.) Through the English-
language publications, his teaching reached
many foreigners. One of them was Van Lysebeth, who began receiving instruction from
Sivananda by correspondence in 1949. (He
was awarded a diploma from the Yoga Vedanta
Forest Academy in 1963, when he met Sivananda for the first time, shortly before the
guru died.) Van Lysebeth's epistolary relationship with Sivananda wasn't unusual; the first
Sivananda centers in Europe were founded by
men and women who'd read Sivananda's books
and corresponded with him but hadn't studied
with him.

During his more than 7,500-mile All-India
Tour (his only major tour of India) in 1950, Sivananda established local and regional branches
of the DLS throughout India. Then, in the
1950s and early 1960s, he sent his disciples,
including the swamis Vishnudevananda, Satchidananda, Satyananda, Venkatesananda, and
Omkarandanda, around India and/or the rest
of the world to form branches of the DLS (or
DLS-inspired but unaffiliated organizations).
Their students, in turn, opened Sivananda yoga
centers.

Sivananda was nicknamed "Swami Propagan-
dananda" by his detractors for his dissemination
of yoga far and wide. Van Lysebeth notes that
"they disapproved of both his modern methods
of diffusion, and his propagation of yoga on
such a grand scale to the general public. . . . He
encouraged a yoga practice which was possible
for everyone: some asanas, a little pranayama,
a little meditation and bhakti; well, a little of
everything."[37] The critics predicted that in the
materialistic West, yoga would "degenerate into
a minor branch of hygienic gymnastics, nothing more. This was considered as a complete
betrayal of yoga and the great rishis."[38]

In actuality, although he always promoted
yoga as health prevention and cure, Sivananda primarily advanced yoga as relief from
the stress brought about by the conditions of
modernity. "Life has become very complex in
these days," he wrote in 1939. "The struggle
for existence is very acute and keen. . . . A

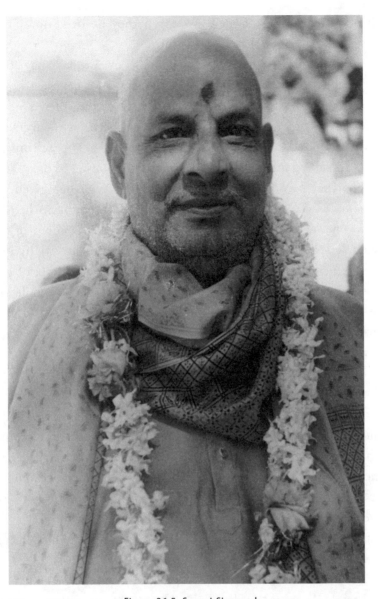

Figure 26.5. Swami Sivananda,
circa 1950

(With the kind permission
of the Sivananda Yoga Vedanta Center, New York)

great deal of continuous mental and physical strain is imposed on modern humanity by its deadening daily work and unhealthy mode of life."[39] To provide a more immersive physical and mental relaxation experience than could be found in sessions at local Sivananda centers, he developed what social historian Sarah Strauss calls a yoga "oasis regime": a "'yoga vacation' . . . that essentially reproduces the European spa experience—another classic 'oasis regime'—with, quite literally, a new twist."[40] In Rishikesh (and later at DLS ashrams around the world), his followers partook in yoga retreats that enabled them to "engage in an ascetic lifestyle for a short while, in order to improve not only their own hectic lives but also the world around them, when they go back home."[41] In taking a break from their worldly social life, they became (at least temporarily) *jivanmukhtas.*

A *jivanmukhta* is one who is liberated while still embodied. "'Liberated in life,'" explains historian of religion Mircea Eliade, "the *jivan-mukta* no longer possesses a personal consciousness—that is, a consciousness nourished on his own history—but a witnessing consciousness, which is pure lucidity and spontaneity."[42] Traditionally, a *jivanmukhta* is distinguished from one who is liberated while separated from the body—that is, when dead. Sivananda was influential in redefining *jivanmukhta* in the 20th century by changing the meaning to one who attains absolute freedom not only while alive but while still involved in the activities of everyday life, distinguished from one who withdraws from society to achieve enlightenment. This new formulation, observes Strauss, "reflects the fact that this ideal was well suited to the lives and goals of the emergent middle classes in India and the West. It did not require them to give up the basic structures and activities of everyday life, but only to reformulate their attitudes and concepts of self and others through the addition of yogic practices."[43] In fact, being this new type of *jivanmukhta* didn't even require students to sacrifice their personality (which is made up of the memories of one's own his-

tory); they needed simply to rejuvenate their spirit.

Some, even today, may consider Sivananda's teachings as a key symptom of yoga's modern decline. But there's no disagreeing with Van Lysebeth, who argues that thanks to Sivananda—his teachings, disciples, and books—"thousands of westerners now practise yoga. Yoga has given meaning to their lives, given them back their health [Van Lysebeth himself was cured of constipation], and helped them to survive in a difficult world."[44] Sivananda's gentle style of yoga with its standard format helps people in India and the West keep their bodies healthy and their minds quiet and calm.

Nevertheless, even Van Lysebeth concedes that the traditionalists weren't entirely wrong in saying that Sivananda's simple messages awakened people's interest in yoga but "completely cut [yoga] off from its deep roots, which lead us back to the origins of our own being and all of the cosmos."[45] Yet Sivananda himself intimated a way to experience exactly this depth of yoga practice within his system. In his 1939 yoga manual, he proposed a guided imagery relaxation exercise—which more accurately should be called a meditation—for *Savasana,* Corpse Pose: "Imagine that . . . your body [is] floating in this vast ocean of spirit. . . . Feel that Lord Hiranyagarbha, the ocean of life, is gently rocking you on His vast bosom. Feel that you are in touch with the Supreme Being"[46] (fig. 26.6).

Any *asana* session (whether practiced in isolation in a room in the basement of a house, in a class at a yoga center down the block, or as part of a four-day retreat that includes *pranayama,*

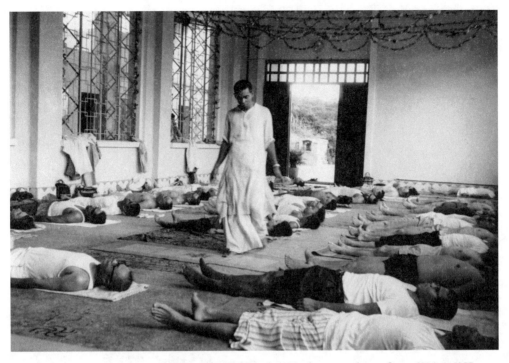

Figure 26.6. Swami Vishnudevananda guiding students in *Savasana*, Corpse Pose, 1956 or 1957
(With the kind permission of the Sivananda Yoga Vedanta Center, New York)

study, presentations, and seated meditation at an ashram in the Bahamas) can be used to practice this or similar meditations. That is, any single *asana* session may be considered as a kind of oasis regime: a period of temporary withdrawal from the concerns of everyday life with its demands set by clocks and calendars, a period of contemplation in which we can live in the eternal present, outside of time, using our body as a vehicle to becoming open to Being.

PART III

Making Yoga Sacred Again

Yogic Embodied Spirituality

27

INDRA DEVI

Becoming
a Western, Female
Yoga Teacher

Sailing to India

Born Eugenie Peterson in 1899 in Riga in Tsarist Russia to sixteen-year-old Sasha Zitovich, a spirited, bohemian Russian noble, and Vasili Pavlovich Peterson, a stodgy, Swedish-born, middle-aged bank director, Indra Devi seemed destined for a theatrical career. She grew up idolizing her mother, who became an actress a few years after her brief marriage ended. Following high school in Petrograd, Devi became a drama student in Moscow. After fleeing with her mother during the Russian civil war that ensued from the 1917 Bolshevik Revolution, she joined a Russian theater troupe in Berlin, the major center of the Russian diaspora, in 1920. She toured Europe with the company to increasing acclaim for six years.

But the course of her life changed in 1926 when Devi, who had been spending her summer vacation with her mother at a Baltic sea resort in Lithuania, attended one of the annual Star Congresses of the Theosophical Society in Ommen, Holland.* Established in 1911, the Order of the Star promoted Jiddu Krishnamurti as the "vehicle" for the Lord Maitreya—in Theosophical doctrine, an advanced spiritual being extremely rare in all of history. Devi was drawn to the gathering despite her skepticism about Krishnamurti being

---

*In another account of her vacation, Devi writes that she was in Latvia.

338

proclaimed by Annie Besant, then president of the Theosophical Society, as (in Devi's words) "a World Teacher, and coming Christ."[1]

The four-day proceedings in mid-August resembled a religious revival. (Although Theosophy is considered by its followers as divine wisdom, culled from all world religions, and not a religion itself, it was founded in 1875 in a wave of religious mania.) Devi was one of over four thousand participants from around the world who pitched tents on the elegant grounds of the Castle Eerde estate, which had been donated to the Order three years earlier by a Dutch nobleman. She gamely slept on a cot in her tent and washed her own dishes. (The Theosophical Society elite stayed in castle chambers or in specially constructed private huts.)

Although many addresses were made to the vast assembly, the talks given by Krishnamurti each evening were the highlights of the gathering. Seekers sat in concentric circles around a huge pile of logs set over kindling and tinder. Krishnamurti arrived, sat for a while, and then rose to set a torch to the wood. As the flames ascended against the night sky, he chanted mantras to the Vedic god of fire, Agni. After returning to his seat, Krishnamurti commenced speaking. He entranced the crowds. Many felt a sense of divine presence, including Devi, who—even later on, after having met Gandhi, Tagore, and Nehru—said that she'd "not come across any other living being whose personality reflected the Divine to such an extent as does Krishnamurti."[2] Meditative silences followed his talks.

The event that was a turning point in Devi's life, though, occurred on the first morning after her arrival. All the attendees assembled for a meditation presided over by Krishnamurti.

Someone explained to Devi that meditation, unlike prayer, is a form of sustained concentration "where the mind and heart are stilled." The effect on her, however, was the opposite. "I received a kind of inner shock. Something within me turned turtle" as soon as Krishnamurti began to chant a Sanskrit mantra. "It came to me like a forgotten call, familiar yet distant. . . . As soon as the meditation was over I rushed to my tent and cried as never before."[3]

When one of her fans in Berlin, Hermann Bolm, a wealthy banker, proposed to her, Devi accepted—on the condition that he pay her expenses for a trip to India before the wedding. (Neither her autobiographical writings nor most photos of her, in which she tends to look drab and defeated, indicate a trait that Devi obviously possessed: she could charm the pants off men, from lovers to statesmen to gurus.) Devi set sail to India on November 17, 1927. She stayed for four months. She visited seventeen locations. Always staying in Indian homes, she adopted Indian customs. "A disappointment to many, India was to me the land of the fulfillment of my dreams," she wrote. "I fell in love with the land and its people and made friends with everyone I met, coolie or prince. Happy beyond measure to be there, I wanted to do something for India, live for India, work for India, die for India."[4]

Devi returned to Europe "only a shadow of my former self. My heart and soul were left behind in my adopted motherland."[5] Estranged from everyone (she broke off her engagement with Bolm), she felt homesick for India. She returned two years later. She stayed in the south for three months, studying Indian classical dance. Then she went to Bombay for the making of *Sher-e-Arab* (Arabian Knight), a film for which she'd been offered a leading part. (Mostly performed by nonprofessional university graduates, the film broke the long-standing tradition of casting films with uneducated, lower-class career actors.) The film premiered in January 1930. Publicity declared the fair-skinned, blue-eyed Westerner as "Indra Devi, the new rising star of the Indian screen." Later in the year, Devi married Jan Strakaty, commercial attaché to the Czechoslovak consulate in Bombay, whom she met at a social gathering. "A new life began for me [in Bombay]," she wrote about her role as a colonial socialite. "A life crowded with engagements, parties, balls and outings."[6]

In 1931 Devi was inveigled by a European friend to go watch a large group of yogins from all parts of India who had just camped on Chowpatty Beach near Bombay on their way to Nashik to attend Kumbh Mela, the religious festival that's the most sacred of all Hindu pilgrimages. Disregarding a warning that it was "simply crazy" for two European women to mix with an Indian crowd, that night Devi and her friend went to the beach, where they saw rows of umbrellas stuck in the ground.[7] Sitting underneath the umbrellas were the yogins. As she and her friend, the only Europeans, wandered among the yogins, Devi felt that "these queer looking, almost completely naked people, their faces and bodies smeared with ashes, resembled a group of jugglers and acrobats in gray tights and make-up." Then she spotted a yogin standing on his head in *Sirsasana*. She was baffled. "Why on earth is he doing that?" she asked. "To please God," replied a bystander. "I could not help commenting ironically on this peculiar idea of pleasing the Heavenly Master," Devi recalled, "and admitted that my conception of Indian yogis was quite different."[8]*

Devi was skeptical of the yogin's motivation because at this time she understood yoga to be a shamanistic-like or magical healing practice, not *asana* practice. However, even when another bystander said that these *sadhus* (ascetics) weren't holy men at all, that they had merely adopted some yoga practices, Devi remained struck by the yogin's singular act. "When returning home, after about half an hour's wandering among these sadhus, we saw the same man still standing motionless on his head. Fraud or no fraud, I was amazed all the same."[9] Devi's witnessing of this yogin standing on his head was to have a powerful and lasting effect on her.

Discovering Yoga

A few years later Devi was dining with a friend who suddenly collapsed at the table, nearly losing consciousness. She took him home. Using what she called yoga healing—concentrating on removing the illness and making "healing passes over his entire body"—she cured him.[10]

Devi learned this pseudoscientific "yoga" treatment in Moscow when she was fourteen

---

*In another account of this event, Devi attributed the weirdness of standing on one's head as a form of worship not to the devotee's choice but to God's preferences: "I couldn't help commenting laughingly on the queer taste of the Heavenly Master" (I. Devi, *Yoga: The Technique*, 19).

years old from reading *Fourteen Lessons in Yogi Philosophy and Oriental Occultism* by Yogi Ramacharaka, the alias of the American William Walker Atkinson, who helped popularize yoga at the turn of the century as Oriental occultism by blithely adapting mesmerism (probably as practiced by Colonel H. S. Olcott, joint founder with Madame Blavatsky of the Theosophical Society in 1875) to yoga. Ramacharaka espoused the power of Human Magnetism.

Human Magnetism, or Pranic Energy, is a most potent therapeutic force, and, in one form or another, it is found in the majority of cases of psychic healing. It is one of the oldest forms of natural healing, and may be said to be almost instinctive in the race. A child who has hurt itself, or who feels a pain, at once runs to its mother who kisses the hurt part, or places her hand on the seat of the pain, and in a few moments the child is better. When we approach one who is suffering, it is very natural for us to place our hands on his brow, or to pass our hand over him. This instinctive use of the hand is a form of conveying magnetism to the afflicted person, who is usually relieved by the act.[11]

In Devi's case, though, something went wrong. The morning after she healed her friend, she herself fell deeply ill. It was as if she had restored her friend's health by incorporating his illness into her own body or by transfusing all of her vitality—her Human Magnetism or Pranic Energy—into him. "As a result of dabbling with something in which I was utterly profane," Devi reasoned, she was to remain sick for nearly four years, suffering from a nervous heart condition with frequent acute attacks of palpitations.[12] "I became very nervous and irritable, often bursting into tears without the slightest provocation. Everything seemed too much for me. I lived in intense weariness and could hardly remember my former singing rhythm of life."[13]

Devi couldn't fathom her misfortune. "After all," she lamented, "I had meant well and had only wanted to help my friend. Why should I have to suffer for it? Was it punishment? If so where was the wrongdoing?"[14] Nothing helped, including pilgrimages to heart specialists—until, on leave with her husband in Prague, she enrolled in a weaving class, where she met a medical student who had studied yogic healing methods. Using the same method (what she described as "prana transmission by passes and concentration") that had caused her illness in the first place, he cured her in only seven days (and without any harm to himself!).[15]

After her miraculous recovery, Devi was consumed with studying yoga. (Years later she would posit a teleological explanation for her illness: it was necessary to put a stop to her frivolous life and start her on the path of yoga.) Upon her return to Bombay in 1937 (or possibly 1936), she asked her Indian friends about yoga, but none of them had practical experience of it. However, her friend Princess Bhuban of Nepal said that her brother could show her some yoga exercises. Prince Mussoorie demonstrated several postures for Devi, including the headstand. Devi told him about the *sadhu* she had seen at Chowpatty Beach. "The Headstand is the best of all exercises," the prince explained. "It is even called the King of Asanas (Yoga postures), because of its manifold valuable effects on our glands, organs, nerves and brains. It works wonders when done with the yogic deep breathing. I know people who were relieved from severe headaches, mental troubles and nervous heart conditions just by standing on the head."[16] When he asked her if she wanted to learn how to stand on her head, she declined, convinced that she would never be able to do it.

On the prince's advice, though, Devi decided to take up yoga at Swami Kuvalayananda's yoga center, Kaivalyadhama Ashram, in Lonavla, the hill station between Bombay and Pune. A friend (whose husband, "a Mohammedan lawyer," first attended classes there to promote the growth of his hair but then took a deeper interest in his training) took her there.[17] Devi enrolled in a class for women. Upon entering the classroom, she found several women already doing exercises. She enviously looked at one standing on her head. The female instructor showed Devi how to do three postures and to breathe deeply and rhythmically, explaining that yoga was different from other systems of physical culture because its exercises are coordinated with deep breathing, resulting in far-reaching physiological and psychological effects. Devi's classes were interrupted by her having to go once again with her husband to Prague.

Discipleship with Krishnamacharya

While in Prague Devi received an invitation to the May 15, 1938, wedding of Crown Prince Jayachamaraja Wadiyar of Mysore to Princess Satya Prem Kumari Ju Deviya, sister of the maharaja of Charkhari, which incited in Devi an overwhelming urge to return to India to attend Krishnamacharya's yoga school. She had been told about the school by a doctor friend who witnessed a yoga demonstration by its students capped by a private demonstration for a small group by Krishnamacharya of one of the *siddhis* (supranormal powers).* Baffling the doctor and the others, Krishnamacharya supposedly stopped his heartbeat for several minutes.

Probably in the late winter or early spring of 1938, Devi set sail for Bombay, stayed only a couple of days, and journeyed south to the Mysore Palace, "arriving long before the wedding preparations had begun."[18] The next day she presented herself to Krishnamacharya to gain admission to his *yogashala*. He told her she couldn't study with him because he had no classes for women. When she offered to take private lessons, he found other excuses to reject her. Devi suspected the true reason for his reluctance was that he believed she wouldn't be able to abide by the demands he made of his students: "He knew that I was a palace guest, who probably came out to India to make a collection of as many thrills as possible; . . . [including] film a sadhu sitting on a nail-bed and by chance to take a few lessons in Yoga. He was not interested in this sort of pupil."[19] He ultimately accepted her, though—after receiving orders from the maharajah, Shri Nalvadi Krishnaraja Wadiyar.†

Unlike her loose participation in classes at Kuvalayananda's school, Devi's involvement

---

*In another (later and therefore probably less reliable) account, Devi claimed that she herself was present for the demonstration.
†In another account of this event, Devi wrote that Krishnamacharya was reluctant to accept her as a student but she persisted until he relented.

in Krishnamacharya's training resembled a traditional discipleship. She gave herself over to a routine of strict discipline. She accepted *yamas* and *niyamas* (yogic ethical guidelines). Her schedule, bathing habits, clothes, and diet were strictly regulated. She practiced *asanas* in the early morning and at noon on her own and in the evening at school with one of Krishnamacharya's assistants. "All of these rules and regulations do not apply to those who take up Yoga exercises for their health," she wrote, "but only to those who undergo the training of discipleship."[20]

To Krishnamacharya's surprise, Devi continued to strictly follow this regime even during the temptations of the daily cocktail parties and dances held as part of the eight-day marriage ceremony. After the great rejoicing was over, she stayed on. Impressed by her determination and progress, Krishnamacharya began to take an interest in her training. In fact, he seems to have developed a soft spot for her. He began "giving me instructions personally instead of leaving me to one of his assistants," Devi reminisced.[21]

When, to Devi's alarm, her body ballooned up, Krishnamacharya reassured her that after a month or so it would find its proper shape because yoga postures normalized the functions of the organs, especially the endocrine glands. "Inside of a few months," she wrote, "I regained my former girlish figure . . . and my youthful appearance. I felt as light and carefree as a school girl on a summer vacation."[22] What was most revelatory to her in her discipleship was the value of yoga as health cure. "I had never taken too literally the Yoga claims as to the effects of their exercises, and placed more faith in the Yoga healing methods," she acknowl-

edged. "Now that I had learned the miraculous results that could be produced by the Yoga postures and deep breathing, I came to realize the profound importance of this system of physical culture."[23]

A few weeks later, encouraged by the oldest student, a sixty-six-year-old man, Devi finally accomplished the act for which she had formerly lacked courage: performing *Sirsasana*, Headstand (see fig. 27.1 on page 344). "Soon," she wrote, "I was able to keep this posture unaided in the middle of the room." Standing on her head in *Sirsasana*—what she would later consider "the most basic and valuable of all postures"—was a transformative experience for Devi.[24] Turned precariously upside down, she experienced for the first time a firmly held sense of self.

After a few months Devi informed Krishnamacharya that she was going to join her husband, who had been transferred to Shanghai while she had stayed behind to continue her yoga studies. To her great surprise, Krishnamacharya told her that he wanted her to teach yoga in China. When she expressed doubts about her abilities to teach, he firmly told her: "You can and you will."[25]

In Bombay for a few months before sailing for Shanghai, Devi fell into a "state of black despair and utter loneliness,"[26] brought on, it appears, by her apprehension at "leaving India, my adopted motherland, being sure that I would always remain a forlorn stranger in any other land."[27] "I understood then why people commit suicide."[28] Devi had long feared isolation. After her parents' marriage dissolved when she was barely out of infancy, her father soon disappeared. When she was a very young child,

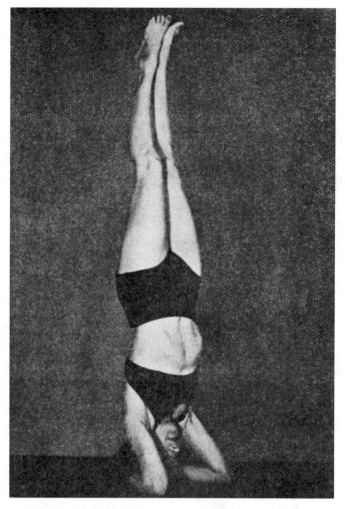

Figure 27.1. Indra Devi demonstrating *Sirsanana* in India, 1946

(From *Yoga: The Technique of Health and Happiness,* by Indra Devi)

her mother ran off to join a touring theater company, leaving Devi with her maternal grandparents. No matter that she led a privileged life at their house (she was tutored at home until she was ten, tended to by servants, lavished with presents, including dolls and dresses, by her doting grandfather, and exposed to the gaiety of frequent parties and receptions)—she nevertheless lived in constant fear that her mother, whom she adored, would never return. During the times when her mother did return home (when she wasn't touring), Devi, like a fan, bathed in her glamour. But when her mother left to go back to the theater troupe, Devi, as if she were unable to store new memories, felt just as abandoned and anxious as if her mother had never visited.

Fortuitously, Krishnamurti—who, after dramatically rejecting any plan to promote him as a World Teacher and withdrawing as the figurehead of the Theosophists at the 1929 Order of the Star assembly, had become an unaffiliated inspirational writer and speaker on philosophical and spiritual subjects—happened to be in Bombay, where he was holding a study group in the mornings at the residence of Ratansi Morarji, a wealthy mill owner.*

Devi attended the group, but "dulled by the pain of [her] sufferings, [she] could not even follow [Krishnamurti's] words."[29] She arranged to meet with Krishnamurti for private counseling. Readily comprehending her desperation, he gave her advice for dealing with what he diagnosed as the cause of her sorrow: her fear of being alone. "It was necessary, according to Krishnaji, to acquire a detached point of view, to see things from a different angle." After enduring a few more days of hopelessness, she was unexpectedly overwhelmed with a feeling of bliss. She had found what Krishnamurti described to her as "the ecstasy of solitude."[30] "Everything changed at once the moment the fear was gone, the moment I was not afraid of losing anything, whether it was life, love, friends or possessions."[31] Devi had undergone her second transformation: loss of self.

Teaching in China

During her sea voyage on a luxury liner to China in late 1938, Devi learned that her new form of self-realization, while not as complete a transformation as attained by those who achieve *moksha,* release, but optimal for someone with her fragile psychic makeup, manifested itself in new attitudes and actions.

The very first evening on the boat, while dressing for dinner, I discovered that I didn't care anymore to decorate myself with jewels and make up my face with lipstick and rouge; neither did I want to wear my tight-fitting and low-cut "smart" evening gowns and was glad to have a few *sarees* with me. It felt strange to think that I was once a good companion for those who enjoyed gaiety, cinemas and dancing, that I was interested in expensive jewels and smart clothes, and could spend my time in going about from one party to another. . . .

It wasn't that I turned all of a sudden into a bore or a prig, but simply that I needed no special distraction or company to "kill the time" because I never felt lonesome or restless any more.[32]

Defined more starkly because in contrast with the haut monde high life she was rejecting aboard the ship, Devi's new sense of existence—her movement toward integration with Being—was symbolized by her replacing the evening gown with the sari (which would later become her iconic garb) (see fig. 27.2 on page 347).

---

*Morarji had been party to a landmark court case involving his wife's will, which was contested because she wasn't born into Hinduism. The Austrian-born Englishwoman, Mena Renda, a Theosophist, who had lived in India for about twelve or thirteen years, converted to Hinduism, took the Hindu name Sulochana, and married Morarji according to Vedic rites on May 21, 1922; honeymooned in Venice, Paris, and London; made a will bequeathing her entire property to Morarji; died on August 14, 1923; and was posthumously declared a Hindu by the Madras High Court on August 20, 1928, thus officially settling the specific question, "Is it open to a lady of European origin to become a Hindu by conversion?" and the general question, "Is it legally permissible for a non-Hindu to become a Hindu?" As a consequence, the will was declared valid.

Upon arriving in Shanghai, which was under Japanese occupation, Devi announced to Strakaty that she "did not mean to continue the empty social life and intended to do something." Her husband was far from supportive. "This statement greatly amused Joe, as he was convinced that I was capable of doing nothing, but when I mentioned the Yoga class, he got a little alarmed: 'Do anything you want, but not this nonsense, please.'"[33]

Over her husband's opposition, Devi persisted in her "nonsense," opening Shanghai's first yoga school, which was variously located on the roof of the French Club; in a friend's gymnasium; in her apartment; in the bungalow (more specifically, in the spacious bedroom, large enough to hold twenty-five pupils at a time) of Madame Chiang Kai-shek, wife of the nationalist leader; and, during the last frantic months of World War II, in three successive houses. Her first students were friends. After she promoted herself (a talk and demonstrations resulted in articles and interviews), her first paying pupil arrived in February 1939. Soon afterward, the American consul's wife and other American women joined the class. The class grew to twenty-five pupils. Devi taught under her maiden name Petersen, in part because her husband was afraid that he'd become a laughingstock if people learned that his wife taught yoga.

Despite her husband's continued disapproval and belittlement (he always maintained that running her own yoga school was "no more than a crazy idea of an idle society woman, who happened to be his wife"), Devi taught yoga in her school in China for seven and a half years to 617 students, mostly Americans.[34] During this time, she facilitated health cures not through yogic sha-manistic healing but through yogic exercise and diet. Her grateful students, in her account, were cured of headaches, weak hearts, rheumatism, nervousness, insomnia, suicidal tendencies, blindness caused by menstruation, stunted growth, asthma, myopia, anemia, and obesity.

Return to India

A few months after the end of the war, in early 1946, Devi and Strakaty left Shanghai. He returned to Czechoslovakia, and she returned to her beloved India. She lectured and taught yoga (the lectures generated teaching jobs) in various locations, becoming the first Occidental woman to teach yoga in India.

Then Devi settled for a while in picturesque Narendra Nagar, a city with an easy mix of the cosmopolitan and spiritual, nestled in the outer foothills of the Himalayas, overlooking Rishikesh, in order to study with Swami Som-nathasbram. While staying as a guest at the palace of the maharajah of Tehri Garhwal, she motored down to the swami's abode near the Ganges for instruction. The rest of the day she practiced yoga and wrote her first book, *Yoga: The Technique of Health and Happiness,* in which she reflected on her struggles with emptiness, loneliness, and despair. "Don't we all know of so many well-to-do people who resort to alcohol and drugs, or even to suicide, because they are unable to stand that inner emptiness, which at first they try to fill with 'wine, women and laughter,' or at best, with some kind of hobby or diversion?" Devi knew such people very well indeed: they were her friends, her husband, and herself. "It goes without saying that none of these external things can give a feeling

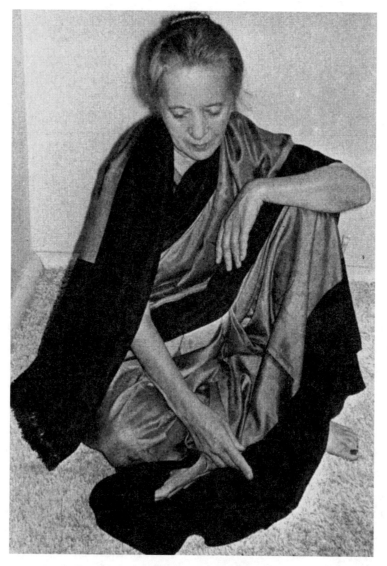

Figure 27.2. Indra Devi in her trademark sari, 1963

(From *Renew Your Life through Yoga*, by Indra Devi)

of lasting happiness or satisfaction, when there is disharmony within."[35]

What alleviates suffering, Devi had discovered, was the turning inward of yoga. She gave a nod to the spiritual aspect of yoga: "It is in India alone that a philosophy exists which takes into consideration the whole man—his spiritual, mental and physical aspects. Yoga, unadulterated, still stands the test of centuries."[36] But what she primarily meant by the turning inward of yoga was calming the mind: "Relaxation of mind and body as well as deep breathing play a very important part in Yoga. Children, savages and animals need no instructions on this subject, so long as they do not acquire the bad habits of civilized men."[37]

She continued:

People who are often worried and depressed, who easily lose their temper and who live under constant nervous tension and fear, are simply wasting away their Prana, i.e., health, energy and vitality. If they only knew how to relax at will, most of their troubles and worries would disappear and be replaced by a calm and comprehensive attitude.

So many patients hear their doctors telling them not to worry and to take things easy, but they are not taught them [sic] how this is done.[38]

Devi had found an eminently practical way to cure psychic pain: yogic postures and deep breathing.

In late 1946, after returning to Shanghai to sell her belongings, Devi was set to return to India to head the yoga therapy treatment in a nature cure home in Kashmir headed by a Buddhist monk. But her friends, "fearing that [she] might become a Buddhist nun and get lost to the world," persuaded her to go to America instead.[39]

Devi docked in San Francisco, California, on January 21, 1947, and immediately went to Los Angeles, where she soon opened a yoga studio in an office complex at 8806 Sunset Boulevard, in West Hollywood. Within a few years, her students included luminaries in the entertainment business.

Devi never saw Strakaty again. He was in Czechoslovakia when the communists took over in 1948 and died in early 1953. "With him a rare man and dear friend were gone," Devi graciously said.[40] On March 14, 1953, she married her companion, Sigfrid Knauer, a renowned doctor who was regularly consulted by people in the film industry on matters of health and happiness. He was a far more suitable husband than Strakaty. Although a staunch Christian, he supported Devi in all her yogic endeavors. In 1960 he bought her a twenty-four-room house, which she called Rancho Cuchuma Ashram, on an eighty-acre ranch in Tecate, Baja Mexico, where she lived and gave teacher training courses twice a year to yoga teachers from around the world.

In 1957, when she became a United States citizen, Eugenie Peterson legally changed her name to Indra Devi.

28

INDRA DEVI

Treating Anxiety with Yoga

Relieving Anxiety: Yoga as Relaxation Technique

Indra Devi listened to the famous (diplomatically unnamed) comedian slumped in an armchair across from her talk about his breakdown. "I was forced to stop working because my nerves were so bad," he said gloomily. "Now I couldn't get a smile from a three-year-old." When Devi asked him what he had tried to help him relax, he replied: "What haven't I tried these past few years! Everything—doctors, psychoanalysts, therapists, walks, drink, pills galore. Now I'm on a 40-pills-a-day routine and it still doesn't do any good. I can't sleep and I can't relax even though I spend my days doing absolutely nothing."[1] Devi didn't ask him when or why things began to fall apart, respond to him with platitudes, reproach him for being privileged and self-indulgent, or tell him that his complaints sounded like one of his comedy routines. She simply related her history of overcoming anxiety through practicing yogic postures and deep, rhythmic breathing. When he asked her how he might go about the breathing exercises to help him relax, she gave him a lesson in deep breathing right then and there. The following week he announced to her that he'd thrown away his pills. A month later she saw him on television "clowning, running around, dancing. Gone was . . . his case of 'nerves.'"[2]

Although she displayed empathy and took action to alleviate the misery of a man at the end of his rope, Devi also saw the larger context of his plight: "His suffering was a sample for what was happening to hundreds of thousands of people across the United States. In this country which offers more material comforts . . . than any other in the world, this distraught man was afflicted by the combination of tension and fear which keeps countless men and women from leading full, rich, productive lives."[3] To relieve the suffering of all Americans "beset with anxiety, unable to relax," Devi sought to introduce yoga to America on a mass scale.[4] During the 1950s and 1960s she taught, lectured, and published three books: *Forever Young Forever Healthy* (1953), *Yoga for Americans* (1959), and *Renew Your Life through Yoga* (1963).

Like the pioneer yogins in India in the 1920s, Devi knew that for yoga to be widely accepted in America, she had to dispel prevalent misconceptions about yoga held by the middle class. She learned this imperative from her own experience. When she first arrived in America in 1947, she was often rebuffed by people at the mere mention of the word *yoga*. "'I am not interested in a weird cult; nor do I care to learn the rope trick, snake charming, fire-eating, or other similar things,'" they told her. "'I can very well live without them.'"[5] This conception of yoga was so prevalent that friends advised her to call yoga by some other name if she wanted to teach it.

"There are a number of unscrupulous adventurers and charlatans in this country who mystify and exploit the gullible public under the cloak of Yoga," Devi warned in *Forever Young Forever Healthy*. But yoga "is in no way related to fortune-telling, palmistry, spirit-dabbling and other such things intended primarily to attract wealthy and frustrated dowagers." She promised to give her readers "a true picture of what Yoga has to offer to the weary, tense and nervous Western world."[6]

Devi's primary strategy for selling yoga to the American public was publicizing its popularity with her show business and high-culture celebrity clientele. She especially made good use of her famous Hollywood followers in promoting her books. In the breezy manner of a gossip column, the copy for the inside flap of the book jacket (probably provided by the publisher) for *Forever Young Forever Healthy* revealed that "Hatha Yoga has been the method used successfully [at Devi's studio] to combat modern day stress, strain and fatigue by such celebrities as Greta Garbo, Jennifer Jones, Ruth St. Denis, Gloria Swanson, Serge Koussevitsky, Robert Ryan and many others."[7] The fact that film stars and other celebrities "have been studying with me," Devi explained in a 1957 address, "made an average man think that there must be something to Yoga after all if it has been taken up by so many prominent personalities"[8] (fig. 28.1).

Westerners living in the post–World War II period weren't the first people to experience anxiety en masse. Throughout history, broad groupings of people experienced anxiety—from generalized nervousness to bouts of terror—in times of revolution, rapid urbanization, famine, warfare, a crisis of faith, large-scale migration, and other turmoil. Yet in no previous era had people analyzed, dwelled on, and defined themselves by anxiety to as great a degree as in the modern era, in general, and the post–World War II years, in particular. This self-aware anxiety was apotheosized in W. H. Auden's Pulitzer Prize–winning dramatic poem "The Age of Anxiety: A Baroque Eclogue," published in 1947. After it appeared, Auden's title phrase was used to describe the characteristic emotional state of the times. Leonard Bernstein wrote about his *Age of Anxiety, Symphony No. 2 (after W. H. Auden)*, compulsively composed

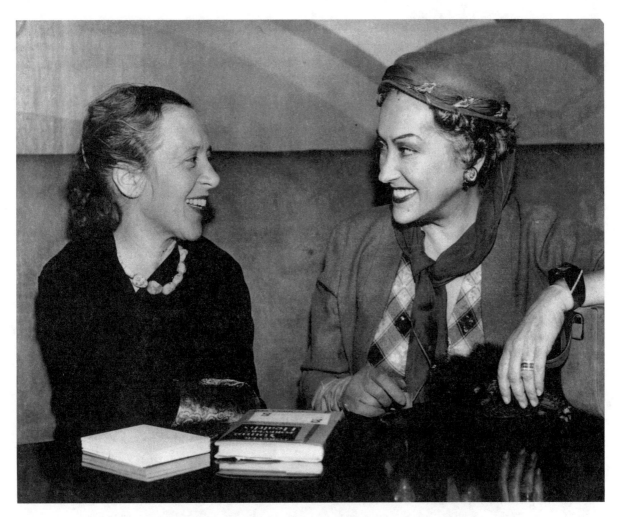

Figure 28.1. Indra Devi (left) with her biggest celebrity booster, Hollywood star Gloria Swanson, 1953
(With the kind permission of Larry Payne, Ph.D., Samata International)

on planes, in hotel lobbies, and in apartment rooms in the years 1948 and 1949 and first performed in 1949: "The essential line of the poem (and the music) is the record of our difficult and problematic search for faith."[9] The Protestant theologian-philosopher Paul Tillich wrote in *The Courage to Be* in 1952:

Sociological analyses of the present period have pointed to the importance of anxiety as a group phenomenon. Literature and art have made anxiety a main theme of their creations, in content as well as in style. The effect of this has been the awakening of people to an awareness of their own anxiety, and a permeation of the public consciousness by ideas and symbols of anxiety. Today it has become almost a truism to call our time an "age of anxiety." This holds equally for America and Europe.[10]

Although we today may be no less anxious than people living in mid-20th-century America and Europe, we no longer live in the Age of Anxiety, because we no longer primarily define ourselves as anxious. The height of the Age of Anxiety was the late 1940s to the early 1960s, when Americans were seeking ways to ameliorate the pressures of career, marriage, and child rearing with cocktails, tranquilizers, psychotherapy, television, vacations, hobbies, and other means.

During this period Devi's classes, lectures, and books generated interest in yoga not only throughout America but around the world. Her three books were best sellers in America and were translated into ten languages. In *The Subtle Body: The Story of Yoga in America*, Stefanie Syman argues that Devi's success at popularizing yoga was due to the fact that she pitched it as a beauty secret, youth elixir, and health tonic: Devi was "good at packaging Hatha Yoga as a defense against illness and aging," making "this maddeningly complex discipline . . . accessible and relevant to postwar Americans."[11] In the 1950s Devi did teach yoga to wealthy women at cosmetics titan Elizabeth Arden's upscale spas in Maine (the first destination spa in America, opened in 1934) and Arizona, where yoga was promoted as a product that could make women trim, youthful, and vital. One of the wealthiest women in the world, Arden built her cosmetics empire (consisting of salons, the first of which was opened on Fifth Avenue in New York City in 1910, and a line of beauty products) by persuading women to wear makeup, which was previously used primarily by prostitutes and the lower class. She convinced middle- and upper-class women that makeup was de rigueur for looking refined and well bred; plain women that makeup made them look beautiful; and middle-aged women that makeup made them look younger. But Devi rejected Arden's offer to join her staff in part because she strenuously rejected such superficial notions of beauty and youth.

In the chapter "The Woman Beautiful" in 1953's *Forever Young Forever Healthy,* Devi advised women, "Remove all your clothes and begin a thorough examination of your entire body. Is there anything you do not like about it?"[12] Then, after asking several more questions about making a self-assessment, she posited (perhaps with a swipe at Arden) that our emotional core manifests itself on our face: "No make-up can hide a hard line around the mouth, a selfish expression on the face, a spiteful glance in the eyes. Now, remain absolutely quiet for a while and then ask yourself this last question: 'Am I as beautiful as I can be?'"[13] Yoga makes us beautiful, Devi argued, by helping us attain peace of mind. And in the chapter "Old Today and Young Tomorrow," Devi encouraged her readers to give up their foolish desires to be young: "Look back at your own life. What did you do with your youth? For myself, I can say that life didn't have any particular meaning to me at that age [the teenage years], and I wouldn't exchange it for my present one if I could. Perhaps this is due to the fact that I am now living a very full, harmonious and happy life, and am at peace with myself and the world. And Yoga has a great deal to do with all of this."[14] In making these down-to-earth arguments, Devi turned the then current notions of beauty and youth on their head, rejecting—not reinforcing—the narcissistic desires of women to be beautiful and youthful.

As early as the 1940s in China, Devi had been vigorously touting yoga as natural health cure. In the 1950s her followers eagerly testified to the beneficial effects of her teachings not on their appearance but on their debilitating ailments (especially constipation and "female disorders"). "It was a great pleasure . . . to have you lecture at the Brooklyn Lodge of the Theosophical Society," a woman from Brooklyn wrote. "After hearing your lecture and seeing you demonstrate some of the genuine Yoga exercises, I decided to join one of your classes. . . . I had been suffering for several years from constipation of a most stubborn nature, exaggerated perhaps by the menopause. After the first exercises on Monday, I had real relief."[15] "Your book [*Forever Young Forever Healthy,* translated into Sindhi] has made even us Indians more keenly aware of the great benefits of the Yoga Asanas," a man from Bombay wrote. One of his close friends, the wife of a university professor, "suffered for many years from nervous stomach troubles, arthritis, and female disorders. After a few months of Yoga practice and following your diet, she has completely recovered from all her troubles."[16]

Yet Devi primarily advertised yoga as a means of calming a troubled mind, and the most pressing reason that people gave for turning to her yoga at midcentury was to have their nervousness assuaged. Her yoga teachings, her followers testified, picked up their lagging spirits and dispelled their desperation. Jack Macfadden (the son of Bernarr Macfadden, the self-proclaimed "father of physical culture") wrote from Hollywood: "Your classes have changed my outlook on life so completely that I anxiously await each new glorious day with enthusiasm and optimism."[17] "The headstand and other exercises actually saved my husband's life when he was suffering a severe form of nervous depression," a former student wrote from Tel Aviv.[18]

In fact, her success in Hollywood (which she parlayed into becoming a yoga celebrity) is owed to her use of yoga as a treatment for anxiety and depression. The tormented actress Jennifer Jones began classes with Devi in her Los Angeles studio, probably in 1948, in order to find relief from feeling hopeless and worthless. Jones was sent to Devi by May Romm, the most famous Hollywood psychoanalyst of the era. Several of her patients (with whom Romm hobnobbed—a not unusual practice of the times) were members of the movie industry, most significantly producer David O. Selznick, with whom Jones was having an affair. (He had even hired Romm to work on *Spellbound,* his 1945 mystery about a female psychoanalyst, for which Romm received a screen credit: "Psychiatric Adviser, May E. Romm, M.D.") Romm probably met Devi at a social gathering, in all likelihood at a party given by the cosmopolitan hostess Bernardine Fritz, whose "Hollywood salon" brought together leading cultural figures (including numerous actors and filmmakers), many of whom were expatriates. (Perhaps Romm and Devi even met at the party Fritz threw to introduce newcomer Devi to members of her glittering crowd.) Romm and Devi would've found commonalities: both were healers and Russian émigrés of the same generation.

According to journalist Adriana Aboy, "Devi, also once an actress, felt an immediate empathy" toward Jones.[19] By teaching

Jones *asanas* and meditation (sitting for five minutes a day while concentrating on the *ujjayi* breath as a means of emptying the mind of all thoughts), Devi was able to alleviate Jones's depression (at least temporarily). Jones became a dedicated votary of yoga, incorporating it into her daily life. During the filming of *Gone to Earth,* which started August 1, 1949, in England on a set at Shepperton Studios in Surrey and on location at sites around Shropshire, Jones, who was "much given to yoga as a means of relaxation," recalls cameraman Christopher Challis in his memoir, "had the disconcerting habit of standing on her head for several minutes just before a take while the assembled company waited in expectation."[20] Jones's praise of Devi led to others in the movie industry attending her classes, thus leading to Devi's reputation as the yoga teacher of Hollywood stars.

Dubbed the "First Lady of Yoga," Devi became the spokesperson for yoga in America. From her, Americans learned of yoga as an ancient—and therefore time-tested—natural protection against and remedy for stress. Devi presented yoga as sensible preventive mental health care (without even mentioning its spiritual essence) most cogently in "Anxiety—The Problem of Our Age," the introduction to *Renew Your Life through Yoga:* just as you protect yourself against drowning by learning to swim, against various hazards by purchasing insurance, and against infectious disease by getting vaccinated, by practicing yoga, she persuasively argued, "you will learn how to protect yourself against tension, anxiety, and fear."[21]

Moksha

In India some older men, after fulfilling the demands and enjoying the satisfactions of caring for their family and earning a living, reject their ordinary life to seek inner calm, the prerequisite for self-realization. And some younger men, upon sensing that the ephemeral concerns of the everyday world cause suffering, renounce all worldly desires and, possessed by a calling, dedicate their life to spiritual pursuits. Typically the older men, remaining at home, and the younger men, going off to a hermitage, turn to a yoga guru for mentorship. The guru instructs them in meditation as the vehicle for attaining *moksha*—variously taken to mean, as Indian psychoanalyst Sudhir Kakar explains, "self-realization, transcendence, salvation, a release from worldly involvement, from 'coming' and 'going.' Yet in Hindu philosophy it is also described as the state in which all distinctions between subject and object have been transcended, a direct experience of the fundamental unity of a human being with the infinite."[22]

In order to transcend the opposition between subject and object and experience unity with Brahman (the world) the yoga aspirant, whether old or young, must not only renounce obligations to family and work but also, through practicing meditation, systematically dissolve the very ego functions that we use in most aspects of our everyday life to attain happiness and success, that we dedicate ourselves to instilling in our children (so they can enjoy happiness and success), and that we sometimes conscientiously examine (in order to solidify) in psychotherapeutic treatment.

The most difficult and critical ego function

that must be dissolved is the complex sense of reality of self and world on which our ability to maintain boundaries between "inside" and "outside," "I" and "others," and "I" and "the world" is founded. "The developmental process by which an infant moves from a state of nonawareness of the world to one in which he becomes a separate and unique person in transaction with distinct others around him," writes Eda G. Goldstein, author of a classic textbook on ego psychology, "is inextricably connected to the development of a sense of reality."[23] When we have a good sense of reality, we experience ourselves as distinct from the world. Yet we feel connected to the world. It seems real. There's no sense that we're walking in a dream. Even when we feel most uncomfortable with our body, finding it grotesque or ludicrous, our body doesn't seem disconnected (from our self) or dissolving or shifting. We experience our body as intact and belonging to us. And when we fall in love, we don't experience a literal merging with another. We keep our own identity.

This undistorted sense of everyday reality is the last of the dozen or so ego functions that the yogin must reject during meditation. Based on a subject (e.g., fire), yogic meditation proper begins with concentration on an object (e.g., glowing coals placed before the yogin). Penetration into the essence of reality occurs during the final three steps of the (commonly) eight-stepped meditation process—*dharana, dhyana,* and *samadhi,* collectively called *samyama.* It cannot occur without concurrently and utterly undoing all accommodations to everyday reality.

This quest for spiritual liberation—the pursuit of replacing quotidian perceptions of reality with divine consciousness, an assimilation of

reality unmediated by the ego—is not without its risks. For the spiritual seeker whose ego isn't autonomous, there's a danger of a vertiginous descent into what is known in Western psychology as "depersonalization": feeling unreal, losing connection with the body, and coalescing with the external world. To ensure against psychotic breakdown, during the meditation session the guru, who has previously (perhaps over a period of years) instructed the *chela* in the subtle mental continuum of *samyama,* monitors the *chela*'s progress and provides support through look, touch, and silence (but not, as in Western psychotherapies, words)—that is, by his presence.

Under the guidance of the guru, the yoga votary eventually achieves a state in which "I" and "Brahman" ("I" and the world) are one. This experience of the dissolution of the separation between subject and object, leading to a feeling of unity with the world, may seem to Westerners to be an alarming break with reality. But for the yogin with a fully integrated self, becoming one with Brahman doesn't damage or weaken his or her sense of self and isn't a hallucination or delusion or regression to the phase of late infancy (when we don't see the world as something outside ourselves); it is, instead, in Kakar's words, a "fully aware activity of a mature adult"[24]—it is, in fact, "an intensely creative approach to external reality . . . and recognized as such with (what [visionary poet William] Blake would call) *delight.*"[25]

In the mid-20th century, Devi, through her classes, lectures, demonstrations, and books, popularized yoga for Americans as a technique for relaxation, or stress reduction. In so doing, she redirected yoga in the service of strengthening the ego instead of dissolving the ego. Whereas traditionally a guru would guide his disciple's withdrawal (from involvement in quotidian life) and disassembling of ego functions (developed to navigate that involvement in quotidian life), Devi was shoring up the ability of her students to tolerate anxiety—a critical function of the ego—in order for them to better cope with the pressures of their lives.

The chirpy pitch on the inside flaps of the jacket to her *Yoga for Americans* perfectly expresses Devi's adaptation of yoga as a technique for stress reduction:

> Ancient India's science of Hatha Yoga gives you a vital, confident approach to the converging pressures and tensions of modern living. Practicing Yoga daily will relax and rejuvenate you in mind and body. You'll face each day with a fresh, buoyant energy that will make you feel years younger. . . .
>
> As you combine these postures with the proper deep breathing, you will start to enjoy sounder sleep, a keener mind and a happier disposition.[26]

Not that Devi didn't know that yoga is essentially soteriology. But she was eminently realistic. She knew that if she were going to help Americans at all, then she'd have to accept that most of them wanted to change—but not all that much. They weren't hankering after a transcendent experience; they just wanted to feel better about themselves. They wanted to be happier. Besides, she realized, totally dedicating oneself to yoga as a system of contemplation with the aim of spiritual liberation isn't suitable for most Americans. "The advanced stages of Yoga require many years of special preparation—practices for which the American mode of living, its tempo and surroundings, are not well suited."[27]

Devi also knew that advanced yogic practices—postures and meditation—could cause harm. "Under existing circumstances these advanced practices may even prove dangerous and detrimental to your physical and mental well being and balance." She was wise to be so cautious, especially considering that her followers—whom, she knew, included many lost souls—were likely to be suffering from anxiety. The higher-level practices of yoga—those that lead to *moksha*—are dangerous to even the slightly mentally unbalanced. "It is better, therefore, to leave [the advanced practices] alone," she concluded, "and to limit yourself to the practice of the Yoga postures and deep breathing and relaxation exercises, with some of the time devoted to concentration and meditation."[28]

Devi understood the dangers of total release of the self for most Westerners because, I think, she understood the dangers for herself. She knew that with her fragile psychic makeup (her battles with anxiety and depression), total abandonment of the self would lead to a breakdown. So, while she never failed to give obligatory reminders that yoga is a spiritual endeavor, she largely presented yoga to her students, audiences, and readers as an Eastern alternative to psychotherapy and pharmaceuticals for allaying anxiety.

Some might consider Devi's undertaking a balm; others, a sacrilege. Some might argue that Devi carried on the yoga tradition by adapting it to the age. She forged yoga into a way to help people "manage," "deal with things," "handle whatever comes up," "muddle through," "get by"—to better cope with everyday reality. And yet, others might argue, what could be more subversive of the classical yoga tradition, whose core principle through time and across lands since Indian antiquity (roughly the 2nd century BCE to the 5th century CE) is that knowledge of ultimate reality, the reality behind everyday appearances, is the key to our salvation, the solution to our suffering?

It turns out, though, that Devi can't receive the praise or blame for originating the concept of yoga as stress relief. While rightly credited with having refined and heavily promoted the concept, she picked up the notion of yoga as stress relief from Krishnamacharya, who taught it to her at the Jagan Mohan Palace in India in 1938.

Krishnamacharya's Legacy

It seemed preordained that Krishnamacharya's fanatical pursuit of yoga philosophy and other related subjects would lead him to a career as an academic (see chapter 17 for a detailed description of his education). When he was a boy in Mysore, in South India, in the late 1800s, he learned yoga (whose goal is union of the human spirit with the Supreme Brahman) and Vaishnavism (whose goal is a life of bliss in service to Vishnu) from his father. Beginning in 1906 he spent ten years earning degrees in various branches of Indian philosophy from six different Indian universities. Eager to learn more about yoga, he traveled to Lake Manasarovar in Tibet in 1915 (so he said, at least) to study for nearly eight years with a guru with expertise in

Patanjali's *Yoga Sutra*, Rammohan Brahmacari, under whose tutelage he absorbed the philosophy of yoga, as well as the practice of *asana* and *pranayama*.

After returning to Mysore in 1925, marrying, and living in poverty for five years, in 1931 Krishnamacharya was given a position teaching Mimamsa and yoga philosophy at the Sanskrit College in Mysore by the maharajah of Mysore, Shri Nalvadi Krishnaraja Wadiyar. Krishnamacharya seemed to have fulfilled his destiny at last. But two years later the maharajah assigned him a new position teaching hatha yoga to members of the royal family in a *yogashala* at the Jagan Mohan Palace. His chief duties there were teaching *srsti krama* to the younger boys and *siksana krama* to the older boys—categories of yoga practice that focus on, respectively, the acquisition and the perfection of skills in *asana*, *pranayama*, and other tools of hatha yoga. In addition, he taught *raksana krama* to the adults.

"The focus of *raksana krama*," explains Kausthub Desikachar, Krishnamacharya's grandson, "is maintenance of health, relief of stress, and rejuvenation. This practice is ideal for most adults with families and busy social and professional lives. At this stage of life, our primary need is to maintain our health, so that we can fulfill our responsibilities."[29] Krishnamacharya taught vigorous *asanas*—sequences of dynamic yogic postures smoothly linked together—to the boys. But as Desikachar makes clear, "Krishnamacharya did not teach the same things to the healthy adults and the Royal Family at the *Yoga Shala* that he taught to his young students and trainee teachers. When working with the healthy adults, he focused more on *raksana krama,* teaching some simple *asanas,* but mainly *pranayama,* and also some meditative practices."[30] ("The essence of my father's teachings," states Krishnamacharya's son [and Kausthub's father] T. K. V. Desikachar, "is this: it is not that the person needs to accommodate him- or herself to yoga, but rather the yoga practice must be tailored to fit each person."[31])

Krishnamacharya's main area of interest, though, was *adhyatmika krama,* the category of yoga practice that nourishes spirituality. He never lost sight of the fact that spiritual liberation is the goal of yoga. "Once you stop the oscillating nature of mind," he wrote in *Yoga Makaranda,* "you can reach the level of dhyana, nididhyasanam, and samadhi, and through that you can see the atma."[32] *Atman* (the more common spelling than *atma*), the first principle of the Vedanta school of Hinduism, is the true self. As Krishnamacharya made clear, while "the body and mind are changing constantly and take on different forms every moment," *atman* "is that which can never be destroyed. That is, it is unchanging and does not take different forms every moment."[33] To attain salvation, one must realize that one's *atman,* true self, is identical with the transcendent self, *brahman.*

Atman/brahman, Krishnamacharya explained, "completely pervades all gross and subtle objects. Moreover, it gives identity and form to all objects and yet it is not affected by their activities." He compared *atman/brahman* to space, and our experience of *atman/brahman* consciousness to our experience of space. "Space contains so many different objects and has so many forms packed into it. Yet we can directly perceive that space exists distinct from these objects and is not associated with any of the objects contained within it, and that its nature is not affected by the properties of any of the objects contained in it."[34]

But despite his immense learning and great interest in the spiritual aspect of yoga, and probably to his great disappointment, Krishnamacharya (in his grandson's telling) seems to have taught few, if any, of the adults *adhyatmika krama* (for this reason, it may be said that he never had any true disciples, except for his son, whom he taught the meditative components of yoga in depth in the late 1980s); what Krishnamacharya taught most adults at the Jagan Mohan Palace wasn't obliteration of the everyday self, with its stable, unique, and separate identity, but shoring up the self using defense mechanisms; not transcendence of everyday life, but accommodation with everyday life; not reintegration with Being, but stress relief—not, in other words, *adhyatmika krama,* but *raksana krama.* The latter, at least, was the category of yoga teaching that Devi received from Krishnamacharya when she studied with him in 1938.

In *Renew Your Life through Yoga,* Devi distilled her *asana* teaching from the "12 basic Yoga postures" described in her three previous books, selecting the seven exercises that "specifically relax the body and the mind. I have not included the Yoga postures which do not directly affect relaxation."[35] She recommended beginning the yoga session by performing *surya namaskar,* which she translated as "the Sun-greeting Exercise," as a warm-up exercise.* "The *Surya Namaskar* is actually a series of nine exercises grouped together which make it a fully rounded routine that affects and revitalizes most of the vital parts and organs of our body."[36] "After you have finished the *Surya Namaskar,* lie down and relax for a while."[37] The yoga postures proper began with (using her spelling of the Sanskrit names and her translations) *Bhujangasana,* Cobra Posture, moved on to *Paschimatanasana,* Stretch, *Viparita Karani,* Reverse Posture, Lotus Pose (unidentified by Devi by its Sanskrit name *Padmasana*), *Yoga Mudra,* Stoop, and *Uddyiana Bandha,* Abdominal Lift (a lock but considered by Devi to be a posture), and ended with *Shirshasana,* Headstand.

The two primary portable yogic relaxation techniques (those that could be easily transferred from the classroom to the everyday world) that Devi promoted were recommended by Krishnamacharya. The first was deep breathing. "Sri Krishnamacharya often used to say," Devi remembered, "'Do the deep breathing whenever you are feeling tired, nervous, tense, hungry, too hot or too cold. Do it when you need extra energy, vitality and strength; or when your hopes are low and your faith failing.'"[38†] This advice was certainly a far cry from historian of religion Mircea Eliade's description of the traditional use of yogic breathing: "Through *pranayama* the yogin seeks to attain direct knowledge of the pulsation of his own life, the organic energy discharged by inhalation and exhalation."[39]

Krishnamacharya recommended to Devi that she use deep breathing to allay her anxiety "whenever [she] faced addressing an audience, especially if [she] had reason to believe it might be an unsympathetic one. 'First take a few deep breaths,' he suggested. 'Then during the last inhalation "take in" the vibrations of the audience, hold the breath for a few seconds, then exhale with the first spoken word.'"[40]

The second portable yogic relaxation technique recommended by Krishnamacharya was *Sirsasana* (see fig. 28.2 on page 360). "Sri Krishnamacharya used to tell me: 'Do the Headstand when you are tired and in need of a tonic; when you are unable to fall asleep; when you are hungry, nervous, and unhappy. Do it when in need of relaxation, when the brain is clouded, when you are in low spots.'"[41]

---

*Although probably taught *surya namaskar* by Krishnamacharya, Devi first learned about *surya namaskar* from Apa Pant. Pant's father, the rajah of Aundh, the great advocate of *surya namaskar,* published two books about the discipline: *Surya Namaskars,* in 1928, and *The Ten-Point Way to Health,* in 1938. "It was his son, Prince Appa, who showed [*The Ten-Point Way to Health*] to me in India several years before I started on my own Yoga training," Devi wrote in 1963 (I. Devi, *Renew Your Life,* 163). She's mistaken, however, about which book she was shown. She took up yoga in earnest in 1938, the year *The Ten-Point Way to Health* was published, so the book she saw several years previously must've been *Surya Namaskars.* Further evidence is that *Surya Namaskars* is the book on *surya namaskar* listed in the bibliography of her first book, *Yoga: The Technique of Health and Happiness,* published in India in 1948, when her memory was no doubt fresher.

†Some skepticism must be voiced about Devi's verbatim quotations of Krishnamacharya's beliefs. Could Devi (or anyone) recall in such detail advice given twenty-five years previously, and could Krishnamacharya, who, by Devi's own admission, "spoke very little English" (Youngman, "Dame of Yoga," 76), have expressed such well-thought-out and articulate advice? Even if she made the wording more elaborate and eloquent, though, the essence of his remarks is no doubt accurately conveyed.

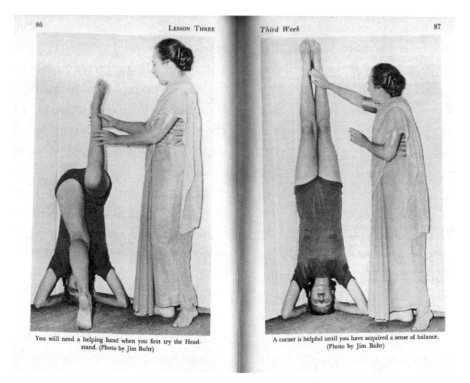

You will need a helping hand when you first try the Headstand. (Photo by Jim Buhr)

A corner is helpful until you have acquired a sense of balance. (Photo by Jim Buhr)

Figure 28.2. Indra Devi helping a student with the Headstand, 1959

(From *Yoga for Americans*, by Indra Devi)

Instead of addressing herself to the few spiritual aspirants (retirees, perhaps, with a disquieting sense of spiritual emptiness) willing to devote their lives to yoga in order to find self-realization, Devi addressed herself to Americans in the prime of their lives who had attained material success but nevertheless felt like failures. In the post–World War II Age of Anxiety, she set about dealing not with a problem of spiritual emptiness among Americans but with a psychological and, to a lesser extent, philosophical malaise by offering hatha yoga as an alternative to psychoanalysis and existentialism—an alternative that insisted on the exploration of identity through the body as much as the mind.

Krishnamacharya, who had been addressing the needs of anxious middle-class Indians, transmitted to his disciple Devi the means—the techniques of hatha yoga—for her to alleviate the anxiety of her classroom students, lecture audiences, and readers. Through her great impact, Krishnamacharya became the main purveyor of yoga as relaxation technique for a fretful American middle class in the mid-20th century. For this reason it can be argued that Krishnamacharya's most significant contribution to modern yoga is his turning yoga away from its traditional role as soteriological quest—as a discipline for liberation—to its role as reliever of stress.

Seeing Things from a Different Angle

When Krishnamurti counseled her "to see things from a different angle," Devi didn't realize that a means of seeing the world from a different angle on a daily basis was readily available to her: her *asana* practice. If she had understood this, she might've grasped the true worth of *Sirsasana,* her venerated Headstand. She perceived the chief benefit of the headstand as physical relaxation that results in mental relaxation—a more complete relaxation than even that derived from *Savasana,* Corpse Pose. "Lie down as if lifeless on the floor; allow no thoughts to pass through your mind; stay that way for a few minutes," she said in her instructions for Corpse Pose. "Even better is the headstand posture, provided, of course, you are already familiar with it and can assume it without difficulty. . . . Why is this posture so relaxing that it acts like a tonic or a pickup? The answer is that when you are upside down the flow of nerve energy is reversed and the constricting pull of gravity diminished, so that the whole body is given a better chance to relax."[42]

Throughout the heyday of Devi's influence, from the early 1950s to the mid-1960s, *Sirsasana,* the yogic exercise par excellence for stress relief, replaced *Padmasana,* Lotus Pose, the yogic exercise par excellence for contemplation, *Sarvangasana,* Shoulder Stand, the yogic exercise par excellence for health, and *Savasana,* the yogic exercise par excellence for relaxation, as the representative yoga exercise. Yet, although responsible for it becoming the apotheosis of yoga, Devi didn't grasp the spiritual nature of the *Sirsasana.* She wasn't interested in exploring the bystander's explanation for the reason the yogin at Chowpatty Beach near Bombay in 1931 stood on his head: "To please God." Then one day she had a revela-tion, experienced as a kind of possession.

"A few years ago," she related in 1975, "when I was conducting a class" at her training center for yoga teachers, Rancho Cuchuma Ashram, in Mexico, "and students were about to assume the Yoga Mudra, I found myself telling them what they should be experiencing [on a spiritual level] while assuming and maintaining this posture."[43]

I cannot say how or where the words came from, but they seemed to flow of their own volition, and I had only to voice them. When I had finished, the class sat still, spellbound.

"Mataji, we have never experienced anything like this. What is it?

"Sai Yoga," I answered without hesitation, surprising myself with this explanation.[44]

In 1966 Devi had found a second spiritual guide (after Krishnamurti) whom she believed was divine: Sai Baba, a guru with the mop of hair that formed "a black halo around His head." At their first meeting she observed, "He looked so gentle, so compassionate, so human, and yet there was something about Him that set Him apart from everybody."[45] Baba evidently felt the same way. When he was a fourteen-year-old boy named Sathya Narayana Raju, he proclaimed himself to be the reincarnation of Sai Baba of Shirdi (a famous saint of the late 19th and early 20th centuries), "announcing that he had come," according to Devi, "to bring people to the realization of their spiritual origin." Sai Baba of Sathya would go on to become a beloved guru and acclaimed philanthropist.[46]*

---

*Devi explains that *Sai* means "Lord, Protector" and *Baba* means "father in the universal sense" (I. Devi, *Sai Baba and Sai Yoga,* 7).

Baba's influence on Devi's spirituality would become the deepest and most lasting of her life. "I feel He is with me all the time," she said, "guarding, teaching and guiding me step by step."[47] When a student asked if Sai Baba had taught her this new approach to *asana* practice, she responded, "Yes."[48] "When?" the student asked. "Right now, this very moment," she answered.[49]

In 1984 Devi led the journalist Virginia Lee through a series of meditations on *asana* to demonstrate the transformational path disclosed to her that day. "Imagine that your body is a temple of the living spirit, and that you are a high priest or priestess of the temple. It has been given into your custody. You have to look after it. . . . Imagine that the time of offering has approached."[50] In the cross-legged seated posture with your hands clasped in back, "you inhale deeply," Devi said,

> then bend down to touch the floor with your forehead. Then you stay in this position for as long as you can. This is the Yoga Mudra. Imagine now that you are offering the little light of your heart to the giver of light. . . .
>
> In Cobra you are a snake lying on the ground of everyday life, seldom lifting yourself up towards the light. And then you suggest that as you rise higher and higher, you get closer to the light.
>
> In the twist, you first look at your past. If there's anything you feel you have done wrong, decide right now what to do to correct it. When you do the twist to the other side, you look at your future. What would you like it to be? And a little voice says to you, "I am the light. I have been waiting for you all these years. So come to me." And in

this way, you do the asanas with a spiritual consciousness.[51]

Devi had discovered that "asanas can, are and should be a step into the spiritual realm. They are not purely physical. If they are purely physical, they are not yoga. They are gymnastics."[52] But in her page-long passage about her signature *asana, Sirsasana,* in the book she wrote after her conversion, *Sai Baba and Sai Yoga,* published in 1975, Devi exposed the limitations of her teachings on embodied spirituality.

> Get into the Headstand. . . . Close your eyes and imagine yourself as a tree . . . your head representing the roots . . . and your body the trunk, growing straight up towards the skies. You are a tree with many branches that are covered not only by leaves but also by beautiful white flowers. . . . Each one of them has a light in its heart . . . flowers of light. You are standing on a hill, so that everyone can see you, even from a distance. . . . At night you look like a bright Christmas tree . . . and people come from near and far to look at you in amazement. . . . And their hearts begin to open up to the Light . . . you have given them a ray of hope.[53]

This sentimental, shallow, and silly guided meditation does not show the way to inhabit our inverted body as a vehicle for reaching the spiritual realm. Compare it to the suggestion for serving God by standing on our head made by G. K. Chesterton (1874–1936), an English writer of Christian apologetics (as well as journalism and detective fiction), in his book *St. Francis of Assisi,* published in 1924. If St. Francis, in one of his strange dreams, had "turned head over heels and stood on his head"[54] and seen

the town of Assisi upside down, it need not have differed in a single detail from itself except in being entirely the other way round. But the point is this: that whereas to the normal eye the large masonry of its walls or the massive foundations of its watchtowers and its high citadel would make it seem safer and more permanent, the moment it was turned over the very same weight would make it seem more helpless and more in peril. . . .

He might see and love every tile on the steep roofs or every bird on the battlements; but he would see them all in a new and divine light of eternal danger and dependence. Instead of being merely proud of his strong city because it could not be moved, he would be thankful to God Almighty that it had not been dropped; he would be thankful to God for not dropping the whole cosmos like a vast crystal to be shattered into falling stars.[55]

Chesterton understood how standing on our head makes us literally see the world differently: "If a man saw the world upside down, with all the trees and towers hanging head downwards as in a pool, one effect would be to emphasise the idea of *dependence*. . . . It would make vivid the Scriptural text which says that God has hung the world upon nothing."[56]

Although her guided meditations based on *Sirsasana* and other *asanas* lack the eloquence, originality, and wisdom of Chesterton's insight about the headstand, Devi did come to understand and proselytize *asana* practice as embodied spirituality. "Asanas are not exercises," she

declared in a distillation of her newfound yoga philosophy, "they are spiritual postures."[57] Unlike Iyengar yoga (developed by B. K. S. Iyengar), Kripalu yoga (developed by Swami Amrit Desai), Ashtanga yoga (adapted by K. Pattabhi Jois from T. Krishnamacharya's Vinyasa yoga, popularized in America as power yoga by Beryl Bender Birch, and now commonly called Vinyasa yoga), hot yoga (developed by Bikram Choudhury), and Sivananda yoga (promoted by Swami Vishnudevananda), Sai yoga never became one of the styles of postural yoga widely practiced in America. Devi's lasting influence on yoga in America, the result of her promotion in the 1950s and '60s of yogic gentle stretching and deep breathing as a balm for the agitated mind, is the mainstream acceptance of yoga as a relaxation technique for relieving stress. Sai yoga (or better yet, some refinement of it), which reflects Devi's mature approach to *asana,* deserves to be actively championed.

Coda

Sigfrid Knauer, Devi's second husband, died on December 21, 1984. Devi moved to Buenos Aires, Argentina, on February 15, 1985. With the assistance of disciples, she established the Indra Devi Foundation there in March 1988. She died on April 25, 2002, at the age of 102. Her body was cremated, and her ashes were scattered over the Rio de la Plata. The long journey of her life would make a riveting Hollywood biopic, a saga crammed with many notable personalities and set in many lands, often against a backdrop of major historical events of the 20th century—albeit a tale not of daring exploits but of a spiritual quest.

29

B. K. S. IYENGAR

Enduring Cruelty

A Yoga Student

Home Life with Krishnamacharya

In 1924, after teaching for thirty-three years at a primary school in the small town of Narsapur, Bellur Krishnamachar retired. He moved his family from Bellur to one of the most populous cities in India, Bangalore, known for being a pensioner's paradise, where he worked as a clerk in a grocery store owned by a Muslim. Four years later he died from appendicitis, leaving his widow (who lived until 1958) with four young children, including Bellur Krishnamachar Sundararaja Iyengar (1918–2014), aged nine. (There had been thirteen children. By 1928 three sons and three daughters were married and out of the house and three children had died, leaving the four children at home.) Fifty years later Iyengar, who had become a famous yoga master, fondly remembered his father: despite the pressures of bringing up a large family in grim poverty, "he was very kind to all of us and never ill-treated us. If anyone questioned him about his fortune, he answered that his children were his fortune."[1]

The burden of bringing up the youngest children fell to the three elder brothers, who all earned a living. Throughout the school year in 1934 Iyengar was living in Bangalore with his eldest brother, Doreswami, an accountant, in order to attend high school. Constantly feeling weak (he was diagnosed by a doctor as having consumption), the four-foot ten-inch, seventy-pound, fifteen-year-old boy struggled with school. His future didn't appear auspicious.

In the late winter/early spring of 1934 the maharajah of Mysore, Shri Nalvadi Krishnaraja Wadiyar, commanded T. Krishnamacharya, the yoga teacher at the royal family's *yogashala* (yoga school) in the Jagan Mohan Palace, to go to Lonavla and Bombay "to see," as Iyengar attested, "the scientific progress that was going on there in the field of Yoga" carried on by Swami Kuvalayananda.[2] (Being sent on this undertaking surely must've rankled the arrogant Krishnamacharya. Kuvalayananda's ambitious endeavor was not only to prove the scientific efficacy of hatha yoga but also to provide the most up-to-date techniques in yogic therapeutics and physical culture—Krishnamacharya's supposed areas of expertise at the palace.) Krishnamacharya, who had married one of Iyengar's sisters, Namagiriamma, in 1925, asked his sickly, teenage brother-in-law to come to nearby Mysore to look after her while he was gone. "Shri Krishnamachar came to Bangalore on his way to Bombay," Iyengar recalled. "He asked me to stay with my sister till his return from Bombay. As there were summer holidays I agreed to go to Mysore. He paid my railway fare and I proceeded to Mysore. I was very keen to see the palace of the Maharaja."[3]

After Krishnamacharya returned from his mission, Iyengar requested to be sent back to Bangalore. But Krishnamacharya convinced him to remain in Mysore by offering to teach him a few *asanas* to improve his health. "As I had not experienced what [good] health really was since birth," Iyengar explained, "I accepted this tempting offer to stay on."[4] When Iyengar agreed to live in Mysore, Krishnamacharya became, in effect, Iyengar's father. In his later years Iyengar sang Krishnamacharya's praises. But in his autobiographical writings and talks of the 1970s and 1980s—especially in the first drafts of an untitled autobiographical sketch written for publication in 1978 and "My Yogic Journey," given as a talk on Iyengar's seventieth birthday in 1988, both raw, unruly recollections—Iyengar revealed his life with Krishnamacharya as a virtual fairy tale of misery in which he became a servant to a sadistic usurper parent who ruled over every aspect of his life.[*]

After a few months Iyengar's daily routine was set. Woken up by Krishnamacharya at 4:00 a.m., Iyengar began the day by having to water a large garden, which took two hours. He studied for school from 6:00 to 7:30, practiced yoga at home from 7:30 to 8:30, taught yoga to "some of the aged persons who were coming" to the *yogashala* from 8:30 to 10:00, went home for lunch, attended classes at the Maharajah High School from 11:00 to 4:30, returned home, and then took a yoga class taught by an advanced student at the *yogashala* from 5:15 to 7:30. The day ended with dinner at home at about 8:00 p.m. with Krishnamacharya, his wife, and his one- and three-year-old daughters, followed by

---

[*]Edited versions of these documents appear in three published collections. The version of Iyengar's untitled autobiographical sketch can be found as "The Body Is My Temple" in *Body the Shrine, Yoga Thy Light* (1978), made available to coincide with Iyengar's 60th birthday. A published expanded version of "My Yogic Journey" can be found as "How Yoga Transformed Me" in *Astadala Yogamala* (Garland of the Eight Petals of Yoga), volume 1 (2000), and a published abbreviated version can be found as "Reflections of My Life" in *Yoga Wisdom and Practice* (2009).

a period meant for homework. "Immediately after food I used to sleep, skipping my studies. The lights were burning, the books were kept open, but I was going to deep sleep. My sister or Guru see me sleeping and wake me up, abusing me for going to sleep."[5]

Exhausted, Iyengar would fall asleep in school. On top of being deprived of sleep, he was underfed, leading him to take desperate actions. "I was ever hungry. I had no guts to ask even my sister for something to eat. We were to eat when called for, and to eat only what was served. I used to steal some money. Pangs of hunger drove me to steal some money to appease it. A hungry man will commit any sin."[6]*

Often when family life is hard, teenagers turn to schoolmates for solace. But Krishnamacharya kept Iyengar isolated from them. "Not one friend could call at my place, nor was I permitted to go to meet friends," Iyengar lamented. "This deprived me of friendship with my school friends, and even to this day [around 1976] I cannot recollect a school friend with whom I can talk now."[7] Iyengar wasn't even allowed to get together with friends after school. Although school closed at 4:30 p.m. and Iyengar didn't have to be at the nearby *yogashala* until 5:15, Krishnamacharya, driven for some reason to control every aspect of Iyengar's life, insisted upon Iyengar returning home to drop off his books before going to the *yogashala,* creating an unnecessary six-mile round trip.

"Thus," Iyengar dolefully recollected of his life with Krishnamacharya, "I lost freedom both in my physical and mental actions."[8]

Even worse for a youth who already had little sense of self-worth because of his poor health ("My appearance in childhood was repulsive and the smell of the sweat was unpleasant"), Krishnamacharya found fault with everything Iyengar did.[9] He was "harsh, wild and hot tempered. He used to get upset even on petty things. His anger knew no bounds. He used to find fault in each and every action."[10]

> If he said one thing at one time, he used to contradict the same at other [sic] time. We were made to accept and obey him in toto without questioning. If I sit in the ordinary cross legs with left leg first, he would say take the right first. If right is placed first, he would say, take the left leg first. If I stand, he would say "Is that the way to stand?" If I change, he would say "Who asked you to change?" If I used to take my food, using certain fingers, he would say "Use other fingers." Next day, he would again admonish me if I followed his yesterday's advice. Life became perplexing to me.[11]

Krishnamacharya had Iyengar coming and going. "I grew nervous even to stand or sit in his presence," Iyengar remembered.[12] As a consequence, home life became a place of torment

---

*In later life Iyengar replaced his anger toward Krishnamacharya for keeping him constantly hungry with its near opposite: praise for Krishnamacharya for being "an excellent cook and it is difficult to say which of his preparations is the best" (Iyengar, *Body the Shrine,* 4). In a more detailed account, Iyengar wrote that Krishnamacharya was "a wonderful cook. . . . He would cook only one or two dishes (during my sister's monthly periods), but they used to be so tasty that I could never decide which one was the best. I used to call his preparations *Madhupakam*—it was like honey" (Iyengar, *Astadala Yogamala,* 52).

for him. "Fear set in in place of affection and I was afraid to face him. He was like that on his pupils, but on his relatives he was even more wild. I dare not oppose or talk to him direct. It was impossible to stand before him when he gets exasperated."[13]

Iyengar and his sister were always on edge. "His moods . . . were very difficult to comprehend and often unpredictable. Hence, we were always alert to his presence." Krishnamacharya routinely slapped them about the back "as if with iron rods." Iyengar pointedly made clear: "My sister also was not spared from such blows."[14] Yet, while he was less inhibited in his abusive behavior toward those close to him, including his wife, it seems that Krishnamacharya was more cruel to Iyengar simply because Krishnamacharya couldn't stand him. Everything the boy did got under his skin.

Yoga Training

Iyengar had only agreed to stay in Mysore because Krishnamacharya promised to teach him yoga. After giving Iyengar some instruction for only a few days at home, Krishnamacharya reneged. "As my body was stiff like a poker, he neglected me and lost interest to teach me."[15] Krishnamacharya wouldn't even permit Iyengar to take lessons given by students at the *yogashala*. "For several months," Iyengar recalled, "I did not even know where the Yogashala was located."[16] Then, as was his wont, Krishnamacharya abruptly changed his mind. "One day he called me and said to me to do yogic exercises with one of his pupils. At that time my body was so stiff that none, not even my Guru, could believe that I could mas-

ter the subject. It was stiff as a poker, and it took months to reach the floor with my fingers in my forward movements."[17]

Iyengar submitted to the severely painful postures day after day for months (see fig. 29.1 on page 368). Already burdened with Krishnamacharya's daily manipulation and intimidation in his family life, how did he survive the harsh yoga lessons under the tutelage of the advanced yoga student? Iyengar was simply too scared to protest. "Due to fear of my Guru, I kept going in Yoga. It was a very painful process when I began. Circumstances came in chains creating restlessness, discomforts, disappointments and despair."[18]

In early 1935 a prestigious criminal judge from Madras, V. V. Srinivas Iyengar, came to visit the *yogashala* and asked to see a yoga demonstration. After gathering his students, Krishnamacharya sat with the judge before them. He asked each student to perform a particular *asana*. He told Iyengar to perform *Hanumanasana*, Hanuman or Monkey Pose, knowing (according to Iyengar) that his senior students would refuse to do this difficult pose. (What in gymnastics is called a split—with one leg stretched straight in front and the other stretched straight in back, while holding the trunk erect—*Hanumanasana* evokes the Monkey God's leap across the thirty-three to fifty-mile strait to Sri Lanka, where he discovered the whereabouts of Sita, Rama's kidnapped wife.) The timid Iyengar went over to Krishnamacharya and discreetly whispered that he didn't know how to perform *Hanumanasana*. Krishnamacharya stood up and explained how to do the pose. To get out of doing the pose, Iyengar then told Krishnamacharya that his underpants

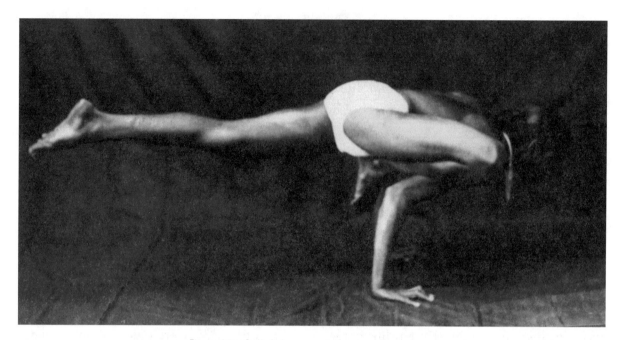

Figure 29.1. B. K. S. Iyengar, at about age seventeen,
demonstrating a variation of *Hamsasana,* Swan Pose, circa 1935
(With the kind permission of B. K. S. Iyengar, Ramamani Iyengar Memorial Yoga Institute)

were too tight to stretch his legs fully out. (All the students were wearing *chaddi,* a form of underpants so tightly stitched that even a finger couldn't be placed between them and the body. Wrestlers wore them so their opponents couldn't grip the cloth.)

Submitting Iyengar to a kind of ritual of obeisance to the father that involves taking away the son's vital force, Krishnamacharya had a senior student cut the underwear on both sides with scissors and ordered Iyengar to perform the posture. As if still in that yoga schoolroom, the seventy-year-old Iyengar vividly recalled his capitulation: "Not to be an instrument of his wrath, I surrendered to him."[19] Iyengar performed the pose, but not without incurring an excruciating hamstring tear (he'd excessively stretched the muscle fibers in the back of one of

his thighs), which took years to heal.

It was Krishnamacharya's rule, Iyengar explained, "that we should present the asana the moment he demands without comments." Krishnamacharya's punishment for (what he perceived as) disobeying this rule deviated from what is commonly accepted as normal: "If we refused, we were served with no food, no water, no sleep, but to massage his legs until he orders as enough. If fingers stop moving, the marks of his powerful hands were on our cheeks."[20] Iyengar didn't say which of these sadistic punishments was most disagreeable to him—being deprived of bodily necessities, rubbing his guru's legs, or getting slapped across the face.

Cavalierly excused by some yoga teachers and students as the manifestation of a teacher's pursuit of perfection in the classroom, Krishnamacharya's temper tantrums were exposed in the home for what they were: bullying. While Krishnamacharya was barely less cruel to others than to Iyengar, they, unlike Iyengar, weren't under Krishnamacharya's thumb in all realms of their life. Iyengar couldn't ignore, avoid, or deflect the continual abuse. He couldn't outwit, disobey, or confront Krishnamacharya. He was helpless to change Krishnamacharya's behavior or get away from it. He couldn't run away. (He had no means of making a living. He was dependent on Krishnamacharya for food and housing.) He couldn't turn to anyone for help.

Perhaps a wise man could've remained untouched by Krishnamacharya's abuse. But Iyengar couldn't recontextualize it as meaningful suffering. He couldn't forgive it. He couldn't be indifferent to it, as if it had nothing to do with him. He couldn't even comprehend it. How could he? How could any child?

As a result, Iyengar was close to having a breakdown. "Fear of Guruji created in me confusion after confusion and whatever he wanted me to do, I was doing wrong. This fear complex and confusion in turn created an instable mind."[21] No matter what actions Iyengar took, they were always wrong. Even to do nothing was wrong. The notion of correct behavior became meaningless. As a result, Iyengar lost his bearings. *Life became perplexing to me.*[22] The simplest way to escape would've been to go crazy—or kill himself.

One morning Krishnamacharya arbitrarily slapped Iyengar. When Iyengar asked why he was being slapped, Krishnamacharya slapped Iyengar again for questioning his behavior. "I walked ten miles to the river to commit suicide," Iyengar revealed to writer Elizabeth Kadetsky. Sensing Iyengar's despair, Krishnamacharya drove after him. But not out of remorse or compassion. "He was proud. He didn't want people leaving. He pushed me to the car and took me home."[23]

Then something happened that made things even worse and—as these things sometimes happen—better. In June or July 1935 Krishnamacharya's favorite student, Keshavamurthy, suddenly and mysteriously left. (He's the handsome, intense, regal-looking boy who illustrates the most contortion-like *asanas* in Krishnamacharya's manual *Yoga Makaranda*.) "His departure," Iyengar said, "was a turning point in my life."[24] Not only because the loss left Iyengar utterly alone but also because "as soon as my only . . . companion left my Guruji, never to return, naturally Guruji's eyes turned on me."[25]*

Krishnamacharya needed Iyengar to fill in for Keshavamurthy at a demonstration before the maharajah at the Mysore town hall in September 1935. "My Guruji said that he would teach me a group of asanas for a few days," Iyengar recounted, "which I should practise daily and prepare for the demonstration." Krishnamacharya tutored Iyengar for three days (the totality of time that Krishnamacharya would

---

*Contradicting his account of complete isolation from his fellow students, Iyengar fondly related how he and Keshavamurthy, the "very lovable student," performed chores together and, more importantly, consoled each other when Krishnamacharya castigated them (Iyengar, "My Yogic Journey," 6). Perhaps Iyengar's total isolation only began after his comrade left, which was about a year after Iyengar moved in with Krishnamacharya.

ever teach Iyengar, aside from the few lessons he gave early on when he lured the boy to remain in Mysore).*

Those 3 lessons are the most memorable days as my body refused to get liberated from stiffness even after hours of hard work. This made me to master the poses but the pains also remained with me for 3 to 4 years.† My Guruji's frightful eyes and fear of his presence kept me silent, even to express what I was undergoing. Though I learnt Yoga, I had no genuine interest in it. It was his anger that kept me going. The pain of the body was unbearable. Often I found difficulty in passing urine or in evacuation.[26]

Some yoga teachers and students have a deeply caring, almost familial relationship. Even before the student falters, the teacher is there to help. And the student—oddly enough, in his or her obeisance and sacrifice—looks after the welfare of the teacher. They are both parent and child. Between Krishnamacharya and Iyengar—who were *literally* family!—there was no caring relationship. To the contrary. Krishnamacharya acted out of uncontrolled anger. It made no difference to him whether he forcefully got Iyengar (literally) into shape or broke Iyengar's body and spirit. And Iyengar, in turn, acted out of fear.

Krishnamacharya never oversaw Iyengar's progress. "He never asked me to rehearse before him. Only, he told me to be ready." Iyengar not only had to prepare his *asana* presentation on his own, he had to overcome his stage fright: "Being weak, I was nervous to appear in public."[27] Despite being "shy, weak and shaky," Iyengar, a natural showman, pulled off a good performance at the demonstration.[28] "Believe me or not," Iyengar told the guests at his seventieth birthday celebration, "I did as asked."[29] All the students who participated in the demonstration received fifty rupees from the hands of the maharajah. Krishnamacharya directed them to deposit the money into a post office savings account. Despite his anxiety that Krishnamacharya would find out, Iyengar secretly withdrew all his money and used it to eat in restaurants.

Tradition of Cruelty

By all accounts, the early modern hatha yoga teachers (even the hotheaded Yogendra), who were primarily responsible for bringing the conditioning postures to the fore of hatha yoga practice, taught the correct performance of *asanas* in a kindly and patient manner. Krishnamacharya, alone among them, severely criticized his students—at least, the young and helpless boys—for their inadequacies in assuming a yogic posture. But then, Krishnamacharya harshly

---

*In an alternative version of these events, Iyengar told how after a year of yoga practice, "my Guru asked me to show him what I had learnt. While watching my movements, he pressed me and handled me consecutively for 3 days" (Iyengar, *Body the Shrine,* 2). Krishnamacharya didn't tell Iyengar that he was instructing him in preparation for the demonstration. "Within a month's time after my Guruji's touch, I was asked to join his advanced pupils in a public demonstration in Mysore" (ibid., 3).
†If Iyengar was referring to new *asanas* that Krishnamacharya taught him, then he was saying that Krishnamacharya's teachings gave him the basis to master the poses over the next month or two before the demonstration. If Iyengar was referring to *asanas* that he'd previously learned from student teachers, then he was saying that Krishnamacharya's teachings enabled him to master these poses during the three days.

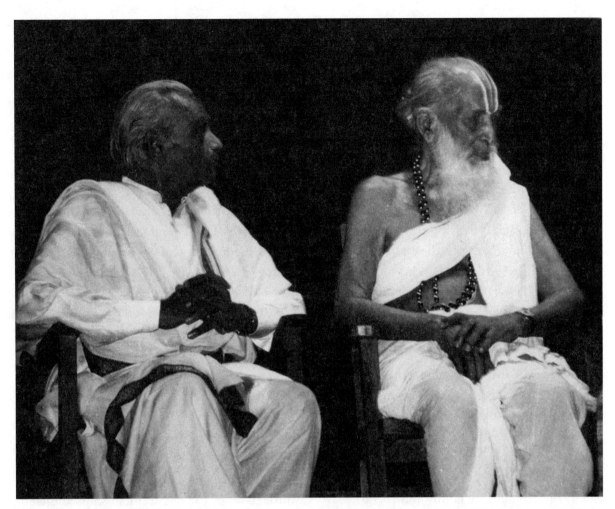

Figure 29.2. B. K. S. Iyengar (left) and T. Krishnamacharya sitting on a dais at an event honoring Krishnamacharya, in which Iyengar gave a lecture on yoga and an *asana* demonstration in tribute to his guru, in Mylapore, Chennai, June 1980

(With the kind permission of Paul Harvey, Centre for Yoga Studies)

criticized Iyengar in all aspects of his life. Krishnamacharya's behavior at home was the same as that in the classroom: his bad temper was dispensed to intimates as well as students.

In his last years Iyengar, who used to brood over Krishnamacharya's abuse—summoning it up as if reliving it—rationalized it (fig. 29.2). When I asked him about Krishnamacharya's

cruelty toward him, Iyengar replied: "He was not only my Guru, but was like a father to me. [His treatment of me] may appear cruel, but if you have read the book of Milarepa of Tibet, he was like the Guru of Milarepa."[30]

Milarepa (1052–1135) was born into a wealthy family in a village in Tibet.* He was originally

<hr>

*Scholars place Milarepa's birth and death in various years. What's certain is that he lived during the late 11th and early 12th centuries.

named Mila Topaga, literally "delightful to hear," after his father's exclamation upon learning the news of his birth. He lived in a splendid two-story manor house supported by four columns and adjoined by a large stable in the back. When he was seven, his father became gravely ill. In preparation for his approaching death, the father assigned his sister and brother as caretakers of his estate, a patrimony that would be turned over to Milarepa when he reached adulthood. But after their brother's death, Milarepa's aunt and uncle took the estate for themselves and forced Milarepa and his mother and sister into labor as their servants. Once adoring friends and family now ridiculed Milarepa.

At fifteen, after his mother tried to restore his inheritance, Milarepa, along with his mother and sister, was thrown out into the streets to beg. Filled with rage (fueled by his mother who threatened to kill herself if he didn't take action), Milarepa apprenticed to a lama to learn sorcery in order to wreak revenge.

A year later a wedding feast for the uncle's eldest son, attended by family and friends, was taking place in the manor house. When the aunt and uncle stepped outside to the portico to discuss their speeches, Milarepa, harnessing occult forces, caused the stallions to mount the mares in the stable, which adjoined the large house. The mares began kicking the stallions. The rearing and kicking horses struck one of the columns of the stately house with such force that it snapped, initiating a chain of structural failings that caused the entire house to collapse. All thirty-five people inside were crushed. Milarepa had spared his aunt and uncle so that they would lead a life of suffering.

Soon afterward, overwhelmed with remorse over the massacre, Milarepa fell into despair. He set out on a quest for redemption, which brought him to Marpa (1012–1097), a Tibetan Buddhist teacher famous for his fierce temper. Milarepa asked Marpa to instruct him in Buddhist teachings to purify his sins. Instead, Marpa flew into a rage and slapped him. Over the next few years Marpa ordered Milarepa to build four immense stone towers on high rocky ledges—and then tear them down and return all the rocks and boulders to where he had found them. The years of strenuous, superhuman effort to construct and destroy these structures wore his body down.

While accepting other students for teaching, Marpa continued to reject Milarepa's requests for sacred instruction by berating and slapping him. Feeling that Marpa turned him away because he didn't deserve to undergo initiation, Milarepa, a broken man, was about to hang himself when Marpa stopped him and told him that he was now ready to receive instruction.

Marpa explained that he had put Milarepa through all of the physical hardships and emotional trials to make him a suitable vessel for the teachings of Buddhism. The aim of Marpa's (seeming) rage was to incite unworthiness as a means of spiritual development. If he could plunge Milarepa into utter despair nine times, Marpa would be able to cleanse him completely of all his sins. (Milarepa completed only eight great ordeals, leaving him with a faint stain of defilement, but Marpa considered the suffering that Milarepa had endured sufficient for his sins to be largely erased.) Upon finally being accepted as a disciple, Milarepa wept. His hair was cut off and he was given a monk's robe. Milarepa spent most of the rest of his life practicing meditation in seclusion. But he also taught groups of disciples, mainly through singing hauntingly beautiful songs of realization.

One can easily see why this historical fable appealed to Iyengar, not least of all (and probably unconsciously) for its fantasy of revenge taken by a boy on his oppressive father figure. But Iyengar was incorrect in saying that its pedagogical moral justifies Krishnamacharya's cruelty. Marpa (at least, according to legend) only appeared to be tyrannical and self-absorbed. In actuality, he set Milarepa to hard labor building structures, denied him initiation into Buddhist practice, and abused him in order to absolve him of his sins. Krishnamacharya's abuse of Iyengar, which left the boy bewildered, distressed, and despairing, wasn't a strategy used by a yoga master to improve his disciple's level of *asana* performance, build his character, or engender his enlightenment (through teaching the concept of non-self by *reductio ad absurdum*). Krishnamacharya seemed to take pleasure in his cruelty. His goal seemed to be to obliterate Iyengar's spark of life.

The lessons that Krishnamacharya gave to Iyengar during those three days of preparation for the 1935 demonstration in Mysore were essentially the only lessons that Iyengar received from Krishnamacharya. No matter that the time was so short. "This was the turning point of my life," Iyengar declared. "Till that time Shri Krishnamachar did not think of teaching me Yoga asanas. Whenever I asked him to teach me some asanas he used to answer that

it all depended upon one's *Karmas* in previous birth. It was my good fortune that due to Keshavamurthy's absence my brother-in-law taught me for a few days and he thus became my Guruji."[31]

It's usually very difficult to pinpoint the incident that accounts for our good or bad fortune. Iyengar could just as well have said that his good fortune lay in the maharajah of Mysore sending Krishnamacharya off to learn about yoga health treatment from Kuvalayananda, which occasioned Krishnamacharya to bring Iyengar to Mysore in 1934. Or, if taking into consideration events that took place after the demonstration, in Iyengar being sent by Krishnamacharya to teach in Pune in 1937, where Iyengar found a haven for the rest of his life. Or in Iyengar marrying sixteen-year-old Ramamani in 1943, who, according to two of Iyengar's brothers, "was largely responsible in moulding his career in face of great adversities of life."[32] Or in Iyengar reluctantly making the long journey to give the famous violinist Yehudi Menuhin a five-minute session that stretched out into three and a half hours, which resulted in Iyengar finding his most receptive audience, Westerners. Or perhaps there was no one turning point in Iyengar's life but instead a causal chain of events.

However these events are shaped into a narrative, though, I think we'd all agree that good fortune wasn't the inevitable result of Iyengar's entire encounter with Krishnamacharya. The outcome could just as well have been Iyengar's physical and mental breakdown or death.

30

B. K. S. IYENGAR

Making Yoga Fierce
A Yoga Teacher

Pune

In November 1935, on an extended trip to India to spend time with his guru and others, the renowned Swami Paramhansa Yogananda was a guest of the maharajah of Mysore, Shri Nalvadi Krishnaraja Wadiyar, at the palace in Mysore. (Yogananda had been living in America since 1920. He established an international center for self-realization in Los Angeles, California, in 1925. He would go on to publish *Autobiography of a Yogi,* an account of his spiritual journey that inspired Westerners to embark on their own Hindu-oriented spiritual searches, in 1946.) When he went to visit the nearby *yogashala,* the yoga school run by T. Krishnamacharya, to see the work being carried on there, "his eyes fell on me," B. K. S. Iyengar recalled, "and he asked me whether I would accompany him to America." Not surprisingly, Krishnamacharya intervened, telling Yogananda that "he might take [the boy] with him on his next visit."[1] Yogananda's flattering request was part of a series of experiences, which had begun with Iyengar holding his own at the yoga demonstration for the maharajah two months previously, that built the teenager's confidence.

In April and May 1936 Krishnamacharya and his students were sent by the maharajah on a lecture and demonstration tour that included a three-week stay at Dharwar. Many women were eager to take up yoga, but in those days, as Iyengar put it, "girls and boys, as well as men and women, were at a distance." It was out of the question for Krishnamacharya to teach them. And the women were too shy to take lessons from the senior students. The women preferred Iyengar because he was the youngest of the group (he was seventeen). "This is the play of destiny," Iyengar recounted, "as my Guru had no other choice but to allow me to teach them." After fifteen days of providing individual instruction to the women, Iyengar had found his lifelong passion: "This is how the ladies of Dharwar ignited interest in me to teach Yoga."[2] (Although he'd already been teaching yoga to the elderly in Mysore, Iyengar considered these sessions in Dharwar to be his first real classes.)

From January 2 to 10, 1937, the Twenty-First World's Conference of YMCAs was held in Mysore. The maharajah asked Krishnamacharya to give a demonstration with some of his pupils at a party for the delegates. "Many watched us," Iyengar reported. Once again he and the other boys performed well. "The Maharaja was impressed."[3]

The YMCA world conference, the first held outside a Western country, was a momentous event in the history of the modern ecumenical movement and, more significantly, of the modern human rights movement. In its preparatory documents, presentations, and discussions, the conference addressed racial problems in the United States, Great Britain, and South Africa. In a special report, the YMCA declared its "belief that discriminations based on race and colour are contrary to the will of God."[4] "Thus, the enlargement of the membership to the non-white population had finally led the YMCA to reflect on its deep values and to define racism as unchristian," writes historian Martti Muukkonen.[5]

Because of this focus on racism, Benjamin Elijah Mays, then president of Morehouse College in Atlanta, was invited to attend the conference. Mays, who would later become a mentor to Morehouse student Martin Luther King, Jr., had a private meeting in Mysore with Mohandas Gandhi on nonviolent civil disobedience as a method to end American segregation.

Even into his final years, Iyengar had no sense of these larger circumstances of the YMCA conference that he participated in or even "whether [the conference] was a local one or an international one." But he still proudly remembered that he "received a gift of fifty rupees from the Maharaja for my demonstration."[6] That a man of Iyengar's great stature remained parochial is easily explained: his youth was such a vale of misery that he never escaped perceiving most incidents in his early life only in the context of being humiliated by or pleasing those (especially Krishnamacharya) with power over him.

Iyengar would never recover from or anywhere near comprehend the damage inflicted on him by Krishnamacharya's abuse. But, even at eighteen, he knew that he needed to find a life free from servitude to Krishnamacharya. During this approximately year-and-a-half period, this series of confidence-building events that he experienced reinforced his determination to gain his liberty.

In the spring of 1937 Iyengar—desperately trying to make a life for himself—arranged to give solo demonstrations in parts of the Kingdom of Mysore. While on tour, he received word from Krishnamacharya about a teaching offer. V. B. Gokhale, who had attended one of Krishnamacharya's yoga lecture/demonstrations in the spring of 1936 in Belgaum, where he was the city's civil surgeon (the doctor employed by the government's medical department), had retired to Pune, the second largest city (after Bombay) in the state of Maharashtra. He asked Krishnamacharya if he would send a senior student to fill a teaching post at the Deccan Gymkhana Club, an upper-class sports club. Because none of the students knew Marathi (the local language in Maharashtra) and only Iyengar spoke some English (the lingua franca in India), Krishnamacharya offered the assignment to Iyengar. Iyengar quickly returned home to consent to taking the position. "I felt that I would be free from the fear of my Gurujee. It was for me like a tiger released from captivity."[7]

On August 30, 1937, eighteen-year-old Iyengar arrived in Pune for the teaching job. He found lodging at a cheap hotel called Café Unique. He was practically broke. His worldly goods consisted of a pair of shirts and *dhotis* (a traditional male garment made of an unstitched rectangular cloth that's wrapped around the waist and legs and knotted at the waist) and bedding. He shaved and bathed without soap. He used one of the *dhotis* for a towel.

Iyengar felt inferior to his students, most of whom were attending nearby colleges. They were "well educated, cultured, civilized and I, as a simpleton, [didn't know] how to speak or behave like them."[8] His puny body "was a laughing stock" to these healthy, strong, well-built young men.[9] And "[he] was treated by Gymkhana authorities as if [he] were a domestic servant."[10] Undeterred, Iyengar "made up

[his] mind not to get agitated or dejected but to work and prove" his worthiness.[11] Determined not to return to Mysore, he embarked on a regime to build his extension and stamina to a level that would impress his students. He regularly practiced ten hours a day. According to Iyengar biographer Kofi Busia:

[Iyengar] could be observed prowling the streets looking, for example, for heavy cobblestones. When he found them he would then sit calmly down in the street, draw his heels in close to his perineum, spread his knees wide out to either side, place the stones upon his knees, and then sit there steadily for hours at a time ostensibly improving his Baddhakonasana [Bound Angle Pose or Cobbler Pose]. Or . . . a road-building crew would pack up for the night or for the weekend and leave a previously innocuous object such as a steamroller parked there until its return. Before anyone knew what had happened, Iyengar would arrive and have worked out some way to drape himself over it in an effort—ultimately successful—to improve his practice and understanding of Urdhva Dhanurasana [Upward Bow Pose or Wheel Pose].[12]

When people came over to Iyengar to ask what he was doing and he proudly told them, "Yoga," they called him "a madcap or a lunatic."[13] But no matter. "I preferred to bear these hurting remarks for the sake of freedom," Iyengar recalled. "I was [more] afraid of my Guruji's moods than to be called as a madcap. The freedom had come to me by chance which I did not like to lose at any cost. If I go back, I have to join my Guruji only. That means to live in this web of constant fear. So without tossing within myself, I made up my mind, come what may, I should enjoy this God given freedom."[14] It wasn't inevitable that Iyengar—a teenager, on his own for the first time, tormented by his own social insecurities and under great pressure to display his worthiness as a yoga teacher—would realize that tolerating the ridicule of people on the streets of Pune was a small price to pay for his freedom from Krishnamacharya. Sometimes people do prefer enduring the rage of a familiar tyrant to putting up with the taunts of strangers. So Iyengar's steely forbearance should by no means be seen as an easy and obvious response.

Eventually Iyengar was able to train his students "without showing exhaustion. This was the turning point in winning over their minds."[15] As his endurance, skill, and knowledge improved, so did his teaching abilities. Recognizing the effectiveness of his instruction, the Deccan Gymkhana authorities repeatedly extended his contract to a total of three years. They also asked him to teach in schools, colleges, and physical education establishments overseen by them in the city.

After the terms of his contract ended in August 1940, Iyengar was forced to fend for himself. For the next few years he had almost no work. And his meager income was so erratic, he related, that "there were occasions when I had a plate of rice once in two or three days. The rest of the time I had to fill my belly with tea or with tap water. . . . My heart, nerve and senses were giving way. Sometimes I cried that even God had forgotten me. . . . This was the

darkest hour."[16] He became so desperate that he even sought an alternative career. In September 1941 he met with the world-famous pioneer of Indian modern dance, Uday Shankar, in Bombay. "I told him of my interest in dance and offered to teach him and his troupe Yoga *asanas,* if he in turn could teach me dancing and maintain me during the period of study."[17] Uday Shankar turned him down.

And yet, despite the hardship, this was a very fertile period for Iyengar. He continued to devote long hours each day to mastering his discipline. He improved his skills in enhancing the flexibility of the few students (most prominently, L. M. Motee, a horseracing card publisher, and his family) that he had. Encouraged by Gokhale, he also began to apply yoga therapeutically to heal or alleviate various common ailments: sinus problems, asthma, flatulence, general weakness, backache, headache, and fatigue. He had learned the therapeutic value of *asana* during lectures/demonstrations given with Gokhale. Gokhale had proposed that he and Iyengar join together to give the lectures/demonstrations on the health benefits of hatha yoga. "The body is known to me," Gokhale told him. "You leave it to me, I will explain very accurately. And you do the poses." "Well, it was a really good combination," Iyengar recalled. "I was really happy, and while he was explaining I started getting the anatomical words, which helped me a great deal to develop my subject."[18]

Inspired by Krishnamacharya's use of ropes at the *yogashala,* Iyengar used ropes and subsequently devised other props to enhance *asanas* for his own practice at home. "As I could not get the *asanas* easily," he disclosed to me,

"I started using available things, like drums, stones, bricks and so forth."[19]*

In 1943 Iyengar returned to Bangalore with Krishnamacharya after giving a yoga demonstration in Rajamahendri at his guru/brother-in-law's request. "He looked at me," Iyengar recalls, "and asked me why I am not marrying." Iyengar bluntly replied, "When I can't stand on my own legs, what is the use of marrying?" Rather than accepting this reasonable answer, Krishnamacharya needled Iyengar: "You are teaching lots of girls. You must have fallen in love and so you are not keen to marry." When Iyengar, knowing that Krishnamacharya was goading him, remained firm, Krishnamacharya changed tactics. "He played with my mother . . . brothers and sisters," convincing them "that they should get me married that year . . . so that I may not go astray and be a victim of bad influences" while living alone in Pune.[20] On July 9, 1943, twenty-four-year-old Iyengar, giving in to family pressure, married sixteen-year-old Ramamani in Bangalore. Iyengar had borrowed money from his pupils in Pune to meet his marriage expenses.

The couple struggled. They had six children. In the early years, while she took care of the children, he remained preoccupied with yoga. His practice and teaching "swallowed [his] whole time of the day." "She never quarreled even once, never complained of my carelessness in looking after the family," Iyengar recalled.

"Often we talked to each other [only] while I was doing inverted asanas for an hour."[21]

It was during this period of intense practice, teaching, exploration, and invention, from the late 1930s to the late 1940s, that Iyengar yoga was forged.

Early in 1939 Bhavanarao Pant Pratinidhi, the rajah of Aundh, who had resurrected *surya namaskar* in the early 20th century, visited Iyengar at the Deccan Gymkhana. Iyengar gave a demonstration of yoga postures. (In appreciation, the rajah gave Iyengar a purse, which the Gymkhana authorities took away, saying that as long as he worked for the club, he wasn't at liberty to accept presents. "What was gifted by generous hands was grabbed away by greedy hands," Iyengar commented.[22]) In an endorsement letter that Iyengar received in March 1939, Bhavanarao praised Iyengar for "practic[ing] the Yogasanas very skillfully and yet very easily. . . . We hope that many young men and women will take advantage of Mr. Iyengar's class of yogic exercises and learn to keep themselves always healthy."[23] The once sickly boy had come to master difficult yoga postures with such proficiency and grace—attained from hours of daily practice during which he strenuously exerted himself and endured debilitating pain—that any trace of effort was erased. In all likelihood he was performing *asanas* more beautifully than anyone in the world.

---

*Iyengar wouldn't introduce props to his students until the mid-1970s. Before then, he noted, he used his body as a prop to guide students into a position. But when he began to instruct large classes (in which he couldn't get around to each student for each pose), he developed props for students that made "the shape [he] used to guide them in private classes." He customized the props to make them safe by utilizing "sophisticated materials so that they could be used without cutting the skin." "From that [first] wall rope," he recounted, "I developed various methodologies of using ropes, belts and other things. They are my inventions, wooden props, belts, strips and so forth" (Iyengar, e-mail to the author, December 23, 2010).

As scholar of South Asian religions David Gordon White notes, "Every group in every age has created its own version and vision of yoga."[24] A 4th-century yoga promoted deliverance through a series of steps that culminate in *samadhi,* a process that replaced religious rites and metaphysical knowledge alone. A tantric and alchemistic yoga, developed in the 8th century, proclaimed the body, previously considered in the yoga tradition as the source of suffering, to be the instrument for liberation in this life. Hatha yoga, a practice developed in the 10th to 11th centuries, asserted that conditioning *asanas* are necessary to render the body healthy and fit for meditation, which, according to the *Yoga Sutra,* must be practiced at great length in a stable and effortless position (commonly a cross-legged seated posture)—the first of the series of forceful yogic techniques that lead to emancipation.

The first generation of modern yogins foregrounded the conditioning *asanas* in the early 20th century in order to teach them as exercise. Until then, the yogic conditioning postures, no matter how demanding, were probably performed casually, if not haphazardly. They were probably first practiced by older men who left behind the householder stage of their lives (the phase of active involvement in the everyday realities of work, family, and community) to seek comprehension of realities behind everyday life. For this soteriological purpose, these men didn't need to excel at the yogic conditioning exercises. As K. V. Iyer, who taught both strength training and yogasana, speculated: "[The ancient] savants knew well enough of the importance of health and fitness as a vehicle for mental and spiritual training. . . . The founders of the Yogic School of Physical Training were men, past middle age, and they lived the life of recluses. They needed only that sort of physical training which could keep them agile and light, physically fit and healthy. . . . [This school] was meant for the man who was in hotquest [*sic*] of self-realisation."[25]

Although the showy display of *asanas* in public places—usually performed by the Naga people—proliferated during the 19th century, the pioneering modern yogins brought previously nonexistent precise and exacting standards (in line with those of modern gymnastics and other sports) to the performance of the yogic conditioning postures. Krishnamacharya further elevated the performance standards, making the *asanas* more refined and elegant. Driven to perfect *asana* as if his life depended on it, Iyengar brought *asana* practice to a level of supreme excellence.

Stepping onto the World Stage

In December 1943 F. P. Pocha, a wealthy Parsi seed merchant, asked Iyengar to train him and his daughter at his residence. Happy with the results, Pocha induced many of his friends to train with Iyengar. Whereas the parochial and proud Maharashtrians tended to scorn the South Indian yogin, the cosmopolitan Parsi community eagerly accepted him.

In 1944 Iyengar used his improved income to make a photo album of himself performing *asanas.* His friend S. Ram, who had a camera, agreed to take the photographs; Iyengar paid for all the materials. Over two days Ram photographed Iyengar performing about 150 poses. The photo shoot was so exhausting that both men fell ill, were nursed by Iyengar's wife, and ended up in the hospital anyway. But Iyengar now had a photo album to promote himself.

In mid-1948 the philosopher Jiddu Krishnamurti came to Pune to give lectures over a three-month period at the Tilak Smarak Mandir, a theater auditorium and exhibition hall, attended each evening by hundreds of admirers. Pocha arranged for Iyengar to meet him. Iyengar, who never read newspapers or books, had no idea who Krishnamurti was. "Somebody told me that he is the greatest thinker of the century, and a personality of the world."[26] Iyengar demonstrated *asanas* for Krishnamurti. Krishnamurti then asked Iyengar to watch him perform *asanas*. Iyengar corrected them. For the first time, in Iyengar's account, Krishnamurti "saw freedom in action."[27] He requested that Iyengar teach him every morning for the rest of his stay in Pune. They wrangled about the time. Krishnamurti wanted to take the lessons at 6:00 a.m. but the proud twenty-nine-year-old, who didn't want to dislodge his regular students from their times, insisted on 4:00 a.m. At 4:00 the next morning, Krishnamurti "was waiting in time to open the doors."[28] Thereafter, Iyengar attended all the talks.

Iyengar would go on to teach Krishnamurti at various times in various locations over the next twenty years. During one of those sessions, when he was teaching *Urdhva Dhanurasana,* Upward Bow Pose or Wheel Pose (a backbend), Iyengar asked Krishnamurti "to feel the vibration of his inner knees."[29] When Krishnamurti said that he didn't know how vibrations could be felt in the knees, Iyengar responded, "Sir, don't you say in your talks whether any of us ever heard the sound of the tree? As the sound of the tree is in its vibration, so too, vibrations in the knees are produced when you do backbends with firm legs. Vibration in the tissues and fibres of the body is a sure sound to feel the right action."[30] Through discussions like these, Iyengar not only developed intimate relationships with his clients but also deepened and clarified the philosophical nature of his teachings.

Word of his teaching Krishnamurti brought Iyengar new contacts in the Parsi community interested in taking lessons with him. In June 1948 one of these new students, an elderly woman, introduced him to the socialite Mehra Jal Vakil. Not only did she become his student and get her family (including her husband, a prominent cardiologist, her mother, Lady Karanjia, and her mother-in-law) to become his students, but Vakil also became Iyengar's most ardent supporter.

On March 2, 1952, Vakil met American violin virtuoso Yehudi Menuhin at a tea party in Bombay. Knowing that he'd recently taken up yoga, she showed him her copy of Iyengar's photo album (which, according to Iyengar, she always carried around with her). Impressed, Menuhin wanted to meet Iyengar. The next morning Vakil called Iyengar to arrange a meeting for him with Menuhin in Bombay. She offered to pay Iyengar's expenses. Iyengar took the noon train and made the seven-hour journey to Bombay.

The next day, March 4, Vakil escorted Iyengar to a 7:00 a.m. session with Menuhin at the Government House, where he was a guest. Plagued by fatigue and anxiety, Menuhin told Iyengar that he would only be able to watch a short demonstration. Iyengar proposed a relaxation exercise instead, to which Menuhin agreed. "I suggested to him to lie down flat and I sat near his head." Iyengar then "regulated his breath by two fingers [presumably the ring finger and thumb of one hand at the nostrils] and controlled his eyes by closing them from the other two fingers of both hands." After two or three minutes, Menuhin fell into a deep sleep. When he awoke forty-five minutes later, he proclaimed that "he had never felt so well in his life even after hours of deep sleep." He embraced Iyengar and requested a demonstration. Iyengar performed a one-hour demonstration, after which he asked Menuhin to show him *asanas* that he'd learned. Iyengar adjusted the positions, "remov[ing] the unnecessary strains." "This 15 minutes instruction," Iyengar recalled, "turned into hours each day for three days."[31] Modern yoga historian Elizabeth De Michelis speculates: "The fact that Iyengar had familiarized himself with the culture of the Anglo-Indian cultic milieu [in which conventional (i.e., orthodox) religious beliefs are attacked] within which Krishnamurti operated probably also paved the way for easier, more successful relations with Menuhin . . . as well as the many Western students with whom he would eventually associate."[32]

Menuhin returned to Bombay for more lessons in 1954. Realizing that with his busy performance schedule it wasn't practical to keep returning to India for yoga lessons, he hired Iyengar as his private tutor to accompany him back to Europe (where he spent most of his career; he would become a citizen of Switzerland in 1970 and the United Kingdom in 1985). Leaving India for the first time, in 1954 Iyengar

traveled with Menuhin to Great Britain, where Iyengar gave private lessons to Menuhin and his friend the Polish pianist Witold Malcuzynski. At the invitation of another of Menuhin's friends, Standard Oil heiress Rebekah Harkness, Iyengar visited the United States in 1956, where he gave private lessons to Harkness and her friends and family and gave demonstrations in New York and Washington, D.C. But it was in Great Britain where he would first achieve renown.

After giving yearly private lessons to students (mainly artists and musicians whom he met through Menuhin) in London, Iyengar held his first class with regular students—what might be deemed his first official class—in a private home there in June 1961. He authorized the six students to teach in 1962. The popularity of their classes greatly increased with the publication in 1966 of his book *Light on Yoga,* acclaimed by Wilfred Clark, founder of the Wheel of British Yoga (which, as the later renamed British Wheel of Yoga, would become the largest yoga organization in England), as the "Bible of Yoga."[33] (Upon being presented with the book by Iyengar, Krishnamacharya, who never passed up an opportunity to undermine Iyengar's self-confidence by disparaging his achievements, said of the poses, "Everything is wrong. Where did you get these?"[34]) In 1969 Iyengar's method of yoga was officially introduced into the adult education curriculum in London—the first yoga classes provided by the Inner London Education Authority (ILEA). (In the 1960s and 1970s, unlike in America, where yoga was established primarily in the marketplace, in England yoga took hold largely through the adult education system.)

Iyengar's teaching had now spread beyond the upper crust. "If Mr. Menuhin was responsible to introduce me and my art to the cream of the western world, particularly Europe," Iyengar explained, "Mrs. Beatrice Harthan, Mrs. Silva Mehta and others helped me to take this subject to the common people of Europe, and Mrs. Mary Palmer became the key person to popularise my Yoga through [the] Ann-Arbor [Michigan] 'Y' in the United States. In course of time, it spread to the other parts of the world, covering all the six continents."[35]

Iyengar had stepped onto the world's stage. However, even though his achievement—Iyengar yoga—was revered, his actual teaching rubbed some people the wrong way.

Iyengar's Teaching

By the early 1960s the shy boy who first taught about twenty-five years earlier to the "ladies of Dharwar" had developed his mature teaching style. He was impatient and quick to find fault. Jon Claxton, an Iyengar teacher in the ILEA from 1974 to 1983, recalls in an interview conducted by yoga social historian Suzanne Newcombe that Iyengar's teaching approach didn't even spare those who became most devoted to him—his students training to be teachers. Their classes were "a strange experience because—he taught in a way that was very un-English really. . . . He wasn't afraid to express his anger. He wasn't afraid to show real disapproval of what was going on—and to humiliate the teachers for not teaching the practice properly."[36]

Although claiming to preserve "what you might call shock treatment" for his pupils who were teachers, Iyengar treated all his early students in England harshly (fig. 30.1).[37] He barked out orders. He yelled at students who were performing poses incorrectly. And he made rough adjustments, grabbing arms and legs and yanking and shoving torsos into their correct positions. Students groused that his initials "B. K. S." (the initials for Iyengar's given names) stood for "bang, kick, slap." Iyengar was especially tetchy about the criticisms of what he calls his "creative adjustment." "This creative adjustment is seen by some people as violence, and I am described as a violent or aggressive teacher!" His forceful adjustments were necessary, he contended, because they "make the person understand subjectively the process which is taking place in his or her body."[38]*

Newcombe describes an incident in 1972 at a demonstration in London: "The concentration

---

*Little is known about the history of the manual adjustments used by yoga teachers to transmit knowledge of conditioning *asanas* to students. Did these adjustments originate centuries ago or only recently as part of the yoga pedagogy necessitated by the advent of the hatha yoga class around 1920? If the latter, were they directly influenced by gymnastics corrections, chiropractic manipulations, Alexander technique subtle tappings, physical therapy positionings, or the like? Whatever the case, hatha yoga was part of the widespread appearance from the late 19th to the mid-20th centuries of diverse bodywork (touch therapy) modalities, based on new or updated traditional techniques. Although sharing the detached intimacy of such corporeal services as a doctor examining a patient, a barber giving a customer a haircut and shave, a lady's maid dressing a mistress, or a mortician beautifying a corpse with cosmetics, the bodywork treatments (hatha yoga, chiropractic, shiatsu, Feldenkrais method, and the rest), in their application of manual contact to make a person's body limber, fluid, aligned, or the like (even more than in their claims to treat medical conditions), are distinctly modern.

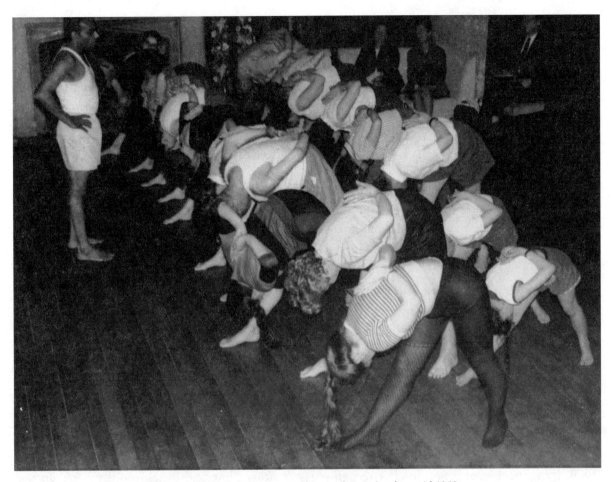

Figure 30.1. B. K. S. Iyengar teaching a class in London, mid-1960s
(With the kind permission of B. K. S. Iyengar, Ramamani Iyengar Memorial Yoga Institute)

and precision that Iyengar demanded from his students' yoga *asana* was sometimes perceived as authoritarian and motivated by anger. In 1972, Iyengar gave a major demonstration at the Friends' House on Euston Road. Some people associated with the Wheel of British Yoga left the demonstration in anger at the perceived violence of Iyengar's approach. This emphasis on discipline was perceived to conflict with the Wheel of British Yoga's promotion of "Gentle Yoga With A Smile."[39]

It was not only traditionalists who found Iyengar's behavior unacceptable. Hector Guthrie, a teacher at the Sivananda Yoga Centre from 1968 to 1972 when it was the "happening" yoga center in London, recalls that there was "a widespread aversion to Iyengar's approach, mainly because he was perceived as an authoritarian bully, and that didn't sit well with the hippie consciousness of the sixties and early seventies."[40] Needless to say, Iyengar had a different take on why his yoga didn't appeal to laid-back flower children. When asked in 1973 if he had any hippie followers, he replied: "No. When they see the discipline that I demand in my class, they go away."[41]

Benefiting from the significant increase in interest in physical exercise (manifested by the fitness revolution) and in personal growth (manifested, in part, by the late 20th-century New Age movement), the popularity of yoga surged during the mid- to late 1970s. As a result, Iyengar was finally able to open a studio, the Ramamani Iyengar Memorial Yoga Institute (RIMYI), across the courtyard from the Iyengar family home in Pune in 1975. "This was a momentous event for the Iyengar movement," notes De Michelis. "The school's founder had now a purpose-built base from which to propagate his teachings, and where pupils from all over the world could come to study and train. . . . Before 1975, [in the words of an early student, Beatrice Harthan] 'early enthusiasts [had] muddled along' by following Iyengar to his varied travel destinations, or by undergoing instruction in his cramped family residence."[42] With the founding of his institute in Pune (and the London Iyengar Institute in 1983), Iyengar achieved a new level of recognition and success. Yet his harsh teaching methods largely remained unchanged. In her memoir Elizabeth Kadetsky describes his behavior at the Yoga Teachers Guidance Course, attended by his 250 most experienced teachers from around the world, at the celebration of the silver jubilee of his Pune institute in January 2000.

His technique was to chide, to hold poses until students buckled, to complain about his quarry in the third person [to his daughter and son]. . . .

"Take pose again! I am not satisfied with your work that is why. I see some people are so lazy. They haven't stayed. . . ."

"No! There is no integration," Iyengar picked up. "Don't ask me to repeat. You never make an attempt! I said bend the leg. I never said stretch the leg. Bend the left leg. Can you see they are all twenty years, thirty years teachers, and still they cannot catch?"

Iyengar looked for his students' weaknesses and rather than softening to them, he berated.[43]

Iyengar rationalized his humiliation of his followers as a necessary consequence of his demand for high standards. What under ordinary circumstances is unacceptable behavior, Iyengar implied, is the acceptable cost of learning true yoga from a master. But his classroom behavior was of a piece with his private behavior acquired in childhood in response to Krishnamacharya's abuse: quick to take offense, suspicious of people's motives, and easily feeling betrayed, he belittled others. In other words, he sometimes behaved like Krishnamacharya. But at other times he mischievously took on the role of tyrant in order to hide a compassion of which Krishnamacharya was never capable.

Many students, especially those who became senior teachers, were captivated by Iyengar. Joan White, who first studied with Iyengar in 1973 in Ann Arbor, Michigan, grants that he was "mercurial and unpredictable": "At times his temper would flash out" and "he would give sharp little hits if he thought we were sleeping (not paying strict attention) that really woke us up." But she also found him "playful," and even "fun." She remembers her early classes with him as "strenuous" and "a bit scary" but "exhilarating." "We really worked extremely hard . . . but I couldn't get enough of it."[44] Echoing White's sentiments,

Bobby Clennell, who first studied with Iyengar in 1973 in London, found him "charismatic," "poetic" and "inspir[ing]." "He helped me find my own strength—you found yourself doing things you wouldn't have imagined you could do, just by the force of his personality. I absolutely thrived under his teaching."[45]

Iyengar's classroom instruction is "a direct and vigorous teaching," writes Ronald Hutchinson in "Iyengar Teaches," a 1971 article in *Yoga & Health,* the magazine that he founded. "Arms in the wrong positions are quickly pulled into their correct positions, while bottoms which are stuck out get a hearty shove to show where they should be tucked in. It is not everybody's way of teaching Yoga, but from the undoubted devotion of many of his pupils, for some it is *their* way."[46]

Iyengar expected his students to be alert to his instructions and to carry them out with full effort—"or else. And in this case,"

Hutchinson explaines, "'or else' means that you are liable to get clobbered, but literally!" While acknowledging that this response was unlikely to happen to a beginner, "it is quite on the cards for an old hand because, if you *are* an old hand, you are not supposed to make the sort of mistake that triggers off the volatile Mr. Iyengar into administering a resounding smack." Yet, Hutchinson writes, qualifying his remark, "there is nothing hard or vicious about it, and it's really egos that get bruised rather than flesh, but if Iyengar trainee teachers learn nothing else, they should surely learn humility."[47] One can easily understand how Iyengar's teaching methods frequently inspired extreme responses. While asserting that Iyengar's impact on the English-speaking West in the field of yoga is unparalleled, Hutchinson admits that people "love him or loathe him—and there is a certain amount of evidence that people often feel either way."[48]

31

B. K. S. IYENGAR

Making Yoga All-Encompassing

Typical Routine

Twenty-eight-year-old Belgian André Van Lysebeth (who would later become a yoga teacher, the founder and director of the Integral Yoga Institute in Brussels, and the publisher of a monthly yoga magazine) was filled with excitement to receive, "on a beautiful day in 1948," a package of books (ordered months previously from difficult-to-obtain catalogs) that arrived by sea mail from India. The first book he opened was Swami Sivananda's *Yogic Home Exercises: Easy Course of Physical Culture for Modern Men and Women,* first published in 1939. Although he had practiced yogic meditation and studied yogic philosophy for the previous three years, Van Lysebeth had never performed conditioning *asanas.* "Receiving that book had such an immediate effect on me that the following morning I spread a carpet for my first session of asanas." By introducing him to *asana* practice, this small book, Van Lysebeth fondly recalls, was responsible for "changing the course of my life." For many years, *Yogic Home Exercises* (supplemented by a correspondence with Sivananda) was sufficient to sustain his practice. "This book covered every aspect of yoga, including all the postures, with photographs and commentaries on their beneficial effects."[1]

Like most Westerners, Van Lysebeth assumed that Sivananda's routine included "all the postures." But the twenty *asanas* in *Yogic Home Exercises* were hardly inclusive: a modified version of Kuvalayananda's streamlined canon (adapted by Sivananda from Sundaram's adaptation of Kuvalayananda's regime), the routine omitted dozens and dozens of other *asanas.*

To accommodate his growing number of disciples, in 1936 Sivananda founded the Divine Life Society, headquartered in an ashram in Rishikesh, picturesquely nestled in a Himalayan hill on the banks of the Ganges. The society also served as his base for spreading his brand of yoga. His missionary ambitions were far reaching. "It is wrong to suppose that Yoga-Asanas are purely meant for the Indians and that they are ideally suited to Indian conditions," he emphatically stated in 1938. In fact, the "remarkable efficacy of Yoga-Asanas as the means of building up a radiant and healthy body" in Westerners has already been proven by his smattering of devoted followers in Europe and America. "Yoga-Asanas can be practiced and are intended not only for India and the Indians but for the whole world and the humanity at large."[2] From the late 1930s to the late 1960s Sivananda yoga became the prominent hatha yoga export around the world. Its importance in the spread of hatha yoga to the West, in particular, is inestimable.

Branches of the Divine Life Society opened in the West in four stages. In the first stage (late 1930s to late 1940s) Western disciples (including Harry Dikman in Riga, Latvia; Louis Brink Fort and Edith Enna in Copenhagen, Denmark; Boris Sakharov in Berlin, Germany; David Ledberg in Stockholm, Sweden; and Ernest Hackel in Los Angeles, California), who learned Sivananda's style of yoga by reading his books and corresponding with him, founded yoga centers.

In the second stage (late 1940s to early 1960s) Westerners (such as the German-born Canadian Sylvia Hellman, who received the Divine Light invocation, a standing meditation in which one accepts that one is a channel of Divine Light, and was given the name Swami Sivananda Radha in 1956) journeyed to the Sivananda's burgeoning complex, where, after being systematically trained (in a course including meditation and lecture courses as well as *asana* practice), they received certification in Sivananda's method and returned home to teach.

In the third stage (mid-1950s to late 1960s) Sivananda sent Indian disciples throughout India and to other countries to disseminate his method of yoga. His two best-known missionaries were Swami Vishnudevananda and Swami Satchidananda. Vishnudevananda was dispatched to the West by his master in 1957 with a ten-rupee note (less than a dollar) and the words: "Go, people are waiting. Many souls from the East are reincarnating now in the West. Go and reawaken the consciousness hidden in their memories and bring them back to the path of Yoga."[3] He founded a Sivananda Yoga Vedanta Centre in Montreal in 1959 and in Quebec in 1962 and established a retreat in the Bahamas in 1967. Satchidananda founded Integral Yoga (the trademark name given by him to Sivananda's yoga) in New York in 1966. In *Yoga Journal's Yoga Basics,* yoga teacher Mara Carrico and the editors of *Yoga Journal* credit these men's efforts, especially the "brilliant and innovative promotional skills" of Vishnudevananda, for the "Sivananda organization blossom[ing] into an international entity."[4]

In the fourth stage (1960s and 1970s) students of Sivananda's first generation of Indian disciples opened their own Sivananda centers. For example, in the United States Marcia Moore and her husband opened the Sivananda

Yoga Vedanta Centre in Boston, Massachusetts, in 1962, and Sita Frenkel and her husband founded a branch of the Divine Life Society in Harriman, New York, in 1964. In Great Britain Barbara Gordon and Judy Stalabrass opened the Sivananda Yoga Centre in London in 1968.

By the early 1960s almost all Sivananda teachers taught the same basic yoga class, which followed Sivananda's selection and sequence of postures. Sivananda had further distilled the yoga regime of twenty postures that Van Lysebeth had learned into the famous Rishikesh series of nine postures, which unfold in a perfect rhythm of pose and counterpose. The main concern, as cultural anthropologist Sarah Strauss points out, was that "everyone know what the trademark sequence of postures is, so that they will be able to join classes at any one of the centers worldwide, without feeling that they are outsiders."[5]

Sivananda's style of yoga wasn't by any means the only hatha yoga taught in the West in the 1970s, although it seems to have been the most prominent, even in England (or, at least, in London), where Iyengar yoga had taken hold (beginning in 1968 Iyengar yoga had a monopoly on all the adult education venues) and author, lecturer, and television instructor Richard Hittleman's style of yoga was very popular. Having met and become fast friends while taking the teacher trainer course with Vishnudevananda at his yoga camp in Val Morin, about fifty miles north of Montreal in the Laurentian Mountains, Gordon and Stalabrass decided to open the first English ashram of the Sivananda Yoga Society in Great Britain. In early 1971 they found a Victorian terraced house on quiet Ifield Road in Earl's Court,

London, for its home. Wanting to ensure that no prospective students would be discouraged, they placed a sign over the doorbell that read: "Ring hard, there is always somebody in."[6] The first class had two students. But after a mere six weeks several classes were being held to accommodate twelve to fifteen students each in the downstairs rooms, with overflow shunted upstairs to take a class in one of the bedrooms. Hector Guthrie recollects that the period when he taught yoga at the London Sivananda Vendanta Yoga Centre in the early 1970s "was a very heady time. We were the busiest yoga centre in the city."[7] The ashram was a mix of exhilarating Eastern spirituality (chanting and meditation sessions, Hindu worship, lectures on varied religious topics), hippie counterculture (people used the center as a "crash pad with drugs in the background"), and trendiness (large numbers of students came and went, celebrities dropped in, the center was featured on BBC television). Although the goings-on were heretical, Guthrie points out, the actual yoga instruction was "orthodox within the Sivananda yoga context. Practitioners of the Sivananda style from around the world, including the mainstream 'Sivananda types' passing through on their ways to points East, were completely familiar with the regimen."[8]

Whatever their circumstances, experiences, and training, most yoga instructors in the 1960s were teaching a streamlined yoga regime. In this, they were following in the footsteps of the first generation of modern hatha yoga teachers (most prominently, Yogendra, Kuvalayananda, and Sundaram). To make hatha yoga palatable to the Indian middle class in the 1920s, the pioneers needed to create a hatha yoga exercise routine that was as different as possible from the hatha yoga performed by renunciate yogins as part of severe ascetic practices (such as standing in *Ekapada Sirsasana,* One Leg behind the Head Pose, while meditating for hours, or standing on the head during *panch-agni tapasya,* five-fire practice, circled by pieces of burning cow dung while meditating during the height of summer heat). So these teachers developed and taught *asana* routines absent arduous poses that couldn't be endured for long and strange poses that bent the body into highly unnatural shapes—poses that demanded great effort and/ or evoked the "self-penance" and "self-torture" practiced by unkempt yoga ascetics.

It's no wonder that B. K. S. Iyengar's encyclopedic manual *Light on Yoga,* which describes (in the minutest detail) and illustrates (often showing stages) two hundred yogic postures (many of which are variations within a posture), electrified the yoga world when it was published in 1966, far eclipsing in impact such esteemed hatha yoga manuals as Theos Bernard's *Hatha Yoga: The Report of a Personal Experience* (1944) and Swami Vishnudevananda's *The Complete Illustrated Book of Yoga* (1960). Even experienced Western yoga teachers didn't know that there were so many ways to configure the trunk and limbs—such strange and startling ways to twist them out of their natural shapes!

Some were drawn to *Light on Yoga* for reasons other than its comprehensiveness. Yoga scholar Norman Sjoman remembers thinking, "I had found something of extreme technical interest—no nonsense." What was mostly available at the time was "Sivananda's books, which made everything seem so easy but left

you somewhat suspended in an unsatisfying fervour."[9] Others, however, were put off by what they perceived as the cold emphasis on correct form in *Light on Yoga.* While respecting its information and even occasionally using it as a reference, Guthrie considered the book to be a blueprint for an inflexible, disagreeable, and emotionally empty yoga experience—one in contrast to the spirited and freewheeling milieu, filled with joy and camaraderie, at the London Sivananda yoga center at the time (before it was forced to conform to the worldwide Sivananda Yoga Vedanta Centre model). "Iyengar's rigid approach didn't sit well with our expansive view of yoga," Guthrie recalls.[10]

Whatever one's opinion's about *Light on Yoga,* though, there was no doubt that Iyengar's wide-ranging, in-depth, systematic presentation of *asana* practice was a monumental undertaking similar in ambition to Andreas Vesalius's mapping of the anatomical structure of the human body, Charles Le Brun's codification of facial expressions that represent human emotion, Carolus Linnaeus's hierarchical classification of plants, or Samuel Johnson's comprehensive documentation of the English lexicon. *Light on Yoga*'s implied case for vastly broadening the typical yoga regimen of the day, as well as for deepening performance proficiency, not only inspired people to take up Iyengar yoga but also increased interest in hatha yoga practice in general.

In teaching the full range of yoga poses to the populace, Iyengar overthrew the mainstream yoga canon developed by the pioneer modern yogins and refined by their immediate successors. But he owed them all a great debt. Kuvalayananda and the other first-generation modern yogins expunged from their teachings those postures considered difficult and off-putting in order to overcome the prejudices held by the Indian middle class, who perceived hatha yoga as a form of street theater or excessive penance (performed largely by disreputable itinerant mendicants) or ascetic spiritual discipline or training for the acquisition of supernatural powers (practiced by renunciates in secluded places). Sivananda focused on making hatha yoga inviting to non-Indians, especially Westerners, who believed that hatha yoga couldn't meet their needs because it was created for Indians to meet their unique needs.

By the 1960s the pioneer modern yogins and their successors had vanquished the bugaboos about hatha yoga as self-torture, magic, and the like, and made a convincing case for hatha yoga's universality (at least among a devoted vanguard). The success of their campaign to frame *asana* practice as physical culture and as physical culture beneficial to all made possible Iyengar's reintroduction of difficult and unnaturally shaped traditional postures—and introduction of difficult and unnaturally shaped recent postures. Through his stubborn determination, Iyengar greatly expanded the repertoire of *asanas* in mainstream modern hatha yoga. Over the subsequent decades the very postures that had repulsed the Indian middle class in the 1920s began to dazzle the yoga world.

Difficult Postures

Iyengar had learned the full repertoire of yoga postures from his teacher, T. Krishnamacharya. Recognizing years later that certain of the *asanas* don't have provenance in early hatha yoga

lore or text, Iyengar, proudly acknowledging the evolving nature of the yoga tradition, readily attributed the addition of contortion stunts into yoga to Krishnamacharya: "New asanas are added [to the yoga repertoire] and Natarajasana is one, like Ganda Bherundasana, Shirsha Padasana, Tiriang Mukhattanasana and so forth," he told me.[11] "The origin [of these poses] is Krishnamacharya"[12] (see chapter 18).

In a scale that measures the intensity of the *asanas* illustrated in *Light on Yoga,* Iyengar assigned 1 to the easiest postures and 60 to the most difficult postures. The new *asanas* that Iyengar attributed to Krishnamacharya were among the more difficult (the number in brackets is their intensity ranking, as determined by Iyengar).

- *Natarajasana* [58] is a standing posture that includes balance and backbending. Beginning in *Tadasana,* Mountain Pose, one brings a leg up behind the back and rests the foot on the head.
- *Ganda Bherundasana* [56] is a prone backbending posture. Beginning with the chin, chest, palms of the hands, knees, and tops of the feet on the floor, the elbows bent, and the buttocks tipped up, one brings the legs up and overhead until the feet, now pulled by the hands, rest on the floor aside the head.
- *Sirsa Padasana* [52] is an inverted backbending posture, considered by Iyengar to be "the hardest of all the back-bending poses."[13] Beginning in *Sirsasana,* Headstand, with the forearms on the floor, one brings the legs over the back until the feet rest on the back of the head.

• *Tiriang Mukhottanasana* [60] is a standing backbending posture. Beginning in *Tadasana*, Mountain Pose, one bends back and grasps the ankles.

Krishnamacharya taught all yoga poses—including the advanced poses that he borrowed from contortion—to children at the Jagan Mohan Palace in Mysore in the 1930s. In the 1960s Iyengar brought this unexpurgated regimen to the West via his book and demonstrations, but it wouldn't be until much later that he actually taught the contortionist-inspired postures.

In the 1960s and early 1970s Iyengar didn't offer beginning, intermediate, and advanced classes to his students. Since even those experienced in yoga were new to his teachings and hence considered beginners, they were all thrown together. (Because Iyengar's classes were far more challenging than those taught by his earliest students who became teachers, even those who took classes with these anointed teachers could be considered virtual beginners.) "In those years, when we were young in body and young in our practice, perhaps we were like children to him," recollects yoga teacher Patricia Walden, who first took classes with Iyengar in 1976.[14]

Instead of being assigned particular poses commensurate with their ability and experience, students in Iyengar's classes all performed the same poses; they just performed them with varying degrees of extension. While the very first classes of a week focused exclusively on standing poses and inversions, by the end of the week classes included all categories of pos-

tures. Students might've performed *Parivrtta Trikonasana*, Revolved Triangle Pose [5], *Adho Mukha Vrksasana*, Handstand [10], *Urdhva Dhanurasana* I, Upward Bow Pose [7], *Padmasana*, Lotus Pose [4], *Gomukhasana*, Cow Face Pose [2], *Mayurasana*, Peacock Pose [9], *Supta Virasana*, Reclining Hero Pose [2], and *Salamba Sirsasana*, Supported Headstand [4] (again, the numbers in brackets are Iyengar's difficulty rankings). These postures were considered difficult, exotic, and contortionist to some, and challenging, clarifying, and exquisite to others. Either way, many loved the precision and dynamism.

Iyengar probably felt that he could teach these fairly difficult *asanas* even to beginners because he provided a progression of increasingly difficult postures that brought the more difficult postures within grasp, and he himself was there to oversee the safety of their execution.

In "Iyengar Teaches," an article in *Yoga & Health*, Ronald Hutchinson describes a class that Iyengar taught at a central London gymnasium (ordinarily used for gymnastics, calisthenics, and basketball) in 1971. While early students warmed up on the floor, Iyengar, "of middle height, with graying hair and deep set luminous eyes," arrived "through a passage of handshakes and smiling greetings" from his senior supporters. He discussed business affairs with them in a corner, while students poured in. After he removed his sandals, "uninhibitedly dispose[d] of his street garments and reveal[ed] himself ready for work in a pair of brightly coloured shorts," he walked to the head of the gymnasium to take charge of the waiting class.[15]

Whereas most yoga classes began from a

seated posture, Iyengar began his class with a series of standing postures, held for long periods of time, with no relaxation periods in between. "Not everybody can stand the pace." He first demonstrated a posture at the front of the class and then, once students, who were preponderantly women, assumed the posture, he moved up and down the rows, "intoning his exhortations in a sonorous voice and adjusting pupils' arms and legs here and there." Occasionally he rushed over to a student to loudly dress her down about her dreadful performance of an *asana,* but "not necessarily because she [was] not trying hard enough, but sometimes because she [was] trying too hard." "'That is all right for me,'" he said, while correcting her position by restricting her strained extension, "'but it is no good for you, yet.'"[16]

Hutchinson illustrates (but doesn't describe) another critical element of Iyengar's teaching methods: abruptly stopping the group activity in order to address common mistakes. While students gathered around, he would have one student demonstrate the posture. He then made adjustments and gave advice to the student so his audience of students could collectively learn how to correct the posture (fig. 31.1).

We see from Hutchinson's account that Iyengar was, as he was reputed to be in the West, "an exacting taskmaster [who] insists on a scrupulously perfect performance of the asanas by his students."[17] Yet we also see that he was a teacher who demanded that his students understand their possibilities tempered by their limitations. He felt a strong responsibility to ensure that no students were injured by overreaching.*

Demonstrations

Along with transforming him from a sickly youth into a healthy man and giving him a profession, notes modern yoga scholar Elizabeth De Michelis, *asana* also provided Iyengar with an outlet for a "personality [that always exhibited] a strong artistic and theatrical component." He performed "hundreds of 'yoga demonstrations' consisting of seamlessly interlinked sequences of *asanas,* some highly acrobatic," while providing a calm and lucid commentary. "Throughout his career Iyengar has remained a master of postural performance with great stage presence."[18] At these demonstrations to promote yoga worldwide, audiences were enthralled with Iyengar's performance of the "highly acrobatic" *asanas,* especially those showy poses borrowed from contortion (see fig. 31.2 on page 394).

Not all, however, were spellbound. "Iyengar's 1970s displays were met with anger by many involved with other forms of yoga in Britain," says sociologist and social historian of modern yoga Suzanne Newcombe. "They felt Iyengar was exhibitionist . . . and violent towards his

---

*In a letter dated October 19, 1975, Diane Clifton, who in 1961 had been one of the first three Western students whom Iyengar taught regularly and in 1962 became one of the first six teachers whom he authorized, sent Iyengar a graduated syllabus for adult education students for his approval. She wrote, "Education Authorities are mainly interested in the safety angle for beginners. I think I mentioned in a previous letter that in Oxford 2 people were taken to hospital from yoga classes and the authorities now realize that the teachers are not fully trained—in spite of their Wheel of Yoga Certificates!" Clifton had created three courses (for beginning, intermediate, and advanced students) based on the Iyengar-designed courses presented in *Light on Yoga.* She cautioned that "for I.L.E.A. [Inner London Education Authority] one should not go beyond these courses" (Clifton, letter to B. K. S. Iyengar, October 19, 1975).

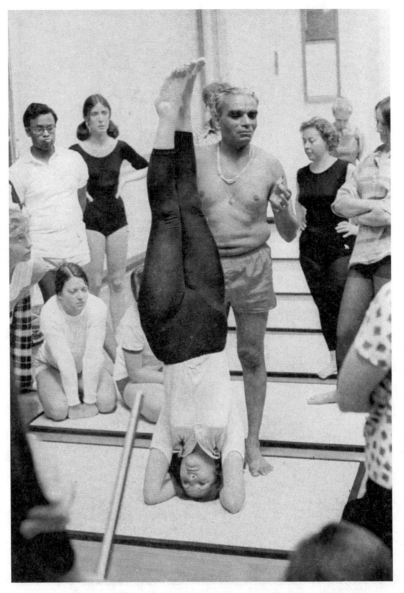

Figure 31.1. B. K. S. Iyengar teaching *Salamba Sirsasana*,
Supported Headstand, in London, 1971

(From *Yoga: A Way of Life*, by Ronald Hutchinson)

own and [potentially] other's bodies."[19] "His displays were seen as one of 'contortionism' and not 'true yoga,' which is about an internal understanding, not external showmanship. (Or so the Wheel [i.e., British Wheel of Yoga] would have argued.)"[20]

Iyengar wasn't holding these demonstrations simply to inspire people to take up yoga; he was also using them as an act of defiance. Flying in the face of both detractors who dismissed yoga as contortionist and yoga practitioners who denied the contortion element in yoga, Iyengar

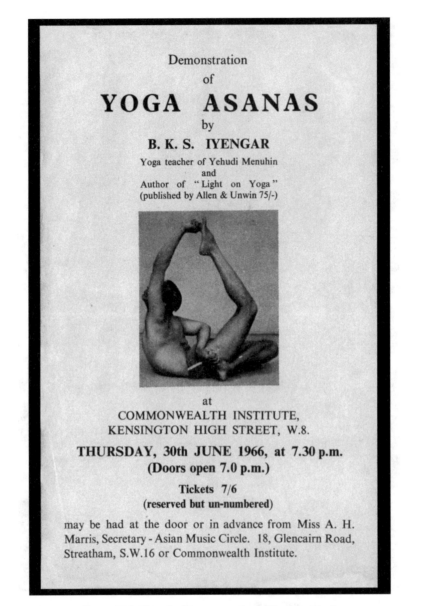

Figure 31.2. Flyer for "Demonstration of Yoga Asanas,"
showing B. K. S. Iyengar performing *Gherandasana* II, Sage Gheranda II Pose, 1966

(With the kind permission of B. K. S. Iyengar, Ramamani Iyengar Memorial Yoga Institute)

emphasized the contortion element in yoga by demonstrating the most extreme yoga poses. A member of a marginalized group, disdained by others as a weirdo yoga contortionist, he turned the tables and took proud ownership of his identity as contortionist. He even flaunted one of the contortion poses, *Natarajasana*, Lord of the Dance Pose, by making it the emblem of his practice, used on his letterhead, as an illustration in his first autobiographical sketch, for publicity photos, and on the cover of later editions of *Light on Yoga* (fig. 31.3).

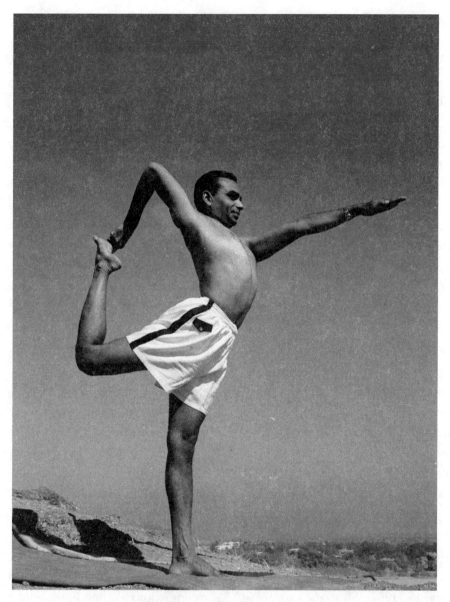

Figure 31.3. B. K. S. Iyengar demonstrating *Natarajasana,* Lord of the Dance Pose, mid-1950s

(With the kind permission of B. K. S. Iyengar, Ramamani Iyengar Memorial Yoga Institute)

Natarajasana

Nataraja, Iyengar explains in *Light on Yoga,* is a name of Siva. "Siva is not only the god of mystical stillness, death and destruction, but also Lord of the Dance." *Nata* means "dancer," and *raja* means "lord" or "king." "In His Himalayan abode on Mount Kailasa and in His southern home, the temple of Chidambaram," Iyengar continues, "Siva dances. The God created over a hundred dances, some calm and gentle, others fierce and terrible. . . . This vigorous and beautiful pose is dedicated to Siva, Lord of the Dance, who is also the fountain and source of Yoga."[21]

Natarajasana is also found in *The Complete Illustrated Book of Yoga,* the yoga manual authored by Vishnudevananda, one of Sivananda's principle disciples, published six years before Iyengar's *Light on Yoga.* Where did Vishnudevananda, who, unlike Iyengar (and K. Pattabhi Jois, another practitioner of the pose), never studied with Krishnamacharya, learn the pose?

When Sivananda visited Pune in 1950 during his All-India Tour, Iyengar requested a meeting to "show him what I knew." According to Iyengar, Sivananda refused to meet with him "due to my poverty."[22] (Quick to feel slighted, Iyengar's explanation for why Sivananda wouldn't meet with him reflects on Iyengar, not Sivananda, who was known for his beneficence.) But after being told by a friend about Iyengar's practice, Sivananda requested photos of Iyengar's complete set of yoga postures. Iyengar sent him a copy of his photo album. Sivananda subsequently invited Iyengar to perform for him in Rishikesh. "Sivananda was impressed by Iyengar's proficiency at yoga," writes Strauss, "and asked him . . . to live in Rishikesh and be part of the DLS [Divine Life Society]. Iyengar declined, saying that he had his family and did not want to renounce his householder lifestyle; however, after the meeting, Iyengar began to make regular visits to Rishikesh."[23]

On January 15, 1952, Sivananda awarded Iyengar with the title "Yogi-Raja." Almost certainly, one of the postures displayed by Iyengar that made such an impact on Sivananda was *Natarajasana.* Considering that Sivananda's *Yogic Home Exercises,* published in 1939, shows only about fifteen poses (the basic canon seems to have been the extent of his *asana* practice), Vishnudevananda probably picked up *Natarajasana* from watching Iyengar.

As the signature pose of Iyengar, the most acclaimed master of postural yoga, *Natarajasana* became the representative yoga pose of the late 20th century. Previous key 20th-century *asanas* were *Padmasana,* Lotus Pose, a seated pose that embodies repose (because it enables the yoga practitioner to remain in the same position with steadiness and ease); *Sarvangasana,* Shoulder Stand, an inversion that brings good health (by stimulating the yoga practitioner's thyroid glands); and *Salamba Sirsasana,* Headstand, an inversion that bestows confidence (through empowering the yoga practitioner to overcome the fears of falling and disorientation). If these *asanas* epitomized, respectively, calm, health, and daring for their times, what did *Natarajasana* epitomize for its time?

Iyengar saw himself as Nataraja's avatar. And he clearly (sometimes desperately) wanted us to see him as the incarnation of Nataraja. So he came close to conflating the yogin and the dancer. "Without shape and form, without grace and without strength, one can neither be a yogi nor a dancer."[24] Actually, a yogin is more like a contortionist: they both bend and twist the body into a set number of freakish positions to full extension. Iyengar was the greatest yogin bender—or "rubber man" or "limber jim" in the jargon of professional contortionists—of them all.*

---

*Even Iyengar, though, couldn't match the skill and suppleness of true contortionists, such as Ivanka, the extraordinary German contortionist who first performed in 1972, at age seven, and retired in 1992. "She could . . . achieve the closest backbend ever, shoulders against buttocks!" oohs Michel Poignant, a French collector of contortion photos and videos. "Not even a beam of light could pass through!" (Michel Poignant, sales letter to the author, August 2009).

Iyengar infused yoga with the élan of contortion. So one might say that *Natarajasana* epitomizes spiritedness—if not flamboyance—in yoga. And he infused yoga with the athleticism of contortion. (People who saw him perform this difficult pose with ease in the 1960s must've been bowled over by his extraordinary athletic abilities, just the way fans were upon first seeing Jesse Owens, Sugar Ray Robinson, or Ted Williams.) But I think that the essential characteristic that this pose embodies arises from another aspect of contortion: the work required to place the body in extreme and unnatural configurations. In adapting the contortion work aesthetic, Iyengar made hatha yoga hard. Which brought a new approach to hatha yoga practice. We can't do a difficult posture by rote; we must think our way into the pose. And we must remain intensely focused on it. This, I think, is what *Natarajasana* epitomizes most of all: total absorption in *asana*.

32

B. K. S. IYENGAR

Making Yoga Precise

Yogic Means of Expressing Sacred Truths

Symbol

"Whilst performing asanas the yogi's body assumes many forms resembling a variety of creatures," B. K. S. Iyengar tells us in a lovely homily found in his mostly dry treatise on *asanas, Light on Yoga.* "His mind is trained not to despise any creature, for he knows throughout the whole gamut of creation, from the lowliest insect to the most perfect sage, there breathes the same Universal Spirit, which assumes innumerable forms."[1] Exploration of the symbolic representations inherent in *asanas* (commonly reflected in their names) as a means of expressing sacred truths is a prominent feature of some contemporary yoga practices.

In her memoir of her yoga journey that eventually led to studying with Iyengar at the Ramamani Iyengar Memorial Yoga Institute (RIMYI), his yoga center in Pune, India, writer Elizabeth Kadetsky gives an account of her earliest yoga classes in the mid-1980s that nicely echoes and extends Iyengar's lesson about embodying the symbolic nature of *asanas*:

Yoga class was a place to torque our bodies into shapes with Sanskrit names, into triangles, fish, herons, pigeons, planks, trees, wombs. When we finally became those shapes, we were something other than ourselves. I felt my body click into a shape, as if for each asana there was a Platonic model in the heavens. Table, rod, chair, crow, lotus. That was when I could squint my eyes and recognize not myself but a pose in the mirror. My body became a medium through which the universe flowed, a chink in the divine. In this way, yoga felt liberating; it distracted us from our preoccupations, suggested we were more than what we were. When we took on the outline of a banyan or a tortoise, we could believe that we were connected to a deep history, that we belonged to a vast universe.[2]

Although including a geometric shape, man-made objects, and a part of the body, the shapes that Kadetsky symbolically assumed were largely vegetation and wildlife. Through embodying flora and fauna, she experienced going backward in time (perhaps back to the 17th century when Indian merchants sold goods under the shade of banyan trees and then to the primordial past when banyans arose in rain forests) and an expansion of space (perhaps out to Earth's habitats teeming with tortoises and other animals and then to celestial objects swirling in space).

In his brief account in *Light on Yoga* of the derivation of the two names, *Tadasana* and *Samasthiti,* for the yogic standing pose, Iyengar gives a hint of the yogic transformation made possible by creative imagery: "Tada means a mountain. Sama means upright, straight, unmoved. Sthiti is standing still, steadiness. Tadasana therefore implies a pose where one stands firm and erect as a mountain. This is the basic standing pose."[3]

Kadetsky provides a sketch of a class in which her first teacher initiated a visualization exercise that expanded on this imagery:

We sat in a semicircle as Julie took a yogic version of military posture. She seemed merely to be standing still. But in her very

stillness, she said, was the embodiment of the mountain. Solid. Strong. Singular. Watching her, I too felt motionless.

"In the beginning of all yoga," she said, staring at a spot on the window behind us, "there is Tadasana—mountain pose. In mountain pose, you feel like a mountain. The human form in the posture of a mountain is dense, rooted, the heels and toe-balls descending into the earth—like the millions of shoots from a thickly growing patch of postdiluvian dandelions—the crown in the head ascending like a redwood, the diaphragm flat and wide, like a vast savanna." The similes rushed forth.[4]

This accretion of images is silly. The teacher should've simply said that the body in *Tadasana* is like a redwood (an especially apt comparison because the class took place in a redwood dojo on a college campus in Santa Cruz, California) or some other tree with a particularly sturdy and straight trunk, or even better, as the unsentimental Kadetsky discerns, like a soldier at attention—or, it can just as well be said, like a garment (a housedress, say, or a monk's frock or a suit) draped on a hanger, a Christian crucified on a wooden cross, a skeleton hanging from a hook in an anatomy class, or a corpse in rigor mortis lying on a metal slab in a morgue.

In *Hatha Yoga: The Hidden Language— Symbols, Secrets, and Metaphor,* Swami Sivananda Radha advocates another approach to inhabiting the symbolic nature of *asanas:* as a means of psychological, not spiritual, transformation. "The name of the asana is the place to begin looking for its symbolic meaning," she explains. "For example: *Mountain*—strong, massive, immovable, insurmountable, high. What have mountains meant to peoples of different cultures? What does mountain mean to me? My inner strength, my immovability (stubbornness?), my strivings, my insurmountable obstacles, my lofty ideals? As I stand in this posture and view it as a symbol, my struggles to reach the top, the stretching of my body and the effort of my muscles help me to see different aspects of myself and gain new insights."[5]

In a letter that Radha displays to open her book, Iyengar politely endorses Radha's interpretation of yoga: "It is a good way of explaining the asanas symbolically so that each asana prepares the sadhaka's [the practitioner's] mind to see the asana in its true perspective."[6] However, when he goes on to explain that homologizing our body with other forms leads to "the transfiguration of true self," he, like Kadetsky, seems to be advocating a traditional (i.e., spiritual, not psychological) goal: hatha yoga is a technique for withdrawing from profane human life to find a deeper, truer life.[7] Yet, with few exceptions, Iyengar had no place in his writings, lectures, and classroom teaching for using symbolic interpretations of *asanas* based on their forms (reflected in their names) as a means of sacred transformation.

Geometric Shape

Around the time that Iyengar was learning *asana,* Wassily Kandinsky, one of the first Western artists to create completely abstract pictures, was expressing an interest in geometric shapes. In his 1931 article "Reflections on Abstract Art," he places the geometric in art in the context of the history (beginning around 1600) of the painter's quest for essence—what

he also called "silence." Abandoning landscapes, Renaissance painters turned to still lifes because they "needed discreet, silent, almost insignificant objects. How silent is an apple beside Laocoön!" For the modern painter, "a circle is even more silent!" he exclaims.[8] The painter of geometrical forms is developing "a newly acquired faculty that enables him to go beneath the skin of nature and touch its essence, its content," he contends.[9] "The contact between the acute angle of a triangle and a circle has no less effect than that of God's finger touching Adam's in Michelangelo."[10]

Kandinsky's rationale for the geometric in art was decidedly spiritual. In his treatise *On the Spiritual in Art: Especially in Painting,* published in 1912, he explains that he doesn't use representation to depict reality because the material world is illusory. Reality is found in "the 'nonmaterial,' or matter that is not perceptible to our senses." He credits Indian philosophy, knowledge of which he gained from occultist and fellow Russian Helena Petrovna Blavatsky, as influential in the formation of this soteriological metaphysics. The wisdom she acquired "after years spent in India,"[11] he writes, sparked her creation of Theosophy, which, "according to Blavatsky, can be equated with eternal truth." Although he, unlike some of his best friends, wasn't a member of the Theosophical Society, Kandinsky praises Theosophy as "a powerful agent in the spiritual climate, striking . . . a note of salvation that reaches the desperate hearts of many who are enveloped in darkness and night."[12]

Abstraction, art critic Hilton Kramer explains in a 1995 review of a Kandinsky exhibition, wasn't, as it's commonly perceived, merely one of a succession of styles in modern art but "represented for its pioneer creators a solution to a spiritual crisis; . . . a categorical rejection of the materialism of modern life; and . . . [a] redefining [of] our relationship to the universe."[13] "The philosophy of art," art historian Meyer Shapiro recognizes in his 1937 discussion of the birth of abstract art, "was also a philosophy of life."[14]

In the 1980s Iyengar dallied with choosing geometric shape as his formal organizing principle. In his major philosophical work, *The Tree of Yoga,* published in 1988, Iyengar ignores naturalistic representation in *asanas*—the notion that in assuming the pose of a tortoise, warrior, plow, et cetera, we become them. Instead he draws attention to the fundamental geometric essence of *asanas*—the notion that in assuming a pose, we partake of an ideal geometric shape:

> The structure of the asana cannot change. . . . One has to study each asana . . . geometrically so that the real shape of the asana is brought out and expressed in the presentation. . . . Study the aspect of an asana. It may be triangular, round, rainbow-shaped [semi-circled] or oval, straight or diagonal. Note all these points by observation, and study and act within that field, so that the body may present the asana in its pristine glory.[15]

As a yogin, Iyengar held that his philosophy of *asana* was also a philosophy of life: through *asana* practice we learn that the stuff of ordinary life is an illusion and that the goal of the spiritual seeker is to attain to absolute reality. Yet unlike Kandinsky, Iyengar didn't explain

his directives for assuming geometric shapes as spiritualized metaphysics. In fact, in his classroom teaching, he didn't direct students to assume geometric shapes at all. What possessed him was establishing precision as the critical element of yogic exercise.

Yoga as Exercise

Precision

A far cry from the familiar, soothing sessions of "gentle yoga with a smile" (the temperate performance of yogic postures to release tension by simultaneously relaxing and energizing the body) championed by the Wheel of British Yoga, Iyengar's early classes in London, writes social historian Suzanne Newcombe, "are remembered by participants as being 'tough' and 'highly charged.'"[16] This tense atmosphere was due in part to Iyengar's ill-tempered instructions, severe criticisms, and rough adjustments. For some students, though, the problem wasn't Iyengar's behavior but an essential element of his teaching: his insistence on precision in performance. They bristled not only at his harsh measures of enforcement but also at what they perceived as his nitpicking. "I have also been branded in England as rough, violent, proud, and so on, a yogi without yogic manners," Iyengar said in 1972, "but they claim as well that I am the only best teacher. How can all that go together? Precision and perfection are ruthless. In that ruthless teaching and practice, the fineness shines. Very few understand the severity of yoga."[17] Actually, many did. While causing consternation and anger in some students, Iyengar's rigorous approach to *asanas* electrified far more students. They found his endless demands for detailed execution of the postures overwhelming but also revelatory and thrilling.

Not only did he bring attention to the details of *asana* to an unprecedented degree, but Iyengar also refined the postures (especially the standing postures, incorporated into yoga earlier in the century, shortly before he took up yoga) in order to facilitate greater range of motion in stretching, which, in turn, demanded more precision. What's more, he emphasized the placement of not only the primary parts (spine, pelvis, and hips) for bending or twisting into a posture but also the ancillary parts (legs and feet, shoulders, arms and hands, head and neck, and fingers and—most famously— toes), which balance and stabilize the posture; in other words, he required precision in the entire body for each unique configuration of *asana*. (One of Iyengar's innovations was having Western students work barefoot because in the many standing postures that he taught, feet in stockings, ballet slippers, or socks would slip on a polished floor. In gripping the floor, the toes, in Iyengar yoga, become prehensile. But even in the nonstanding poses, Iyengar demanded that all parts of the body become actively involved, including the feet.)

Although the postures are performed dynamically, because of this exacting attention to detail the pace of an Iyengar class tends to be slow and even digressive, not flowing and propulsive. Class rhythm is sacrificed for the time-consuming struggle of each student (often with the assistance of the teacher) to perform the postures precisely. Yoga teacher Patricia Walden, who first studied with Iyengar in 1976, said in 2005, "When we studied with Guruji in the 1970s, we did many, many poses in each class. He rained instructions on us with a torrent of intensity."[18] "As the years have passed," she continues, "he has added new dimensions to his teaching. We do fewer poses per class, but he takes us deeper into each."[19]

Iyengar's emphasis on quantity over quality in the mid-1970s may have been a response to the loss of his beloved wife, Ramamani, at the age of forty-three in 1974. During this time he threw himself into his practice, perhaps to escape his grief; in his teaching he drove his students in the same way he drove himself. For the next few years "the classes in India were a marathon of doing, doing and doing," recalls yoga teacher Joan White. "We would do the vast quantity of poses that he himself was doing." By 1978, perhaps because his grief had subsided, Iyengar began "teaching fewer poses in a great deal more detail," says White.[20] He was himself again.

In a differing account of the trajectory of Iyengar's teaching, yoga teacher Angela Farmer, who first studied with Iyengar in the early 1960s in London, describes his deliberative approach as having evolved over decades. "It was difficult to catch what he was doing," she recalled in 1983 about her classes with Iyengar in the 1960s and into the 1970s. "He taught the postures very rapidly and it was sort of like Lord Shiva's dance. . . . Now he's been refining a method which is very safe and can be given out step by step to large numbers of people."[21]

Whether his frantic teaching was an anomaly of the mid-1970s or the norm since the 1930s (or at least the 1960s), in slowing down in the late 1970s Iyengar wasn't accommodating his students; in fact, he was demanding that they adapt to even greater standards of precision. Yet he was accommodating them, perhaps in the most important way possible: by helping them perfect the poses (as best they could) without injuring themselves by precipitously overreaching. To further these ends, in the 1970s in Pune and in the 1980s in London he introduced props (such as wood blocks, blankets, straps, and bolsters) in classes to allow students to achieve greater extension and harmony of form without strain.

Yoga teacher Karin Stephan identifies Iyengar's "interpretation of how to execute the postures, not the postures themselves," as the feature that makes his method unique. His "flair for precision, a sense of perfection in each movement," distinguishes his yoga from "standard Hatha Yoga."[22] The yoga teacher and scholar Norman E. Sjoman, who studied with Iyengar in India from about 1970 to 1976, similarly concludes: "It is only recently, through the work of B. K. S. Iyengar, that this direction [toward precision in *asanas*] has been taken up. . . . He has . . . insisted on a principle of precision that is not found or cannot be determined from the older texts on yoga or even in the modern books of his contemporaries."[23]

The innovative nature of Iyengar's yoga clearly lies, in part, in his celebrated (and sometimes reviled) obsessive attention to detail in *asana*. But what exactly is the biomechanical principle upon which this demand for precision in *asana* rests? Iyengar needed to know in order for him to understand *asana* on its material level, as exercise.

Anatomy

What Iyengar imparted to his students as the foundation of his teaching wasn't the imperative to homologize the body with *asana* shapes— whether they resemble natural or human-made forms (reflected in their names) or geometric forms but the need for strict adherence to the anatomical demands inherent in *asana*. Take, for example, the instructions in *Light on Yoga* for *Tadasana,* the basic posture in Iyengar's yoga regime, and hence the posture that best exemplifies his implacable insistence on precision in *asana* (see fig. 32.1 on page 404):

1. Stand erect with the feet together, the heels and big toes touching each other. Rest the heads of metatarsals [the five bones in the foot between the ankle and toes] on the floor and stretch all the toes flat on the floor.

2. Tighten the knees and pull the knee-caps up, contract the hips and pull up the muscles at the back of the thighs.

3. Keep the stomach in, chest forward, spine stretched up and the neck straight.

4. Do not bear the weight of the body either on the heels or the toes, but distribute it evenly on them both.

5. Ideally in Tadasana the arms are stretched out over the head, but for the sake of convenience, one can place them by the side of the thighs.[24]

Iyengar's actual classroom teaching confirmed that instead of verbally encouraging students to draw on the symbolic meaning of a pose or adjusting them so their bodies conformed more closely to a shape (e.g., mountain or tree, peacock or serpent, bow or plow, hero or god, triangle or circle), he commanded students to pay attention to the anatomical details of a

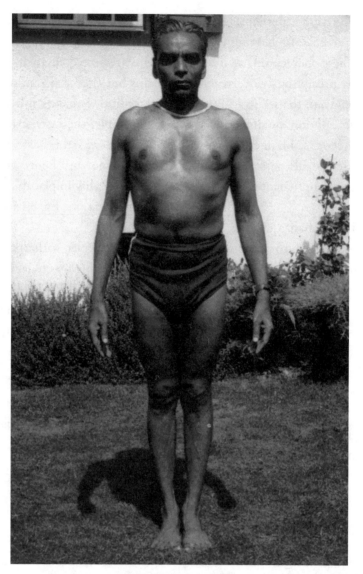

Figure 32.1. B. K. S. Iyengar
demonstrating *Tadasana*, Mountain Pose, circa 1970

(With the kind permission of B. K. S. Iyengar,
Ramamani Iyengar Memorial Yoga Institute)

pose. Stephan recalls a classroom instruction at Iyengar's institute in 1983: "'What's happening in your right foot? What's happening in your left? Your right thigh, left thigh, spine, right side of the back, left side of the back?' he challenged us. We immediately became totally aware of our bodies, descending our awareness to each and every part. . . . The posture was *tadasana*, which means mountain, and it is the very first posture he teaches. 'How can you learn to stand on your head if you can't even stand on your feet?' he chided us."[25]

Just as a new imaginary line, the prime meridian, was added to longitude, latitude, and the equator at the International Meridian Conference in Washington, D.C., in 1884 to answer the question, Where am I? (thus enabling us to chart our location and direction on the surface of Earth), a reference posture, called the anatomical position, was established by the German Anatomical Society at a meeting in Basel, Switzerland, in 1895 to answer the question, Where are the parts of my body? A part of the Basle Nomina Anatomica (BNA), the international standard on human anatomic nomenclature, the anatomical position enables us to describe and categorize the relationship of the body's bony parts to one another (orientation) and their movement in space (direction).

In the anatomical position one stands erect, facing forward, the arms at the sides, the palms of the hands facing forward (the thumbs are extended peripherally), and the feet parallel and close. All movement is a deviation from this reference position. For example, when the forearm is drawn from the anatomical position toward the shoulder, decreasing the angle between the forearm and upper arm, this simple bending movement is classified as flexion of the elbow joint in the anteroposterior plane. The anatomical position has been disturbed. When a leg that's been raised to the side is brought down toward the axis of the trunk, this simple lowering movement is classified as adduction in the lateral plane. The anatomical position has been restored.

In Iyengar's yoga system, *Tadasana* is the primary position from which all other yoga positions are defined. (The main difference between the anatomical position and *Tadasana* is the placement of the hands. In the anatomical position the hands are placed palms forward. In *Tadasana* the hands are placed palms inward. One can move back and forth between East and West—between two cultures, as it were—with just the flick of a wrist.) Just as in sports and medicine, where any movement is defined as a variance of the anatomical position, in Iyengar's yoga system each *asana* is considered a variance of *Tadasana*. It's the ideal: all the other *asanas* are imperfect, earthly variations of it and, as such, create a yearning to return to it.

Iyengar, in effect, applied the principles of postural alignment—standard posture as exemplified by the anatomical position—to each pose. In his system postural alignment is maintained as much as possible within the variations demanded by the unique configurations of each pose. Each pose is a variation of *Tadasana*; in each pose, no matter how small the trace, *Tadasana* is maintained as much as possible. It's in this futile, grand attempt to maintain standard posture in all *asanas* that Iyengar's precision rests—and his basic biomechanical principle was revealed to him.

Symmetry and Alignment

Although he'd been refining poses for forty years, Iyengar only started to consider the basic biomechanical principle underlying his *asana* practice in 1975: "I began to look at photographs of people, drawing lines between their way and my way of doing [yoga], chest to chest, hand to hand, elbow to elbow. The poses [of other yogins] were there, but not aligned. In head balance [*Sirsasana,* which, to a great extent, is *Tadasana* upside down], the head was in one place, the nose another place, the chest another place; one leg was turning."[26] What he realized was that he, in contrast to the other yogins, had been orienting his poses in accordance with the central line of the body. "Maybe you have read the *Bhagavad Gita*," he said to his admirers, directly addressing them, "where we are asked to keep the body in a rhythmic, harmonious state without any variations between the right and the left, the front and the back, measuring from the central line of the body which runs from the middle of the throat to the middle of the anus." Then, after drawing them in, he challenged his audience members, modeling their thoughts: "Can I adjust the various parts of my body . . . to be parallel to that central line?"[27]

No matter that Iyengar, as is the wont of some creative people, made up this source in the *Bhagavad Gita;* he had found the basic biomechanical principle underlying the precision of his *asana* practice: alignment, which consists of symmetry of body segments from left to right and balance of body segments from front to back. Viewed from the front or back, the body is symmetrical when its right and left sides correspond (as Iyengar stated, they are, essentially, without variations). Viewed from the side, the body is balanced when its front and back sides are in accord with gravity (contrary to what Iyengar stated, they have total variations—for example, the concave curve of the cervical spine, the convex curve of the thoracic spine, and the concave curve of the lumbar spine in the back and the opposing spinal curvature in the front, or the flatness of the shoulder blades in the back and the protrusion of the sternum and ribs in the front). When body segments are aligned, they're positioned (at the joints) in an arrangement that calls for the least muscular effort. Thus, alignment is the key to maintaining and achieving not only precision, rigor, balance, and full extension but also relaxation in *asana*. Iyengar finally understood the basic exercise principle of his system, which enabled him to deepen both his teaching and his own practice.

Iyengar's analysis of yogic postures was also part of another 20th-century movement, the same one that produced athletic coaches, physical educators, fitness trainers, physical therapists, dance instructors, and others: the application of research in human movement (studies on the workings of human muscles, bones, and joints) to improve physical performance in sports, exercise, rehabilitation, and dance.

Iyengar was influenced not only by the cross-fertilization from these fields but also by the improved *asana* performance standards developed by previous yogins, from the extremely demanding teachings of Krishnamacharya back to the groundbreaking work of the modern hatha yoga pioneers, especially Swami Kuvalayananda, in the 1920s. Before the early 20th century, there were no detailed instructions for assuming conditioning *asanas* because these limbering-up exercises were of secondary importance. Precision in performance only became necessary when the pioneer yogins moved the yogic conditioning postures to the forefront of hatha yoga practice. If they were to succeed in getting people to take up hatha yoga, they knew they had to come up with detailed instructions for assuming *asanas*. They turned to Western physical culturists, not traditional yogins, for their understanding of muscles and joints.

(And the Western physical culturists, in turn, drew on the accumulation of knowledge of the musculoskeletal system that originated with the ancient Greek physician Galen.) So Iyengar didn't transform previous modern *asana* practice; he refined it. He elevated its performance standards.

Contemporary yoga teachers, even those not trained in his method, have, in turn, adopted Iyengar's pedagogy. As a result, his teaching practices—extremely detailed instructions for taking poses, minute adjustments for correcting poses, and the use of props (blankets, blocks, straps, pillows, bolsters, and such) to aid alignment in poses—are now common features of most yoga classes. (Some enterprising cultural anthropologist might want to conduct fieldwork on the dissemination of these practices, charting their lineage to Iyengar.)

Among Iyengar's followers, the application of the latest knowledge of joint and muscle movement to yoga continues. As Sjoman points out, "[Iyengar's] western students have gone even further with the concept of precision, drawing on the understanding of movement, muscle function and anatomy built up in the physiotherapy and functional anatomy schools of the West."[28]

If Iyengar had drowned himself when he was a tormented youth, some other second- or third-generation modern yogin would've analyzed yoga's underlying dynamics to bring about higher standards of performance. Like the application of the line to art, the application of knowledge of muscle and joint movement to yoga was inevitable and evolutionary, especially considering the sweep of the performance revolution of the last forty years (making astoundingly high performance levels the norm in sports, fitness, chess, classical music, automobile manufacturing, and other fields). Which doesn't take away from the extraordinariness of Iyengar's achievement, gained through his solitary, unshakable (and perhaps unhinged) decades-long pursuit of perfecting *asana*.

Yoga as Performing Art

Geometric forms were introduced into modern art by Pablo Picasso and Georges Braque in 1907 in their Cubist paintings, which reduced reality to fragments—especially basic geometric structures—viewed from various angles, thus depicting reality in flux. Their portrait paintings influenced graphics and the performing arts. Historian and philosopher of modern dress Anne Hollander comments that during the 1920s, "the clothed figures in fashion drawings were designed to resemble hard-edged and streamlined cubes and cylinders, or to look like flat arrangements of geometric pattern."[29] In his theatrical experiments at the Bauhaus, Oskar Schlemmer "advanced to what he called 'the fully plastic art of the human body,'" writes culture critic Peter Conrad, by "allowing . . . rectangles to clad themselves in flesh."[30] In his 1925 dance *Crescendo,* Léonide Massine, the principal choreographer of Ballets Russes, "summed up modernity as a geometrical dance," Conrad adds. "A programme note explained that the purpose was to exhibit 'the angular tendencies of the time.'"[31]

This impulse toward the geometric also played a role in the birth of abstract art. Rejecting the five-hundred-year role of the Western painter to represent reality (traditionally by using planar recession and chiaroscural modeling to create the illusion of three-dimensionality), Kandinsky, Kazimir Malevich, Piet Mondrian, and others introduced geometric shapes in abstract paintings in the 1910s.* With the Haus am Horn, an exhibition house built in Weimar in 1922, the Bauhaus, the legendary arts, crafts, design, and architecture school founded in Germany in 1919, "took on the look we now associate with it: sleek chairs, metal fixtures, white exteriors," writes filmmaker Judith Pearlman. "The roof was flat and there were 90-degree angles everywhere."[32]

Both the Cubist and Bauhaus movements "were propelled by the same geometric appetite," observes art critic James Gardner in his discussion of the inception of geometric abstraction in art in the early 20th century, "the same willful need to reject the organic curvature of all earlier European art, from the cave paintings of Lascaux to the last, absinthial gasps of representation in the studios of the Symbolists."[33]

"Something about right angles and straight lines seemed so quintessentially modern, so redolent of the machine age," Gardner continues.[34] Indeed, nothing in the impulse toward the geometric in art, graphics, theater, dance, industrial design, and architecture epitomizes the modern so much as rectilinear forms, from skyscrapers (where, at their heights, their soaring vertical lines of steel are met by horizontal lines of intense winds) to the Vienna Method pictorial charts (five lines of pictograms of battleships allow one to compare at a glance the five biggest naval powers in 1938) to the Great War ceme-

teries in Flanders and northern France designed by British architect Edwin Lutyens (with their abstract lines formed by identical rows of headstones, they are the first modernist memorials). And there's no more powerful example of modernist geometricization than simple drawings of the human body composed of just a few dashed-off lines.

When visiting twenty-four-year-old expressionist dancer Palucca (Margarethe "Gret" Paluka) in Dresden in 1926, the sixty-year-old Kandinsky saw four staged dance photographs of Palucca, wearing a toga-like garment, taken by her close friend, the dance photographer Charlotte Rudolph. Kandinsky made analytical drawings directly based on these photographs (when placed over the photographs, his ink-on-tracing-paper drawings precisely overlay Palucca's shape), which he used to illustrate an article, "Dance Curves: The Dances of Palucca," published in *Das Kunstblatt* (The art paper) in March 1926 (fig. 32.2).

In her photographs, Rudolph heightened reality. She dramatically portrayed Palucca's fully realized positions through the use of theatrical lighting, shallow studio space, and claustrophobic framing. (Palucca barely emerges out of darkness in two images and casts shadows in the other two.) And she vividly captured Palucca's emotional state (although it's hard to tell if it's joyous or possessed). Kandinsky, in contrast, radically simplified reality. He dynamically represented Palucca's positions with a few (mostly)

---

*Although geometric art is a seminal innovation of modernism, 20th-century avant-garde artists didn't invent geometric art. It's present in many cultures throughout history. For example, centuries-old Islamic art, with its prohibition against the depiction of religious figures, is based on geometric patterns.

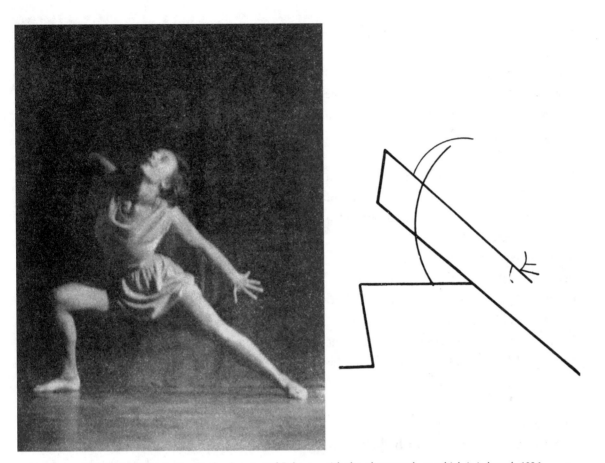

Figure 32.2. Wassily Kandinsky drawing of Palucca, with the photograph on which it is based, 1926
(From "Dance Curves: The Dances of Palucca," *Das Kunstblatt* 10, no. 3 [March 1926], with the kind permission of the Photo Service office of the Bauhaus-Archiv/Museum für Gestaltung, Berlin)

geometric lines that indicate the main axes of her trunk, limbs, and head. What he wished to emphasize in his "translation" of the four photographs into diagrammatic form, he explained, "is not only the extraordinarily precise construction of the dances in their temporal development, but also, first and foremost, the precise structuring of individual moments."[35] His caption for the third drawing reads: "Two large, parallel lines, supported upon a right angle.

Energetic development of the diagonal. Observe the exact position of the fingers as an example of precision in every last detail."[36] One could easily mistake these drawings of dance movements (if they were a bit less quirky and expressive) as graphic notations for yoga postures as taught by Iyengar.*

In his instructions (paraphrased below with his key directional terms intact) in *A Physiological*

---

*One should keep in mind, as Kramer notes, that "the straight line never became for [Kandinsky], as it did for Mondrian, either a sign of his spiritual mission or an exclusive component of his aesthetic" (Kramer, "Kandinsky," 3).

Handbook for Teachers of Yogasana for preserving the alignment of *Tadasana* in *Trikonasana*, Triangle Pose, Iyengar yoga teacher Mel Robin reveals the underlying rectilinear nature of *Trikonasana* when performed according to Iyengar's strictures (fig. 32.3):

- With the legs outspread, rotate and bend the trunk so that elements of the back of the body (e.g., the scapulae and buttocks) are "in a vertical plane."
- Keep the legs "straight."
- Place the axis of the pelvis "perpendicular" to the axis of the spine and "parallel" to the axis of the shoulders.
- Make the distance between the right front pelvis and lowest right rib "equal" to the distance between the left front pelvis and the lowest left rib.
- Maintain the normal spinal curvatures so that the neck is "in line" with the rest of the spine.[37]

In making known the powerful hidden patterns characterized by straight lines in Iyengar's version of *Trikonasana,* Robin establishes Iyengar's biomechanical principle of alignment as a manifestation of the modernist impulse for the rectilinear—which means to say, adumbrates Iyengar's system of hatha yoga as a modernist aesthetic endeavor.

Like a choreographer or gymnastics coach, Iyengar demanded that his students enter, hold, and exit a pose with precision, ease, grace, and élan. (All these fleeting attributes disappear at the end of a session, when, like a ballerina skittering off stage, we walk off the yoga studio floor to head to the changing room, which means to say, return to our quotidian lives.) When the inherent "beauty and harmony of the asanas" is manifested, Iyengar declaimed, hatha yoga becomes "a performing art" that can be "appreciated by onlookers."[38]

Iyengar's view of yoga as an art form may have derived from an early interest in physical disciplines that emphasize beauty—for example, bodybuilding (when he was a boy, bodybuilding was newly in vogue in India, and he met the most prominent Indian bodybuilder, K. V. Iyer, then at the height of his fame, in the Bangalore neighborhood where they both lived) and Indian modern dance (when he was a young adult struggling to make ends meet as a yoga teacher, he wanted to become a dancer). Almost surely, though, Iyengar learned to apply aesthetic criteria to yoga from his guru, T. Krishnamacharya. Like Sundaram, Krishnamacharya demonstrated *asanas* to drum up interest in yoga among the general population, but he also gave *asana* demonstrations at festivities to impress and amaze spectators—the beginnings of yoga perceived as an art (and the harbinger of yoga as a competitive sport). With his zeal to refine *asana* practice, Iyengar brought an even higher aesthetic standard to yoga than Krishnamacharya. "In fact," Sjoman argues, "[Iyengar's] work is a reformation of the asana system that he was originally taught."[39] And indeed, Krishnamacharya's poses appear almost lumpy, soft, unstable, and listless compared with Iyengar's angular, crisp, grounded, and dynamic poses.

But the element of performing art in yoga, if it exists at all, is quite limited; it can't compare to the towering art of dance created by

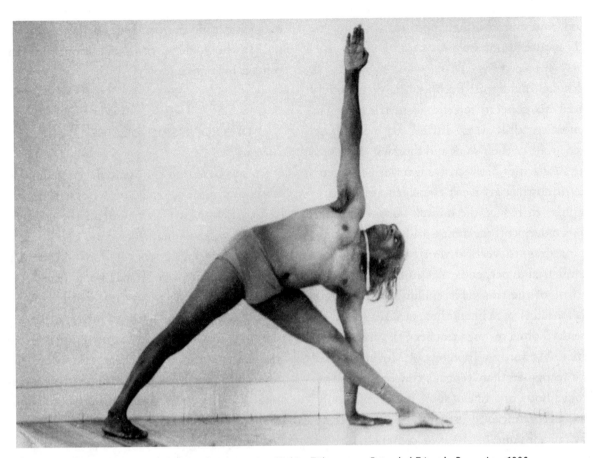

Figure 32.3. B. K. S. Iyengar demonstrating *Utthita Trikonasana*, Extended Triangle Pose, circa 1990
(Photo by Silvia Prescott, with the kind permission of B. K. S. Iyengar, Ramamani Iyengar Memorial Yoga Institute)

modern choreographers such as George Balanchine, Martha Graham, Merce Cunningham, Paul Taylor, Yvonne Rainer, and Mark Morris. Doubtless, yoga and dance share what dance critic Jennifer Homans considers the essence of ballet: "the linear and mathematically and geometrically proportioned organization of the human body."[40] But unlike dance, with its infinite movement, yoga is restricted to a set number of ideal positions, thus rendering yoga movement—even when performed at the highest level, as Iyengar nearly did even in his old age—unimaginative and inexpressive,

whereas dance movement touches our souls (sometimes in small ways, such as when one dancer leans on the other). In this constraint, yoga is more similar to the narrow beauty of gymnastics. Iyengar-style yoga primarily entails slow, controlled movement and stillness, whereas gymnastics entails a high degree of momentum, agility, and balance; nevertheless, both are formulaic.

Perhaps it's best said that modern hatha yoga can be artistic when in the hands (and feet) of a graceful and serene performer like Iyengar. But like gymnastics (or, for that matter, clothes, food, and conversation), postural yoga, by its very nature, is not art.

Although modernist European painters anticipated his concern for the geometric, Iyengar almost certainly wasn't influenced by them or even aware of their work and theories. However, the similarities between Iyengar yoga and geometric abstract art aren't coincidental. Iyengar's impulse to reduce the human body—perhaps, in its movement, the most unruly manifestation of nature—to vertical, horizontal, diagonal, parallel, and perpendicular lines was characteristic of the times. He couldn't have created his formalist yoga in another era. "At the end of the day," observes yoga teacher Eric Shaw in his article "Towards a Topology of Moving Yoga," "we recognize that Iyengar's conception of the [yogic] body as a vale of force lines [could only have been conceived in] this age [and not in] any previous one."[41]

Nevertheless, like other performance outliers (such as 1940s–1950s American golfer Ben Hogan, who spent years analyzing and experimenting with his golf swing and practiced far more than his competitors) considered to be oddballs early in their career for their fanatical devotion to study and practice and attention to the details of execution, Iyengar was a great original. Not only for his revival of the old (and advocacy of the new) weird *asanas* and for his perfection of *asana* but also, most significantly, for his recognition that the arduous, exacting,

and exuberant performance of *asana* doesn't nullify the yogic spiritual tradition but reinvents it for our times.

Yogic Means of Expressing Sacred Truths

Line

If it's not based on the symbolic or geometric configurations of *asanas,* on what is the spirituality in Iyengar yoga based? In the dynamic rectilinear line—manifested in the body as alignment—Iyengar was able to find the spiritual dimension in yoga that he couldn't find in shape: "There is a Universal Reality in ourselves that aligns us with a Universal Reality that is everywhere else. . . . Alignment from the outermost body or sheath (kosa) to the innermost is the way to bring our own personal Reality into contact with Universal Reality. The Vastasutra Upanishad says, 'Setting limbs along proper lines is praised like the knowledge of Brahman (God).'"[42] Iyengar had accessed the nonmaterial in yoga through the unlikeliest yet most obvious path: his decades-long fanatical refinement of the material in yoga.

This kind of insight into the nature of hatha yoga as embodied spirituality became possible for Iyengar late in life as a result of a transformative inward journey shaped by applying traditional yogic philosophy to his experience of his body in *asana*—a journey that was made under duress.

33

B. K. S. IYENGAR

Spiritualizing the Domain of Acrobatics

Asana *Practice as the Eight-Limbed Path*

Attacks on Hatha Yoga

In the 1970s and 1980s the yoga devout sought to rehabilitate yoga—to reclaim its traditional spiritual values—by exposing the common misconceptions of the hatha yoga vogue. "As soon as we leave the basic 'cross-legged' [position] and its variants," warned French Orientalist Jean Varenne in 1973, "we are entering the domain of acrobatics, and it is obvious that this means losing view of yoga's single goal, which is that of achieving samadhi [union with the divine] by meditation"[1] (see fig. 33.1 on page 414).

Varenne granted that these yogic "acrobatic" positions are salutary. For example, *Sirsasana,* Headstand, "ensures good irrigation of the brain and prevents the hair going white (some even claim that white hair will become black again as a result of practicing it regularly!). Clearly we are dealing here with an adventitious exercise that can have a beneficent effect on the yogi's health." Nevertheless, this conditioning *asana* "is not, properly speaking, part of yoga technique in the full sense of the term, since there can evidently be no question of meditating normally and for long periods in this position."[2] (Never mind that many yogins find *Sirsasana* the best pose for meditation.)

In stressing the centrality of seated meditation as the primary technique for spiritual liberation, Varenne was following the injunction ordained in the

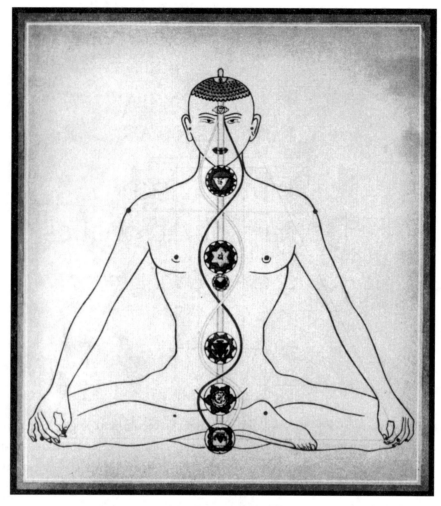

Figure 33.1. Illustration of a yogin sitting in meditation

(From *Yoga: The Method of Re-Integration*, by Alain Danielou)

authoritative yoga treatise *Yoga Sutra* (a Sanskrit compilation probably last redacted in the 4th century but attributed to Patanjali in the 10th century) and the yoga-influenced Hindu scripture *Bhagavad Gita* (probably composed in stages between the beginning of the Common Era and the 2nd century). In the former, an aphorism teaches: "Sitting should be steady and easy. This is done by loosening of effort and meditating on the endless."[3] In a passage in the latter, Lord Krishna, in explaining to Arjuna his duties as a prince and warrior, commands:

Having set in a clean place his firm seat, neither too high nor too low, covered with sacred grass, a deerskin, and a cloth, one over the other,

There taking his place on the seat, making his mind one-pointed and controlling his thought and sense, let him practise yoga for the purification of the soul.

Holding the body, head and neck erect and still, looking fixedly at the tip of his nose, without looking around (without allowing his eyes to wander),

Serene and fearless, . . . subdued in mind, let him sit, harmonized, his mind turned to Me and intent on Me alone.[4]

Varenne and others wanted to restore human salvation (whether by expanding consciousness to the level of limitless time and space or by focusing on God/Krishna alone) as the core principle of yoga—a principle subverted, they believed, by the 20th-century upstart yogins and their followers who popularized a hatha yoga focused almost exclusively on conditioning postures.

In his talk at the celebration for his seventieth birthday in 1988, B. K. S. Iyengar recalled that what he learned most from attending philosopher Jiddu Krishnamurti's lecture series given in Pune in 1946 is "do not criticize and do not justify."[5] Learning this lesson explains why "yogis all over the world criticised me that I do physical Yoga, but I do not criticise anybody," Iyengar said. "You don't find me attacking or criticizing others or their systems. . . . I am not keen to justify that what I do is right. . . . I do not bother about others' remarks."[6] Scholar of modern yoga Elizabeth De Michelis naively takes Iyengar's remark at face value. She even gives it the import of a life-changing revelation: "This [Krishnamurti's homily] would indeed have been momentous input for a man struggling . . . between the contradicting dictates of 'tradition' and 'modernity.'"[7] In actuality, when he was assailed in the 1970s and early

1980s by the righteous for teaching some sort of gymnastics, calisthenics, or acrobatics, the thin-skinned Iyengar vigorously justified his *asana* practice, capped by the 1988 publication of *The Tree of Yoga,* a compilation largely drawn from recordings and transcripts of a series of meetings and lectures with students and teachers from 1985 to 1987. In feeling compelled to defend himself against accusations by pious yogins of desacralizing traditional hatha yoga, Iyengar was preceded by the first-generation yogins who forged hatha yoga into an indigenous form of exercise and the second-generation yogins who exported hatha yoga as exercise.

Shri Yogendra, who, in 1918 in Bombay, was the first yogin to teach yoga physical culture as an end itself, argued that in his system a preliminary bout of spirituality sanctifies the corporeal: during his routine, instead of the conditioning exercises preparing for a long seated meditation, a brief seated meditation at the start ensures that the conditioning exercises that follow are performed "in perfect peace." "Mentally watch the breath going in and out just for one full minute," he advised, until "you are fully self-possessed."[8] "By "establishing inner harmony" and "elation through poise and composure," an initial preliminary seated meditation—as if casting a spell—provides "the most favourable condition for the practice of other exercises to follow."[9]

The feisty yogin-lawyer S. Sundaram, who was the author of the first (or, at least, the first extant) modern hatha yoga manual, *Yogic Physical Culture,* published in 1929, used a different strategy to defend yoga as physical culture. On the first page of the first chapter of his book, he described the goal of the

Vedantin: "His object is to realize Brahman—to achieve the hardest—Self-Realisation—to complete the cycle of evolution." However, the instrument of achievement, Sundaram pointed out, "is the God-given one, the human body. If this goes wrong, the ambition, material or spiritual, is retarded."[10] Therefore: "It is no sin to care for the body. The *pseudo*-Vedantin may say, 'forget the body.' This would only mean blaspheming Vedanta or just like Satan quoting scriptures to serve his ends. There is no signal injunction in the Shastras to perpetuate drains and sewages in the human system. It has to be respected and treated as a God-like gift, which it really is."[11]

Having made his stirring case for the need to tend to the body, Sundaram found no need to mention the body as the vehicle for self-realization again his book.

Swami Kuvalayananda, who, in 1924, founded Lonavla, the first laboratory to scientifically study yoga, deftly disarmed his religious critics by shrewdly agreeing with them. The scientific investigations of yogic physical culture that he proposed to carry out and report on may give people "the impression that Yoga is only a system of physical culture and therapeutics," he declared in his mission statement in the inaugural (October 1924) issue of his journal *Yoga-Mimansa*. "But nothing can be farther from the truth than this impression. The physical side is only a minor aspect of Yoga which is chiefly mental and spiritual."[12] After conceding the inconsequential nature of the physical aspect of yoga, Kuvalayananda embarked unfettered on his lifework to promote the physical aspect of yoga—in particular, the conditioning postures—as health cure.

No yogin was more assailed by the yoga orthodoxy than the second-generation yoga innovator Swami Sivananda, who exported his style of hatha yoga around the world beginning in the 1930s. One of his followers, the Belgian yoga teacher, author, and publisher André Van Lysebeth, concedes in his tribute to Sivananda that the traditionalists were not entirely wrong: "Hatha yoga for health and physical fitness is only a caricature of yoga in its totality. Often yoga is completely cut off from its deep roots, which lead us back to the origins of our own being and of the cosmos."[13] Of the thousands of Westerners who have taken up yoga, most practice only *asanas* and some relaxation or meditation, and they "will be happy to cure their constipation, insomnia and backaches." But Van Lysebeth makes a sensible justification for Sivananda's brand of yoga. "This may not be traditional yoga. Would it be better to let people suffer? If any technique may be of some use to someone, . . . who could refuse him help in the name of orthodoxy? Besides, those hundreds of thousands of beginning practitioners form the nursery from which will emerge the full-fledged yogic aspirants of the future."[14] Not that Sivananda cared about what his critics thought of him. "Indifferent to adverse opinions, Swami Sivananda just went on teaching, writing and publishing."[15]

But none of these yogins aggressively defended himself against critics as Iyengar did. Only Iyengar defiantly and directly challenged his critics: "How many of you really know how to do an asana? How many of those who say that asanas are [solely] physical know the depth of the way of doing them which I have been describing?"[16]

Iyengar could've simply conceded that his style of yoga is exercise, but—with its breadth (variety of *asanas*) and depth (precision of *asanas*)—a superior form of yogic exercise. He could've even argued that practicing his style of yoga is the perfect set of limbering-up exercises to prepare for going off to a quiet place to sit in meditation. Instead Iyengar defiantly argued that his practice—composed of conditioning postures—is infused with spirituality, while the traditional practice of his accusers, carried out over centuries—composed primarily of meditative postures in which one sits to achieve a contemplative state—is totally absent spirituality. "You may all have practiced meditation," he scornfully told his accusers. "You may be doing meditation sitting in a corner and becoming empty within yourselves with that emptiness which comes also in sleep. . . . I meditate, not sitting in a corner, but . . . in every position I perform, in every asana."[17]

As was his habit, Iyengar defended the singular *asana*-based yoga that he created by scathingly attacking his doubters—in effect, accusing them of being the yoga heretics. But in making his argument that seated meditation is like sleep, he wasn't just attacking his attackers; he was being dismissive of anyone who sits to meditate. It isn't easy in our hectic lives (in which many of us must be continually active just to keep things barely under control) to set aside time during the day to sit and observe our fleeting or ruminative thoughts and attempt to quiet our mind. It was reckless and unkind of Iyengar to say otherwise. Especially considering that his previous writings on seated meditation showed him to be its most passionate and eloquent adherent.

Seated Meditation

Iyengar's guru, Tirumalai Krishnamacharya, taught that meditation should be practiced in a seated position. He recommended that under the ideal conditions one should build a private ashram in a fenced-in area in a solitary place near a holy river. Inside the building, one should "spread a seat of grass on the ground in a clean space not facing the front door. Over that spread a tiger skin or deer skin and over that put a white blanket or a clean white cloth. Prepare such a place for sitting."[18] In the 15th-century *Hatha Yoga Pradipika*, Svatmarama described exactly how to go about this meditative sitting in his instructions for *Siddhasana*, Accomplished Pose, which is similar to *Padmasana*, Lotus Pose: "Press firmly the heel of the left foot against the perineum, and the right heel above the male organ. With the chin pressing on the chest, one should sit calmly, having restrained the senses, and gaze steadily at the space between the eyebrows. This is called Siddha Asana, the opener of the door of salvation."[19]

In *Body the Shrine, Yoga Thy Light,* published in 1978, Iyengar presents his instructions for the seated posture as a "common sense" technique for cultivating the physical steadiness and effortlessness needed for meditation.[20]

When the ancients, however, counseled, "Sit in any comfortable position with the spine straight," they certainly did not mean that slouching would do. To sit in a loose, collapsed sort of way induces sleep. Drowsiness is not to be mistaken for meditation. Meditation does not make the mind dull. Rather, in meditation the mind is still, but razor-sharp, silent but vibrant with energy. This state cannot be achieved without a firm, stable sitting posture, where the spine ascends and the mind descends and dissolves in the consciousness of the heart, where the true Self reveals itself. The whole body, far from being ignored, is taken up in this spiritual alertness, till the whole man becomes pure flame. An alert, erect spine creates a spiritual intensity of concentration that burns out distracting thoughts and the brooding over past and future, and leaves one in the virginal, fresh present.[21]

In this movingly expressive and startling description of seated yogic postures, Iyengar upends their traditional supporting role and assigns them a new starring role as the agent of transcendence: "an alert, erect spine *creates* a spiritual intensity of concentration" [italics added]. Yet in his actual yoga practice, he performed little or no seated meditation, even that which was in accord with his writing. In fact, he had been belittling the practice for at least nearly twenty years. In 1960 he said to his students, "To sit in Lotus Pose and gaze at one's nose is said to be a spiritual practice; to do Lotus Pose and concentrate on the coccyx or elsewhere is said to be a physical practice. Where is the difference? How can Hatha Yoga [in which one performs the Lotus Pose as a conditioning posture for the hips and pelvis] be only physical and Raja Yoga [in which one assumes the Lotus Pose for meditation] only spiritual?"[22] In 1965 he said, probably referring to active *asanas,* "Meditation is really to do everything with love, not to sit and close the eyes and utter the name of God mechanically. That is a waste of time."[23]

Iyengar practiced yoga without interruption or troublesome incidents from 1958 to 1978 (though in early 1958 he had periods of dizziness and blackouts). "My practice was smooth and enjoyable," he recalled.[24] Then a minor but shattering incident occurred at his sixtieth birthday celebration (fig. 33.2).

The completion (or sometimes the onset) of the sixtieth year of life in Indian tradition is considered to mark a turning point in a man's life: unfettered by occupation and family, he turns away from the ephemeral and toward the eternal—to matters of the spirit. A sacred Vedic ceremony, called *shashtiabdapoorthi,* commemorated with rituals and attended by colleagues, friends, and family, is held. At Iyengar's sixtieth birthday celebration, held on the commencement of his sixtieth year on December 14, Krishnamacharya delivered the *mangalasish,* invocation of blessings, which he'd composed in Sanskrit for this special occasion. "One who has defeated his opponents, one who is adept in manifold yogic asanas (who has dived deep in the ocean of Yoga)," Krishnamacharya intoned about Iyengar, "may he live long." Then Krishnamacharya reminded those who had gathered for the celebration that Iyengar was not one to neglect the spiritual side of yoga. "Sometimes he is engaged in teaching Yoga without giving up the authentic classical way. . . .[25] He himself is also engaged in practising Yoga constantly for his own spiritual experience and he is established in the city of Pune."[26] This effusive public praise of Iyengar's spirituality was actually a dig. After the festivities were over, Krish-

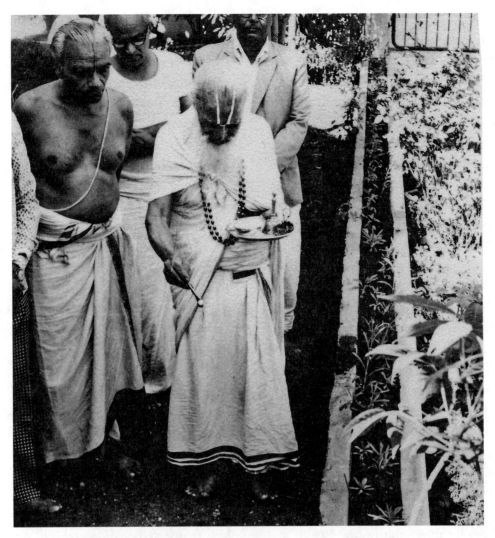

Figure 33.2. T. Krishnamacharya (right) performing a tree-planting ceremony
while B. K. S. Iyengar looks on at Iyengar's sixtieth birthday celebration
at the Ramamani Iyengar Memorial Yoga Institute compound, 1978

namacharya privately told Iyengar "to devote time on meditation and to lessen . . . physical strain"—that is, to meditate in a seated position and, in Iyengar's interpretation of Krishnamacharya's injunction, to greatly reduce—in fact, to eliminate—any practice of conditioning postures.[27]

Although having far surpassed his guru in achievement and fame, Iyengar dutifully obeyed Krishnamacharya's injunction to meditate: he sat on a rug either before sunrise or after sunset "for at early dawn and late evening the Spirit of God pervades over the earth like a healing benediction."[28] (Iyengar recalls that before his *pranayama* practice he'd wake up his doting wife to have her make him a cup of coffee: "After preparing coffee for me, she went back to sleep."[29] So it's likely that he practiced seated meditation—perhaps as an extension of his *pranayama* practice—in the morning as well.)

Iyengar adopted what he considered "the classic meditative pose": "the cross-legged *Padmasana* pose with the spine held straight and rigid."[30] He pressed his hands together, palm against palm, and placed them at his breastbone. ("This classic pose of all prayer is not only symbolic but also practical. Symbolically the palms salute the Lord, Who is within." Practically, "if both palms press equally against each other, both mind and body are in balance and harmony."[31]) He commenced rhythmic movements of inhalation, retention, and exhalation of the breath. Through these techniques he stilled his mind, thereby opening up his heart to the divine. "It has been maintained that yogic meditation is without content, a mere emptying of the mind. . . . The intellect of the mind may cease its roving but the intellect of the heart goes out to the Lord."[32]* Iyengar meditated in this manner for three months (fig. 33.3).

The result, Iyengar lamented afterward, was that his body "lost its grace and elasticity." After a struggle to return to his previous conditioning ("the body was rebelling but the will-power was growing stronger to break the barriers of the body"), he returned to a schedule of four to five hours of *asana* practice each day. His body was mended, but his break with Krishnamacharya was irreparable: "This made me not to respect the words of those whom I revere, but have no experience of their own."[33]†

Iyengar might've been especially irked by Krishnamacharya telling him to meditate because when he was taught *asana* at the *yogashala*, he never received instruction in the spiritual aspects of hatha yoga. "If my brother-in-law also had an eye to my deeper spiritual or personal development, he did not say so at the time," Iyengar remarked.[34] But then Krishnamacharya didn't teach yoga as soteriology—as a sustained, rigorous practice that orients one toward the realization of one's true identity as Self—at the *yogashala*. Modern yoga scholar Mark Singleton reports that Srinivasa Rangacar, one of Krishnamacharya's earliest students and assistant teachers at the *yogashala*, "became disgusted with the methods taught there, concluding that 'but for Yogic exercises [Krishnamacharya] had no idea of the real inner bases of [yoga].'"[35] "The evidence from the period, and oral testimony," Singleton concludes, "suggests that in his role at the *yogasala* Krishnamacharya did certainly focus almost exclusively on the external, physical exercise component of yoga."[36]

Krishnamacharya did conduct classes in yoga theory in his home for his students. "Unfortunately," Iyengar later recalled, "I was not one of them."[37] Evidently he didn't miss much. T. R. S. Sharma, another student, told Singleton

---

*This description of Iyengar's meditation practice is based on his instructions, not his recollections.

†As fate would have it, Iyengar was struck by a scooter in mid-1979 (not in January, as he recollected), severely injuring his left side, and then struck by another scooter within three months, severely injuring his right side. "As Yoga means evenness, these two accidents evenly injured my body," he quipped in 1988. "My practice reached the rock bottom. Since 1979, I am fighting to come back to my 1977 standard." It took him twenty-five years to fully recover (Iyengar, *Astadala Yogamala,* 48).

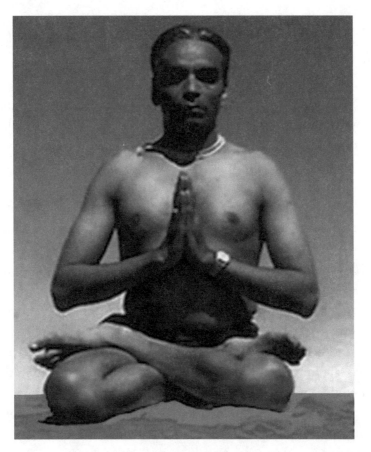

Figure 33.3. B. K. S. Iyengar
sitting in meditation, circa mid-1970s

(With the kind permission of B. K. S. Iyengar,
Ramamani Iyengar Memorial Yoga Institute)

that "Krishnamacharya's nightly teaching at the *sala* was concerned uniquely with *angalaghava* ('lightness of limb') and that 'the spiritual aspects of yoga like *dhyana, dharana* and the *samadhi* states were rarely talked about.'"[38]

Whatever the layers of his resentment, Iyengar was so enraged by Krishnamacharya's command to sit in meditation and its consequences that, like a teenage son who fears if he lets out his full wrath he'd murder his father, he couldn't direct his fury clearly and unambiguously at Krishnamacharya; instead, he diverted it toward a vague group of people who criticized him for not meditating, of whom Krishnamacharya was one. When Iyengar scornfully replied to his critics, "If closing the eyes and remaining silent is meditation, then all of us are meditating every day eight or ten hours in our sleep. Why do we not call that meditation? It is silence, is it not?" he was lashing out at Krishnamacharya.[39] Not only was Iyengar's first enemy his surrogate father and guru Krishnamacharya, but every enemy, it appears, became Krishnamacharya.

But Iyengar didn't merely nurse his resentment of Krishnamacharya's opprobrium (and perhaps his shame over his acquiescence to Krishnamacharya's directive); he used it as a spur to deepen his philosophy of *asana*. De Michelis attributes Iyengar's turning inward in the late 1970s to his having reached a stage in life in which, after having attained worldly success, he could finally focus on *moksha,* spiritual liberation: "Up to 1975 . . . Iyengar was mainly busy elaborating and propagating his style of yoga *practice.* It was only after *Light on Yoga's* success, the establishment of the Ramamani Iyengar Memorial Yoga Institute and the attainment of professional and personal maturity that these influences [his early contacts with Sivananda and Krishnamurti, who espoused the belief that each person has an inner faculty that's receptive to Being] could emerge."[40] While it would be foolish to dismiss this explanation for his increased attention to spiritual matters during this period, it would be even more foolish to ignore in Iyengar's accelerated spiritual development—as in his fierce determination to create an *asana* practice that surpassed his guru's in refinement—the importance of pique.*

Moving Meditation

In the *Yoga Sutra,* Patanjali expounded a yoga that consists of eight limbs: *yama* (abstinences), *niyama* (observances), *asana* (seated postures), *pranayama* (breath control), *pratyahara* (withdrawal of senses), *dharana* (concentration), *dhyana* (absorption), and *samadhi* (contemplation). He described the third limb, *asana,* as sitting yogic postures that cultivate effortlessness and steadiness in meditation. In the *Hatha Yoga Pradipika,* Svatmarama maintained that conditioning *asanas* should be practiced "for gaining steady posture, health and lightness of body" to facilitate, it's implied, maintaining meditative *asanas* for long periods of time by eliminating the distractions of fidgetiness and lethargy, weakness and pain, and heaviness and stiffness.[41]

In *Yoga Makaranda,* published in 1934, Krishnamacharya made the case, in accordance with traditional interpretation of the *Yoga Sutra,* that the steps of the eightfold yogic path to liberation should be carried out sequentially. "Just as in order to climb the Tirupati hill one has to climb step by step and only at the end does one achieve *darsanam* [the beholding of the divine] of the *swami* and experience happiness," he argued, "similarly everyone who follows the path of *yoga sastra* has to climb the eight steps of *yama, niyama, asana, pranayama, pratyahara, dharana, dhyana,* and *samadhi* proceeding according to the given order. Whoever climbs these eight steps proceeding according to the regular order will experience bliss."[42]

In accordance with the *Hatha Yoga Pradipika,* Krishnamacharya also argued that practicing conditioning *asanas* is necessary to supplement meditation in seated *asanas* because from the conditioning *asanas* one "gains strength of the body,"[43] achieves a condition wherein "the

---

*De Michelis seems to be on firmer ground when she speculates that in the 1990s, with Iyengar "entering his seventies, this is . . . a natural time of reflection and of searching deeper into the subject (Self-realization) to which he has dedicated his life" (De Michelis, *History of Modern Yoga,* 209).

various parts of the body . . . function at the perfect, ultimate level," and acquires a "healthy body and good health."[44]

In the mid-1960s Iyengar's thinking about the eight-step path to enlightenment and the role of conditioning postures had not evolved much beyond his teacher's. His introduction to his yoga manual, *Light on Yoga,* published in 1966, is largely an extended, conventional explication of Patanjali's philosophy (retroactively called raja yoga by Svatmarama), informed by Svatmarama's additions of the conditioning postures. He presents the eight limbs as sequential stages. He makes a strong case for performing conditioning postures in preparation for meditation: "The Yoga aspirant need[s] the knowledge and discipline of the Hatha Yoga of Svatmarama to reach the heights of Raja Yoga dealt with by Patanjali."[45] The benefit of the conditioning *asanas,* he argues, is that they've evolved over centuries to secure a "strong and elastic body," "keep the body free from disease," and "reduce fatigue and soothe the nerves."[46]

But Iyengar also was bringing something new to yoga philosophy: a sensitivity to and a deep appreciation of the importance of the body as a vehicle for spirituality. He points out the difference between the goal of the yogin and the goal of those who perform similar disciplines. Actors, acrobats, athletes, and dancers have great control over their bodies, he maintains, but "they often put the body above all else."[47] In contrast,

> the yogi conquers the body by the practice of asanas and makes it a fit vehicle for the spirit. He knows that it is a necessary vehicle for the spirit. . . .

> The needs of the body are the needs of the divine spirit which lives through the body. The yogi does not look heaven-ward to find God for he knows that He is within, being known as the Antaratma (the Inner Self). He feels the kingdom of God within and without and finds that heaven lives in himself.[48]

Compared to the writings of Rainer Maria Rilke and other modern interpreters of the resurrection of the body, Iyengar's description of the spiritually infused body is simplistic and trite. Within the yoga tradition, however, Iyengar's insights were an unprecedented lyrical and profound expression of the role of the body as an instrument of the soul.

In "Yoga and Meditation," an article in *Body the Shrine, Yoga Thy Light,* published in 1978, Iyengar continues his grand defense of the place of the body in the yogic spiritual path, although it's unclear at first whether he's referring to the body in seated *asanas* or conditioning *asanas:* "Meditation must begin with the body. It is the vehicle of the Self. . . . The ancients in their wisdom knew this, but modern make-believe would ignore the body."[49]

Later on in the article, however, in a significant advance of his philosophy of *asana,* he unambiguously declares that meditation begins, continues, and ends with the body configured in conditioning *asanas:* "Body posture is important. The awareness from within of every pore of the body *in the various asanas* is itself meditation. . . . The [conditioning] asanas are not simply important because they strengthen the nerves, lungs and other parts of body but also for their role in meditation. *They are themselves vehicles of meditative action*" [italics added].[50] In Iyengar's newly formulated yoga philosophy, the active *asanas,* which make the dull body fulgent, are the optimal vehicle for meditation.

The late 1970s and early 1980s saw the full blossoming of Iyengar's philosophy of yoga with his application of Patanjali's eight-limbed path of liberation to his hatha yoga practice. In *The Tree of Yoga,* Iyengar uses the symbol of a tree to diagram the eight components of the path: *yama* is the roots; *niyama,* the trunk; *asana,* the branches; *pranayama,* the leaves; *pratyahara,* the bark; *dharana,* the sap; *dhyana,* the flower; and *samadhi,* the fruit. He cautions his followers to experience these components as a whole during their yoga practice: "to see the tree in totality without naming it as flower, fruit, leaf or bark. The moment you see the leaf, you forget the tree." And he cautions his followers to experience all the components: "Similarly, if you say that you want to meditate [practice the inward-turning limbs] and you forget the other limbs of yoga, you are no longer seeing the whole tree."[51]

These arguments are the heart of Iyengar's attack on seated meditation. Seated meditation emphasizes the three inward-turning limbs of meditation, collectively called *samyama*—consisting of *dharana* (single-pointed concentration), *dhyana* (widened concentration), and *samadhi* (prolonged concentration)—to the exclusion of the other limbs. These three steps of spiritual actualization, Iyengar argues, can't be practiced separately from all the previous steps. "[They] are the effects of that practice. They cannot be practiced directly."[52] What can be practiced directly are conditioning *asana* and *pranayama.* (A kernel of this thinking can be found as early as 1966 in a revelatory offhand personal observation in *Light on Yoga:* "My experience has led me to conclude that for an ordinary man or woman in any community of the world, the way to achieve a quiet mind is to work with determination on two of the eight stages of Yoga mentioned by Patanjali, namely, asana and pranayama."[53]) Of all the limbs, though, Iyengar declares the conditioning *asana* central: "All the eight limbs of yoga have their place within the practice of asana."[54]

Traditionally in yoga the object of meditation, assimilated while seated, has been an image (e.g., of the god Vishnu or of our body as a corpse), glowing coals (used for the subject of fire), a mandala, a mantra (e.g., Om), or even a particular area of the body with symbolic value (e.g., the point between the eyebrows, considered the commanding circle, or the solar plexus, considered the lotus of the heart). Iyengar implicitly considers these objects of meditation as arbitrary and ideological accretions. We penetrate into the essence of things, he argues, through concentrating on what is inherent in our *asana* practice: namely, performing *asanas.* In other words, for Iyengar, bending and twisting the body into the shapes of conditioning *asanas* isn't merely the vehicle of meditation; it's the *object* of meditation. Thus, in Iyengar's schema, *dharana* becomes concentration on assuming a pose. *Dhyana* becomes concentration on refining the pose by making adjustments to the whole body. *Samadhi* becomes prolonged concentration on dwelling within the pose. The three inner steps can't be practiced directly because they're mental processes applied to performing a yogic pose.

To some, Iyengar's claim that "within the one discipline of asana all the eight levels of yoga are involved, from yama and niyama through to samadhi," seemed baseless or even outlandish.[55] "A study of classical texts shows that [Iyengar and other teachers'] interpretation of Yoga as the exclusive practice of different postures is not supported by the authority of the ancient texts on Yoga, nor is it in line with the view of asanas as a preliminary foundation of practice in traditional Yoga texts," writes Gudrun Bühnemann, scholar of Sanskrit and South Asian religions.[56] She's correct, of course. There's no precedent in text or performance for a spiritualized yoga practice to revolve around the conditioning postures. Iyengar had overturned the tradition.

Iyengar could've easily made the claim that through a long and difficult internal quest he'd evolved a path to spiritual liberation that uses the conditioning postures as the object of meditation. Instead, as was his wont, he unnecessarily tried to dupe and intimidate his critics (and

his followers!) into believing that his meanings of *asana* and *samyama* were the original meanings and that his *asana*-oriented yoga practice had always been a spiritual discipline. But there was no need for such legerdemain, bullying, and bluster. Like any magician, however, Iyengar didn't want to give away the secrets of his trick. He preferred to astonish. But what could be more astonishing than the radical reinterpretations he used to transform yogic "gymnastics" into meditation?

In the late 1970s and early 1980s, probably in response to Krishnamacharya's harsh criticism that his time passionately devoted to his *asana* practice would be time better spent devoted to meditation, Iyengar felt compelled to forge his *asana* practice (which he had long considered as a spiritual discipline) into a coherent lived philosophy—a meditation—based on Patanjali's eight-step path to liberation. But he couldn't have applied this traditional framework to his *asana* practice if it weren't already highly conducive to being transformed into structured meditation.

34

B. K. S. IYENGAR

Making *Asana* Practice into a Meditation of Insight

Samyama in Iyengar Yoga

Dedicated to the precise and dynamic performance of often challenging *asanas,* the hatha yoga developed by B. K. S. Iyengar seemed particularly ill suited for being made into a spiritual practice, let alone the eightfold path of liberation explicated by Patanjali in the *Yoga Sutra.* What made it the ripest form of late 20th-century hatha yoga to undergo a spiritual transformation, however, was exactly its emphasis on the performance of *asana,* rather than on the benefits of *asana* practice to our lives outside the classroom—even such worthwhile benefits as acquiring good health, maintaining flexibility, relieving stress, becoming a better person, or facilitating steadiness and ease in seated meditation. "In other words," as yoga scholar Norman Sjoman explains, "the asanas [in Iyengar yoga] become complete in their own right, they have their own indigenous 'mystique.' The realization of that 'mystique' [is] in the complexities of the movement itself—a suitable object considering the complex psycho-physical nature of movement, stillness and balance."[1]

Iyengar was by no means the first yogin to analyze *asanas,* separating the poses into their constituent parts and closely examining those parts. Detailed instructions for practicing *asanas* first appeared in book form in the first modern yoga manual, *Yogic Physical Culture,* published in 1929 by S. Sundaram (who based his instructions on those found in articles in Kuvalayananda's *Yoga-Mimansa*), and have appeared in almost all subsequent yoga manuals.

But Iyengar comprehended the complexities of *asana* to a greater degree than his predecessors and contemporaries. And it's the great concentration demanded by his exquisite, intricate instructions to address these complexities that makes performing *asana* in an Iyengar classroom a suitable object of the eight-step meditation, including the three interiorized components, collectively called *samyama,* which Iyengar translated as "total integration."[2]

In *The Tree of Yoga,* Iyengar describes how a continuum of concentration on *asana* in *samyama* can extended from *dharana* (single-pointed concentration) to *dhyana* (widened concentration) to *samadhi* (prolonged concentration). Concentration on the first stage of *asana*—placing the body in the preliminary position and then assuming the basic configuration that defines the pose—embodies *dharana.* Concentration on the second stage of *asana*—refining the pose by subtly adjusting the parts of the body that perfect the pose, then assessing and further adjusting the pose, and lastly extending the pose—embodies *dhyana.* Concentration on the third stage of *asana*—dwelling within the pose—embodies *samadhi.*

Paschimottanasana is commonly translated as Seated Forward Bend but is literally—and poetically—translated as the Stretching from the West Pose, from *paschima* (west), *uttan* (stretch), and *asana* (posture). (Because prayers are traditionally observed facing east, the entire back of the body—from head to heels—faces west.) It's one of the six conditioning *asanas* (of the fifteen *asanas*) described in the first hatha yoga manual, the 15th-century *Hatha Yoga Pradipika:* "Having stretched the legs on the ground, like a stick, and having grasped the toes of both the feet with both the hands," wrote Svatmarama, "when one sits with his forehead resting on the thighs, it is called *Paschima Tana.*"[3]

According to Iyengar, after sitting on the floor with the legs stretched straight in front and putting the palms on the floor beside the hips, we begin *Paschimottanasana* proper by bending forward exclusively from the hips (the region around the joint that joins the pelvis with the upper part of the thighbone/femur), not from the waist (the part of the trunk between the pelvis and ribs). The agonists, the hip flexor muscles (the iliopsoas), contract to draw the lower back and pelvic bowl toward the front thighs. The antagonists, the hip extensor muscles (the gluteus maximus and upper part of the hamstrings), accommodate this forward movement by relaxing. The more they can relax, the more we can bend forward from the hips.

Bending forward from the hips is an unnatural and difficult movement. Despite moving with gravity, the upper body, tipped far off its axis, must work mightily (with the assistance of the abdominal muscles) to internally support its straightness as it slowly progresses downward. This movement can be performed only with a great deal of strain. As yoga anatomist H. David Coulter observes: "If you watch people bending forward in daily life, you will notice that they nearly always bend from the waist. This is the more natural movement. You would look very odd indeed if you kept your back straight and bent forward from the hips to pick up an object from a coffee table. . . . [Bending forward from the hips is] more difficult, not only because there is more weight to control but also because by definition it requires a reasonable measure of hip flexibility, and this can't be taken for granted."[4]

But bending from the hips, Iyengar discovered, is what allows us to have great extension in *Paschimottanasana*. Not wanting to discourage those of us who are beginners, he prepares us in his instructions in *Light on Yoga* for the difficulties of forward bending and provides encouragement: "to start with the back will be like a hump," but we should "try to keep the back concave." Gradually, over the course of our yoga practice, we learn to keep the back straight (with its natural curves) by lifting the chest and sitting as far back as possible on the sitting bones (ischial tuberosities), with the pelvis tipped forward (as it is in the Dog Tilt Pose) and the buttocks stretching away from the posterior thighs. We assist this stretch by pulling the trunk forward using our hold on the toes as leverage. "Then the hump will disappear and the back will become flat"[5] (fig. 34.1).

After bending as far as we can from the hips, we lower our back from the waist—in effect, rounding the back: "Bend and widen the elbows, using them as levers, pull the trunk forward and touch the forehead to the knees. Gradually rest the elbows on the floor, stretch the neck and trunk, touch the knees with the nose and then with the lips."[6] The back edges of the vertebrae of the lumbar, thoracic, and cervical spine are incrementally moved apart as the chin rests on (or as close as we can get to) the shins. The agonists, the trunk flexor muscles (rectus abdominis and external and internal oblique abdominals), contract with gravity while the antagonists, the trunk extensor muscles (erector spinae), relax.

Respecting their limitations as well as recognizing their potential, Iyengar didn't push students to the point of injury. He cautioned them that minutely moving toward perfection (in this case, folding the torso toward the legs) is more important than overreaching to achieve perfection. And he didn't just model a pose and expect students to follow along; he went around to adjust them to ensure proper alignment, often suggesting the use of props (in this case, pulling on a belt placed on the arches and/or sitting on a blanket to tilt the pelvis forward) to modify the pose to fit their skill level. Iyengar had well learned the lesson taught to him, when he was "very stiff and still very new" to yoga, by Krishnamacharya demanding that he perform *Hanumanasana,* Monkey Pose (what in gymnastics is called the split) which resulted in months of pain from a pulled thigh muscle. "This taught me that you had to [push students] far, but without forcing. Brutality is not the same as giving of yourself."[7]

As practiced by Iyengar, *Paschimottanasana* is first refined by making adjustments to the feet, legs, trunk, arms, hands, neck, and head. An Iyengar teacher might make these instructions (formulated by Iyengar and enlarged upon by his followers): Keep the feet close together and squared, as if they were flat against a wall. Lengthen the calves and backs of the thighs and keep the backs of the knees pressed down and firmly resting on the floor (aided by pulling the trunk forward). Lock the knees and tighten the shins and front thighs. Don't let the legs roll outward. Pull up the outer thighs. Relax the buttocks. Stretch the sides of the buttocks and waist evenly. Don't strain the back.

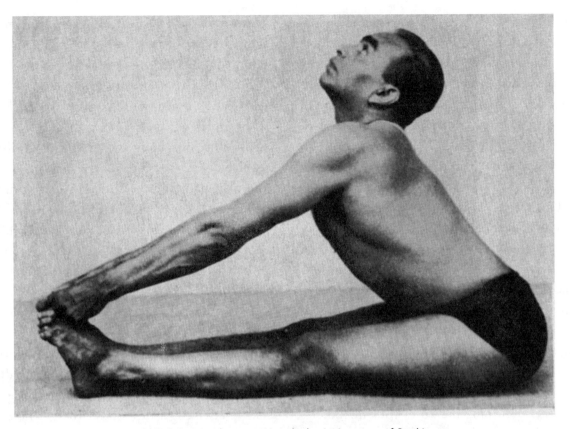

Figure 34.1. B. K. S. Iyengar demonstrating the beginning stage of *Paschimottanasana*,
Seated Forward Bend, 1966

Tighten the abdomen. Let the neck and head drop.[8]

The pose is further refined by what Iyengar, in *Tree of Yoga,* calls "reflection"—determining whether all parts of the body are in their correct position, and if they're not, making any necessary adjustments. "You reason: 'Am I doing this right? Am I doing it wrong?'" Iyengar explains. "'Why I have got this sensation on this side? Why am I getting that sensation there?'"[9] Any pain or discomfort we feel in parts of the body, he's saying, may be an indication that we're doing an *asana* incorrectly.

(Iyengar distinguished between "right pain," which is "usually felt as a gradual lengthening and strengthening feeling," and "wrong pain," which is "often a sharp and sudden cautionary feeling that our body uses to tell us we have gone too far beyond our present abilities." Pain that is "persistent and intensifying" is also "wrong pain."[10]) If we feel discomfort in *Paschimottanasana* "at the top of [a] buttock bone" (the right or left ischial tuberosity), he suggests that we observe whether "one leg [is] touching the floor and the other buttock slightly off the floor," which would result in the hip extensor muscles (the gluteus maximus, supplemented by the hamstrings, adductor magnus, and gluteus medius) stretching on the inside (lateral part) of the lowered buttock side and on the outside (medial part) of the raised buttock side.[11] "Are you aware of all these things?" he asks. "Perhaps you are not, because you don't meditate in the poses. You do the pose, but you don't reflect in it."[12]

Lastly, the pose is refined through extension. Though Sundaram (in *Yogic Physical Culture or the Secret of Happiness,* 1929), Kuvalayananda (in *Asanas,* 1931), Krishnamacharya (in *Yoga Makaranda,* 1934), and subsequent yogins gave instructions for extending *Paschimottanasana,* Iyengar (in *Light on Yoga,* 1966) far surpasses them with his exhaustive instructions for extending the pose.

> When [touching the knees with the nose and lips] becomes easy, make a further effort to grip the soles and rest the chin on the knees. When this also becomes easy, clasp the hands by interlocking the fingers and rest the chin on the shins beyond the knees. When [this position] becomes easy, grip the right palm with the left hand or the left palm with the right hand beyond the outstretched feet and keep the back concave. . . . Rest the chin on the shins beyond the knees. If [this position] also becomes easy, hold the right wrist with the left hand or the left wrist with the right hand and rest the chin on the shins beyond the knees. . . . Advanced pupils may extend the hand straight, rest the palms on the floor, join the thumbs beyond the outstretched feet and rest the chin on the shins beyond the knees.[13]

An essential aspect of Iyengar yoga, extensions are performed until the final pose is achieved (fig. 34.2).

Paschimottanasana is completed when our head is resting on our shins (or as close as possible) without further effort. We are still. With our body in a state of equilibrium between tension and relaxation, work and play, pain and pleasure, past and future, our mind is emptied. There's no more thinking. "To remain positively and thoughtfully thoughtless [in this way]," Iyengar explains in a daft but illuminating formulation, "is samadhi."[14]

In the absence of thought, the illusion of ego-identity is dissolved. We stop misidentifying our self with the "I." The "I" is no longer doing the pose. "The moment the object dissolves into the subject and the subject forgets itself, . . ." Iyengar expounds, "there is no difference between me and the object of my contemplation."[15] The meditator (the "I") and the object (the body in *asana*) are one. We are the pose. Startlingly inverting the common adage "mind over matter," Iyengar concludes that because "the various . . . parts of the body are positioned in their places in a proper order and feel rested and soothed . . . the mind experiences the tranquility and calmness of bones, joints, muscles, fibres and cells."[16] We're at peace.

The Meditation of Insight

In her discussion of the presentation in the *Bhagavad Gita* of yoga as a doctrine of liberation, Indology scholar Angelika Malinar describes two goals of yogic meditation:

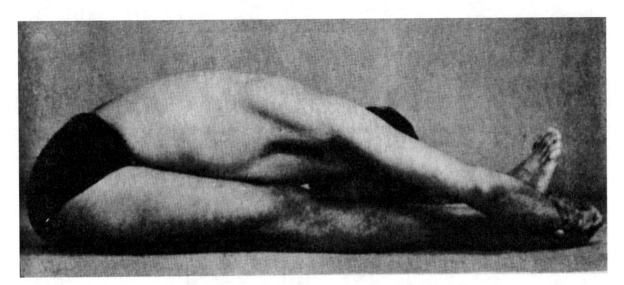

Figure 34.2. B. K. S. Iyengar demonstrating one of the extensions of the end stage
of *Paschimottanasana,* Seated Forward Bend, 1966

The state of *brahmanirvana* is defined as the complete cessation of mental activity (*nirodha*). This aligns with a well-established concept of yogic meditation as a liberating practice that emphatically requires the stoppage of all thought processes. This is to be distinguished from the yoga that results in the vision of the self, or of God, as this self (as is the case when Krsna is declared to be the object and goal of yoga). In this way the Bhagavadgita includes not only what may be distinguished as "theistic" and "non-theistic" yoga, but also two types of yoga and meditation found in Buddhist texts as well: first, yoga as a practice that aims at *nirodha,* complete cessation of mental activity followed by ultimate happiness; and second, as a practice of meditation that culminates in insight (*prajna*) or vision (of the self, god, etc.).[17]

Iyengar placed himself in the first tradition of attaining quiescence through emptying the mind of all thought—a quiescence marked not by inactivity, though, but by motion that leads to stillness (repose). As he explains in *The Tree of Yoga,* extraneous thinking is excluded through total absorption in assuming the various yoga conditioning poses.

In my method of teaching, because I take you through a lot of poses, I keep you for two or three hours, or sometimes four hours, without allowing your mind to go elsewhere. . . . Do the pupils know that four hours have passed? No. So I have kept them in a spiritual state for four hours. . . .

Suppose I were to ask you to do a meditation, to close your eyes and remain in silence. . . . Could I know what was going on in your mind? Perhaps you would call that spiritual, but I would say there is no spirituality there because your mind will be wandering elsewhere. That is not my method of teaching. . . . So I don't need a certificate to say whether this is physical yoga or spiritual yoga. When I am teaching I know that for four hours your mind has not been allowed to wander. And when I teach I make you full—fully aware of your body, your mind, your senses and your intelligence.

. . . You may meditate sitting in a corner, but I am moving everywhere and I am meditating.[18]

Students concur. In 1983 yoga teacher Karin Stephan writes about her experience studying with Iyengar in Pune in the 1970s and early 1980s: "There is an almost electrifying atmosphere in the classroom which lasts from beginning to end. It keeps students so tuned to the moment that though the mind may wander from time to time, caught by the piercing cry of the chick pea vendor in the street or the sight of the brilliant red flowers on the trees outside the classroom, the energy itself brings one constantly back to the present."[19]

Iyengar had placed himself in the cessative meditation tradition at least since 1959, when he said to students, "Meditation is oneness, when there is no longer time, sex, or country. The moment when, after you have concentrated on doing a pose (or anything else) perfectly, you hold it and then forget everything not because you want to forget but because you are concentrated: this is meditation.[20] But he also placed himself in the yogic meditative tradition of reflecting on an object as a means of being

washed over with comprehensions of reality. In *Light on Life: The Yoga Journey to Wholeness, Inner Peace, and Ultimate Freedom,* written with contributions by John J. Evans and Douglas Abrams and published in 2005, he explains: "Samadhi is an experience where the existence of "I" disappears. . . . We can see that we are divine. . . . We truly understand at the core of our being that our individual soul is part of the Universal soul."[21]

Expansive yogic meditation, as yoga scholar Mircea Eliade explains in *Yoga: Immortality and Freedom,* is an elaborate, formalized, coherent process solely orientated by lucidity. "For the 'mental continuum' never escapes from the yogin's will. It is never enriched laterally, by uncontrolled associations, analogies, symbols, etc. At no moment does this meditation cease to be an *instrument* for penetrating into the essence of things—that is, finally, an instrument for taking possession of, for 'assimilating,' the real."[22] Focusing on the object yields insight into reality ordinarily hidden during everyday life. This final step, *samadhi,* of a series of yogic techniques is so dense and pure that it seems not that we're focusing on the object but that, as described in Patanjali's aphorism (translated by Chip Hartranft), "the essential nature of the object shines forth, as if formless."[23]

In his commentary in *Practical Yoga: Ancient and Modern* on the *Yoga Sutra,* the out-of-fashion English-born American philosopher of yoga Ernest E. Wood, who accommodated his primarily American general audience by making yoga practices accessible to them and yoga philosophy applicable to their lives, provides a perceptive reflection, based on his personal experience, on meditating on a rose: "That rose—we have now lost our personal angle. We are conscious of it, as a young child is conscious before it has developed an idea of its own personality—with the full vividness and reality of experience. . . . It is as Patanjali says: 'There is the shining of the mere object alone, as if devoid of one's own form.' As if we were not there. But we are entranced."[24] (Wood translates Patanjali's aphorism differently from Hartranft, which means to say, interprets Patanjali's aphorism differently.)

But this shining forth of an object is also an opening up to Being. Wood, a philosopher of humble objects, also meditates on the "exquisite pattern" of a teapot lid (all that's left of a teapot that was broken long ago). In his usual blend of knowledge and feeling, he recounts: "I have long admired the beauty of [the lid], but just now I took it up and looked at it afresh—very closely. I realized that I have not seen it properly before." He then sees the beauty of objects everywhere, and, by extension, is overwhelmed with a sense of "belong[ing] therefore to the whole of things." "Yes, I look at one tiny piece of the pattern. It is something like the edge of a leaf. There meet only two lines and a bit of color," he concedes, "but with this meditation

they become my window into infinity. This beauty is life of which I can never tire."[25]*

Eliade presents a similar unfolding of revelations in his description of a traditional formal yogic meditation on glowing coals placed before a yogin. The yogin connects "the physiochemical process taking place in the coal with the process of combustion that occurs in the human body"; connects "the fire before him with the fire of the sun"; and obtains "a vision of existence as 'fire.'"[26] Patanjali lists other suitable paths of meditation—for example, concentrating on the sun yields insight about the vastness of the universe; on the navel, the arrangement of the parts of the body; and on the heart, the play of ideas in the mind.

For Iyengar, the sole object of meditation is the configuration of the body in the diverse conditioning *asanas*. But how can we grasp the immaterial, eternal, and numinous through placing our body in the various weird configurations of conditioning *asanas*? In other words, how can meditation on the conditioning *asanas* be part of the yoga tradition of (what scholar of South Asian religions David Gordon White identifies as) the open model of the human body that links the mind-body complex to phenomena outside itself?[27]

---

*Symbolic activities, such as making patterned pots, it should be noted, may be the defining difference not only between humans and animals but between *Homo sapiens* and the species they replaced in Europe about forty thousand years ago, *Homo neanderthalensis*—that is, symbolic activities may be what make us human. Wood's meditation might've taken him in the direction of pondering the facets of humanness.

35

B. K. S. IYENGAR

Teaching *Asana* as Embodied Spirituality

Recollecting the Body

After having scraped together the money to pay for her travel, living expenses, and tuition, thirty-three-year-old Noëlle Perez-Christiaens left France on July 1, 1959, to study one-on-one with B. K. S. Iyengar as part of her spiritual search, first inspired by reading *Voyage d'une Parisienne à Lhassa (My Journey to Lhasa)* at an early age.* After a week stay in Bombay, where she had disembarked on July 7, she arrived at Iyengar's cramped home in Pune on July 13. Her first class was on July 14. To her disappointment, she found it "just a special gymnastics without any spirituality."[1] In the classroom, where he was most supremely himself, Iyengar often seemed to be more imperious gymnastics coach than wise spiritual teacher. He insisted on long, grueling sessions of arduous yogic bends, twists, and balances (not, of course, the acrobatic flips and high, explosive leaps of gymnastics) and demanded precision, correcting the smallest imperfections in performance. "This girl is bushed," Perez-Christiaens wrote in her journal on July 15.[2]

Perez-Christiaens considered leaving but stayed on because of her attraction to the "precise and refined technique."[3]† "Although kind," she noted upon

---

*Voyage d'une Parisienne à Lhassa may have been the source of James Hilton's depiction of Shangri-La in *Lost Horizon* (see chapter 22).

†Becoming virtually part of the household, she would stay with Iyengar and his family for the next two and a half months. Her last class was September 27. She never returned to India but later attended Iyengar's classes in Switzerland and France.

first observing Iyengar giving a class, "he does not tolerate the halfway manner of teaching we have in Europe. Everything has to be done right, into the smallest details."[4] "Believe me," she breathlessly wrote her parents after only five lessons, "he sees all and lets you know that you just relaxed a tiny little muscle in the big toe of the left foot while he was adjusting your right knee." Gradually, though, she came to a realization: Iyengar's teachings were far more than "a marvelous kind of gymnastics."[5] "Even if contemplation was not ostensibly part of the practice," write her devoted students Georgia and Phillipe LeConte, "what she found there was a confrontation with the self."[6]

In the tradition of wisdom teachers, Iyengar facilitated—or, more accurately, stirred up—a student's confrontation with the self by sprinkling his classroom teaching with arresting aphorism-like sayings. What made some of them especially startling, provocative, poetic, and humorous, as well as sometimes seemingly quixotic, unclear, and impenetrable, was that they were of a piece with his *asana* instructions.

As evidenced by a collection of his 1959–1975 sayings, titled *Sparks of Divinity,* compiled by Perez-Christiaens from her notes along with the notes of other students, including Beatrice Harthan and Silva Mehta in England, Iyengar regularly made character building a critical part of his *asana* teachings, often by delivering a sage punchline that completed a setup line. "You feel in your own body what it is to suffer," he said, perhaps in response to a student who complained about having pain. "Your personal experience provides you with great love and compassion."[7] "Will power is here," he said, slapping a young man's buttocks. "If you know how to contract the muscles, if they are strong, you get will power."[8] "The standing poses are meant to strengthen the ankles and knees," he said. "These postures help you to maintain stability in times of catastrophe."[9] "Everyone has a side which is better than the other," he said, while showing one student the differences between the sides of another student carrying out a pose. "Balance between *Ha,* the right, and *Tha,* the left, is yoga."[10] Explaining the duality of "I" and "body" that occurs when a student becomes afraid to assume *Sirsasana,* Headstand, he said, "The moment you raise your feet from the floor, you experience the identity of 'I.' Take that away and retain the oneness, the total awareness which must remain throughout the posture."[11]

Some of the truths (though they bore his personal mark, they were universal truths) that Iyengar uttered in his *asana* instructions during this period were of a spiritual nature. He said: "Yoga is Self-realization through the understanding of the body."[12] And: "One who lives totally in the body lives totally in the Self."[13] But these spiritual truths were generalizations. In the 1980s, as he became increasingly concerned with shoring up the self only as a means of ultimately losing the self in preparation for opening up to Being (what he called "Self"), he realized that each *asana* (or set of similar *asanas*) resonates with its own revelations. As a result, he began to draw his students' attention to the particular configurations—the peculiarities—of each *asana* as distinct and unique paths to liberation.

Stripped of its everyday utilitarian functions, the body in yoga is divested of its limitless movements (e.g., reaching up to take a plate from the cupboard, rushing toward a shop to purchase chocolates, heartily embracing an old friend, pointing the direction to a subway station, kneeling to tie a shoe, shrugging to express dismay). Restricted to a repertory of preordained postures, the body in hatha yoga thus becomes of a piece with the other essential elements of yoga practice: staying in one small, delineated place; erasing expressions and eliminating gestures; breathing rhythmically; and ending the fluctuation of the mind. This extreme simplification of life is the basic yogic condition for meditation. Most people would consider that placing the body in a still yogic position (whether a seated posture or a resolved moving posture) held with steadiness and ease is a means of temporarily forgetting the body to facilitate meditation. For the embodied revelations of Iyengar yoga to occur, however, the body isn't forgotten but recollected. Or, perhaps more accurately said, the body is forgotten in its usual sense—the physical form that's assailed by opposites (such as restlessness and lethargy, pride and shame, and pleasure and pain) to which we constantly adapt—in order for the body to be recollected as a means of opening ourselves up to Being. As philosopher of phenomenology David Michael Levin points out, our openness to Being, made possible through having a deep sense of our body, is *always already* ours, so that, in the recollection, we are progressively realizing what we were *given* to understand all along."[14]

Iyengar guided his students in recollecting their body in particular *asanas* by calling on them to cultivate an awareness of what yoga philosopher Karl Baier describes as the three basic dimensions of *asana:* its "relation to the spatiality, the temporality, and the rootedness of human existence."[15] Iyengar invited his students to extend the continuum of mental effort from perfection of the pose to attunement to Being: the immensity and intimacy of space; the vastness and eternal present of time; and the grounding in and resistance to the pull of Earth. Examples of these classroom teachings may be found in Iyengar's *Light on Life,* published in 2005:

- "Those of you modestly struggling to join your hands behind your back (as well as round your knee!) after several years of practice of twistings [such as *Marichyasana* III, Marichi's Pose], may well exclaim, 'What can samadhi possible [*sic*] have to do with me?' . . . Penetration [to the center of our being, the soul] is possible in any asana that you can perform with reasonable proficiency."[16]
- In *Tadasana,* Mountain Pose, we have "our feet on the earth and our head in the heavens."[17] To Iyengar, *heavens* denotes the perfect, unified, omnipresent, and eternal—characteristics of the real that are revealed to us through experiencing the powerful presence of our aligned upright body.
- "Extend the energy of the asana out through your extremities" in *Virabhadrasana,* Warrior Pose. "Everywhere you extend, you are going toward the cosmos."[18]
- In *Trikonasana,* Triangle Pose, "our body seems to be trying to collapse forward to the floor. . . . So we apply ourselves and learn the adjustments that will cause the

whole body to open. We extend and redress our arm, lengthen the chest, and open the pelvis. . . . When you do the asana correctly, the Self opens by itself; this is divine yoga."[19]

- "For the yogi, the physical body corresponds to one of the elements of nature, namely the earth. We are mortal clay, and we return to dust. . . . As you explore your own body, you are in fact exploring this element of nature itself."[20] Twisting poses, such as *Marichyasana* III, "make us aware of the density, strength, and scent of the body's clay."[21]
- "*Savasana* is about shedding . . . many skins, [including] memories and projects for the future. . . . Only present awareness without movement and [past and future] time is there. Present awareness is the disappearance of time in human consciousness."[22]

What, we might wonder, would a guided meditation on the body in *Paschimottanasana* be like?

In a commentary that's meant to be scientific medical advice but is more a mix of quackery and fable in the "Effects" section of his entry for *Paschimottanasana* in *Light on Yoga,* Iyengar unwittingly intimates a path for comprehending the real by concentrating on the body in this pose. First he valorizes animal anatomy (at least that of quadrupeds) over human anatomy: "The spines of animals are horizontal and their hearts are below the spine. This keeps them healthy and gives them great power of endurance. In humans the spine is vertical and the

heart is not lower than the spine, so that they soon feel the effects of exertion and are also susceptible to the heart diseases." Performing *Paschimottanasana,* Iyengar argues, literally puts us in the position of animals: "In Paschimottanasana the spine is kept straight and horizontal and the heart is at a lower level than the spine. A good stay in this pose massages the heart, the spinal column and the abdominal organs, which feel refreshed." As a result: "the mind is rested" (see fig. 35.1 on page 438).[23]

Iyengar seems to be presenting a literal account of the origin of mankind's heavyheartedness. His edifying point is that we should act—or, at least, position ourselves—like four-legged animals in order to attain peace of mind. Inasmuch as we're sitting on the floor with our legs stretched in front of us and leaning forward with our arms reaching out (not, quadruped-like, getting down on all fours, as we do during the appropriately named Dog Tilt Pose), we must find other paths of meditation for recollecting the body in *Paschimottanasana*. Experiences that occur to many of us in the course of performing *Paschimottanasana* may, I suggest, be used as these paths of meditation:

- Seated on the floor, with our legs stretched out in front of us, we're relatively secure. Although there's a slight chance of tipping over, there's no danger of falling. We're grounded on the floor, on the earth, on Earth under the heavens.
- We bow and stretch out our arms in a gesture of supplication to the divine. In so doing, we express appreciation for having been given life. We give thanks for

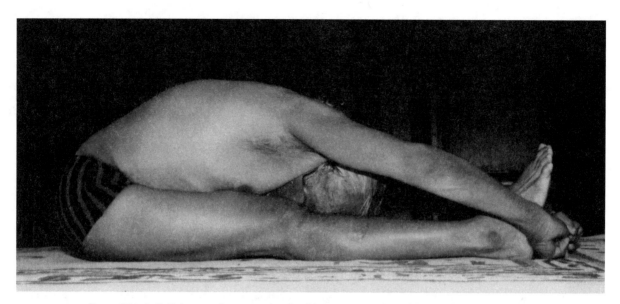

Figure 35.1. B. K. S. Iyengar demonstrating *Paschimottanasana,* Seated Forward Bend, circa 1992

(With the kind permission of B. K. S. Iyengar, Ramamani Iyengar Memorial Yoga Institute)

what spiritual psychotherapist Stuart Sovatsky calls "our finite 'segment' of the eternal."[24]

- Folded in on ourselves, with our internal organs tucked beneath us, we enclose ourselves. We protect ourselves. We're our own shelter. We're at home in our body and in the universe.

- Leaning forward and, like an infant, catching hold of our big toes, we smile with delight. We're complete unto ourselves. We provide for ourselves. We're the divine power, Kundalini, coiled round upon herself, holding her tail in her mouth and lying half asleep at the base of the spine.

- Bent forward with our head on or near our legs, our sight is restricted. At first we have a hint of panic over the loss of (perceived) control over our surroundings. But then our blinkered view of the phenomenal world opens us up to the inner world, where, conscious of our being, we gather our wits and find calm.

- In bending forward and grasping our feet, the current of energy that flows through our electrical (nervous) system, which is ordinarily dispersed in various directions, completes a circuit: the dull and torpid body becomes vital and vibratory, in harmony with the vibration of the universe.

- We're attentive to the most subtle and subversive interference with our spiritual progress: complaining (silently to ourselves!) about our pain (especially in the hamstrings) and exhaustion. When we stop complaining, we find ourselves surrendering to the pain and exhaustion of our body and, in doing so, come to accept the inevitable suffering of our lives entangled in impermanence.

- Insofar as our sense of direction in this pose is based on the posterior of the body turned to the west and the anterior of the body turned to the east, we find ourselves lost. The back faces up, and the chest faces down. But in our disorientation we apprehend that up and down, front and back, the cardinal directions—all orientation in space—is nonsense. We're part of the divine cosmos.

According to Iyengar, immersion in *asana* unsullied by intrusive thoughts results in a feeling of great calm and, sometimes, in comprehensions like these of realities hidden from us during our quotidian lives—in other words, in revelation.

Scholar of the religions and philosophies of India Gerald James Larson likens the insight into reality gained by yogins to a level of aesthetic/sensing awareness attained by people with highly developed knowledge and refined sensibilities: "when a disciplined mathematician, for example, comes upon a new proof and describes it as 'elegant,' or when a disciplined connoisseur hears a great performance of music or sees a great painting and describes the experiences as 'noble' or 'sublime.'"[25] The egalitarian Iyengar, in contrast, believed that the *samadhi* of insight or vision is accessible to ordinary people—those without specialized knowledge or cultured tastes—engaged in common pursuits.

What do I mean when I say "everyone seeks samadhi"? Not just through yoga, the slow, sure, safe, and proven method. People seek samadhi through drugs, alcohol, the danger of extreme sports, the romanticism of music, the beauty of nature, and the passion of sexuality. There are a thousand ways, and they all involve the transcendence of the suffering ego in a blissful fusion with an entity much greater than ourselves. When we shed a tear for the two lovers united at the end of a film, or for a character reformed and redeemed, we are expressing our own longing to flee the confines of self, to unite with the greater, to discover through loss of the known, the endless, gorgeous horizon of the unknown.[26]

In this startlingly insightful and generous passage about the inclusiveness of ways of transcendence—with an emphasis on a popular art, the movies, with its tales of hard-won love and redemption—Iyengar described the path to *samadhi* as a deeply emotional experience.* In making a connection between yoga practice and these other powerful experiences, he grasped that the understanding gained through our yogic spiritual practice shakes and transforms us. As Geoffrey Samuel, scholar of Eastern religions, explains: "The point is not to assert the logical proposition that one is Siva, or that all is Buddha-nature, but to directly experience the truth in which those words refer. The liberating insight is thus not a logical proposition but something intrinsic to a patterning or attunement of the mind-body system as a whole to the wider universe of which it forms an indissoluble part." In other words: "The liberating insight is both understanding and inner transformation."[27]

---

*Iyengar's interest in the arts, high or low, was minimal. And his writing style, tone, and sentiments in *Light on Life* are unlike those of his previous books. So one can't but suspect that the view he expresses here—and much else in this book—was made with critical input by his coauthors John J. Evans and Douglas Abrams. But at the very least Iyengar endorsed this view.

While pointing out that secular paths to transformation may be equally as valid pursuits as yoga, Iyengar recognized that he is only qualified to teach the yogic path: "Some methods of escape are obviously harmful and unsustainable, like drugs or alcohol. Great art, great music, or great works of literature can also begin the work of transformation in the heart of humankind. But I can honestly teach only from what I know. Asana was my school and university, pranayama was where I earned my doctorate, and it is these yoga practices that I have learned for the path to the blissful fusion."[28]

Iyengar's application of Patanjali's eight-step path of liberation to the yogic conditioning postures in the late 20th century (approximately 1,600 years after the *Yoga Sutra,* which sets forth the eight limbs of yoga practice, was composed) is the great yoga philosophy of our times. The dynamic meditation that Iyengar created from his *asana* practice is new, brash, relevant, coherent, wise, and exalted. Not that it can't be placed within a powerful religious and philosophical current that originated in the West in earlier centuries: New Age spirituality.

Influences on Iyengar's Spirituality

The Brahmo Samaj was founded in Calcutta in 1828 to reform Hinduism; its members abandoned the authority of the Vedas, the sacred Hindu texts; rejected Hindu rituals; and discarded Hindu beliefs in avatars, karma, and rebirth. The society formulated a Hinduism that derived, in part, from Harmonial Religion, originated by the Christian mystic Emanuel

Swedenborg in the 18th century and carried on by transcendentalists, such as the nondenominational Ralph Waldo Emerson, and mesmerists in the 19th century. Swedenborg believed that we have an inner connection to the cosmos (the universe or the infinite). Sociologist of religion Robert C. Fuller explains: "Swedenborg's doctrines gave the nineteenth century its most vivid articulation of a form of piety in which 'harmony,' rather than contrition or repentance, is the sine qua non of the regenerated life. . . . The deity—here conceived as an indwelling cosmic force—is approached not via petitionary prayer or acts of worship, but through a series of inner adjustments. . . . The barriers separating the finite personality from the 'divinity which flows through all things' are gradually penetrated."[29]

In *A History of Modern Yoga: Patanjali and Western Esotericism,* yoga scholar Elizabeth De Michelis chronicles the incorporation of Swedenborgianism, transcendentalism, and mesmerism—key components of 19th-century New Age religion—into Brahmo ideology. In 1875 the Brahmo leader Keshubchandra Sen, she relates, "introduced the modern reading of individualistic 'God-realization' as 'direct perception,' a concept that will become pivotal in Vivekananda's understanding of 'realization,'" to Hindu devotees.[30] The young, impressionable Swami Vivekananda, she speculates, was exposed to and adopted this teaching in the early 1880s when he was involved in Brahmo activities. Vivekananda's belief in Self-realization, she further speculates, was refined and reinforced in the early 1890s by "what Vivekananda came in contact with as he settled into the Western cultic lifestyle" (that is, as he was welcomed into the circle of the educated elite who were exploring alternatives to standard Christianity) during his time in America:[31] "In a way, all that Vivekananda was coming in contact with were more advanced elaborations of beliefs that were based on, and thus confirmed, his earlier worldview."[32]

In his first book, *Vedanta Philosophy,* published in 1896, Vivekananda famously proclaimed, "Each soul is potentially divine. The goal [of the spiritual seeker] is to manifest this divinity within."[33] He promoted Patanjali's eight-limbed path as the scientific means of accessing the divine. By redefining yoga as a "'Harmonial' technique detailing the 'inner adjustments' necessary for approaching the indwelling deity, thus attaining 'Self-realization,'" Vivekananda made yoga modern.[34]

Even proponents of hatha yoga as physical culture and health cure (including Iyengar's guru, T. Krishnamacharya) were quick to take up Vivekananda's formulation and use it to promote *asana* practice to the populace as an easily accessible way to attain a state of spirituality. "Adopted and cultivated in conditions of marked privatization and relativization of religion [associated with the decline of institutionalized religion], modern postural yoga [her term for the modern yoga that foregrounds the postural exercises] is successful, like other Harmonial belief systems," De Michelis argues, "because it provides [in Fuller's phrase] 'experiential access to the sacred.'"[35]

The influence of Vivekananda's beliefs on Iyengar's beliefs is evidenced at least as early as 1966 in Iyengar's first book, *Light on Yoga,* where Iyengar states in his explication of the *Yoga Sutra* that the goal of yoga is "to unite the individual soul with the Divine Universal Soul."[36] Iyengar biographer Kofi Busia attributes Iyengar's belief in the union of individual self and Self to the religious tradition into which he was born: "As a follower of Ramanuja's brand of Visisthadvaita . . . , Iyengar believed that the Supreme was expressed in a much more personalized form than was the case with most other schools of Vedanta. His view was therefore that each individual contained an in-dwelling spirit."[37] But no matter what the origin of his belief in this concept, the emphasis that Iyengar placed on accessing the divine through yogic technique reveals the influence of Vivekananda's Neo-Vedantism—an emphasis underscored by the near total absence of Hindu rites, sacred texts, and traditional beliefs in Iyengar's practice. The primary reason why Iyengar "bow[ed] before the noblest of sages Patanjali"[38] was because "he gives methods of concentrating on the universal spirit of God."[39]

In 1988, in *The Tree of Yoga,* Iyengar repeats: "Yoga means union. The union of the individual soul with the Universal Spirit is yoga."[40] What made Iyengar's spiritual practice unique, though, even within the modern form of Hinduism influenced by 19th-century New Age religion, is the high degree to which it assigns the concrete, personal experience of the body (in *asana*) as the vehicle of transcendence—the means of attuning the inner faculty to the cosmos. "You and I have to use finite means—body, [and the three mental faculties of] mind, intelligence and consciousness [which, respectively, gather information on, make discriminating adjustments to, and bring awareness to the body]—to reach the infinite seat of the soul which is the mother of all these things."[41] In this, Iyengar had a close affinity to the quest for a direct sensuous intuition—an unmediated vision—of reality espoused by the 19th-century philosopher Friedrich Wilhelm Joseph Schelling and carried on by 19th-century Romantics, such as William Wordsworth.

Schelling believed, as literary critic Geoffrey Hartman writes, that a transcendental synthesis "grants the possibility of perceiving the essential harmony of man and nature through an intuitive voluntaristic act." In the 1850 version of *The Prelude,* Wordsworth presented a boy's account of swiftly skating at night, then stopping short: "yet still the solitary cliffs / Wheeled by me—even as if the earth had rolled / With visible motion her diurnal round!" Hartman comments about this famous passage: "The mystical suspense is gained after [bodily] exertion, when the will is at rest, and Nature is empowered to take over."[42] This observation, perhaps with "the Universal Spirit" replacing "Nature," could've been made about Iyengar in the repose stage of a conditioning *asana.*

Ritual in Iyengar Yoga

The modern hatha yoga session has evolved into a three-part ritual, a patterned, compressed spiritual journey. In the brief introductory phase, the teacher commonly initiates chanting and breathing exercises. In the long middle phase, the teacher gives instruction in *asana* practice through explanation, example, and adjustment. In the brief final phase, the teacher guides students in relaxation. Insightfully applying the concept of liminality in ritual (first developed by anthropologist Arnold van Gennep in the early 20th century and rediscovered by anthropologist Victor Turner in the mid-20th century) to modern postural yoga in general and to Iyengar yoga in particular, De Michelis describes the chanting at the start of the session as the separation (preliminal) phase; the vigorous conditioning *asanas,* which constitute the yoga practice proper, as the transition (liminal) phase; and *Savasana,* Corpse Pose, the final relaxation, as the incorporation (postliminal) phase. Although Iyengar adapted this tripartite structure to his philosophy, his classroom teaching failed to take full advantage of the rhythm of the ritual.

Phase I

Some of Iyengar's yoga sessions began with chanting an invocation to Patanjali. Like the chanting of "OM," this chanting is a declaration of the sacred nature of the yoga session. But Iyengar could've made explicit in this first phase that the ensuing session was a process of withdrawal from normal modes of being, of casting off the concerns and illusions of the everyday life, in order to make way for spiritual awakenings achieved by embarking upon the eight stages of Patanjali's yoga—"stages of the mental ascetic itinerary," as Eliade describes them, "whose end is final liberation"—in *asana.*[43]

Admittedly, as presented in *The Tree of Yoga,* Iyengar's application of the eight-step path is more theoretical than experiential: it isn't mulled over (yet struggled over), self-reflective, or particularly lived in. (That's not to say that Iyengar wasn't engaged in a long spiritual journey. He explored the spiritual dimensions of yoga through deeply inhabiting *asanas* for decades.) So it's no wonder that he didn't introduce his class—perhaps with a short reading, personal anecdote, or philosophical reflection—by plainly defining it as quiet, receptive, inward-turning work, in general, or the eight-step path, in particular.

Phase II

During the second phase, Iyengar ground down his students. He attempted to destroy their previously taken-for-granted identities (which means to say, their modes of being) as members of society: "As I shout at them to straighten their legs in *Sirsasana* (headstand), they cannot be wondering what is for dinner or whether they will be promoted or demoted at work. For those who habitually flee the present, one hour's experience of 'now' can be daunting, even exhausting."[44]

While providing practical instructions for performing *asanas,* Iyengar also guided students to open up to Being. By these means, the disorientation of this phase became a passage from one's commonly experienced secular identity to one's rarely experienced sacred identity—to one's divine nature. However, Iyengar applied his classroom sayings—which, like prayers, incantations, and hymns, invite devotees to appropriate a mode of being that transcends the human condition—spottily and haphazardly. He could've made them the vital part of a sustained spiritual teaching during this middle phase. Each *asana* (or a series of *asanas*) would've still inspired a separate meditation, for the object of the meditation changes with each configuration; nevertheless, the session would've unfolded to students as a series of revelations, gradually deepening their feeling of reverence. In this way, practicing conditioning *asanas* would've truly become a kind of worship.

Phase III

De Michelis interprets *Savasana* in Iyengar yoga "as an exercise in sense withdrawal and mental quietening, and thus as a first step towards meditative practice" and, through its symbolic death and resurrection, as "the key step in a secular . . . ritual of initiation into our [quoting Bob and Linda Boudreau Smith in *Yoga for a New Age*] 'heritage . . . of cosmic consciousness.'"[45] In Iyengar's radical reinterpretation of modern hatha yoga, though, it's the numerous arduous conditioning *asanas,* which demand great effort and release, not *Savasana,* that are the primary gateway to transformation.

To be sure, *Savasana* is not mere relaxation in Iyengar's scheme. Like all the conditioning *asanas* in Iyengar yoga, each in its own way, *Savasana* begins with the practitioner at the threshold between the quotidian structuring of time, space, and groundedness and ends with an expanded sense of time, space, and groundedness; it connects the self to the Self. What sets *Savasana* apart is its particular configuration and lack of great effort and release: the entire body lies supine on the ground and is totally passive from beginning to end, making it particularly conducive to the surrender and thankfulness apposite to the conclusion of a demanding session. As Iyengar explains in *Light on Pranayama,* in *Savasana* the practitioner should "surrender . . . his all—his breath, life and soul—to his Creator."[46] "His being then gets merged in the Infinite (Paramatma)."[47]

This phase is also defined as a period of

consolidation of what has been undergone—an imprinting of the previous experience—followed by a transition back to the everyday world with its necessary concerns and commitments. Iyengar could've made clearer to his students that they're now prepared to reemerge into the profane world with their life regenerated by contact with the sacred.

Iyengar's Legacy

No matter that Iyengar's philosophy and practice fall short of perfection. In the explication of his philosophy and practice in his writings and his transmittal of knowledge in the classroom, Iyengar gave us ample guidance to attune our body within each pose of our yoga practice to the openness of Being.

Of course, some students remained indifferent to Iyengar's application of spirituality to hatha yoga. They used their practice to cultivate beauty (a slim physique and youthful looks); to obtain fitness (flexibility and grace); to alleviate the pain and hardship of injury and illness; or to achieve a sense of emotional healing (sometimes experienced as euphoria or calm or a mixture of euphoria and calm that ensues from being totally absorbed in strenuous exercise). And others, seeking spiritual meaning in their hatha yoga practice, found his preoccupation with perfection in *asana* so misguided (it set them to becoming preoccupied with struggling to overcome a sluggish body) and his tactics—his insults and rebukes, not to mention his bangs, kicks, and slaps—so offensive that any consideration of his spiritual teachings was precluded.

But for those who were receptive, Iyengar's spiritual teachings changed their lives. Yoga teacher Joan White, who first took classes with Iyengar in 1973, recalled in 2013: "I had never met a teacher with such passion and dedication and [even though his English wasn't yet up to snuff] such a creative way of communicating with his students. . . . I found (and do find) that his sayings made (and continue to make) a huge difference in my life. He introduced me to new ways of thinking about things, both on the physical and on the spiritual plane."[48]

These days, aspects of Hinduism (images of deities, sacred music, readings of doctrine, prayers, chanting, or rituals) are commonly grafted onto postural yoga classes so students can pretend (to themselves!) that in practicing *asana* they're partaking of a spiritual act, not merely exercising to get in shape. Absent all trappings of religion, the Iyengar yoga class is a path to spiritual exaltation that is based solely in the bodily experience of dwelling within the *asanas*.

In forging his conditioning *asana* practice into a vehicle for an embodied spirituality, Iyengar erased the distinction between the physical and the spiritual in yoga. "[*Asanas*] should be performed in such a way as to lead the mind from attachment to the body towards the light of the soul," he said, "so that the practitioner may dwell [in the body as a means of dwelling] in the abode of the soul."[49] In Iyengar's formulation, in which "the practitioner is the subject and the asana is the object . . . , the instrument (body) and the asana become one."[50] The body, spiritually illuminated in *asana*, becomes radiant (fig. 35.2).

Figure 35.2. (opposite). Illustration of the identification and unification of the macrocosm in the body of a yogin
(From *Yoga Art*, by Ajit Mookerjee)

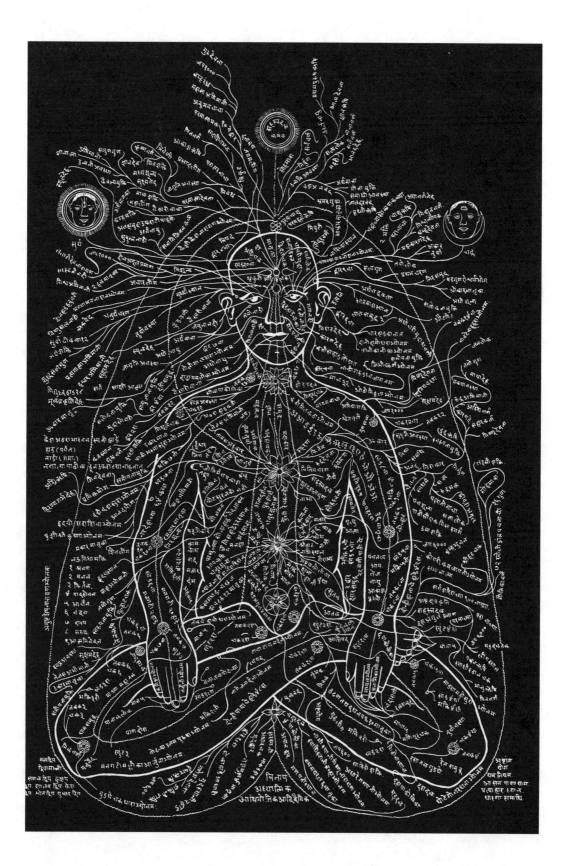

Notes

Chapter 1. Shri Yogendra:
Rejecting the Role of Yoga Guru

1. Santan Rodrigues, *Householder Yogi,* 15.
2. Ibid., 27.
3. *Mundaka Upanishad,* in Swami Prabhavananda and Frederick Manchester, *Upanishads,* 44.
4. Prabhavananda and Manchester, *Upanishads,* xi.
5. Rodrigues, *Householder Yogi,* 27.
6. Shri Yogendra, "Paramahamsa ni Prasadi," unpublished account, 1916, in Rodrigues, *Householder Yogi,* 33.
7. Ibid.
8. Rodrigues, *Householder Yogi,* 27.
9. Ibid., 19.
10. Ibid., 33.
11. Ibid., 34.
12. Ibid.
13. Ibid., 37.
14. Paramahamsa Madhavadasaji to Yogendra, Sept. 3, 1916, in Rodrigues, *Householder Yogi,* 38–39.
15. Madhavadasaji to Yogendra, Sept. 4, 1916, in Rodrigues, *Householder Yogi,* 40–41.
16. Madhavadasaji to Yogendra, Sept. 5, 1916, in Rodrigues, *Householder Yogi,* 41–42.
17. Rodrigues, *Householder Yogi,* 40.
18. Ibid., 41.
19. Madhavadasaji to Yogendra, Sept. 4, 1916, in Rodrigues, *Householder Yogi,* 40.
20. Rodrigues, *Householder Yogi,* 40–41.
21. Sudhir Kakar, *Inner World,* 127.
22. Ibid., 128.

23. S. Yogendra, "Yoga Institutes," 10.
24. Kakar, *Inner World,* 139.
25. Eastern and Western Disciples, *Life of the Swami Vivekananda,* 255.
26. Ibid., 290.
27. Paramhansa Yogananda, *Autobiography,* 89–91.
28. Rodrigues, *Householder Yogi,* 44.
29. Ibid., 45.
30. Ibid., 46.
31. Ibid., 48.
32. Ibid., 46.
33. S. Yogendra, "Yoga Institutes," 10.
34. Ibid., 11.
35. Ibid., 10.
36. Yogendra to Madhavadasaji, Feb. 12, 1920, in Rodrigues, *Householder Yogi,* 110.
37. Yogendra to Popat, Dec. 20, 1920, in Rodrigues, *Householder Yogi,* 111.
38. Rodrigues, *Householder Yogi,* 198.
39. Yogendra to Dayaram, May 31, 1929, in Rodrigues, *Householder Yogi,* 198.
40. Yogendra, *Prabhubhakti,* in Rodrigues, *Householder Yogi,* 52.
41. Ibid., 53.
42. Ibid., 52.
43. Swami Vivekananda, *Vedanta Philosophy,* 16.
44. Yogendra to Madhavadasaji, Dec. 8, 1920, in Rodrigues, *Householder Yogi,* 113.
45. Ibid., 112.
46. Yogendra to Popat, March 10, 1922, in Rodrigues, *Householder Yogi,* 184.
47. Ibid., 184–85.

Chapter 2. Shri Yogendra: Creating the Profession of Yoga Teacher

1. B. B. Misra, *Indian Middle Classes,* 307.
2. Rodrigues, *Householder Yogi,* 72.
3. Ibid.
4. S. Yogendra, *Yoga Asanas Simplified,* 20.
5. Ibid., 18.
6. Rodrigues, *Householder Yogi,* 218.
7. S. Yogendra, *Yoga Asanas Simplified,* 26.
8. Ibid., 48.
9. Yogendra to Dayaram, May 31, 1929, in Rodrigues, *Householder Yogi,* 198.
10. S. Yogendra, *Yoga Asanas Simplified,* 44.
11. Ibid., 58.
12. David Gordon White, *Sinister Yogis,* 212.
13. S. Yogendra, "Yoga: Its Antiquity," 2.
14. Ibid.
15. S. Yogendra, "Yoga Physical Culture," 7.
16. S. Yogendra, *Yoga Asanas Simplified,* 52.
17. Ibid., 44–45.
18. Elizabeth De Michelis, *History of Modern Yoga,* 248.
19. George L. Mosse, *Image of Man,* 47.
20. S. Yogendra, *Yoga Asanas Simplified,* 71.
21. Ibid., 47.
22. Ibid., 46.
23. Ibid., 81.
24. Ibid., 55.
25. Ibid., 133.
26. S. Yogendra, *Yoga Hygiene Simplified,* 122 n.
27. S. Yogendra, *Yoga Asanas Simplified,* 29–30.
28. Ibid., 31–32.
29. Ibid., 28.
30. Ibid., 18.
31. Ibid., 27–28.
32. Ibid., 29.
33. Ibid., 28.
34. Geoffrey Samuel, *Origins of Yoga,* 8–9, 177; and Karen Armstrong, *Buddha,* 24.
35. *Shiva Samhita,* quoted in Ernest S. Wood, *Yoga Dictionary,* 66.
36. Rodrigues, *Householder Yogi,* 73.
37. S. Yogendra, *Yoga Asanas Simplified,* 79.
38. Ibid., 84 and 85.
39. Karl Marx, *Theories of Surplus Value,* 166.
40. David L. Chapman, *Sandow the Magnificent,* 3.
41. Ibid., 101.
42. Rodrigues, *Householder Yogi,* 19.
43. S. Yogendra, *Yoga Asanas Simplified,* 82.

Chapter 3. Shri Yogendra: Making Yoga into Calisthenics

1. Johann Christoph Friedrich Guts Muths, *Gymnastics for Youth,* 190.
2. Friedrich Ludwig Jahn, *German Nationality,* quoted in Ellen W. Gerber, *Physical Education,* 128.
3. Thomas Wentworth Higginson, "Saints, and Their Bodies," 23.
4. Ibid., 19–20.
5. Per Henrik Ling, *General Principles of Gymnastics,* quoted in Geo. H. Taylor, *Exposition of the Swedish Movement-Cure,* 53.
6. Edward Mussey Hartwell, "On Physical Training," 743–44.
7. Gerber, *Physical Education,* 160.
8. Ibid., 161.
9. J. P. Müller, *My System,* 11.
10. Sarah Wildman, "Kafka's Calisthenics," para. 4.
11. Müller, *My System,* 22.
12. Ibid., 9.
13. Ibid., 7.
14. Ibid., 38.
15. Ibid., 25–26.
16. S. Yogendra, *Yoga Asanas Simplified,* 81.
17. Ibid., 124.
18. Ibid.
19. Ibid., 127.
20. Ibid., 125.
21. Rodrigues, *Householder Yogi,* 204.
22. Müller, *My System,* 22.
23. S. Yogendra, *Yoga Asanas Simplified,* 154–55
24. Ibid., 58.
25. Ibid., 60.
26. Ibid., 145.
27. Ibid., 150.
28. Ibid., 129.
29. Ibid., 60.
30. Ibid., 139.
31. Gudrun Bühnemann, *Eighty-four Asanas,* 27.
32. Müller, *My System,* 76.
33. S. Yogendra, *Yoga Asanas Simplified,* 133–34.
34. Ibid., 135.
35. Ibid., 91.
36. Bühnemann, *Eighty-four Asanas,* 28.
37. S. Yogendra, *Yoga Asanas Simplified,* 91.
38. Müller, *My System,* 47.
39. Ibid., 71.
40. S. Yogendra, *Yoga Asanas Simplified,* 96.
41. Rodrigues, *Householder Yogi,* 204–5.
42. S. Yogendra, *Yoga Asanas Simplified,* 151.
43. Müller, *My System,* 86.
44. Ibid., 16.
45. S. Yogendra, *Yoga Asanas Simplified,* 117.
46. Ibid., 115.
47. Ibid., 146.
48. Higginson, "Gymnastics," 144–45.
49. Ibid., 171.
50. Ibid., 172.
51. Jan Todd, *Physical Culture,* 81.
52. Dio Lewis, *New Gymnastics,* 5.
53. Ibid., 62 (sentences reordered).
54. Ibid., 62–63.
55. Ibid., 102–15.
56. Ibid., 112.
57. Ibid., 14.
58. Higginson, "Gymnastics," 145.
59. S. Yogendra, *Yoga Asanas Simplified,* 18.

Chapter 4. Shri Yogendra: Taking Practical Yoga to the New World

1. Rodrigues, *Householder Yogi,* 74.
2. Morarji Jeram Trikamji to Yogendra, March 3, 1919, in Rodrigues, *Householder Yogi,* 76.
3. Henry Lindlahr, *Philosophy of Natural Therapeutics,* 18.
4. Ibid.
5. S. Yogendra, *Yoga Hygiene Simplified,* 63.
6. Lindlahr, *Philosophy of Natural Therapeutics,* 19.
7. Ibid., 322.
8. Joseph S. Alter, *Gandhi's Body,* 53.
9. S. Yogendra, *Yoga Hygiene Simplified,* 87.
10. Ibid., 102.
11. Ibid.
12. Ibid., cover.

13. Rodrigues, *Householder Yogi,* 75.

14. S. Yogendra, *Yoga Hygiene Simplified,* 10.

15. Rodrigues, *Householder Yogi,* 79.

16. Ibid.

17. Vivekananda, "Miracles," interview with a *Memphis Commercial* reporter, Jan. 15, 1894, in *Complete Works of Swami Vivekananda,* 5:183.

18. Ibid., 183–84.

19. Vivekananda, "Concentration," lecture delivered at Washington Hall, San Francisco, March 16, 1900, in *Complete Works of Swami Vivekananda,* 4:225.

20. Vivekananda, *Vedanta Philosophy,* 18.

21. Ibid., 19.

22. Ibid., 18.

23. Vivekananda, "Science of Yoga," lecture delivered at Tucker Hall, Alameda, California, April 13, 1900, in *Complete Works of Swami Vivekananda,* 7:437.

24. Mark Singleton, *Yoga Body,* 71.

25. Vivekananda to Mary Hale, Feb. 1, 1895, in Vivekananda, *Complete Works of Swami Vivekananda,* 5:73.

26. Vivekananda to Sara Bull, Feb. 14, 1895, in Vivekananda, *Complete Works of Swami Vivekananda,* 6:300.

27. Josephine MacLeod, quoted in Mary Louise Burke, *World Teacher,* 25.

28. Sara Ellen Waldo, in Sister Devamata, *Reminiscences of Swami Vivekananda* 2nd ed., (Mayavati: Advaita Ashrama, 1964), 115, quoted in Swami Tathagatananda, "Glimpses of Swamiji's Life," 476.

29. Laura Glenn, in S. N. Dhar, *A Comprehensive Biography of Swami Vivekananda,* vol. 1 (Madras: Vivekananda Prakashan Kendra, 1975), 709, quoted in Tathagatananda, "Glimpses of Swamiji's Life," 477.

30. Burke, *World Teacher,* 39–40.

31. Vivekananda, *Vedanta Philosophy,* 17.

32. Ibid., 18.

33. Ibid., 19.

34. Ibid.

35. Ibid.

36. Ibid., 17.

37. *New York Herald,* "Balm of the Orient."

38. Ibid.

39. Ibid.

40. Swami Kripananda, "Just What Yoga Is."

41. *New York Herald,* "Balm of the Orient."

42. Leon Landsberg to Sara Bull, April 16, 1895, in Burke, *New Gospel,* 148–49.

43. Ibid., 149.

44. Burke, *New Gospel,* 151.

45. Ibid., 149.

46. Swami Abhedananda, *How to Be a Yogi,* 54.

47. Ibid., 54–56.

48. Stefanie Syman, *Subtle Body,* 69.

49. Abhedananda, *How to Be a Yogi,* 53–54.

50. Ibid., 61–62.

51. Ibid., 50.

52. Ibid.

53. Vivekananda to Pramadadas Mitra, Feb. 7, 1890, in Vivekananda, *Complete Works of Swami Vivekananda,* 6:221.

54. Vivekananda to Balaram Bose, Jan. 30, 1890, in Vivekananda, *Complete Works of Swami Vivekananda,* 7:444.

55. Vivekananda, conversation with a disciple, 1902, in *Complete Works of Swami Vivekananda,* 7:242.

56. Ibid., 243.

57. Vivekananda to Akhandananda, March 1890, in Vivekananda, *Complete Works of Swami Vivekananda,* 6:233.

58. Vivekananda to Pramadadas Mitra, Feb. 7, 1890, in Vivekananda, *Complete Works of Swami Vivekananda,* 6:221.

59. Ibid., 222.

60. Vivekananda to Pramadadas Mitra, March 3, 1890, in Vivekananda, *Complete Works of Swami Vivekananda,* 6:230.

61. Vivekananda, *Vedanta Philosophy,* 19–20.

62. Vivekananda, conversation with a disciple, 1902, in *Complete Works of Swami Vivekananda,* 7:242.

63. Vivekananda, *Vedanta Philosophy,* 19.

64. Vivekananda, conversation with a disciple, March 16, 1900, in *Complete Works of Swami Vivekananda,* 4:225.

65. Vivekananda, conversation with a disciple, 1901, in *Complete Works of Swami Vivekananda,* 7:206.

66. Vivekananda, "Concentration," in *Complete Works of Swami Vivekananda,* 4:225.

67. Vivekananda, conversation with a disciple, 1901, in *Complete Works of Swami Vivekananda,* 7:206.

68. De Michelis, *History of Modern Yoga,* 181–82.

69. Vivekananda, *Vedanta Philosophy,* 17.

70. Ibid., 19.

71. Ann Louise Bardach, "How Yoga Won the West."

72. S. Yogendra, *Yoga Asanas Simplified,* 24.

73. Vincent Anderson, "India—The Land of Miracles," in *World Magazine,* Sept. 11, 1921, quoted in Rodrigues, *Householder Yogi,* 97.

74. Rodrigues, *Householder Yogi,* 98.

75. Ibid., 105.

76. Yogendra to Popat, Feb. 26, 1920, in Rodrigues, *Householder Yogi,* 90.

77. Yogendra to Popat, circa. Feb. 1920, in Rodrigues, *Householder Yogi,* 91.

78. Rodrigues, *Householder Yogi,* 175.

79. Ibid., 126.

80. Ibid., 175.

81. Ibid., 126.

82. Anand, "Genesis of Modern Yoga," *Journal of the Yoga Institute,* Feb. 1967, quoted in Rodrigues, *Householder Yogi,* 131.

83. Rodrigues, *Householder Yogi,* 153.

84. Ibid., 157.

85. Ibid., 155.

86. Ibid., 158.

87. Ibid., 173–74.

88. Ibid., 174.

89. Ibid., 176.

90. Ibid., 188.

Chapter 5. Shri Yogendra: Making Yoga Gentle

1. Leela Fernandes, *India's New Middle Class,* 12.

2. S. Yogendra, *Hatha Yoga Simplified,* 124.

3. Ibid.

4. Laura Williams Iverson, "Conscious Home Exercise," 43.

5. S. Yogendra, *Yoga Asanas Simplified,* 156.

6. Ibid., 155–56.

7. Genevieve Stebbins, *Dynamic Breathing,* quoted in S. Yogendra, *Yoga Asanas Simplified,* 156.

8. Stebbins, *Dynamic Breathing,* 91.

9. S. Yogendra, *Hatha Yoga Simplified,* 127.

10. S. Yogendra, *Yoga Asanas Simplified,* 158–59.

11. S. Yogendra, *Hatha Yoga Simplified,* 127.

12. Stebbins, *Dynamic Breathing,* 79.

13. Swami Svatmarama, *Hatha Yoga Pradipika,* chapter 1, verse 34.

14. Stebbins, *Dynamic Breathing,* 91.

15. S. Yogendra, *Hatha Yoga Simplified,* 113.

16. S. Yogendra, *Yoga Asanas Simplified,* 128.

17. Ibid., 128–29.

18. Ibid., 128.

19. Ibid., 158.

20. S. Yogendra, *Hatha Yoga Simplified,* 125.

21. S. Yogendra, *Yoga Asanas Simplified,* 99.

22. Ibid., 104.

23. Ibid., 105.

24. Ibid., 104

25. Ibid., 101.

26. Ibid., 105.

27. M. K. Gandhi, "Anasakti Yoga," in *Selected Writings of Gandhi,* ed. Ronald Duncan, 37.

28. S. Yogendra, *Yoga Asanas Simplified,* 102.

29. Ibid., 103.

30. Ibid., 81.

31. Ibid., 44.

32. Rodrigues, *Householder Yogi,* 21.

33. Yogendra to Madhavadasaji, Dec. 8, 1920, in Rodrigues, *Householder Yogi,* 112.

34. Ibid., 113.

35. Ralph Waldo Emerson, "Nature," in *Works of Emerson,* 2:415.

36. *Sadhakas* of the Yoga Institute, *Celebration,* 24.

37. Jayadeva Yogendra, dictation to Armaiti N. Desai, as noted in Desai's e-mail to the author, Sept. 9, 2013.

38. J. Yogendra, *Yoga Cyclopaedia*, vol. 3, 3 (unnumbered).

39. *Sadhakas* of the Yoga Institute, "Man and Mind," 14.

40. Desai, e-mail to the author, May 23, 2013.

Chapter 6. Swami Kuvalayananda: Claiming Yoga Is Science

1. Swami Sivananda, *Yogic Home Exercises,* 12–13 (sentences rearranged).

2. Eugen Sandow, *Strength,* 15.

3. Müller, *My System,* 12.

4. Ibid., 20.

5. Bhavanarao Pant Pratinidhi, *Surya Namaskars,* i.

6. K. V. Iyer, *Muscle Cult,* 42.

7. S. Yogendra, *Yoga Asanas Simplified,* 60.

8. Ibid., 61.

9. Ibid., 52.

10. Vivekananda, *Vedanta Philosophy,* 5.

11. Ibid., 6.

12. De Michelis, *History of Modern Yoga,* 176.

13. Abhedananda, *How to Be a Yogi,* 43.

14. Ibid., 45.

15. E. H. Starling, "Croonian Lectures," 339.

16. Sheila M. Rothman and David J. Rothman, *Pursuit of Perfection,* 19.

17. S. Sundaram, *Yogic Physical Culture,* 7.

18. Ibid., 9.

19. Ibid., 16.

20. Manohar L. Gharote and Manmath M. Gharote, *Swami Kuvalayananda,* 11.

21. Swami Kuvalayananda, "Recollections of Kuvalayananda," July 29, 1956, in K. B. Mahabal, *Guruvarya Prof. Manikrao Yanche Charitra* (Nasik: K. B. Mahabal, 1957), 112, quoted in Gharote and Gharote, *Swami Kuvalayananda,* 20.

22. Kuvalayananda, "Recollections of Kuvalayananda," in R. K. Bodhe and G. Ramakrishna, *Yogi and Scientist,* 46.

23. Ibid.

24. Kuvalayananda, "Rationale of Yogic Poses" (July 1926), 212 (editorial "we" in original quotation).

25. Kuvalayananda, "Recollections of Kuvalayananda," in Bodhe and Ramakrishna, *Yogi and Scientist,* 46.

26. Gharote and Gharote, *Swami Kuvalayananda,* 14.

27. Kuvalayananda, "Recollections of Kuvalayananda," in Mahabal, *Prof. Manikrao,* quoted in Gharote and Gharote, *Swami Kuvalayananda,* 23.

28. Gharote and Gharote, *Swami Kuvalayananda,* 23.

29. Kuvalayananda, "Recollections of Kuvalayananda," in Bodhe and Ramakrishna, *Yogi and Scientist,* 23.

30. Gharote and Gharote, *Swami Kuvalayananda,* 23.

31. Kuvalayananda, "Towards Foundation and After," 312.

32. Ibid., 312–13.

33. Ibid., 313.

34. Kuvalayananda, "Training Facilities at the Kaivalyadhama," 75.

35. Kuvalayananda, "Kaivalyadhama" (Oct. 1925), 311.

36. Kuvalayananda, "Towards Foundation and After," 314.

37. Svatmarama, *Hatha Yoga Pradipika,* chapter 1, verse 1.

38. William J. Broad, *Science of Yoga,* 25.

39. Kuvalayananda, "Note on Ductless Glands," 132.

40. Ibid., 135.

41. Ibid.

42. Kuvalayananda, "Mechano-Yogic Therapy," 248.

Chapter 7. Swami Kuvalayananda: Promoting Yoga as Health Cure

1. Svatmarama, *Hatha Yoga Pradipika,* chapter 11, verse 29.

2. Ibid., 1:31.

3. Ibid., 1:33.

4. Ibid., 1:46.

5. Alter, *Gandhi's Body,* 57.

6. Bernarr Macfadden, *Building of Vital Power,* 263.

7. Macfadden, *Keeping Fit,* 18.

8. Macfadden, *Encyclopedia of Physical Culture,* 1236.

9. Macfadden, *Building of Vital Power,* 4.

10. Macfadden, *Keeping Fit,* 18.

11. Macfadden, *Building of Vital Power,* 45.

12. Macfadden, *Macfadden's Physical Training.*

13. Robert Ernst, *Weakness Is a Crime,* 12.

14. Macfadden, *Building of Vital Power,* 232.

15. Ibid., 78.

16. Kuvalayananda, *Asanas,* 72.

17. *The Maharashtra,* Oct. 22, 1924, in Kuvalayananda, "A Few Press Notices" (Feb. 1925), 155 (sentences reordered).

18. *The Kesari,* Oct. 21, 1924, in Kuvalayananda, "A Few Press Notices" (Feb. 1925), 155.

19. *Tatvajnana Mandira,* Jan. 1925, in Kuvalayananda, "A Few Personal Appreciations," 235.

20. *Nava-Sangha,* Dec. 21, 1924, in Kuvalayananda, "A Few Press Notices" (Feb. 1925), 153.

21. *Prabuddha Bharata,* Oct. 1925, in Kuvalayananda, "A Few Press Notices" (Oct. 1925), 302–3.

22. Svatmarama, *Hatha Yoga Pradipika,* chapter 1, verse 19.

23. Ibid., chapter 4, verse 7.

24. Kuvalayananda, "Kaivalyadhama: A Review," inside back cover.

25. Kuvalayananda, "Rugna-Seva-Mandira," 75.

26. Kuvalayananda, "Kaivalyadhama: A Review," 80.

27. Kuvalayananda, prescription for M. K. Gandhi, May 5, 1927, in Kuvalayananda, *Vision and Wisdom,* 32–33.

28. M. K. Gandhi to Kuvalayananda, April 17, 1927, in Kuvalayananda, *Vision and Wisdom,* 31.

29. Kuvalayananda to M. K. Gandhi, June 4, 1927, in Bodhe and Ramakrishna, *Yogi and Scientist,* 169.

30. Kuvalayananda to M. K. Gandhi, June 8, 1927, in Bodhe and Ramakrishna, *Yogi and Scientist,* 169–70.

31. Kuvalayananda to M. K. Gandhi, June 22, 1927, in Kuvalayananda, *Vision and Wisdom,* 37.

32. M. K. Gandhi to Kuvalayananda, June 17, 1927, in Kuvalayananda, *Vision and Wisdom,* 35.

33. Kuvalayananda to M. K. Gandhi, July 4, 1927, in Kuvalayananda, *Vision and Wisdom,* 40–41.

34. Ibid., 41.

35. Ibid.

36. Ibid.

37. Ibid., 40.

Chapter 8. Swami Kuvalayananda: Investigating the Yogic Phenomena

1. Kuvalayananda, "Sarvangasana Part I," 59–60.

2. Ibid., 64.

3. Ibid., 63.

4. Sundaram, *Yogic Physical Culture,* 19–20.

5. Macfadden, *Exercising for Health,* 28.

6. Sundaram, *Yogic Physical Culture,* 19–20.

7. B. K. S. Iyengar, *Light on Yoga,* 212–13.

8. Ibid., 213.

9. Gary Kraftsow, *Yoga for Wellness,* 259.

10. Kuvalayananda, "Sarvangasana Part I," 68.

11. Ibid., 69.

12. Ibid., 70.

13. Ibid., 73.

14. Kuvalayananda, "Sarvangasana Part II," 219.

15. Ibid., 220.

16. Kuvalayananda, "Sarvangasana Part II (cont.)," 296–97.

17. Kuvalayananda, "Sarvangasana Part III," 65.

18. Ibid., 67.

19. Ibid., 65.

20. Ibid., 66.

21. Ibid.

22. Ibid., 65–66.

23. Ibid., 66.

24. Ibid., 71.

25. Ibid.

26. Ibid., 72.

27. Ibid., 67.

28. Kuvalayananda, "Sarvangasana Part I," 74.

29. Mel Robin, *Physiological Handbook,* 400–401.

30. Broad, *Science of Yoga,* 40.

31. Kim E. Innes, Cheryl Bourguignon, and Ann Gill Taylor, "Risk Indices," 491.

Chapter 9. Swami Kuvalayananda: Standing Up Straight

1. Peter Gaskell, *Manufacturing Population,* 162.

2. Christian Wilhelm Braune and Otto Fischer, "Center of Gravity of the Human Body," 17.

3. Ibid., 15.

4. Christian Wilhelm Braune, *Atlas of Topographical Anatomy,* 1.

5. Braune and Fischer, "Center of Gravity of the Human Body," 17.

6. Ibid., 81.

7. Ibid., 74.

8. Kuvalayananda, "Some Practices for Increasing Stature," 143.

9. Ibid., 146.

10. Ibid., 147.

11. Ibid., 148.

12. Ibid., 147.

13. Ibid., 148.

14. Ibid., 149.

15. Ibid., 148.

16. G. Stanley Hall, *Adolescence,* quoted in Kuvalayananda, "Some Practices for Increasing Stature," 149.

17. Ibid.

18. Ibid.

19. Ibid.

20. Hall, *Adolescence,* 192.

21. Kuvalayananda, "Some Practices for Increasing Stature," 146.

22. Ibid., 147.

23. Ibid., 146.

24. Kuvalayananda, *Asanas,* 139.

25. Iyer, *Physical Training,* lesson 3, 6.

26. Ibid., 9.

27. Ibid., 2–3.

28. Ibid., lesson 5, 11.

29. Ibid., lesson 3, 5.

30. Ibid., 17.

31. Ibid., 18.

32. Ibid., 18–19.

33. Ibid., 4.

34. Gene A. Logan and Wayne C. McKinney, *Anatomic Kinesiology,* 269.

35. Hall, *Adolescence,* 193.

36. Hall, *Adolescence,* quoted in Kuvalayananda, "Some Practices for Increasing Stature," 149.

37. Kuvalayananda, "Some Practices for Increasing Stature," 147.

38. Mircea Eliade, *Yoga,* 55.

Chapter 10. Swami Kuvalayananda: Youthifying the Spine

1. Herman Melville, "Bartleby, the Scrivener," 39.

2. Ibid., 39–40.

3. Wharton Hood, "On the So-Called 'Bone-Setting,'" 336.

4. A. T. Still, *Autobiography,* 325.

5. Ibid., 111–12.

6. D. D. Palmer, *Chiropractor,* 5.

7. Ibid.

8. Ibid., 51.

9. D. D. Palmer and B. J. Palmer, *Science of Chiropractic,* 23.

10. Ibid., 30.

11. Ibid., 23.

12. Ibid., 58.

13. Ibid., 59.

14. Sundaram, *Yogic Physical Culture,* 39.

15. Ibid., 39–40.

16. Kuvalayananda, "Rationale of Yogic Poses" (Oct. 1926), 261.

17. Kuvalayananda, *Asanas,* 160.

18. Kuvalayananda, "Rationale of Yogic Poses" (Oct. 1926), 258 (sentences reordered).

19. Ibid., 258–59.

20. Ibid., 259.

21. Kuvalayananda, *Asanas,* 159.

22. Kuvalayananda, "Rationale of Yogic Poses" (Oct. 1926), 264.

23. Ibid., 265.

24. Iyer, *Physical Training,* lesson 3, 12.

25. Ibid., 13.

26. Ibid.

27. Kuvalayananda, *Asanas,* 82.

28. Iyer, *Physical Training,* lesson 3, 13.

29. Ibid.

30. André Van Lysebeth, *Yoga Self-Taught,* 78.

31. Ibid., 80.

32. Kuvalayananda, *Asanas,* 138–39.

33. Ibid., 139.

34. Kuvalayananda, "Matsyasana," 58.

35. Sundaram, *Yogic Physical Culture,* 25.

36. Ibid.

37. Van Lysebeth, *Yoga Self-Taught,* 78.

38. Kuvalayananda, "Towards Foundation and After," 316.

39. Indra Devi, *Forever Young,* 17.

40. De Michelis, *History of Modern Yoga,* 211.

41. Vanda Scaravelli, *Awakening the Spine,* 10.

42. Kuvalayananda, "Kaivalyadhama: A Review," 86.

43. Kuvalayananda to M. L. Gharote, Dec. 6, 1965, in Kuvalayananda, *Blended to Perfection,* 85.

44. Kuvalayananda to M. L. Gharote, Dec. 13, 1965, in Kuvalayananda, *Blended to Perfection,* 87.

45. Gharote and Gharote, *Swami Kuvalayananda,* caption to illustration facing 144.

46. Arthur Koestler, *Lotus and Robot,* 102.

47. Manmath Gharote, e-mail to the author, Feb. 16, 2012.

Chapter 11. K. V. Iyer:
Mixing Bodybuilding and Yoga

1. Iyer, "Beauties," 160.

2. Iyer, *Perfect Physique,* 4.

3. Iyer, "Beauties," 160.

4. Mark H. Berry, "If You Had a Bar Bell—,"34.

5. Ibid., 82.

6. Iyer, "Beauties," 163.

7. Ibid., 164.

8. Ibid., 159.

9. Alter, *Wrestler's Body,* 97.

10. Iyer, "Beauties," 160.

11. Ibid., 161.

12. Ibid., 164.

13. Iyer, *Physical Training,* lesson 4, 2.

14. Ibid., lesson 4, 1.

15. Ibid., lesson 4, 4.

16. Iyer, *Muscle Cult,* 41.

17. Ibid., 42.

18. Ibid., 43.

19. Iyer, "Beauties," 164.

20. Iyer, *Chemical Changes in Physical Exercise,* iii.

21. Ibid., 3.

22. Ibid., 39.

23. Ibid., 58.

24. Ibid., 65.

25. Tamar Garb, *Bodies of Modernity,* 55.

26. Iyer, *Perfect Physique,* 42.

27. Iyer, *Muscle Cult,* 39.

28. Jack La Lanne, *For Men Only,* 14.

29. Ibid., 13.

30. Ibid., 15.

31. Iyer, *Muscle Cult,* 44.

32. Berry, "If You Had a Bar Bell—," 82.

33. Kuvalayananda, *Asanas,* 139.

34. Sundaram, *Yogic Physical Culture,* 109.

Chapter 12. S. Sundaram:
Publishing a Yoga Manual

1. Sundaram, *Yogic Physical Culture,* i.

2. Suddhananda Bharatiar, "Diamond Jubilee," 6.

3. Members of the Committee, "Biographical Sketch," 13.

4. Ibid., 18.

5. Ibid.

6. Ibid. (sentences reversed).

7. Ibid., 19.

8. Ibid., 20.

9. Ibid., 21.

10. Bharatiar, "Diamond Jubilee," 5–6.

11. Members of the Committee, "Biographical Sketch," 21.

12. Sundaram, *Yogic Physical Culture,* preface, i.

13. Ibid., i–ii.

14. Singleton, *Yoga Body,* 136.

15. R. S. Gherwal, *Practical Hatha Yoga,* 1–2.

16. Ibid., 7.

17. Kuvalayananda, "Sarvangasana Part I," 67.

18. Gherwal, *Practical Hatha Yoga,* 24.

19. Iyer, foreword to *Yogic Physical Culture,* by S. Sundaram, i.

20. Sundaram, *Yogic Physical Culture,* Preface, ii.

21. Ibid., iii.
22. Bharatiar, "Diamond Jubilee," 6.
23. Sundaram, *Yogic Physical Culture,* 52.
24. Members of the Committee, "Biographical Sketch," 23.
25. Ibid., 22.
26. Sri Venkataseshan, "Yogacharya Sri Sundaram," in *Yogacharya Sri Sundaram,* 12.
27. Sundaram, *Yogic Physical Culture,* 61.
28. Sundaram, *Yogic Physical Culture,* preface ii.
29. Kuvalayananda, "Halasana," 228.
30. Sundaram, *Yogic Physical Culture,* 40.
31. Ibid., 36 and 37.
32. Ibid., 35.
33. Iyengar, letter to the author, Sept. 28, 2007.
34. Georg Feuerstein, *Yoga Tradition,* 325.
35. Patanjali, *Yoga-Sutra of Patanjali,* II:46, II:47, II:48.
36. Wood, *Practical Yoga,* 114.
37. Norman Sjoman, *Yoga Tradition,* 45.
38. Norman Sjoman and H. V. Dattatrey, *Yoga Touchstone,* 21–22.
39. Bühnemann, *Eighty-four Asanas,* 22.

Chapter 13. S. Sundaram: Meditating on the Body in Yoga

1. Maxick, *Muscle Control,* 7.
2. *Health & Strength,* circa. Jan. 1910, quoted in Maxick, *Muscle Control,* 17.
3. Maxick, *Muscle Control,* 13.
4. Ibid., 12.
5. Kuvalayananda, "Rationale of Yogic Poses (Cont.)," 50.
6. Kuvalayananda, "Rationale of Yogic Poses (Concluded)," 121.
7. Sundaram, *Yogic Physical Culture,* 61.
8. Maxick, *Muscle Control,* 20 and 22.
9. Alter, *Yoga in Modern India,* 25.
10. Iyengar, *Light on Yoga,* 422.
11. Sundaram, *Yogic Physical Culture,* 62.
12. Alter, *Yoga in Modern India,* 24.
13. Ibid., 25.
14. Iyengar, *Light on Yoga,* 422.
15. Ibid., 424.

16. Sundaram, *Yogic Physical Culture,* 61–62.
17. Ibid., 62.
18. Ibid., 62–63.
19. Ibid., 62.
20. Ibid., 62–63.
21. Ibid., 63.
22. Ibid.
23. Ibid.
24. W. Somerset Maugham, *Writer's Notebook,* 291.
25. Singleton, "Salvation through Relaxation," 289.
26. Bharatiar, "Diamond Jubilee," 6.
27. Ibid., 6–7.
28. Members of the Committee, "Biographical Sketch," 29.
29. Ibid., 30.
30. Maugham, *Writer's Notebook,* 292.
31. Members of the Committee, "Biographical Sketch," 14.
32. Ibid., 15.
33. Maugham, *Writer's Notebook,* 291.
34. Members of the Committee, "Biographical Sketch," 21.
35. Ibid., 16.

Chapter 14. Bhavanarao Pant Pratinidhi: Reviving *Surya Namaskar*

1. Pratinidhi, *Surya Namaskars,* 51.
2. Chapman, *Sandow the Magnificent,* 104.
3. Sandow, *Strength,* 41.
4. Ibid., 15–16.
5. G. Mercer Adam, *Sandow on Physical Training,* 114–15.
6. Sandow, *Strength,* 16.
7. Pratinidhi, *Surya Namaskars,* 51.
8. Chapman, e-mail to the author, March 3, 2006.
9. Pratinidhi, *Surya Namaskars,* 51.
10. Pratinidhi, *Ten-Point Way to Health,* 78–79.
11. Roxanne Gupta, e-mail to the author, July 5, 2006.
12. This description is based on Roxanne Gupta's 2005 video of the sun worship ritual.
13. This description is based on Roxanne Gupta's

1989 video of Iyengar's demonstration of *surya namaskar.*

14. Gupta, e-mail to the author, July 5, 2006.

15. Kuvalayananda, "Rationale of Yogic Poses" (July 1926), 210.

16. D. C. Mujumdar, *Encyclopedia of Indian Physical Culture,* 453.

17. Pratinidhi, *Surya Namaskars,* 47.

18. Bhagvat Sinh Jee, *Aryan Medical Science,* 61.

19. Mujumdar, *Encyclopedia of Indian Physical Culture,* 453.

Chapter 15. Bhavanarao Pant Pratinidhi: Promoting *Surya Namaskar* as Health Cure and Strengthening Exercise

1. Pratinidhi, *Surya Namaskars,* 43.

2. Ibid., 44.

3. Ibid., 5.

4. Ibid., 13.

5. Ibid., 48.

6. Ibid., 46.

7. Ibid., 48.

8. Ibid., 34.

9. Ibid., 12.

10. Ibid., 16.

11. Wood, *Yoga Dictionary,* 28–29.

12. Pratinidhi, *Surya Namaskars,* 19.

13. Ibid., 30.

14. Alter, *Gandhi's Body,* 95.

15. Pratinidhi, *Surya Namaskars,* 12.

16. Ibid., 1.

17. Ibid., 10–11.

18. Alter, *Gandhi's Body,* 95.

19. Pratinidhi, *Surya Namaskars,* 51.

20. Ibid., 4.

21. Pratinidhi, foreword to *Encyclopedia of Indian Physical Culture,* ed. Mujumdar, xxiii.

22. Pratinidhi, *Surya Namaskars,* 51.

23. Ibid., 1–2.

24. Ibid., 49.

25. Ibid., 43.

26. Ibid., 49.

27. Ibid., 22.

28. Ibid., 16.

29. Ibid., 22.

30. *Yajurveda* (The Texts of the White Yajurveda), trans. by Ralph T. H. Griffith, quoted in Pratinidhi, *Surya Namaskars,* 22.

Chapter 16. Bhavanarao Pant Pratinidhi: Making *Surya Namaskar* a Part of Physical Education

1. Aundh State Constitution Act of 1939, in appendix 4 of *Aundh Experiment,* by Indira Rothermund, 133.

2. Apa Pant, foreword to *Aundh Experiment,* by I. Rothermund, xv.

3. Rothermund, *Aundh Experiment,* 25–26.

4. Alter, *Gandhi's Body,* 94.

5. Ibid., 99.

6. Pratinidhi, *Ten-Point Way to Health,* quoted in Alter, *Gandhi's Body,* 98.

7. Alter, *Gandhi's Body,* 94.

8. Alter, *Wrestler's Body,* 98.

9. Pant, *Surya Namaskars,* quoted in Alter, *Wrestler's Body,* 98.

10. Alter, *Wrestler's Body,* 98.

11. Pratinidhi, *Surya Namaskars,* foreword, I.

12. Pant, *Surya Namaskars,* 15.

13. Pratinidhi, *Surya Namaskars,* 85.

14. Ibid., 85–86.

15. Ibid., 61.

16. Ibid., 89.

17. Indira Gandhi, foreword to *A Moment in Time,* by A. Pant, unnumbered page facing 10.

18. Gharote and Gharote, *Swami Kuvalayananda,* 107.

19. Pratinidhi, foreword to *Encyclopedia of Indian Physical Culture,* ed. Mujumdar, xxiii.

20. Ibid., xxiv.

21. Susan Sontag, "Fascinating Fascism," 26.

22. Pratinidhi, *Surya Namaskars,* 62–63.

23. Ibid., 61.

24. Sontag, "Fascinating Fascism," 26.

25. Mujumdar, *Encyclopedia of Indian Physical Culture,* 452.

26. Ibid., 450.

27. Pratinidhi, *Surya Namaskars,* 5.

28. Mujumdar, *Encyclopedia of Indian Physical Culture,* 456.

29. Pratinidhi, *Surya Namaskars,* 1.

30. Pratinidhi, foreword to *Encyclopedia of Indian Physical Culture,* ed. Mujumdar, xxiii.

31. Kuvalayananda, "Rationale of Yogic Poses" (July 1926), 212–13.

32. Ibid., 213.

33. Pratinidhi, foreword to *Encyclopedia of Indian Physical Culture,* ed. Mujumdar, xxiii.

34. I. Gandhi, foreword, unnumbered page facing 10.

35. Pant, *Moment in Time,* 94.

36. Ibid., 48.

37. Ibid., 13.

38. Pant, *Mandala,* 18.

39. Pant, *Moment in Time,* 14.

Chapter 17. T. Krishnamacharya: Keeping the Flame

1. T. K. V. Desikachar and R. H. Cravens, *Health, Healing, and Beyond,* 42.

2. T. Krishnamacharya, narrative, in Desikachar and Cravens, *Health, Healing, and Beyond,* 42.

3. Desikachar and Cravens, *Health, Healing, and Beyond,* 43.

4. Elizabeth Kadetsky, e-mail to the author, Dec. 10, 2012.

5. White, *Sinister Yogis,* 244.

6. Iyengar, *Body the Shrine,* 4.

7. Fernando Pagés Ruiz, "Krishnamacharya's Legacy," 100.

8. Iyengar, *Astadala Yogamala,* 52.

9. Ruiz, "Krishnamacharya's Legacy," 100.

10. Iyengar, *Astadala Yogamala,* 53.

11. Kuvalayananda, "Rationale of Yogic Poses" (July 1926), 214–15.

12. Sundaram, *Yogic Physical Culture,* 2.

13. Ibid., 3.

14. Ibid.

15. Singleton, *Yoga Body,* 178–79.

16. Ibid., 179.

17. Kuvalayananda to Nalvadi Krishnaraja Wadiyar,

April 2, 1934, in Bodhe and Ramakrishna, *Yogi and Scientist,* 371.

18. Sjoman, *Yoga Tradition,* 53.

19. Kuvalayananda to Nalvadi Krishnaraja Wadiyar, April 2, 1934, in Bodhe and Ramakrishna, *Yogi and Scientist,* 371.

20. *Jaganmohan Palace Administrative Records, 1931–1947,* for the year 1932–1933, quoted in Singleton, *Yoga Body,* 179.

21. Iyengar, *Astadala Yogamala,* 53.

22. Sundaram, *Yogic Physical Culture,* 4.

23. Ibid., 4–5.

24. *Report of the Physical Training Committee of the Government of Bombay, 1927–1929,* quoted in Gharote and Gharote, *Swami Kuvalayananda,* 38.

25. *Report of Dr. A. Souza,* quoted in Gharote and Gharote, *Swami Kuvalayananda,* 39.

26. I. Devi, *Forever Young,* 18.

27. Ibid., 18–19.

28. Ibid., 17.

29. *Life,* "Speaking of Pictures . . . This Is Real Yoga," 10.

30. Ibid.

31. Ibid.

32. John Campbell Oman, *Mystics,* 66–67.

33. Singleton, *Yoga Body,* 58.

34. Pratinidhi, foreword to *Encyclopedia of Indian Physical Culture,* ed. Mujumdar, xxi.

35. Ibid., xxiv.

36. Sjoman, *Yoga Tradition,* 107.

37. S. A. Krishnaiah, "Acrobatics," 1.

Chapter 18. T. Krishnamacharya: Incorporating Contortion into Yoga

1. Nelson Hall, *Stage Tricks,* 96.

2. Ibid., 94.

3. Iyengar, *Light on Yoga,* 409.

4. N. Hall, *Stage Tricks,* 98.

5. Ibid., 94.

6. Ibid., 14.

7. Ibid.

8. Karl Toepfer, "Twisted Bodies," 104.

9. G. Strehly, *L'Acrobatie et les acrobats* (Acrobatics

and the acrobats), quoted in Michel Louis, *Contortionists,* 3 (unnumbered).

10. Bobbie Trebor, "Acrobatics?," 19.
11. Ibid., 21.
12. Ibid.
13. Ibid., 56.
14. Robert L. Jones, "Stunts?," 44.
15. Sreedharan Champad, *Album of Indian Big Tops,* 3.
16. Singleton, *Yoga Body,* 59.
17. Toepfer, "Twisted Bodies," 105.
18. Trebor, "Acrobatics?," 21.
19. Jones, "Stunts?," 43.
20. Ibid.

Chapter 19. T. Krishnamacharya: Infusing Yoga with *Surya Namaskar*

1. Iyengar, *Body the Shrine,* 6.
2. Kuvalayananda to Nalvadi Krishnaraja Wadiyar, April 2, 1934, in Bodhe and Ramakrishna, *Yogi and Scientist,* 371.
3. Kuvalayananda, *Asanas,* 137.
4. Singleton, *Yoga Body,* 199.
5. Gharote and Gharote, *Swami Kuvalayananda,* 92.
6. Kuvalayananda, *Yaugic Sangha Vyayam* (Yogic group exercise), 22–27.
7. Gharote and Gharote, *Swami Kuvalayananda,* 93.
8. Singleton, *Yoga Body,* 204.
9. Ibid.
10. Ibid., 206.
11. Ibid., 204.
12. Gharote and Gharote, *Swami Kuvalayananda,* 117.
13. Ibid., 119.
14. Singleton, *Yoga Body,* 206.
15. Ibid., 200.
16. Ibid., 201.
17. Ibid., 203.
18. Ibid., 203–4.
19. Ibid., 206.
20. Ibid., 180.
21. Ibid., 181.
22. Ibid., 180.
23. *Jaganmohan Palace Administrative Records, 1931–1947,* for the year 1934–35, quoted in Singleton, *Yoga Body,* 180.
24. T. Krishnamacharya, *Yoga Makaranda or Yoga Saram (Essence of Yoga),* 26.
25. Singleton, e-mail to the author, Dec. 14, 2005.
26. Singleton, *Yoga Body,* 179.
27. Ibid., 176–77.
28. Ruiz, "Krishnamacharya's Legacy," 100.
29. Iyengar, *Light on Life,* xix.
30. Singleton, *Yoga Body,* 195.
31. Iyengar, *Light on Life,* xix.
32. Linda Sparrowe, *Yoga,* 52.
33. Ruiz, "Krishnamacharya's Legacy," 98 (sentences rearranged).
34. Singleton, "Yoga Makaranda," 337.
35. Ruiz, "Krishnamacharya's Legacy," 99.
36. Sjoman, *Yoga Tradition,* 50.
37. Van Lysebeth, *Pranayama,* 118.
38. Ibid., 135.
39. Eddie Stern, foreword to *Yoga Mala,* by K. Pattabhi Jois, xvi.
40. Ruiz, "Krishnamacharya's Legacy," 101.

Chapter 20. K. V. Iyer: Mixing Bodybuilding and Yoga at the Palace

1. Fazlul Hasan, *Bangalore through the Centuries,* 215.
2. John Lord, *Maharajahs,* 86.
3. Ibid., 188.
4. Iyer, *Perfect Physique,* 2.
5. V. Sitaramiah, "Personal Portrait," 21.
6. Garb, *Bodies of Modernity,* 55.
7. Singleton, "Notes from an Interview with Dr. K. V. Karna (K. V. Iyer's Son)," Sept. 17, 2005, e-mail to the author, Sept. 18, 2005.
8. Singleton, *Yoga Body,* 191.
9. Ibid.
10. Sundaram, *Yogic Physical Culture,* i.
11. Singleton, *Yoga Body,* 191.
12. H. Anantha Rao, "Prof. Iyer's Gift," 71.
13. H. A. Rao, interview with Singleton, Sept. 19, 2005, in Singleton, *Yoga Body,* 194.
14. H. A. Rao, "Prof. Iyer's Gift," 71.

15. Alter, "Yoga and Physical Education," quoted in Singleton, *Yoga Body,* 191.

16. Singleton, *Yoga Body,* 191.

17. Madhava Rao, e-mail to the author, Feb. 22, 2004.

18. Shivarama Karanth, "Imprint in Memory," 6.

19. Sitaramiah, "Personal Portrait," 15.

20. Vasantha Karna, "My Father-in-Law," 63.

21. H. K. Ranganath, "Embodiment of Exalted Ideals," 30.

22. H. A. Rao, "Prof. Iyer's Gift," 73.

23. K. G. Nadagir, "Prof. K. V. Iyer," 81.

24. V. Karna, "My Father-in-Law," 60.

25. Iyer, *Physique and Figure,* 90.

26. Iyer, *Physical Training,* lesson 9, 8.

27. Iyer, *Physique and Figure,* 85.

28. Iyer, *Physical Training,* lesson 3, 13–14.

29. Alter, *Wrestler's Body,* 96.

30. Iyer, *Physical Training,* lesson 5, 8.

31. Iyer, *Physique and Figure,* 50.

32. Ibid., 81.

33. Ibid., 46.

34. K. V. Karna and Vasantha Karna, *Prof. K. V. Iyer,* 1.

35. Iyer, *Physique and Figure,* 50.

36. Ibid., 51.

37. Iyer, *Physical Training,* lesson 1, 18.

38. Karl Baier, "Yoga Tradition," 24.

39. Feuerstein, *Yoga Tradition,* 327.

40. M. H. Krishniah, "Short Story," 140.

41. H. A. Rao, "Prof. Iyer's Gift," 77.

Chapter 21. K. V. Iyer: Presenting *Surya Namaskar* as Stretching Exercise

1. Karanth, "Imprint in Memory," 5.

2. Iyer, *Surya Namaskar,* 3.

3. Pratinidhi, *Surya Namaskars,* 12.

4. Iyer, *Surya Namaskar,* 26.

5. Ibid., 30.

6. Iyer, *Physical Training,* lesson 3, 13.

7. Iyer, *Surya Namaskar,* 18.

8. Iyer, *Surya Namaskar,* 18–19.

9. Ibid., 4.

10. Ibid., 5.

11. Daniel Freund, e-mail to the author, April 3, 2006.

12. Iyer, *Surya Namaskar,* 8–9.

13. Ibid., 3.

14. Ibid., 10.

15. Mark Lewis, "Warm Up," 132.

16. Ibid., 132–33.

17. Iyer, *Surya Namaskar,* 4.

18. H. A. Rao, e-mail to the author, Feb. 27, 2004 (sentences reordered).

19. Iyer, *Surya Namaskar,* 12, 15.

20. Ibid., 15.

21. Ibid., 1.

22. John Grimek, "K. V. Iyer—A Tribute," 55.

23. Iyer, *Surya Namaskar,* 4.

24. R. S. Balsekar, "Surya Namaskar," 66.

25. B. S. Narayana Rao, "Iyer and His Stage Activities," 94.

26. Iyer, *Physique and Figure,* 86.

27. Sumana, "Memories," 42.

28. Ibid., 42–43.

29. Ibid., 51.

30. Ibid., 53.

Chapter 22. Louise Morgan: Making *Surya Namaskar* into an Elixir for Western Women

1. Louise Morgan, introduction to *Ten-Point Way to Health,* by B. P. Pratinidhi, 7.

2. Ibid.

3. Ibid.

4. Morgan, "Secret of Health," 7.

5. Ibid.

6. J. M. Barrie, *Peter and Wendy,* 1.

7. Donald Gray, "Science," 56.

8. Andrew Sarris, *Ain't Heard Nothin' Yet,* 48.

9. *Health & Strength,* "Tibetan Legend," 640.

10. Morgan, "Secret of Health," 7.

11. Morgan, "Surya Namaskars," 5.

12. Morgan, introduction, 10.

13. Morgan, "Surya Namaskars," 5.

14. Morgan, introduction, 10.

15. Morgan, "Surya Namaskars," 5.
16. Ibid.
17. Morgan, "Have You Learnt," 4.
18. Morgan, "Cure Bad Temper," 5.
19. Morgan, "Final Lesson," 5.
20. Morgan, "Surya Namaskars," "Have You Learnt," "Cure Bad Temper," and "Final Lesson."
21. Morgan, "Surya Namaskars," 5.
22. Morgan, "Have You Learnt," 4.
23. Ibid.
24. Ibid.
25. Morgan, introduction, 12.

Chapter 23. Louise Morgan: Pointing the Way to Health through *Surya Namaskar*

1. Louise Morgan to Apa Pant, Aug. 12, 1962, Louise Morgan and Otto Theis papers (sentences reversed).
2. Pant to Morgan, May 9, 1962, Louise Morgan and Otto Theis papers.
3. Morgan to Pant, May 20, 1962, Louise Morgan and Otto Theis papers (misdated, probably from early or mid-June 1962).
4. Pant to Morgan, June 22, 1962, Louise Morgan and Otto Theis papers.
5. Pratinidhi, *Ten-Point Way to Health,* photo caption I:1.
6. Ibid., photo captions I:2, 4, 8; II:2, 4, 8.
7. Pratinidhi, *Surya Namaskars,* 42.
8. Pratinidhi, *Ten-Point Way to Health,* 59–60.
9. Pratinidhi, *Surya Namaskars,* 37.
10. Pratinidhi, *Ten-Point Way to Health,* 36.
11. Ibid., 54.
12. Ibid., 110.
13. Ibid., 43.
14. Ibid., 51.
15. Ibid., 52.
16. Ibid., 110.
17. Ibid., 109.
18. Ibid., 61.
19. Ibid., 110.
20. Ibid., 51.

21. Ibid., 109–10.
22. Ibid., 47.
23. Ibid.
24. Ibid., 62–63.
25. Ibid., 61.
26. Ibid., 48.
27. S. Devi, *Easy Postures for Woman* [*sic*], 22.
28. Ibid.
29. Ibid., 24.
30. Ibid., 23–24.
31. Ibid., 23.
32. Pratinidhi, *Ten-Point Way to Health,* 42.
33. Ibid.
34. Morgan, introduction, 14.
35. Ibid., 14–15.
36. Ibid., 15.
37. Joan Acocella, "Once upon a Time," 73.
38. Eliade, *Yoga,* 85.
39. Pratinidhi, *Ten-Point Way to Health,* 25–26.
40. Morgan, introduction, 15.

Chapter 24. Louise Morgan: Becoming Aware of the Body in *Surya Namaskar*

1. Charles S. Sherrington, *Nervous System,* 130.
2. Ibid., 317.
3. Ibid., 130.
4. Matthias F. Alexander, *Use of the Self,* 3.
5. Morgan, *Inside Yourself,* 33.
6. Sherrington, *Endeavour of Jean Fernel,* 89.
7. Ibid.
8. Morgan, *Inside Yourself,* 169.
9. Ibid., 42.
10. Pratinidhi, *Ten-Point Way to Health,* 54.
11. Ibid., 44–45.
12. Ibid., 38.
13. Ibid., 39.
14. Morgan, "Surya Namaskars," 5.
15. Pratinidhi, *Ten-Point Way to Health,* 39.
16. Morgan, "Surya Namaskars," 5.
17. Morgan, "Cure Bad Temper," 5.
18. Morgan, "Have You Learnt," 4.
19. Morgan, "Cure Bad Temper," 5.

20. Morgan, "Final Lesson," 5.

21. Morgan, introduction, 15.

22. Pratinidhi, *Surya Namaskars,* 14.

23. Pratinidhi, *Ten-Point Way to Health,* 36–37.

24. Aldous Huxley, foreword to *Inside Yourself,* by L. Morgan, 8–9.

25. Scaravelli, *Awakening the Spine,* 80.

26. Morgan, "Final Lesson," 5.

27. Morgan, *Inside Your Kitchen,* 20.

28. Pratinidhi, *Ten-Point Way to Health,* 48.

29. Ibid., 41–42.

30. Morgan, "Cure Bad Temper," 5.

Chapter 25. Apa Pant: Making *Surya Namaskar* into a Meditation

1. Pant, *Moment in Time,* 94.

2. Pant, *Surya Namaskars,* 1.

3. Pant, *Moment in Time,* 104.

4. Ibid., 103.

5. Ibid., 104–5.

6. Pratinidhi, *Surya Namaskars,* 5.

7. Ibid., 47.

8. Morgan, introduction, 8.

9. Morgan, "Cure Bad Temper," 5.

10. Morgan, introduction, 11–12.

11. M. K. Gandhi, in *Harijan,* Nov. 12, 1938, quoted in Rothermund, *Aundh Experiment,* 2.

12. Rothermund, *Aundh Experiment,* 6.

13. Pant, *Moment in Time,* 7.

14. Ibid., 43–44.

15. Pant, *Unusual Raja,* 95.

16. Ibid., 96.

17. Pant, *Moment in Time,* 47.

18. Pant, *Unusual Raja,* 96.

19. Ibid.

20. Pant, *Surya Namaskars,* 2.

21. Sivananda, *Yogic Home Exercises,* 17.

22. Lee Khoon Choy, *Diplomacy,* 66.

23. B. I. Taraporewala, "Iyengar—The Artist," 438.

24. Pant, *Moment in Time,* 181.

25. Pant, *Surya Namaskars,* 12.

26. Pant, *Moment in Time,* 34.

27. Ibid., 94.

28. Morgan to E. F. Bozman, May 24, 1962, Louise Morgan and Otto Theis papers.

29. Morgan to Pant, May 20, 1962 (misdated), Louise Morgan and Otto Theis papers.

30. Pant to Morgan, June 22, 1962, Louise Morgan and Otto Theis papers.

31. Ibid.

32. Pant to Morgan, July 13, 1962, Louise Morgan and Otto Theis papers.

33. Pant, "Short Note," Part III:3, Louise Morgan and Otto Theis papers.

34. Ibid., Part III:4.

35. Eliade, *Yoga,* 45.

36. Ibid., 48.

37. Pant, "Short Note," Part III:6.

38. Ibid., Part III:10.

39. Ibid., Part II:9.

40. Ibid., Part III:5.

41. Ibid., Part III:6.

42. Morgan to Pant, Aug. 12, 1962, Louise Morgan and Otto Theis papers.

43. Ibid.

44. Pant, *Surya Namaskars,* 14.

45. Ibid., 2.

46. Ibid., 19.

47. Ibid.

48. Ibid., 18.

49. Ibid.

50. Pant, *Moment in Time,* 189.

51. Ibid., 191.

52. Ibid., 189.

53. Ibid., 191.

54. Ibid., 188.

55. Ibid., 189.

56. Pant, "Short Note," Part III:5.

57. Ibid., Part III:10.

58. Morgan, introduction, 11.

59. Gupta, *Yoga of Indian Classical Dance,* 36.

60. Pant, *Moment in Time,* 181.

61. Ibid., 71.

62. Ibid., 182.

63. Ibid., 184.

64. Ibid., 184–85.

Chapter 26. Swami Sivananda: Using *Surya Namaskar* as a Warm-up Exercise for Yoga

1. Jess Stearn, *Yoga, Youth, and Reincarnation,* 27.

2. Marcia S. Moore to Katharine and Wilmon Brewer, Aug. 8, 1962, Marcia S. Moore Collection.

3. Moore, announcement, Sept. 1962, Marcia S. Moore Collection.

4. Stearn, *Yoga, Youth, and Reincarnation,* 58.

5. Ibid., 13.

6. Ibid., 3.

7. Moore to Katharine and Wilmon Brewer, June 10, 1962, Marcia S. Moore Collection.

8. Stearn, *Yoga, Youth, and Reincarnation,* 46.

9. Ibid., 48.

10. Ibid., 47.

11. Ibid., 48.

12. Ibid., 49–50.

13. Ibid., 50.

14. Ibid.

15. Ibid.

16. Ibid., 51.

17. Ibid.

18. Ibid., 52.

19. Ibid., 53.

20. Ibid., 54–55.

21. Ibid., 54.

22. Ibid., 51.

23. Sivananda, "Message," 2.

24. Sivananda, *Yogic Home Exercises,* 17.

25. Ibid., 51.

26. Ibid., 17.

27. Ibid., 18.

28. Ibid., 17–18.

29. Ibid., 18.

30. Ibid.

31. Sivananda, *Hatha Yoga,* 151.

32. Swami Vishnudevananda, *Book of Yoga,* 69.

33. Ibid., 325.

34. Van Lysebeth, *Yoga Self-Taught,* 229.

35. S. Yogendra, *Yoga Asanas Simplified,* 99.

36. Van Lysebeth, "Yogic Dynamo," 12.

37. Ibid., 11.

38. Ibid., 12.

39. Sivananda, *Yogic Home Exercises,* 60.

40. Sarah Strauss, *Positioning Yoga,* 97.

41. Ibid., 45.

42. Eliade, *Yoga,* 363.

43. Strauss, *Positioning Yoga,* 44–45.

44. Van Lysebeth, "Yogic Dynamo," 13.

45. Ibid.

46. Sivananda, *Yogic Home Exercises,* 65 (sentences rearranged).

Chapter 27. Indra Devi: Becoming a Western, Female Yoga Teacher

1. I. Devi, *Yoga: The Technique,* 53 (author listed as Eugenie Strakaty, Devi's married name).

2. Ibid., 55.

3. I. Devi, *Forever Young,* 5.

4. Ibid., 6–7.

5. Ibid., 8.

6. Ibid., 9.

7. I. Devi, *Yoga: The Technique,* 18.

8. I. Devi, *Forever Young,* 1.

9. I. Devi, *Yoga: The Technique,* 19.

10. I. Devi, *Forever Young,* 10.

11. Yogi Ramacharaka, *Fourteen Lessons,* 118–19.

12. I. Devi, *Forever Young,* 10–11.

13. Ibid., 11.

14. Ibid., 12.

15. I. Devi, *Yoga: The Technique,* 21.

16. I. Devi, *Forever Young,* 15.

17. I. Devi, *Yoga: The Technique,* 25.

18. I. Devi, *Forever Young,* 18.

19. I. Devi, *Yoga: The Technique,* 29.

20. I. Devi, *Forever Young,* 19.

21. I. Devi, *Yoga: The Technique,* 31.

22. I. Devi, *Forever Young,* 19.

23. Ibid., 20.

24. I. Devi, *Renew Your Life,* 12.

25. I. Devi, *Yoga: The Technique,* 57.

26. Ibid., 58.

27. Ibid., 61.

28. Ibid., 58.

29. Ibid.

30. Ibid., 59.

31. Ibid., 60.

32. Ibid., 62–63.

33. Ibid., 63.

34. Ibid., 70.

35. Ibid., 15.

36. Ibid., 11–12.

37. Ibid., 35.

38. Ibid., 37.

39. Audrey Youngman, "Dame of Yoga," 79.

40. Ibid.

Chapter 28. Indra Devi: Treating Anxiety with Yoga

1. I. Devi, *Renew Your Life,* 11.

2. Ibid., 14.

3. Ibid., 11–12.

4. Ibid., 12.

5. I. Devi, "Yoga for You," para. 1.

6. I. Devi, *Forever Young,* ix.

7. Ibid. (jacket copy).

8. I. Devi "Yoga for You," para. 12.

9. Leonard Bernstein, "Age of Anxiety," para. 3.

10. Paul Tillich, *Courage to Be,* 35.

11. Syman, *Subtle Body,* 192.

12. I. Devi, *Forever Young,* 117.

13. Ibid., 120.

14. Ibid., 126.

15. I. Devi, *Yoga for Americans,* 200.

16. Ibid., 207.

17. Ibid., 202.

18. Ibid., 197.

19. Adriana Aboy, "Indra Devi's Legacy," 53.

20. Christopher Challis, *Really So Awful?,* 89.

21. I. Devi, *Renew Your Life,* 14.

22. Kakar, *Inner World,* 16.

23. Eda G. Goldstein, *Ego Psychology,* 49.

24. Kakar, *Inner World,* 27.

25. Ibid., 26.

26. I. Devi, *Yoga for Americans* (jacket copy).

27. Ibid., xxii.

28. Ibid.

29. Kausthub Desikachar, *Yoga of the Yogi,* 74

30. Ibid., 93.

31. T. K. V. Desikachar, *Heart of Yoga,* xix.

32. Krishnamacharya, *Yoga Makaranda,* 19.

33. Ibid., 20.

34. Ibid., 19.

35. I. Devi, *Renew Your Life,* 159.

36. Ibid., 163

37. Ibid., 171.

38. Ibid., 73.

39. Eliade, *Yoga,* 58.

40. I. Devi, *Renew Your Life,* 73.

41. Ibid., 192.

42. Ibid., 50.

43. I. Devi, *Sai Baba and Sai Yoga,* 3.

44. Ibid.

45. Ibid., 12.

46. Ibid., 7.

47. Ibid., 81.

48. Virginia Lee, "First Lady of Yoga," 53.

49. I. Devi, *Sai Baba and Sai Yoga,* 3.

50. V. Lee, "First Lady of Yoga," 53.

51. Ibid., 53–54.

52. Ibid., 54.

53. I. Devi, *Sai Baba and Sai Yoga,* 139.

54. G. K. Chesterton, *St. Francis,* 69.

55. Ibid., 74–75.

56. Ibid., 74.

57. V. Lee, "First Lady of Yoga," 53.

Chapter 29. B. K. S. Iyengar: Enduring Cruelty

1. Iyengar, *Body the Shrine,* 4.

2. Iyengar, "My Yogic Journey," 3.

3. Iyengar, *Body the Shrine,* 6–7.

4. Iyengar, "My Yogic Journey," 4.

5. Iyengar, untitled autobiographical sketch, 3.

6. Iyengar, *Body the Shrine,* 7.

7. Iyengar, untitled autobiographical sketch, 2.

8. Ibid.

9. Ibid., 1.

10. Ibid., 2.

11. Iyengar, "My Yogic Journey," 5.

12. Iyengar, *Body the Shrine,* 7.

13. Iyengar, untitled autobiographical sketch, 2.

14. Iyengar, *Astadala Yogamala,* 52.

15. Iyengar, "My Yogic Journey," 5.

16. Iyengar, *Body the Shrine,* 7.

17. Iyengar, untitled autobiographical sketch, 2.

18. Iyengar, *Iyengar: His Life and Work,* xiii.

19. Iyengar, "My Yogic Journey," 9.

20. Ibid., 10.

21. Ibid., 6.

22. Ibid., 5.

23. Kadetsky, *First There Is a Mountain,* 80.

24. Iyengar, "My Yogic Journey," 6.

25. Ibid., 6–7.

26. Iyengar, untitled autobiographical sketch, 2–3.

27. Iyengar, "My Yogic Journey," 7.

28. Iyengar, *Body the Shrine,* 3.

29. Iyengar, "My Yogic Journey," 7.

30. Iyengar, e-mail to the author, Dec. 8, 2007.

31. Iyengar, *Iyengar: His Life and Work,* 11.

32. Iyengar, *Body the Shrine,* 114.

Chapter 30. B. K. S. Iyengar: Making Yoga Fierce

1. Iyengar, *Iyengar: His Life and Work,* 14.

2. Iyengar, "My Yogic Journey," 11.

3. Iyengar, untitled autobiographical sketch, 4.

4. 1937 report by the commission appointed by the World's Alliance of YMCAs, quoted in Martti Muukkonen, *Ecumenism of the Laity,* 225.

5. Muukkonen, *Ecumenism of the Laity,* 225–26.

6. Iyengar, letter to the author, Sept. 28, 2007.

7. Iyengar, *Body the Shrine,* 4.

8. Iyengar, "My Yogic Journey," 15.

9. Ibid., 19.

10. Iyengar, *Body the Shrine,* 17.

11. Ibid., 15.

12. Kofi Busia, "Blessings of Marriage," section 11 of "Biography of Iyengar," para. 1.

13. Iyengar, "My Yogic Journey," 15.

14. Ibid., 16.

15. Ibid., 15.

16. Iyengar, *Body the Shrine,* 21.

17. Ibid., 21.

18. Anne Cushman, "Iyengar Looks Back," 158.

19. Iyengar, e-mail to the author, Dec. 23, 2010.

20. Iyengar, "My Yogic Journey," 29–30.

21. Ibid., 34.

22. Iyengar, *Body the Shrine,* 17.

23. Pratinidhi, letter to Iyengar, March 3, 1939, quoted in Iyengar, letter to the author, Sept. 28, 2007.

24. White, "Introduction: Yoga," 2.

25. Iyer, *Physical Training,* lesson 3, 13–14.

26. Iyengar, "My Yogic Journey," 44.

27. Ibid., 45.

28. Ibid., 46.

29. Ibid., 49.

30. Ibid., 49–50.

31. Iyengar, untitled autobiographical sketch, 12.

32. De Michelis, *History of Modern Yoga,* 204.

33. Taraporewala, "How 'Light' Was Written," 432.

34. Kadetsky, *First There Is a Mountain,* 154.

35. Iyengar, "My Yogic Journey," 58.

36. Jon and Ros Claxton, interview with Suzanne Newcombe, in Newcombe, "Social History of Yoga," 113.

37. Iyengar, *Tree of Yoga,* 163.

38. Ibid., 44.

39. Newcombe, "Stretching for Health," 43.

40. Hector Guthrie, e-mail to the author, Oct. 9, 2012.

41. Iyengar, in Perez-Christiaens, *Sparks of Divinity,* 127.

42. De Michelis, *History of Modern Yoga,* 200–201.

43. Kadetsky, *First There Is a Mountain,* 240–41.

44. Joan White, e-mail to the author, May 5, 2013.

45. Bobby Clennell, e-mail to the author, March 12, 2013.

46. Ronald Hutchinson, "Iyengar Teaches," 25.

47. Ibid.

48. Ibid., 22.

Chapter 31. B. K. S. Iyengar: Making Yoga All-Encompassing

1. Van Lysebeth, "Yogic Dynamo," 10.
2. Sivananda, *Practical Lessons in Yoga,* 32–33.
3. Vishnudevananda, foreword to *Sivananda Companion to Yoga,* by Lucy Lidell, 7.
4. Mara Carrico, *Yoga Journal's Yoga Basics,* 38.
5. Strauss, *Positioning Yoga,* 100.
6. Hutchinson, "Case of the Instant Ashram," 29.
7. Guthrie, e-mail to the author, Oct. 9, 2012.
8. Guthrie, e-mail to the author, Nov. 19, 2012.
9. Sjoman, e-mail to the author, Oct. 20, 2012.
10. Guthrie, e-mail to the author, Oct. 19, 2012.
11. Iyengar, letter to the author, Sept. 28, 2007.
12. Iyengar, letter to the author, July 23, 2007.
13. Iyengar, *Light on Yoga,* 225.
14. Patricia Walden, voiceover for *Genius in Action,* 2:25–2:31.
15. Hutchinson, "Iyengar Teaches," 23.
16. Ibid., 25.
17. Hutchinson, *Yoga: A Way of Life,* 23.
18. De Michelis, *History of Modern Yoga,* 200.
19. Newcombe, e-mail to the author, Oct. 26, 2007.
20. Newcombe, e-mail to the author, Dec. 3, 2007.
21. Iyengar, *Light on Yoga,* 229.
22. Iyengar, untitled autobiographical sketch, 11.
23. Strauss, *Positioning Yoga,* 66.
24. Iyengar, *Tree of Yoga,* 157.

Chapter 32. B. K. S. Iyengar: Making Yoga Precise

1. Iyengar, *Light on Yoga,* 44.
2. Kadetsky, *First There Is a Mountain,* 37.
3. Iyengar, *Light on Yoga,* 61.
4. Kadetsky, *First There Is a Mountain,* 36.
5. Swami Sivananda Radha, *Hatha Yoga,* xvii.
6. Iyengar, foreword to *Hatha Yoga,* by S. Radha, xiii.
7. Ibid., xiv.
8. Kandinsky, "Reflections on Abstract Art," 759.
9. Ibid., 760.
10. Ibid., 759.
11. Kandinsky, *Spiritual in Art,* 143.
12. Ibid., 145.
13. Hilton Kramer, "Kandinsky," 3.
14. Meyer Shapiro, *Modern Art,* 202.
15. Iyengar, *Tree of Yoga,* 55.
16. Newcombe, *Social History of Yoga,* 113.
17. Iyengar, in Perez-Christiaens, *Sparks of Divinity,* 122.
18. Walden, *Genius in Action,* 1:23–1:37.
19. Ibid., 2:44–2:53.
20. Joan White, e-mail to the author, May 6, 2013.
21. Angela Farmer in conversation with Karin Stephan, quoted in Stephan, "Portrait of Iyengar," 352.
22. Stephan, "Portrait of Iyengar," 351.
23. Sjoman, *Yoga Tradition,* 47.
24. Iyengar, *Light on Yoga,* 61.
25. Stephan, "Portrait of Iyengar," 346.
26. Iyengar, *Iyengar: His Life and Work,* 197.
27. Iyengar, *Tree of Yoga,* 70.
28. Sjoman, *Yoga Tradition,* 47.
29. Anne Hollander, *Sex and Suits,* 154.
30. Peter Conrad, *Modern Times,* 407 (sentence restructured).
31. Ibid., 410.
32. Judith Pearlman, "Revisiting the Bauhaus," 50.
33. James Gardner, "On the Grid Again," 22.
34. Ibid.
35. Kandinsky, "Dance Curves," 520.
36. Ibid., 522.
37. Robin, *Physiological Handbook,* 521.
38. Iyengar, *Tree of Yoga,* 155.
39. Sjoman, *Yoga Tradition,* 47.
40. Jennifer Homans, "Universalist," 25.
41. Eric Shaw, "Topology of Moving Yoga," 5.
42. Iyengar, *Light on Life,* 8.

Chapter 33. B. K. S. Iyengar: Spiritualizing the Domain of Acrobatics

1. Jean Varenne, *Yoga,* 109.
2. Ibid.

3. Patanjali, *Yoga Sutra*, II:46, II.47 (author's translation).

4. S. Radhakrishnan, *Bhagavadgita*, VI:11–14.

5. Iyengar, "My Yogic Journey," 46.

6. Ibid., 47.

7. De Michelis, *History of Modern Yoga*, 204.

8. S. Yogendra, *Yoga Asanas Simplified*, 128.

9. Ibid., 128–29.

10. Sundaram, *Yogic Physical Culture*, 1.

11. Ibid., 2.

12. Kuvalayananda, "Editorial Notes," 3.

13. Van Lysebeth, "Yogic Dynamo," 13.

14. Ibid., 14.

15. Ibid., 12.

16. Iyengar, *Tree of Yoga*, 72.

17. Ibid., 70.

18. Krishnamacharya, *Yoga Makaranda*, 33–34.

19. Svatmarama, *Hatha Yoga Pradipika*, chapter 1, verse 37.

20. Iyengar, *Body the Shrine*, 74.

21. Ibid.

22. Iyengar, in Perez-Christiaens, *Sparks of Divinity*, 50.

23. Ibid., 77.

24. Iyengar, "My Yogic Journey," 57.

25. Krishnamacharya, "Mangalasish," xiii.

26. Ibid., xv.

27. Iyengar, "My Yogic Journey," 57.

28. Iyengar, *Body the Shrine*, 74.

29. Iyengar, "My Yogic Journey," 25.

30. Iyengar, *Body the Shrine*, 74.

31. Ibid., 75.

32. Ibid.

33. Iyengar, "My Yogic Journey," 57.

34. Iyengar, *Light on Life*, xix.

35. Singleton, *Yoga Body*, 196.

36. Ibid., 197.

37. Iyengar, *Astadala Yogamala*, 53.

38. Singleton, *Yoga Body*, 196–97.

39. Iyengar, *Tree of Yoga*, 144.

40. De Michelis, *History of Modern Yoga*, 203.

41. Svatmarama, *Hatha Yoga Pradipika*, chapter 1, verse 19.

42. Krishnamacharya, *Yoga Makaranda*, 8.

43. Ibid.

44. Ibid., 9.

45. Iyengar, *Light on Yoga*, 24–25.

46. Ibid., 42.

47. Ibid.

48. Ibid., 42–43.

49. Iyengar, *Body the Shrine*, 73.

50. Ibid., 74.

51. Iyengar, *Tree of Yoga*, 77.

52. Ibid., 139.

53. Iyengar, *Light on Yoga*, 29.

54. Iyengar, *Tree of Yoga*, 50.

55. Ibid., 46.

56. Bühnemann, *Eighty-four Asanas*, 23.

Chapter 34. B. K. S. Iyengar: Making *Asana* Practice into a Meditation of Insight

1. Sjoman, *Yoga Tradition*, 47–48.

2. Iyengar, *Tree of Yoga*, 139.

3. Svatmarama, *Hatha Yoga Pradipika*, chapter 1, verse 30.

4. H. David Coulter, *Anatomy of Hatha Yoga*, 240–41.

5. Iyengar, *Light on Yoga*, 116.

6. Ibid.

7. Iyengar, in Perez-Christiaens, *Sparks of Divinity*, 208–9.

8. The instructions made by Iyengar yoga teachers derive from three sources. (1) Jean M. Couch with Nell Weaver, *Runner's World Yoga Book* (Mountain View, Calif.: Runner's World Books, 1979); (2) Mira Mehta, Silva Mehta, and Shyam Mehta, *Yoga: The Iyengar Way* (New York: Alfred A. Knopf, 1994); and (3) the classroom teachings of Judy Brick Freedman.

9. Iyengar, *Tree of Yoga*, 68.

10. Iyengar, *Light on Life*, 50.

11. Iyengar, *Tree of Yoga*, 42.

12. Ibid., 43.

13. Iyengar, *Light on Yoga*, 116–17.

14. Iyengar, *Tree of Yoga*, 65.

15. Ibid., 118.

16. Ibid., 54–55.

17. Angelika Malinar, "Yoga Practices," 64.

18. Iyengar, *Tree of Yoga,* 161–62.

19. Stephan, "Portrait of Iyengar," 348.

20. Iyengar, in Perez-Christiaens, *Sparks of Divinity,* 41.

21. Iyengar, *Light on Life,* 215.

22. Eliade, *Yoga,* 73.

23. Patanjali, *Yoga-Sutra of Patanjali,* III:3.

24. Wood, *Practical Yoga,* 141–42.

25. Ibid., 138.

26. Eliade, *Yoga,* 72.

27. White, "'Open' and 'Closed' Models," 12.

Chapter 35. B. K. S. Iyengar: Teaching *Asana* as Embodied Spirituality

1. Iyengar, in Perez-Christiaens, *Sparks of Divinity,* 3.

2. Ibid., 6.

3. Ibid., 3.

4. Ibid., 6.

5. Ibid., 7.

6. Ibid., 3.

7. Ibid., 47.

8. Ibid., 38.

9. Ibid., 115–16.

10. Ibid., 76.

11. Ibid., 146.

12. Ibid., 109.

13. Ibid., 131.

14. David Michael Levin, *Body's Recollection of Being,* 53.

15. Baier, "Philosophical Dimensions of Asana," 18.

16. Iyengar, *Light on Life,* 223.

17. Ibid., 7–8.

18. Ibid., 36.

19. Ibid., 61–62.

20. Ibid., 22.

21. Ibid., 206.

22. Ibid., 232–33.

23. Iyengar, *Light on Yoga,* 170.

24. Stuart Sovatsky, *Words from the Soul,* 26.

25. Gerald James Larson, "Patanjala Yoga," 87.

26. Iyengar, *Light on Life,* 223–24.

27. Samuel, *Origins of Yoga,* 351.

28. Iyengar, *Light on Life,* 224.

29. Robert C. Fuller, *Alternative Medicine,* 51.

30. De Michelis, *History of Modern Yoga,* 138.

31. Ibid., 114.

32. Ibid., 116.

33. Vivekananda, *Vedanta Philosophy,* vii.

34. De Michelis, *History of Modern Yoga,* 115.

35. Ibid., 250.

36. Iyengar, *Light on Yoga,* 30.

37. Busia, "Light in Inner London," section 14 of "Biography of Iyengar," para. 2.

38. Iyengar, *Light on Yoga,* 9 (unnumbered).

39. Iyengar, *Tree of Yoga,* 119.

40. Ibid., 3.

41. Ibid., xi.

42. Geoffrey H. Hartman, *Unmediated Vision,* 19.

43. Eliade, *Yoga,* 48.

44. Iyengar, *Light on the Yoga Sutras,* 221.

45. De Michelis, *History of Modern Yoga,* 257–58.

46. Iyengar, *Light on Pranayama,* 249.

47. Ibid., 251.

48. Joan White, e-mail to the author, May 15, 2013.

49. Iyengar, *Tree of Yoga,* 56.

50. Ibid., 55.

Bibliography

Abhedananda, Swami. *How to Be a Yogi.* New York: Vedanta Society, 1902.

Aboy, Adriana. "Indra Devi's Legacy." *Hinduism Today,* October/November/December 2002, 52–54.

Acocella, Joan. "Once upon a Time." *New Yorker,* July 23, 2012, 73–78.

Adam, G. Mercer, comp. and ed. *Sandow on Physical Training.* Toronto: J. Selwin Tait & Sons, 1894.

Alexander, Matthias F. *The Use of the Self.* Bexley, Kent: Integral Press, 1932.

Alter, Joseph S. *Gandhi's Body: Sex, Diet, and the Politics of Nationalism.* Philadelphia: University of Pennsylvania Press, 2000.

———. *The Wrestler's Body: Identity and Ideology in North India.* Berkeley and Los Angeles: University of California Press, 1992.

———. *Yoga in Modern India: The Body between Science and Philosophy.* Princeton, N.J.: Princeton University Press, 2004.

Armstrong, Karen. *Buddha.* New York: Penguin Group, 2001.

Baier, Karl. "Iyengar and the Yoga Tradition." *BKS Iyengar Yoga Teachers' Association News Magazine,* Winter 1995, 12–32.

———. "On the Philosophical Dimensions of Asana." *BKS Iyengar Yoga Teachers' Association News Magazine,* Winter 1994, 16–23, 27–32.

Balsekar, R. S. "The World's Oldest P. C. System Part One: 'Surya Namaskar.'" *Superman,* December 1937, 64–66.

Bardach, Anne Louise. "How Yoga Won the West." *New York Times,* October 2, 2011.

Barrie, J. M. (James Matthew). *Peter and Wendy.* New York: Charles Scribner's Sons, 1911.

Bell, Martin, dir. *The Amazing Plastic Lady.* A 29-minute documentary produced for the *National Geographic Explorer* television series, 1993.

Bernstein, Leonard. "The Age of Anxiety." Prefatory note to the score for *The Age of Anxiety, Symphony No. 2 (after W. H. Auden),* March 1949. www.orsymphony

.org/concerts/0910/programnotes/cl2_essay.aspx.

Berry, Mark H. "If You Had a Bar Bell—." *Strength,* October 1927, 34–37, 82–83, 85–86, 89–90.

Bharatiar, Suddhananda. "Diamond Jubilee of the Yogacharya." In *Yogacharya Sri Sundaram: In Commemoration of His 61st Birthday* (souvenir booklet), edited by Yogacharya Sri Sundaram's 61st Birthday Celebration Committee, 5–8. Bangalore, India: Yoga Publishing House, 1962.

Bodhe, R. K., and G. Ramakrishna. *Yogi and Scientist: Biography of Swami Kuvalayananda.* Lonavla, India: Kaivalyadhama, 2012.

Braune, Christian Wilhelm. *An Atlas of Topographical Anatomy—After Plane Sections of Frozen Bodies.* Translated by Edward Bellamy. London: J. & A. Churchill, 1877.

Braune, Christian Wilhelm, and Otto Fischer. "The Center of Gravity of the Human Body as Related to the Equipment of the German Infantry." In *Treatises of the Mathematical-Physical Class of the Royal Academy of Sciences of Saxony,* no. 7. Translated by Defense Documentation Center (U.S.). Leipzig, Germany: S. Hirtel, 1889.

Broad, William J. *The Science of Yoga: The Risks and the Rewards.* New York: Simon and Schuster, 2012.

Brunnström, Signe. *Brunnstrom's Clinical Kinesiology.* 4th ed., revised by L. Don Lehmkuhl and Laura K. Smith. Philadelphia: F. A. Davis Company, 1983. First published in 1962.

———. "The Changing Conception of Posture: Method of Dealing with Faulty Posture." *Physiotherapy Review* 20, no. 2 (March–April 1940): 79–84.

Bühnemann, Gudrun. *Eighty-four Asanas in Yoga: A Survey of Traditions.* New Delhi: D. K. Printworld, 2007.

Burke, Marie Louise. *Swami Vivekananda in the West: New Discoveries.* Vol. 3, *The World Teacher,* part 1. 3rd ed. Mayavati, India: Advaita Ashrama, 1985.

———. *Swami Vivekananda in the West: New Discoveries.* Vol. 5, *A New Gospel,* part 1. 3rd ed. Mayavati, India: Advaita Ashrama, 1987.

Busia, Kofi. "A Biography of BKS Iyengar." Accessed September 1, 2015. www.kofibusia.com/iyengarbio.php.

Carrico, Mara, and the editors of *Yoga Journal. Yoga Journal's Yoga Basics.* New York: Henry Holt and Company, 1997.

Challis, Christopher. *Are They Really So Awful? A Cameraman's Chronicles.* London: Janus Publishing Company, 1995.

Champad, Sreedharan. *An Album of Indian Big Tops (History of Indian Circus).* Houston, Tex.: Strategic Book Publishing and Rights Co., 2013.

Chapman, David L. *Sandow the Magnificent: Eugen Sandow and the Beginnings of Bodybuilding.* Urbana and Chicago: University of Illinois Press, 1994.

Chesterton, G. K. *St. Francis of Assisi.* New York: Image Books, 1957. First published in 1924.

Clifton, Diane. Letter to B. K. S. Iyengar, October 19, 1975. Held in the archives of the Iyengar Yoga Institute, Maida Vale, London.

Conrad, Peter. *Modern Times, Modern Places.* New York: Alfred A. Knopf, 1999.

Coulter, H. David. *Anatomy of Hatha Yoga: A Manual for Students, Teachers, and Practitioners.* Honesdale, Pa.: Body and Breath, 2001.

Cushman, Anne. "Iyengar Looks Back." *Yoga Journal,* November/December 1997, 85–91, 156–65.

Dadape, E. V. "Wrestling." *Vyayam* 1, no. 5 (May 1927): 124–27.

Danielou, Alain. *Yoga: The Method of Re-Integration.* New Hyde Park, N.Y.: University Books, 1949.

Day, Harvey. *The Study and Practice of Yoga.* London: Thorsons Publishers, 1953.

De Michelis, Elizabeth. *A History of Modern Yoga: Patanjali and Western Esotericism.* London and New York: Continuum, 2004.

Desikachar, Kausthub. *The Yoga of the Yogi: The Legacy of T. Krishnamacharya.* Chennai, India: Krishnamacharya Yoga Mandiram, 2005.

Desikachar, T. K. V. *The Heart of Yoga: Developing a Personal Practice.* Rev. ed. Rochester, Vt.: Inner Traditions International, 1999. First published in 1995.

Desikachar, T. K. V., and R. H. Cravens. *Health, Healing, and Beyond: Yoga and the Living Tradition of T. Krishnamacharya.* New York: Aperture Foundation, 1998.

Devi, Indra. *Forever Young Forever Healthy.* New York: Prentice-Hall, 1953.

———. *Renew Your Life through Yoga.* Englewood Cliffs, N.J.: Prentice-Hall, 1963.

———. *Sai Baba and Sai Yoga.* Delhi, Bombay, Calcutta, and Madras: Macmillan Company of India, 1975.

——— [Eugenie Strakaty]. *Yoga: The Technique of Health and Happiness.* Allahabad, India: Kitabistan, 1948.

———. *Yoga for Americans.* Englewood Cliffs, N.J.: Prentice-Hall, 1959.

———. "Yoga for You." Presentation at the 15th World Vegetarian Congress, 1957. www.ivu.org/congress/wvc57/souvenir/devi.html.

Devi, Sita. *Easy Postures for Woman.* Bombay and New York: Yoga, 1934.

Eastern and Western Disciples. *The Life of the Swami Vivekananda,* vol. 1. Mayavati, India: Advaita Ashrama, 1914.

Eliade, Mircea. *Yoga: Immortality and Freedom.* 2nd ed., translated by Willard R. Trask. Princeton, N.J.: Princeton University Press, 1969. First published in French in 1954.

Emerson, Ralph Waldo. *The Works of Ralph Waldo Emerson.* Edited by George Sampson. 5 vols. London: George Bell & Sons, 1906.

Ernst, Robert. *Weakness Is a Crime: The Life of Bernarr Macfadden.* Syracuse, N.Y.: Syracuse University Press, 1991.

Fernandes, Leela. *India's New Middle Class: Democratic Politics in an Era of Economic Reform.* Minneapolis: University of Minnesota Press, 2006.

Feuerstein, Georg. *The Yoga Tradition: Its History, Literature, Philosophy and Practice.* Prescott, Ariz.: Hohm Press, 1998.

Freud, Sigmund. *Beyond the Pleasure Principle.* Translated by James Strachey. New York: Bantam Books, 1959. First published in German in 1920.

Fuller, Robert C. *Alternative Medicine and American Religious Life.* New York: Oxford University Press, 1989.

Gandhi, Indira. Foreword to *A Moment in Time,* by Apa Pant. Two (unnumbered) pages between 10 and 11. India: Orient Longman, 1974.

Gandhi, M. K. "Anasakti Yoga or the Gospel of Selfless Action." An extract from Gandhi's commentary on the Bhagavad Gita. In *Selected Writings of Mahatma Gandhi,* edited by Ronald Duncan, 35–41. Boston: Beacon, 1951.

Garb, Tamar. *Bodies of Modernity: Figure and Flesh in Fin-de-Siècle France.* London: Thames and Hudson, 1998.

Gardner, James. "On the Grid Again at New MoMA Gallery." *New York Sun,* June 12, 2008, 1, 22.

Gaskell, Peter. *The Manufacturing Population of England, Its Moral, Social, and Physical Conditions, and the Changes Which Have Arisen from the Use of Steam Machinery; with an Examination of Enfant Labor.* London: Baldwin and Cradock, 1833.

Gerber, Ellen W. *Innovators and Institutions in Physical Education.* Philadelphia: Lea & Febiger, 1971.

Gharote, Manohar L., and Manmath M. Gharote. *Swami Kuvalayananda: A Pioneer of Scientific Yoga and Indian Physical Education.* Lonavla, India: Lonavla Yoga Institute, 1999.

Gherwal, R. S. *Practical Hatha Yoga, Science of Health: How to Keep Well and Cure Diseases by Hindu Yogic Practice.* Place of publication, publisher, date of publication, printer, and copyright holder unknown. Held in the archives of the Department of Special Collections, Donald C. Davidson Library, University of California, Santa Barbara, California.

Goldstein, Eda G. *Ego Psychology and Social Work Practice.* New York: Free Press (a division of Macmillan), 1984.

Gray, Donald. "Can Science Make Us Live Forever?" *Modern Mechanix,* June 1936, 54–56, 125.

Grimek, John. "K. V. Iyer—A Tribute to India's Most Outstanding Developed Man." *Muscular Development* 17, no. 3 (May/June 1980): 46–47, 55–56.

Gupta, Roxanne Kamayani. *A Yoga of Indian Classical Dance.* Rochester, Vt.: Inner Traditions International, 2000.

Guts Muths, Johann Christoph Friedrich. *Gymnastics for Youth: Or, a Practical Guide to Healthful and Amusing Exercises for the Use of Schools— An Essay toward the Necessary Improvement of Education, Chiefly as It Relates to the Body.* Translated by "The Translator." London: J. Johnson, 1800. First published in German in 1793.

Hall, G. Stanley. *Adolescence: Its Psychology (and Its Relations to Physiology, Anthropology, Sociology, Sex, Crime, Religion, and Education).* Vol. 1. New York: D. Appleton and Company, 1904.

Hall, Nelson. *Stage Tricks and Hollywood Exercises: How to Develop Skill in Suppleness and Acrobatics.* New York: Exposition Press, 1957.

Hartman, Geoffrey H. *The Unmediated Vision: An Interpretation of Wordsworth, Hopkins, Rilke, and Valéry.* New Haven, Conn.: Yale University Press, 1954.

Hartwell, Edward Mussey. "On Physical Training." In *Report of the Commissioner of Education for the Year 1903,* vol. 1, edited by William T. Harris, 721–58. Washington D.C.: Government Printing Office, 1905.

Hasan, M. Fazlul. *Bangalore through the Centuries.* Bangalore, India: Historical Publications, 1970.

Health & Strength. "The Tibetan Legend: Recent Confirmations and a Dawn of Hope." June 3, 1933, 640.

Higginson, Thomas Wentworth. "Gymnastics." In *Out-Door Papers,* 131–76. Boston: Ticknor and Fields, 1863.

———. "Saints, and Their Bodies." In *Out-Door Papers,* 1–30. Boston: Ticknor and Fields, 1863.

Hittleman, Richard. *Yoga for Physical Fitness.* Englewood Cliffs, N.J.: Prentice-Hall, 1964.

Hollander, Anne. *Sex and Suits: The Evolution of Modern Dress.* New York: Alfred A. Knopf, 1994.

Homans, Jennifer. "The Universalist." *New Republic,* August 23, 2012, 23–27.

Hood, Wharton. "On the So-Called 'Bone-Setting,' Its Nature and Results." *Lancet,* March 11, 1871, 336–38; March 18, 1871, 372–74; April 1, 1871, 443–41; April 15, 1871, 499–501.

Hutchinson, Ronald. "Case of the Instant Ashram." *Yoga & Health* 1, no. 3 (1971): 27–31, 47.

———. "Iyengar Teaches." *Yoga & Health* 1, no. 7 (1971): 22–27.

———. *Yoga: A Way of Life.* London: Hamlyn Publishing Group, 1974.

Huxley, Aldous. Foreword to *Inside Yourself: A New Way to Health Based on the Alexander Technique,* by Louise Morgan, 7–9. London: Hutchinson & Co., 1954.

Innes, Kim E., Cheryl Bourguignon, and Ann Gill Taylor. "Risk Indices Associated with the Insulin Resistance Syndrome, Cardiovascular Disease, and Possible Protection with Yoga: A Systematic Review." *Journal of the American Board of Family Practice* 18 (2005): 491–519.

Iverson, Laura Williams. "Conscious Home Exercise for Women: Cultivating a New Mind/Body Practice in the Late Nineteenth Century." Thesis, Florida State University, 2007.

Iyengar, B. K. S. *Astadala Yogamala* (Garland of the Eight Petals of Yoga). Vol. 1. New Delhi: Allied Publishers, 2000.

———. *Body the Shrine, Yoga Thy Light.* Bombay: B. I. Taraporewala, 1978.

———. Foreword to *Hatha Yoga: The Hidden Language—Symbols, Secrets, and Metaphor,* by

Swami Sivananda Radha, xiii–xiv. Spokane, Wash.: Timeless Books, 1996.

———. *Iyengar: His Life and Work.* New Delhi: CBS Publishers & Distributors, 2001. First published by Timeless Books, 1987.

———. *Light on Pranayama: The Yogic Art of Breathing.* New York: Crossroad Publishing Company, 1997. First published in 1981.

———. *Light on the Yoga Sutras of Patanjali/Patanjala Yoga Pradipika.* London: Aquarian Press, 1993.

———. *Light on Yoga.* New York: Schocken Books, 1970. First published by George Allen & Unwin, 1966.

———. "My Yogic Journey." Draft of a talk given on his seventieth birthday, December 14, 1988, at Tilak Smarak Mandir in Pune, India. Held in the archives of the Iyengar Yoga Institute, Maida Vale, London.

———. *The Tree of Yoga: Yoga Vrksa.* Boston: Shambhala, 2002. First published as *Yoga Vrksa: The Tree of Yoga* by Fine Line Books in Oxford, 1988.

———. Untitled autobiographical sketch (draft of "The Body Is My Temple" in *Body the Shrine, Yoga Thy Light*), n.d. [c. 1976]. Held in the archives of the Iyengar Yoga Institute, Maida Vale, London.

Iyengar, B. K. S., with John J. Evans and Douglas Abrams. *Light on Life: The Yoga Journey to Wholeness, Inner Peace, and Ultimate Freedom.* Emmaus, Pa.: Rodale Books, 2005.

Iyer, K. V. "The Beauties of a Symmetrical Body." *Vyayam* 1, no. 6 (June 1927): 159–64.

———. *Chemical Changes in Physical Exercise.* Bangalore City, India: Bangalore Press, 1943.

———. Foreword to *Yogic Physical Culture or the Secret of Happiness,* by S. Sundaram, i–ii. Bangalore, India: Gurukula, 1929.

———. *Muscle Cult—A Pro-em to My System.* Bangalore City, India: Bangalore Press, n.d. [c. 1930].

———. *Perfect Physique—A Proem to My System.* Bangalore City, India: Bangalore Press, n.d. [c. 1936]

———. *Physical Training through Correspondence.* Bangalore City, India: Vyayamshala and Physical Culture Correspondence School, n.d. [c. 1942].

———. *Physique and Figure with a Course of Dumb-Bell Exercises.* Bangalore City, India: Bangalore Press, 1940.

———. *Surya Namaskar.* 4th ed. Bangalore City, India: Bangalore Press, 1949. First published in 1937.

Jones, Robert L. "Can Your Child Do These Stunts?" *Strength,* October 1929, 42–44, 69–70.

Kadetsky, Elizabeth. *First There Is a Mountain: A Yoga Romance.* New York: Little, Brown and Company, 2004.

Kakar, Sudhir. *The Inner World: A Psycho-analytic Study of Childhood and Society in India.* 2nd ed. New Delhi: Oxford University Press, 1999. First published in 1978 and revised in 1981.

Kandinsky, Wassily. "Dance Curves: The Dances of Palucca." In *Kandinsky: Complete Writings on Art,* edited and translated by Kenneth C. Lindsay and Peter Vergo, 520–23. Boston: Da Capo Press, 1982. First published as "Tanzkurven: Zu den Tänzen der Palucca," *Das Kunstblatt* (The art paper) 10, no. 3 (March 1926): 117–20.

———. *On the Spiritual in Art: Especially in Painting.* In *Kandinsky: Complete Writings on Art,* edited and translated by Kenneth C. Lindsay and Peter Vergo, 120–219. Boston: Da Capo Press, 1982. First published as *Über das Geistige in der Kunst: Insbesondere in der Malerei* by R. Piper & Co. in Munich, 1912.

———. "Reflections on Abstract Art." In *Kandinsky: Complete Writings on Art,* edited and translated by Kenneth C. Lindsay and Peter Vergo, 756–60. Boston: Da Capo Press, 1982. First published as "Reflexions sur l'art abstrait," *Cahiers d'art* 1, nos. 7–8 (1931): 351–53.

Karanth, Shivarama. "An Imprint in Memory." In *Prof. K. V. Iyer: A Remembrance—Essays on the Life and Works of Prof. K. V. Iyer,* edited by Sumana, 1–9. Bangalore, India: V. Si. Sampada, 1994.

Karna, K. V., and Karna, Vasantha. *Prof. K. V. Iyer*

(1898–1980): A Profile. Bangalore, India: V. Si. Sampada, 1993. One-page handout.

Karna, Vasantha. "My Father-in-Law: As I Saw Him." In *Prof. K. V. Iyer: A Remembrance—Essays on the Life and Works of Prof. K. V. Iyer,* edited by Sumana, 54–66. Bangalore, India: V. Si. Sampada, 1994.

Koestler, Arthur. *The Lotus and the Robot.* London: Hutchinson & Co., 1960.

Kraftsow, Gary. *Yoga for Wellness: Healing with the Timeless Teachings of Viniyoga.* New York: Penguin/Arkana, 1999.

Kramer, Hilton. "Kandinsky & the Birth of Abstraction." *New Criterion* 13 (March 1995): 3.

Kripananda, Swami. "Just What Yoga Is." *New York Herald,* March 27, 1898.

Krishnaiah, S. A. "Acrobatics." In *South Asian Folklore: An Encyclopedia,* edited by Margaret A. Mills, Peter J. Claus, and Sarah Diamond, 1–2. New York: Routledge, 2003.

Krishnamacharya, T. "Mangalasish" (Blessings). In *Body the Shrine, Yoga Thy Light,* by B. K. S. Iyengar, xi–xv. Bombay: B. I. Taraporewala, 1978.

———. *Yoga Makaranda or Yoga Saram (The Essence of Yoga).* Translated by Lakshmi Ranganathan and Nandini Ranganathan in 2006 from the 1938 Tamil translation by C. M. V. Krishnamacharya. First published in Kannada in 1934. https://docs.google.com/file/d/0B7JXC_g3qGl WM2IyOWNlNWEtZmU1NC00NmM0LT g2OTEtNWQxMzg0NDVjMmU4/edit?hl=en &authkey=CJDkxU4&pref=2&pli=1.

Krishniah, M. H. "Short Story, Kailasam Smarane and Mruccha Katika." In *Prof. K. V. Iyer: A Remembrance—Essays on the Life and Works of Prof. K. V. Iyer,* edited by Sumana, 118–40. Bangalore, India: V. Si. Sampada, 1994.

Books by Swami Kuvalayananda

———. *Asanas.* Bombay: Popular Prakashan, 1964. First published in 1931.

———. *Yaugic Sangha Vyayam* (Yogic group exercise). Lonavla, India: Kaivalyadhama, 1936.

Edited articles by Swami Kuvalayananda

———. "Can We Develop Mechano-Yogic Therapy?" *Yoga-Mimansa* 2, no. 4 (October 1926): 246–54.

———. "Editorial Notes." *Yoga-Mimansa* 1, no. 1 (October 1924): 1–5.

———. "A Few Personal Appreciations and Press Notices." *Yoga-Mimansa* 1, no. 3 (July 1925): 234–35.

———. "A Few Press Notices." *Yoga-Mimansa* 1, no. 2 (February 1925): 151–56.

———. "A Few Press Notices." *Yoga-Mimansa* 1, no. 4 (October 1925): 301–4.

———. "Halasana," *Yoga-Mimansa* 1, no. 3 (July, 1925): 228–230.

———. "Kaivalyadhama." *Yoga-Mimansa* 1, no. 4 (October 1925): 309–11.

———. "The Kaivalyadhama: A Review of Its Activities from Oct. 1924 to March 1930." *Yoga-Mimansa* 4, no. 1 (July 1930): 75–86.

———. "Matsyasana or the Fish Pose." *Yoga Mimansa* 1, no. 1 (October 1924): 57–58.

———. "A Note on the Ductless Glands." *Yoga-Mimansa* 2, no. 2 (April 1926): 129–39.

———. "The Rationale of Yogic Poses." *Yoga-Mimansa* 2, no. 3 (July 1926): 207–17.

———. "The Rationale of Yogic Poses." *Yoga-Mimansa* 2, no. 4 (October 1926): 257–65.

———. "The Rationale of Yogic Poses (Continued)." *Yoga-Mimansa* 3, no. 1 (January 1928): 45–52.

———. "The Rationale of Yogic Poses (Concluded)." *Yoga-Mimansa* 3, no. 2 (April 1928): 121–26.

———. "Rugna-Seva-Mandira: Rules and Regulations for Patients." *Yoga-Mimansa* 3, no. 1 (January 1928): 75–77.

———. "Sarvangasana or the Pan-Physical Pose Part I." *Yoga-Mimansa* 1, no. 1 (October 1924): 54–56, 59–75.

———. "Sarvangasana or the Pan-Physical Pose Part II." *Yoga-Mimansa* 1, no. 1 (July 1925): 217–21.

———. "Sarvangasana or the Pan-Physical Pose Part II

(cont.)." *Yoga-Mimansa* 1, no. 4 (October 1925): 292–97.

———. "Sarvangasana or the Pan-Physical Pose Part III." *Yoga-Mimansa* 2, no. 1 (January 1926): 65–72.

———. "Some Practices for Increasing Stature." *Yoga-Mimansa* 2, no. 2 (April 1926): 143–49.

———. "Towards Foundation and After." *Yoga-Mimansa* 1, no. 4 (October 1925): 312–17.

———. "Training Facilities at the Kaivalyadhama." *Yoga-Mimansa* 2, no. 1 (January 1926): 75–80.

Collected letters by Swami Kuvalayananda

———. *Blended to Perfection.* Compiled by Manmath M. Gharote. Lonavla, India: Lonavla Yoga Institute, 2006.

———. *Vision and Wisdom—Letters of Swami Kuvalayananda.* Edited by G. Ramakrishna. Lonavla, India: Kaivalyadhama, 1999.

La Lanne, Jack, with Jim Allen. *For Men Only: With a 30-Day Guide to Looking Better and Feeling Younger.* New York: Prentice-Hall, 1973.

Larson, Gerald James: "Patanjala Yoga in Practice." In *Yoga in Practice,* edited by David Gordon White, 73–96. Princeton and Oxford: Princeton University Press, 2012.

Lee Khoon Choy. *Diplomacy of a Tiny State.* Singapore: World Scientific Publishing Co., 1993.

Lee, Virginia. "First Lady of Yoga." *Yoga Journal,* January/February 1984: 23–25, 48–51, 53–55.

Levin, David Michael. *The Body's Recollection of Being: Phenomenological Psychology and the Deconstruction of Nihilism.* London: Routledge & Kegan Paul, 1985.

Lewis, Dio. *The New Gymnastics for Men, Women, and Children.* Boston: Ticknor and Fields, 1864.

Lewis, Mark. "Mark Lewis Invites You To—Warm Up with Surya Namaskars." *Vigour* 4, no. 5 (December 1948): 132–33.

Life. "Speaking of Pictures . . . This Is Real Yoga." February 24, 1941, 10–12.

Lindlahr, Henry. *Philosophy of Natural Therapeutics.* 3rd ed. Chicago: Lindlahr Publishing Co., 1921. First published in 1918.

Ling, Per Henrik. *General Principles of Gymnastics.* Quoted in Geo. H. Taylor, *An Exposition of the Swedish Movement-Cure* (New York: Fowler and Wells, 1860), and in Edward Mussey Hartwell, "On Physical Training," in *Report of the Commissioner of Education for the Year 1903,* vol. 1, edited by William T. Harris, 721–58 (Washington D.C.: Government Printing Office, 1905).

Logan, Gene A., and Wayne C. McKinney. *Anatomic Kinesiology.* 3rd ed. Dubuque, Iowa: Wm. C. Brown Company Publishers, 1982. First published in 1970.

Lord, John. *The Maharajahs.* New York: Random House, 1971.

Louis, Michel. *Contortionists.* Wuppertal, Germany: Europa Verlag, 1974.

Macfadden, Bernarr. *Building of Vital Power.* New York: Physical Culture Publishing Company, 1904.

———. *Exercising for Health.* New York: Macfadden Publications, 1929.

———. *Keeping Fit.* New York: Macfadden Publications, 1923.

———. *Macfadden's Encyclopedia of Physical Culture.* Vol. 3. New York: Physical Culture Publishing Company, 1912.

———. *Macfadden's Physical Training: An Illustrated System of Exercise for the Development of Health, Strength and Beauty.* New York: Macfadden Company, 1900.

Malinar, Angelika. "Yoga Practices in the Bhagavadgita." In *Yoga in Practice,* edited by David Gordon White, 58–72. Princeton and Oxford: Princeton University Press, 2012.

Marx, Karl. *Theories of Surplus Value.* Translated by G. A. Bonner and Emile Burns. New York: International, 1952. First published in German in 1863.

Maugham, W. Somerset. *A Writer's Notebook*. Garden City, N.Y.: Doubleday & Company, 1949.

Maxick. *Muscle Control or Body Development by Will-Power*. 8th ed. London: Athletic Publications, n.d. First published in 1911 by Ewart, Seymour & Col.

Melville, Herman. "Bartleby, the Scrivener." In *The Piazza Tales,* 31–107. New York: Dix & Edwards, 1856.

Members of the Committee (under the supervision of S. Sundaram). "Yogacharya Sri Sundaram: Biographical Sketch." In *Yogacharya Sri Sundaram: In Commemoration of His 61st Birthday* (souvenir booklet), edited by Yogacharya Sri Sundaram's 61st Birthday Celebration Committee, 13–35. Bangalore, India: Yoga Publishing House, 1962.

Misra, B. B. *The Indian Middle Classes: Their Growth in Modern Times*. London: Oxford University Press, 1961.

Mookerjee, Ajit. *Yoga Art*. Boston: New York Graphic Society, 1975.

Moore, Marcia S. (Marcia Moore Acker). Letters. Marcia S. Moore Collection. Concord Free Library, Concord, Massachusetts.

———. Announcement. Marcia S. Moore Collection. Concord Free Library, Concord, Massachusetts.

Books by Louise Morgan

———. *Inside Your Kitchen: The Source of Good Living*. London: Hutchinson & Co., 1956.

———. *Inside Yourself: A New Way to Health Based on the Alexander Technique*. London: Hutchinson & Co., 1954.

———. Introduction to *The Ten-Point Way to Health,* by Bhavanarao Pant Pratinidhi, 7–16. London: J. M. Dent & Sons, 1938.

Articles by Louise Morgan

———. "Final Lesson in Surya Namaskars." *News Chronicle,* August 20, 1936, 5.

———. "Have You Learnt How to Breathe?" *News Chronicle,* August 6, 1936, 4.

———. "Surya Namaskars." *News Chronicle,* July 30, 1936, 5.

———. "'Surya Namaskars'—The Secret of Health." *News Chronicle,* July 6, 1936, 7.

———. "These Exercises May Cure Bad Temper." *News Chronicle,* August 13, 1936, 5.

Letters by Louise Morgan

———. Louise Morgan and Otto Theis papers. Beinecke Rare Book and Manuscript Library, Yale University, New Haven, Connecticut.

Mosse, George L. *The Image of Man: The Creation of Modern Masculinity*. New York: Oxford University Press, 1996.

Mujumdar, D. C., ed. *Encyclopedia of Indian Physical Culture*. Baroda, India: Good Companions, 1950. A one-volume English translation based on ten volumes published in Marathi from 1935 to 1950.

Müller, J. P. *My System: 15 Minutes' Work a Day for Health's Sake!* Translated by G. M. Fox-Davies. Copenhagen: Tillge's Boghandel, 1905. First published in Danish, 1904.

Muukkonen, Martti. *Ecumenism of the Laity: Continuity and Change in the Mission View of the World's Alliance of Young Men's Christian Associations, 1855–1955*. Joensuu, Finland: University of Joensuu Publications in Theology, 2002.

Nadagir, K. G. "Prof. K. V. Iyer: His Physical Exercise Technique." In *Prof. K. V. Iyer: A Remembrance—Essays on the Life and Works of Prof. K. V. Iyer,* ed. by Sumana, 79–92. Bangalore, India: V. Si. Sampada, 1994.

Newcombe, Suzanne. "A Social History of Yoga and Ayurveda in Britain, 1950–1995." PhD diss., University of Cambridge, 2008.

———. "Stretching for Health and Well-Being: Yoga and Women in Britain, 1960–1980." *Asian Medicine* 3, no. 1 (2007): 37–63.

New York Herald. "Balm of the Orient Is Bliss-Inspiring Yoga." March 27, 1898.

Oman, John Campbell. *The Mystics, Ascetics, and Saints of India.* London: T. Fisher Unwin, 1905.

Palmer, D. D. *The Chiropractor.* Los Angeles: Beacon Light Printing Co., 1914.

Palmer, D. D., and B. J. Palmer. *The Science of Chiropractic: Its Principles and Adjustments.* Davenport, Iowa: Palmer School of Chiropractic, 1906.

Books and papers by Apa Pant

———. Foreword to *The Aundh Experiment: A Gandhian Grass-roots Democracy,* by Indira Rothermund, xi–xix. Bombay: Somaiya Publications, 1983.

———. *Mandala: An Awakening.* India: Orient Longman, 1978.

———. *A Moment in Time.* India: Orient Longman, 1974.

———. "A Short Note on Surya Namaskars—A Yogic Exercise." 1962. Louise Morgan and Otto Theis papers. Beinecke Rare Book and Manuscript Library, Yale University, New Haven, Connecticut.

———. *Surya Namaskars: An Ancient Indian Exercise.* New Delhi: Orient Longman, 1970.

———. *An Unusual Raja: Mahatma Gandhi and the Aundh Experiment.* Hyderabad, India: Sangam Books (India), 1989.

Letters by Apa Pant

———. Louise Morgan and Otto Theis papers. Beinecke Rare Book and Manuscript Library, Yale University, New Haven, Connecticut.

Patanjali. *The Yoga-Sutra of Patanjali.* Translated by Chip Hartranft. Boston: Shambhala Publications, 2003.

Pearlman, Judith. "Revisiting the Bauhaus." *New York Times Magazine,* August 14, 1983, 22–25, 50–57.

Perez-Christiaens, Noëlle, comp. *Sparks of Divinity: The Teachings of B. K. S. Iyengar from 1959 to 1975.* Expanded edition. Berkeley: Rodmell Press, 2012. First published in 1976.

Prabhavananda, Swami, and Frederick Manchester, trans. *The Upanishads: Breath of the Eternal.* New York: The New American Library, 1963. First published by Vedanta Press in 1947.

Pratinidhi, Bhavanarao Pant. Foreword to *Encyclopedia of Indian Physical Culture,* edited by D. C. Mujumdar, xii–xiv. Baroda, India: Good Companions, 1950.

———. *Surya Namaskars (Sun-Adoration) for Health, Efficiency & Longevity.* Aundh State Press, 1928.

———. *The Ten-Point Way to Health.* London: J. M. Dent & Sons, 1938.

Radha, Swami Sivananda. *Hatha Yoga: The Hidden Language—Symbols, Secrets, and Metaphor.* Spokane, Wash.: Timeless Books, 1996.

Radhakrishnan, S., trans. *The Bhagavadgita.* London: George Allen & Unwin, 1948.

Ramacharaka, Yogi. *Fourteen Lessons in Yogi Philosophy and Oriental Occultism.* Chicago: Yogi Publication Society, 1911.

Ranganath, H. K. "An Embodiment of Exalted Ideals." In *Prof. K. V. Iyer: A Remembrance—Essays on the Life and Works of Prof. K. V. Iyer,* edited by Sumana, 27–35. Bangalore, India: V. Si. Sampada, 1994.

Rao, B. S. Narayana. "Prof Iyer and His Stage Activities." In *Prof. K. V. Iyer: A Remembrance—Essays on the Life and Works of Prof. K. V. Iyer,* edited by Sumana, 93–103. Bangalore, India: V. Si. Sampada, 1994.

Rao, H. Anantha. "Prof. Iyer's Gift to the Field of Physical Education." In *Prof. K. V. Iyer: A Remembrance—Essays on the Life and Works of Prof. K. V. Iyer,* edited by Sumana, 67–78. Bangalore, India: V. Si. Sampada, 1994.

Rao, M. R. Raja. *The Secret of Perfect Health: Surya Namaskar.* Bangalore City, India: Bangalore Press, 1960.

Robin, Mel. *A Physiological Handbook for Teachers of Yogasana.* Tucson, Ariz.: Fenestra Books, 2002.

Rodrigues, Santan. *The Householder Yogi: Life of Shri Yogendra.* Santa Cruz, Bombay: Yoga Institute, 1982.

Rothermund, Indira. *The Aundh Experiment: A Gandhian Grass-roots Democracy.* Bombay: Somaiya Publications, 1983.

Rothman, Sheila M., and David J. Rothman. *The Pursuit of Perfection: The Promise and Perils of Medical Enhancement.* New York: Pantheon Books, 2003.

Ruiz, Fernando Pagés. "Krishnamacharya's Legacy." *Yoga Journal,* May/June 2001, 96–101, 161–64, 166–68.

Sadhakas of the Yoga Institute, ed. *Celebration of a Yogic Life.* Santa Cruz East, Mumbai: Yoga Institute, 2011.

———. "Man and Mind." In *Yoga Cyclopaedia,* vol. 3, edited by Jayadeva Yogendra, 9–22. Santa Cruz East, Mumbai: Yoga Institute, 1993.

Samuel, Geoffrey. *The Origins of Yoga and Tantra: Indic Religions to the Thirteenth Century.* Cambridge: Cambridge University Press, 2008.

Sandow, Eugen. *Strength and How to Obtain It.* London: Gale & Polden, 1897.

Sarris, Andrew. *"You Ain't Heard Nothin' Yet": The American Talking Film—History & Memory 1927–1949.* New York: Oxford University Press, 1998.

Scaravelli, Vanda. *Awakening the Spine: The Stress-Free New Yoga That Works with the Body to Restore Health, Vitality and Energy.* San Francisco: Harper San Francisco, 1991.

Shapiro, Meyer. *Modern Art: 19th and 20th Centuries.* New York: George Braziller, 1978.

Shaw, Eric. "Towards a Topology of Moving Yoga: Transcending B. K. S. Iyengar and His Cultural Moment." *JOY: The Journal of Yoga* 7, no. 1 (Fall/Winter 2008), www.journalofyoga.org/towardstopology.pdf.

Sherrington, Charles S. *Endeavour of Jean Fernel.* Cambridge: Cambridge University Press, 1946.

———. *The Integrative Action of the Nervous System.* New Haven: Yale University Press, 1906.

Singleton, Mark. "Salvation through Relaxation: Proprioceptive Therapy and Its Relationship to Yoga." *Journal of Contemporary Religion* 20, no. 3 (2005): 289–304.

———. *Yoga Body: The Origins of Modern Posture Practice.* Oxford: Oxford University Press, 2010.

———. "Yoga Makaranda of T. Krishnamacharya." In *Yoga in Practice,* edited by David Gordon White, 337–52. Princeton and Oxford: Princeton University Press, 2012.

Sinh Jee, Bhagvat. *A Short History of Aryan Medical Science.* New York: Macmillan and Co., 1896.

Sitaramiah, V. "Personal Portrait." In *Prof. K. V. Iyer: A Remembrance—Essays on the Life and Works of Prof. K. V. Iyer,* edited by Sumana, 10–26. Bangalore, India: V. Si. Sampada, 1994.

Sivananda, Swami. *Hatha Yoga.* Rishikesh, India: Yoga Vedanta Forest University (Divine Life Society), 1950.

———. "Message from His Holiness Swami Sivananda." In *Yogacharya Sri Sundaram: In Commemoration of His 61st Birthday* (souvenir booklet), edited by Yogacharya Sri Sundaram's 61st Birthday Celebration Committee, 2. Bangalore, India: Yoga Publishing House, 1962.

———. *Practical Lessons in Yoga.* Bombay: D. B. Taraporevala Sons & Co., 1938.

———. *Yogic Home Exercises: Easy Course of Physical Culture for Modern Men and Women.* Bombay: D. B. Taraporevala Sons & Co., 1939.

Sjoman, Norman E. *The Yoga Tradition of the Mysore Palace.* 2nd ed. New Delhi: Abhinav Publications, 1999. First published in 1996.

Sjoman, Norman E., and H. V. Dattatrey. *Yoga Touchstone.* Calgary, Canada: Black Lotus Books, 2004.

Sontag, Susan. "Fascinating Fascism." *New York Review of Books* 22, no. 1 (February 6, 1975): 23–30.

Sovatsky, Stuart. *Words from the Soul: Time, East/West Spirituality, and Psychotherapeutic Narrative.* Albany: State University of New York Press, 1998.

Sparrowe, Linda. *Yoga.* Westport, Ct.: Hugh Lauter Levin Associates, 2002.

Starling, E. H. "The Croonian Lectures on the Chemical Correlation of the Functions of the

Body, Lecture I." *Lancet* 166 (first published as vol. 2), no. 4275 (August 5, 1905): 339–41.

Stearn, Jess. *Yoga, Youth, and Reincarnation.* Garden City, N.Y.: Doubleday & Company, 1965.

Stebbins, Genevieve. *Dynamic Breathing and Harmonic Gymnastics: A Complete System of Psychical, Aesthetic and Physical Culture.* New York: Edgar S. Werner, 1893.

Stephan, Karin. "Portrait of B. K. S. Iyengar." In *Iyengar: His Life and Work,* by B. K. S. Iyengar, 343–53. New Delhi: CBS Publishers & Distributors, 2001.

Stern, Eddie. Foreword to *Yoga Mala,* by K. Pattabhi Jois, xiii–xvii. New York: North Point Press, 2002.

Still, A. T. *Autobiography of Andrew T. Still, with a History of the Discovery and Development of the Science of Osteopathy.* Kirksville, Mo.: self-published, 1897.

Strauss, Sarah. *Positioning Yoga: Balancing Acts across Cultures.* Oxford and New York: Berg, 2005.

Sumana. "Prof. K. V. Iyer—Memories." In *Prof. K. V. Iyer: A Remembrance—Essays on the Life and Works of Prof. K. V. Iyer,* edited by Sumana, 36–53. Bangalore, India: V. Si. Sampada, 1994.

———. ed. *Prof. K. V. Iyer: A Remembrance—Essays on the Life and Works of Prof. K. V. Iyer.* Bangalore, India: V. Si. Sampada, 1994. Originally published in Kannada; translated for the author's use in 2008 by Ramu Rao.

Sundaram, S. *Yogic Physical Culture or the Secret of Happiness.* Bangalore, India: Gurukula, 1929.

Svatmarama, Swami. *The Hatha Yoga Pradipika.* Translated by Pancham Sinh. Delhi: Sri Satguru Publications, 1981. First published in 1915.

Syman, Stefanie. *The Subtle Body: The Story of Yoga in America.* New York: Farrar, Straus and Giroux, 2010.

Taraporewala, B. I. "How 'Light on Yoga' Was Written." In *Iyengar: His Life and Work,* by B. K. S. Iyengar, 427–32. New Delhi: Timeless Books, 1987.

———. "Iyengar—The Artist." In *Iyengar: His Life and Work,* by B. K. S. Iyengar, 437–44. New Delhi: Timeless Books, 1987.

Tathagatananda, Swami. "Glimpses of Swamiji's Life in New York." *Prabuddha Bharata or Awakened India* 100 (March 1995): 471–77.

Taylor, Geo. H. *An Exposition of the Swedish Movement-Cure, Embracing the History and Philosophy of This System of Medical Treatment, with Examples of Single Movements, and Directions for Their Use in Various Forms of Chronic Disease, Forming a Complete Manual of Exercises; Together with a Summary of the Principles of General Hygiene.* New York: Fowler and Wells, Publishers, 1860.

Tillich, Paul. *The Courage to Be.* New Haven, Ct.: Yale University Press, 1952.

Todd, Jan. *Physical Culture and the Body Beautiful: Purposive Exercise in the Lives of American Women 1800–1875.* Macon, Ga: Mercer University Press, 1998.

Todd, Mabel E. *The Thinking Body: A Study of the Balancing Forces of Dynamic Man.* Princeton, N.J.: Princeton Book Company, 1968. First published by Paul B. Hoeber in 1937.

Toepfer, Karl. "Twisted Bodies: Aspects of Female Contortionism in the Letters of a Connoisseur." *TDR/The Drama Review* 43, no. 1 (T161; spring 1999): 104–36.

Trebor, Bobbie. "Should We Do Acrobatics?" *Strength,* July 1931, 19–21, 56, 58.

Van Lysebeth, André. *Pranayama: The Yoga of Breathing.* London: Unwin Paperbacks, 1979. First published in French as *Pranayama: La dynamique du soufflé* in 1971.

———. *Yoga Self-Taught.* New York: Harper & Row, 1971. First published in French as *J'apprends le yoga* in 1968.

———. "The Yogic Dynamo." *Yoga,* September 1981, 10–14.

Varenne, Jean. *Yoga and the Hindu Tradition.* Chicago: University of Chicago Press, 1976. First published as *Le yoga et la tradition hindoue* in 1973.

Vasu, Rai Bahadur Srisa Chandra, trans. *Gheranda Samhita*. New Delhi: Munshiram Manoharlal Publishers, 2001. First published in 1914–1915.

Venkataseshan, Sri. "Yogacharya Sri Sundaram." In *Yogacharya Sri Sundaram: In Commemoration of His 61st Birthday* (souvenir booklet), edited by Yogacharya Sri Sundaram's 61st Birthday Celebration Committee, 12. Bangalore, India: Yoga Publishing House, 1962.

Vishnudevananda, Swami. *The Complete Illustrated Book of Yoga*. New York: Julian Press, 1960.

———. Foreword to *The Sivananda Companion to Yoga*, by Lucy Lidell with Narayani and Giris Rabinovitch. London: Gaia Books, 1983.

Vivekananda, Swami. *The Complete Works of Swami Vivekananda*. Edited by Mayavati Ashram. 8 vols. Mayavati, India: Advaita Asharama, 2008. First published in 1922.

———. *Vedanta Philosophy: Lectures by the Swami Vivekananda on Raja Yoga and Other Subjects*. 7th ed. New York: Baker & Taylor Company, 1899. First published in 1896.

Walden, Patricia. Voiceover for the film *Genius in Action*, 2005. www.youtube.com/watch?v=6MMw1TDYTOg.

White, David Gordon. "Introduction: Yoga, Brief History of an Idea." In *Yoga in Practice*, edited by David Gordon White, 1–23. Princeton and Oxford: Princeton University Press, 2012.

———. "'Open' and 'Closed' Models of the Human Body in Indian Medical and Yogic Traditions." *Asian Medicine: Tradition and Modernity* 2, no. 1 (2006): 1–13.

———. *Sinister Yogis*. Chicago: University of Chicago Press, 2009.

———, ed. *Yoga in Practice*. Princeton and Oxford: Princeton University Press, 2012.

Wildman, Sarah. "Kafka's Calisthenics." In "Fitness Issue," a special issue of *Slate*, January 21, 2011. www.slate.com/articles/life/fitness/2011/01/kafkas_calisthenics.html.

Wood, Ernest E. *Practical Yoga: Ancient and Modern*. New York: E. P. Dutton & Co., 1948.

———. *Yoga Dictionary*. New York: Philosophical Library, 1956.

Yogacharya Sri Sundaram's 61st Birthday Celebration Committee (under the supervision of S. Sundaram), ed. *Yogacharya Sri Sundaram: In Commemoration of His 61st Birthday* (souvenir booklet). Bangalore, India: Yoga Publishing House, 1962.

Yogananda, Paramhansa. *Autobiography of a Yogi*. New York: Philosophical Library, 1946. Reprint, New Delhi: Sterling Publishers, 2003.

Yogendra, Jayadeva, ed. *Yoga Cyclopaedia*. Vol. 3. Santa Cruz East, Mumbai: Yoga Institute, 1993.

Yogendra, Shri. *Hatha Yoga Simplified*. 20th ed. Bombay: Yoga Institute, 1982. First published in 1931.

———. "His Holiness Paramhansa Madhavadasaji." *Yoga* 1, no. 1 (1933): 8–9.

———. "Right Approach to Yoga." *Yoga* 12, no. 11 (June 1967): 161–63.

———. "Yoga: Its Antiquity and Development." *Yoga* 1, no. 1 (1933): 2–4.

———. *Yoga Asanas Simplified*. Rev. ed. Bombay: Yoga Institute, 1956. First published in 1928.

———. *Yoga Hygiene Simplified*. Rev. ed. New York: Pyramid Books, 1969. First published by the Yoga Institute in Bombay in 1930.

———. "Yoga Institutes." *Yoga* 1, no. 1 (1933): 10–11.

———. "Yoga Physical Culture." *Yoga* 1, no. 1 (1933): 5–8.

Youngman, Audrey. "Dame of Yoga." *Yoga Journal*, September/October 1996, 74–79, 146.

Zumbro, W. M. "Religious Penances and Punishments Self-Inflicted by the Holy Men of India." *National Geographic* 24, no. 12 (December 1913): 1257–313.

Index

Books of Related Interest

The Heart of Yoga
Developing a Personal Practice
by T. K. V. Desikachar

Chakras
Energy Centers of Transformation
by Harish Johari

The Yin Yoga Kit
The Practice of Quiet Power
by Biff Mithoefer

Shiva
Stories and Teachings from the Shiva Mahapurana
by Vanamali

The Yoga-Sūtra of Patañjali
A New Translation and Commentary
by Georg Feuerstein, Ph.D.

Yoga Spandakarika
The Sacred Texts at the Origins of Tantra
by Daniel Odier

Yoga for the Three Stages of Life
Developing Your Practice as an Art Form, a Physical Therapy,
and a Guiding Philosophy
by Srivatsa Ramaswami

Ayurveda: A Life of Balance
The Complete Guide to Ayurvedic Nutrition
and Body Types with Recipes
by Maya Tiwari

Indian Mythology
Tales, Symbols, and Rituals from the Heart of the Subcontinent
by Devdutt Pattanaik

INNER TRADITIONS • BEAR & COMPANY
P.O. Box 388 • Rochester, VT 05767
1-800-246-8648 • www.InnerTraditions.com

Or contact your local bookseller